Introduction *to* Pathology

for the Physical Therapist Assistant

Jahangir Moini, MD, MPH

Professor of Allied Health Sciences
Everest University
Melbourne, Florida

Reviewers

Julie Feeny, MS, PT
PTA Program Director
Illinois Central College

Cosette Hardwick, PT, DPT
Assistant Professor
PTA Program
Missouri Western State University

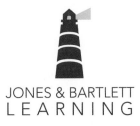

JONES & BARTLETT
LEARNING

World Headquarters
Jones & Bartlett Learning
5 Wall Street
Burlington, MA 01803
978-443-5000
info@jblearning.com
www.jblearning.com

Jones & Bartlett Learning books and products are available through most bookstores and online booksellers. To contact Jones & Bartlett Learning directly, call 800-832-0034, fax 978-443-8000, or visit our website, www.jblearning.com.

Substantial discounts on bulk quantities of Jones & Bartlett Learning publications are available to corporations, professional associations, and other qualified organizations. For details and specific discount information, contact the special sales department at Jones & Bartlett Learning via the above contact information or send an email to specialsales@jblearning.com.

Production Credits

Publisher: William Brottmiller
Senior Acquisitions Editor: Joseph Morita
Managing Editor: Maro Gartside
Production Manager: Tracey McCrea
Marketing Manager: Grace Richards
Manufacturing and Inventory Control Supervisor: Amy Bacus
Composition: Publishers' Design and Production Services, Inc.

Cover Design: Kristin E. Parker
Rights & Photo Research Manager: Katherine Crighton
Rights & Photo Researcher: Sarah Cebulski
Cover Image: © Fabrizio Argonauta/Dreamstime.com
Printing and Binding: Courier Kendallville
Cover Printing: Courier Kendallville

To order this product, use ISBN: 1-978-1-4496-3058-4

Library of Congress Cataloging-in-Publication Data
Moini, Jahangir, 1942–
    Introduction to pathology for the physical therapist assistant / Jahangir Moini.
        p. ; cm.
    Includes bibliographical references and index.
    ISBN 978-0-7637-9908-3 (pbk.)
    I. Title.
    [DNLM: 1.   Pathologic Processes. 2.   Allied Health Personnel. 3.   Physical Therapy (Specialty)   QZ 4]
    615.8'2023--dc23
            2011037934

6048

Printed in the United States of America
16   15   14   13   12   10   9   8   7   6   5   4   3   2   1

Dedication

This book is dedicated to
my granddaughter, Laila Jade Mabry.

Brief Table of Contents

Table of Contents

Preface

After 22 years of teaching pathology for allied health, I realized each allied health profession needs its own specialized pathology textbook. Therefore, I have attempted to write this book to specifically target physical therapist assistants as an introduction to pathology.

Pathology is a core area of knowledge for allied health students. For physical therapist assistants, the material must be easy to understand while focusing on the day-to-day requirements of their jobs. This textbook contains 29 chapters organized into five units. It also features three appendices, a glossary, and an index. Each chapter contains an overview, learning objectives, bolded medical terms, "Red Flag" boxes that alert students to critical material, many tables and figures, a summary, multiple choice review questions, practical scenarios based on actual cases with critical thinking questions, and relevant website addresses. The book is printed in full color.

This book is also accompanied by a student companion website that contains an interactive glossary, chapter quizzes, and other activities to help students understand and reinforce key concepts. An Instructor's Manual, PowerPoints, and Test Bank are available for instructors.

Reviewers/Contributor

Contributor

Karen Coupe, PT, DPT, MSEd
Physical Therapist Assistant Program
Keiser University
Ft. Lauderdale, Florida

Reviewers

Dennis Gavin, PT, MTC, MSc
Physical Therapist, Supervisor
Health First, Inc.
Palm Bay, Florida

Jacqueline Klaczak Kopack, PT, DPT
Program Director, Physical Therapist Assistant Program
Harcum College
Bryn Mawr, Pennsylvania

Jennifer L. Pitchford, PTA, BS
Instructor, Physical Therapist Assistant Program
Jefferson Community and Technical College
Louisville, Kentucky

Barbara "BJ" Simmons, PTA, Med
Instructor, Academic Coordinator for Physical Education
Kellogg Community College, Physical Therapist Assistant
 Program
Battle Creek, Michigan

Stacey Bell Sloas, PT, MSE
Assistant Professor
Arkansas State University
State University, Arkansas

Heather C. Taylor, PT
Academic Coordinator of Clinical Education, Faculty
Surry Community College
Dobson, North Carolina

Wendy M. Zorman, PT
Instructor Physical Therapist Assistant Program
Remington College Cleveland, West Campus
Euclid, Ohio

Acknowledgments

I acknowledge the following individuals for their time and efforts in aiding me with their contributions to this book.

Morvarid Moini, Designer
Nova Southeastern University, College of Dental Medicine

Greg Vadimsky, Manuscript Assistant
Melbourne, Florida

Also, I thank the entire staff of Jones & Bartlett Learning, especially David Cella and Maro Gartside.

I also thank the reviewers who gave their time and guidance in helping me to complete this book.

About the Author

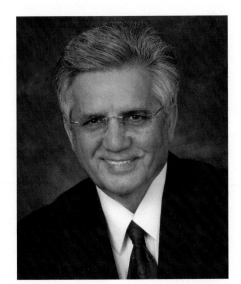

Dr. Moini was assistant professor at Tehran University School of Medicine for 9 years, where he taught medical and allied health students. The author is a professor and former director (for 15 years) of allied health programs at Everest University (EU). Dr. Moini established several programs at EU's Melbourne, Florida campus.

As a physician and instructor for the past 35 years, he advocates that all health professionals must understand the pathology of the human body, which requires understanding of major core subjects such as pharmacology, anatomy, and physiology.

Dr. Moini is actively involved in teaching and helping students prepare for service in various health professions. He has been an internationally published author of various allied health books since 1999.

Introduction to Health and Disease

Health Versus Disease

LEARNING OBJECTIVES

After completion of the chapter the reader should be able to

1. Describe how disease affects homeostasis.
2. Identify the major classifications of human diseases.
3. Discuss how a pathologic condition or disease may develop.
4. List at least 10 vocabulary terms related to pathophysiology that appear in this chapter.
5. Explain the importance of patient history in the treatment of diseases.
6. List the various steps involved in maintaining homeostasis.
7. Describe the differences between acute, subacute, and chronic disease.
8. Describe the various types of diagnostic tests and procedures discussed in this chapter.

KEY TERMS

Angiogram: an x-ray image produced by angiography, which involves injecting a radiopaque substance into the blood vessels.

Arteriogram: an x-ray image produced by arteriography, which involves injecting a radiopaque substance into the arteries.

Autopsy: medical examination of a dead body to discover the cause and manner of death.

Biopsy: a surgical procedure wherein a piece of tissue is removed for further diagnostic study. Some biopsies require general anesthesia, whereas others are minor procedures done with local anesthesia or no anesthesia at all.

Degeneration: deterioration of tissue to a less functionally active form.

Electrocardiogram: a printed readout of the electrical activity of the heart.

Electroencephalogram: a printed readout of the electrical activity of the brain.

Electromyogram: a printed readout of the electrical activity of skeletal muscles.

Endoscopy: a procedure that allows the viewing of internal body structures through the use of tubular devices with cameras and other equipment attached.

Hemophilia: the body's inability to control normal blood clotting or coagulation.

Homeostasis: the regulation and stabilization of a normal internal body environment.

Iatrogenic: pertaining to a disease or condition caused by a physician's treatment. For example, side effects of drugs are sometimes referred to as iatrogenic conditions.

Idiopathic: pertaining to a disease or condition of unknown cause.

Isotopes: substances that emit characteristic radiation, used to label various substances to determine their uptake and excretion.

Laparoscope: a device used for minimally invasive procedures that require small incisions; it allows internal body structures to be viewed either by

KEY TERMS CONTINUED

an attached camera or a remote camera that is connected by cabling.

Mammogram: an x-ray of the breast, used to detect tumors and other abnormalities.

Microscopic: requiring a microscope to be seen.

Probability: the likelihood that something will occur.

Radioactive: capable of giving off alpha, beta, or gamma rays.

Radiopaque: not allowing the passage of x-rays or other types of radiation.

Ultrasound: the use of ultrasonic waves to form images of interior body organs.

Overview

In the understanding of the human body, it is important to comprehend normal body structures and functions and how functional or physiologic changes affect the body. *Pathophysiology* is the branch of science that studies structural and functional changes in tissues and organs that lead to disease. Disease causes either obvious or hidden changes to normal anatomy and physiology. Pathophysiology also encompasses *pathology*, which is the study of changes to cells and tissues associated with disease.

Disease is a term describing any deviation from the normal state of health or wellness. It includes physical, mental, and social conditions. Disease leads to a disruption of **homeostasis** in the body. Minor changes are usually corrected by the body, which eventually returns to its normal state. A "normal" body state is measured with indicators such as pulse or blood pressure, using specific figures that represent an *average* range signifying normal health. Age, gender, family history, environment, and levels of activity all influence an individual's normal state.

In general, maintaining homeostasis involves several different steps:

- Avoid smoking, second-hand smoke, and environmental pollutants
- Be physically active, no less than 3–4 days per week, as indicated by the American Council on Exercise (www.acefitness.org)
- Perform self-screening checks for cancer and have regular medical checkups that include cancer screening
- Follow all instructions at leisure, home, and work that concern health and safety
- Eat 5 to 10 servings of fruits and vegetables per day, as indicated by the American Dietetic Association
- Limit alcoholic beverages to no more than two servings per day
- Limit exposure to the sun to the amount recommended (no more than 15 minutes three times per week), and use sunscreen before any extended exposure
- Visit the doctor or dentist regularly as well as when changes to your normal health occur

Study of Pathophysiology

Based on losses of function or changes in function to normal body structures, pathophysiology uses the knowledge of basic human anatomy and physiology. Disorders that affect each organ or body system usually have specific signs and symptoms. For example, with liver damage, clotting factors are not produced normally, resulting in excessive bleeding.

The skin and sclera of the eyes may become yellowed in color as the liver cannot normally excrete bilirubin. If the liver is inflamed, the capsule surrounding it stretches, causing pain in the *right hypochondriac region* of the abdomen.

This chapter focuses on major diseases. The principles of pathophysiology apply to all disease states. Health care is focused on the prevention of disease. The knowledge of previous cases and their outcomes is used to develop new treatment strategies. For example, before 1981 there were no available treatments for what we now know as AIDS, because the condition was yet to be diagnosed. Since then, knowledge of the disease and its transmission has helped in the development of many drugs that have successfully slowed the activity of the virus.

More significant prevention is attained by the use of routine vaccinations, genetic screening, blood pressure testing, and other programs. Combined, ongoing learning about disease processes is vital because of the difficulties of diagnosis and treatment, the complexity of disease states, and the many different options for testing that are available.

Ongoing study of disease also raises ethical, legal, and social issues. Although genetic research strives to prevent genetic disorders, the altering of genetic factors is controversial. Legal and ethical issues take longer to resolve compared with scientific advances.

Health care practitioners must always strive to recognize disease complications as quickly as possible. Delays may cause a disease to become more severe and even deadly. Detailed discussions between patients, their families, significant others, caregivers, and health care professionals are encouraged to ensure thorough understanding of conditions, treatments, and outcomes. Current technology allows the possibility of better diagnosis and treatment than ever before. Nontraditional therapies outside "conventional" medicine may have complementary benefits when used along with traditional medical treatments.

> ### RED FLAG
> The study of pathophysiology is essential for the physical therapist assistant (PTA) to understand the complexity of diseases and the ongoing study of disease, which raises ethical, legal, and social issues.

Developments in Pathophysiology

The cause of disease may be intrinsic or extrinsic in nature. Examples of intrinsic causes of disease include age, inheritance, or sex. Examples of extrinsic causes include infectious agents or behaviors such as inactivity, illegal drug abuse, or smoking. In certain cases a disease may have no known cause and is referred to as **idiopathic**.

Health care professionals must stay current on medical advances and information because developments in medicine occur very rapidly. As the knowledge of pathophysiology increases, diagnostic tests improve and more effective drugs are developed. Many disorders can now be controlled, prevented, or even cured due to technologic advances. For example, newly developed drugs can now control HIV. Various vaccines can prevent many communicable diseases. Radiation therapy can cure certain types of leukemia.

Continual study of new pathophysiology advances is essential, and developments are ongoing. For example, patients with diabetes can use blood-measuring devices that operate as minicomputers to read blood glucose levels more quickly and accurately, with less pain, than ever before. Although sometimes costly, these developments are balanced against the long-term costs of hospitalization or when patients are unable to maintain employment due to their disease process. Disease information is coordinated throughout the world by agencies such as the World Health Organization, Centers for Disease Control and Prevention, and the U.S. Public Health Service.

RED FLAG

The PTA should always stay current on the discovery of new diseases, diagnostic tools, and patient treatments.

Vocabulary of Pathophysiology

A solid knowledge foundation of anatomy and physiology is critical in understanding the effects of disease on the body. Abnormal conditions usually involve changes that may occur at the cellular (**microscopic**) level. Pathologic conditions begin with cellular changes. In the laboratory, pathology studies attempt to establish or determine the cause of a disease. These studies commonly involve examining tissue specimens from **biopsy** or surgical procedures. Body fluids are commonly analyzed for diagnosis. After death, an **autopsy** may be conducted to fully understand the factors that contributed to a fatal disease. Pathophysiologic changes may indicate the basic causes of disease, regardless of whether it is from genetics, neoplasms, or infections. Common terms used in pathophysiology are listed in **Table 1–1**. **Figure 1–1** illustrates the occurrence of disease.

RED FLAG

The PTA must be familiar with the terminology of many diseases and conditions to understand the concepts of pathology.

TABLE 1–1 Pathophysiology Vocabulary

Term	Definition	Comments
Acute	Short-term, with extreme symptoms	An acute disease lasts for a short time but develops quickly, with marked signs such as fever and pain (such as in acute appendicitis)
Chronic	Long-term, developing gradually with lesser symptoms, usually causing more permanent damage	Often, a chronic disease involves intermittent acute episodes; example: rheumatoid arthritis
Communicable	Infections that can be spread from one person to another	Certain communicable diseases must be reported to health authorities; an example of a communicable disease is *measles*
Comorbidities	Two or more coexisting but unrelated medical conditions	Posttraumatic stress disorder with borderline personality disorder
Complications	New additional (secondary) problems arising after an original disease begins	Example: a heart attack patient develops congestive heart failure as a complication
Diagnosis	Identification of a specific disease via evaluation of signs and symptoms	Laboratory tests or other tools are often used to verify several factors to confirm a diagnosis; for example, pain, swelling, and position may indicate a broken leg bone, but confirmation is via x-rays
Diagnostic tests	Laboratory tests that assist in diagnosing a specific disease	May also be used to monitor responses to treatment or progression of disease; may involve chemical analyses, examination of specimens, identification of microorganisms, or radiologic studies
Epidemics	Outbreaks of disease that occur over a given area, with many cases of the disease	Example: influenza (which also may occur sporadically or as a pandemic)
Epidemiology	The science of tracking the occurrence or pattern of disease	Includes data on transmission and distribution of disease, which is used to detect patterns yearly by major data collection centers such as the CDC and WHO
Etiology	The causative factors of a particular disease; when the cause is unknown, it is termed *idiopathic*; if a treatment, procedure, or error is responsible, it is termed *iatrogenic*	Etiologic agents include congenital defects, genetic or inherited disorders, viruses, bacteria, immune dysfunction, metabolic conditions, degenerative changes, malignancy, burns, etc.

(Continues)

TABLE 1-1 Pathophysiology Vocabulary (*Continued*)

Term	Definition	Comments
Exacerbations	Increased signs of disease	Along with remissions, they mark progression of a disease
Latent	An initial "silent" disease stage, in which no clinical signs are evident	May be referred to as the incubation period, lasting between 1 day and several weeks
Lesion	A specific local change in tissue that may be microscopic or highly visible	Example: blisters or pimples on the skin
Manifestations	Clinical evidence or effects (signs and symptoms) of disease	Examples: redness, swelling, fever
Morbidity	The disease rates within a group	Sometimes indicates the functional impairment that certain conditions cause upon the population
Mortality	Indicates the relative number of deaths from a particular disease	Example: the mortality rates of heart disease and cancer are higher than other diseases
Occurrence	A disease's occurrence is tracked by its incidence (number of new cases) and prevalence (number of existing cases)	Prevalence of disease is always a higher number than incidence
Onset	The speed of development of disease, which may be sudden and obvious (acute) or insidious, with gradual progression and vague or mild signs	Examples: acute onset describes gastroenteritis, whereas insidious onset describes hepatitis
Pathogenesis	Development of a disease	Also refers to the sequence of events involved in tissue changes that relate to the disease process
Precipitating factors	Conditions that trigger acute episodes; they differ from predisposing factors	Example: a high-cholesterol diet may predispose a patient to angina, but the actual angina attack is precipitated by extreme physical activity
Predisposing factors	Those that indicate a high risk for a disease but not certain development	Example: exposure to asbestos is a predisposing factor for cancer
Prevention	Related to disease, prevention is closely linked to predisposing factors and etiology	Preventive measures include dietary changes, lifestyle changes, vaccinations, environmental changes, and quitting smoking or drinking alcohol
Probability	The likelihood that something will occur	Example: the more occlusion that exists in the coronary arteries, the higher the probability of myocardial infarction
Prodromal	The time in early disease development when a patient is aware of a nonspecific change in the body	Examples: fatigue, headache, loss of appetite
Prognosis	The **probability** or likelihood for recovery or other outcomes	Averages are used to determine probability figures used in the prognosis of a disease
Recovery	Period of recuperation or convalescence and return to normal health	It may last for several days or months
Remissions	Subsiding disease symptoms	Along with exacerbations, remissions mark the progress of a disease
Sequelae	Potential unwanted outcomes of a primary condition	Example: paralysis after recovery from a stroke
Signs	Objective indicators of disease that are obvious to others	Examples: fever or a skin rash
Subacute	A state that is neither acute nor chronic but rather in between, having a rather recent onset or relatively rapid change	Example: subacute bacterial endocarditis, in which the condition worsens for up to 1 year before it is fatal; requires the presence of a previous heart valve disease for the bacterium to colonize and develop
Subclinical	A state existing in some pathologic conditions wherein no obvious manifestations occur	Example: kidney damage progressing to renal failure before any signs manifest
Symptoms	Subjective feelings	Examples: pain or nausea
Syndrome	A collection of signs and symptoms occurring together	Usually occurs in response to a certain condition
Therapy	Therapeutic interventions or treatment measures to promote recovery or slow the progress of a disease	May include drugs, surgery, behavior modification, or physiotherapy

CDC, Centers for Disease Control and Prevention; WHO, World Health Organization.

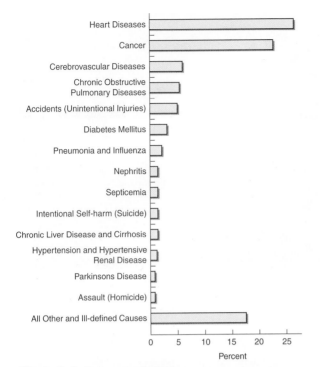

Figure 1-1 Occurrence of disease.

Source: Kung HC, Hoyert DL, Xu J, Murphy SL. Deaths: Final data for 2005. National Vital Statistics Reports; vol. 56, no. 10. Hyattsville, MD: National Center for Health Statistics; 2008.

Classifications of Disease

Diseases are generally classified into broad categories. Those in each category may not be closely related, and many diseases from different categories have similar morphology or pathogenicity. These categories are as follows:

- Congenital and hereditary diseases: Caused by developmental disturbances such as chromosomal and genetic abnormalities, intrauterine injury, or a combination of environmental and genetic factors. Examples include **hemophilia** and congenital heart disease due to German measles (rubella).
- Chronic (or steadily worsening) diseases: Cause **degeneration** of various body parts, often as a result of aging. Degeneration often occurs sooner in the life of the patient and is not linked to aging. Examples of degenerative diseases include certain types of arthritis and arteriosclerosis (hardening of the arteries).
- Inflammatory diseases: Those in which the body reacts to injury or harmful agents with inflammation. Causes include various microorganisms, allergic reactions, hypersensitivity states, and autoimmunity states. Some inflammatory diseases may be of unknown origin. Examples of inflammatory diseases include pneumonia, sore throat, and hay fever.
- Metabolic diseases: Cause disturbances in normal metabolic processes. Examples of metabolic diseases include diabetes, thyroid conditions, endocrine gland disturbances, and fluid and electrolyte imbalances.
- Neoplastic diseases: Characterized by abnormal cell growth. These diseases lead to various benign and malignant tumors.

Patient History

The completion of accurate and thorough patient medical or health histories is vital. When done correctly a patient history can help with planning or treatment, with understanding potential complications of disease, and with assessing related previous conditions, allergies, and drug therapies. Patient histories usually begin with written information provided by the patient. A follow-up discussion with a health care professional allows clarification of the provided information. The question and answer format can help to detect additional problems concerning the patient's health, both past and present.

> **RED FLAG**
>
> The PTA must be concerned with patient history, as obtained by the physical therapist during the initial evaluation, and needs to be aware of the patient's current or past medical history. Acute or chronic disorders may be determined from a detailed patient medical history. Additional information relevant to the patient history that is obtained by the PTA during patient conversation should be reported to the physical therapist and noted in the documentation.

Physical Examination

Specific areas of the body may be examined to determine the initial point or progression of disease or illness. This may involve a physical examination of one or more body regions. If an abnormality is detected, an attempt is made to correlate to the patient's medical history. There may be several potential diagnoses related to the presented signs and symptoms, so a thorough examination and clinical history must be used. In addition, laboratory tests and other diagnostic procedures assist the physical examination as the basis of a diagnosis.

Diagnosis of Disease

The many methods of diagnosing disease available today are classified as either invasive or noninvasive procedures. The PTA must be familiar with all diagnostic methods available. Invasive procedures require the patient's body to be "invaded" and include the use of needles, catheters, and other instruments. With noninvasive procedures, there is either no risk or only minimal risk to the patient. Noninvasive procedures include radiographic procedures and urine testing.

In general, invasive procedures have higher risks for potential damage than noninvasive procedures. The health care professional must weigh the potential benefits versus the potential risks of any procedure before proceeding. Patients must be fully informed about these benefits and risks.

Invasive and noninvasive diagnostic procedures may be classified in a variety of ways. There are eleven major classifications of diagnostic methods:

1. Clinical laboratory tests: Blood and urine testing to check for variations in components such as urea, hemoglobin, cell counts, enzymes, organ function, clearance rates, uptake and excretion rates, amounts of microorganisms, and antibodies.
2. Cytologic or histologic examination of cells and tissues: These tests may reveal the causes of disease based on small samples of tissue removed from affected tissues

or organs. The procedure used in these tests is called a *biopsy*. Instruments used include bronchoscopes, gastroscopes, and other endoscopic instruments.

3. Electrical activity tests: Include **electrocardiogram**, **electroencephalogram**, and **electromyogram**. Electrodes are attached to various body points to measure electrical activity changes in the body. Many heart conditions are determined and assessed with these tests. Brain tumors, strokes, and other alterations to cerebral function are also able to be assessed. Skeletal muscle function may also be determined with these tests.

4. Endoscopy: The use of flexible or rigid tubular instruments to examine various areas of the body. Each instrument is named according to the type of internal examination for which it is used. An **endoscopy** is an examination of the interior of the body, including the esophagus, stomach, trachea, major bronchi, bladder, colon, and rectum. Endoscopes and related instruments use a light source along with a system of lenses. Examples of instruments include
   a. Esophagoscope: to examine the interior of the esophagus
   b. Gastroscope: to examine the stomach
   c. Bronchoscope: to examine the trachea and major bronchi
   d. Cystoscope: to examine the interior of the bladder
   e. Sigmoidoscope: to examine the rectum and sigmoid colon
   f. Colonoscope: to examine the entire length of the colon

5. Laparoscopy: Similar to endoscopy, this procedure uses a **laparoscope** to look inside the abdominal and pelvic organs as well as to remove the gallbladder, appendix, ovary, and for other smaller surgical procedures. During a laparoscopy carbon dioxide is used to inflate the peritoneal cavity, which separates the internal organs so they can be examined more easily. The laparoscope is inserted through a small incision, usually near the umbilicus, in the abdominal wall.

6. X-ray examination: Uses the passage of x-rays through various areas of the body to be examined, with the resulting image exposed on an x-ray film. Lower density tissues absorb little of the x-rays, causing them to appear darker, whereas higher density tissues absorb more, causing them to appear lighter. An x-ray film image is called a *radiograph* or *roentgenogram*. When the breast is examined via this type of procedure, the result is called a **mammogram**. Many internal organs are examined via a combination of x-rays and the administration of a **radiopaque** substance (a *contrast medium*). These substances enhance the visibility of internal organs and structures (**Figure 1–2**).

Radiopaque oil may be instilled to examine structures such as the bronchi (a bronchogram), which is shown in **Figure 1–3**.

Another example is an intravenous pyelogram, wherein a radiopaque substance is injected into a vein. As it is excreted in the urine, it outlines the contour of the urinary tract (**Figure 1–4**). Gallstones can be seen

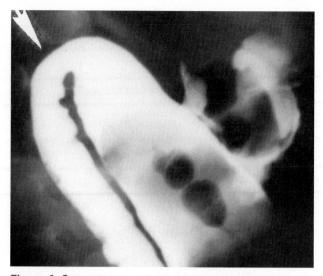

Figure 1–2 X-ray film after injection of radiopaque barium sulfate suspension into colon (barium enema), illustrating narrowed area (arrow) that impedes passage of bowel contents.

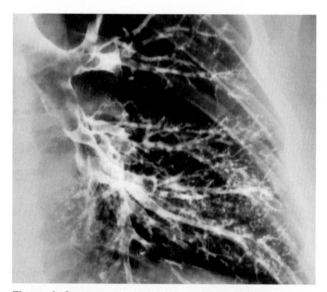

Figure 1–3 Bronchogram illustrating normal branching of bronchi and bronchioles that are normal in caliber and appearance.

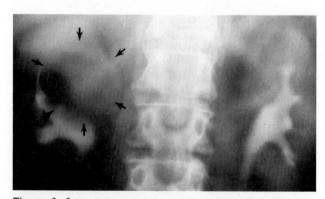

Figure 1–4 Intravenous pyelogram (IVP). Arrows outline filling defect caused by a large cyst in kidney that distorts renal pelvis and calyces. The opposite kidney appears normal.

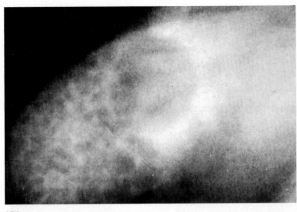

(A)

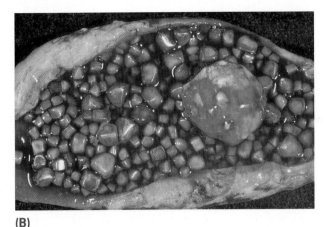

(B)

Figure 1–5 (A) Gallstones demonstrated by means of radiopaque material concentrated in bile. Gallstones occupy space and appear as radiolucent (dark) areas within radiopaque (white) bile. Note the large radiolucent area, indicating a large gallstone, surrounded by smaller radiolucent areas, representing multiple smaller stones. (B) Opened gallbladder removed surgically from the same patient. Compare appearance and location of stones with x-ray appearance.

when they are present in the gallbladder because they show up as irregularities in the radiopaque material that concentrates there (**Figure 1–5**).

When the flow of blood in the arteries is studied, the procedure is called an **arteriogram** or **angiogram**. For example, a common type of angiogram is a *carotid angiogram* (**Figure 1–6**). When blood flow is studied through the heart, it is known as a *cardiac catheterization*. Computed tomography (CT) is used to produce cross-sectional images of the body from various angles.

7. Computed tomography (CT): Uses specialized x-ray machines to produce cross-sectional body images by the rotation of the x-ray tube around the patient at different levels. The patient lies on a table, encircled by

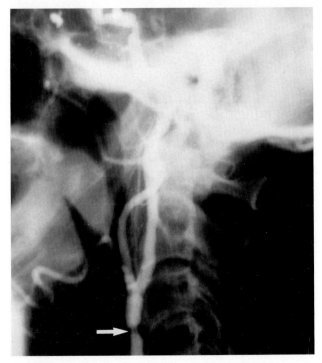

Figure 1–6 Narrowing of carotid artery in neck (arrow) demonstrated by carotid angiogram.

many radiation detectors housed in a movable x-ray tube (**Figure 1–7**). The data from the radiation detectors are fed directly into a computer that creates images that are displayed on a monitor and can be recorded on film (**Figures 1–8** and **1–9**).

CT scans appear similar to traditional x-rays. Substances that are denser appear lighter, and those that are less dense appear darker. Organs are very distinct because the fat separating them appears only slightly. When a standard x-ray cannot detect an internal abnormality, a CT scan usually can.

> **RED FLAG**
>
> A CT scan subjects the patient to approximately 200 times as much radiation as a traditional x-ray. However, this type of scan allows very detailed three-dimensional imaging, which is essential in specific circumstances such as internal injuries resulting from trauma.

8. Magnetic resonance imaging (MRI): Produces computerized images of organs and tissues, similar to the technology used in CT scans. MRI uses strong magnets and radiofrequency waves to produce images via computerized scanners. MRIs do not use ionizing radiation as do CTs, however. They use the response of hydrogen protons inside water molecules to produce images by causing them to move out of and then return to their original positions. Therefore, MRI is an excellent method of examining body tissues with high water content. MRIs are considered safer than x-rays, CT scans, and similar techniques. MRIs are preferred over CTs for areas with higher bone content such as the spinal cord, eye orbit, or lower skull conditions (**Figure 1–10**). In MRI the patient lies on a table that is slowly moved into the scanner, similar to a CT scan.

> **RED FLAG**
>
> Because MRIs use magnetic waves, they do not expose patients to ionizing radiation as do CTs.

9. Positron emission tomography (PET): First developed in the 1970s, PET scans are techniques used to study body functions by injecting glucose (or other compounds) that have been labeled with positron-emitting

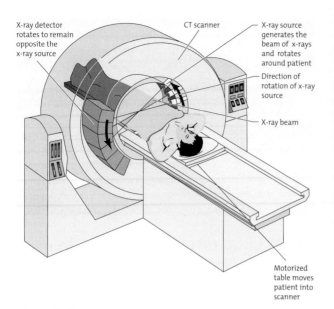

X-ray detector rotates to remain opposite the x-ray source

CT scanner

X-ray source generates the beam of x-rays and rotates around patient

Direction of rotation of x-ray source

X-ray beam

Motorized table moves patient into scanner

Figure 1–7 Computed tomographic (CT) scan. The patient lies on a table that is gradually advanced into the scanner. X-ray tube mounted in scanner rotates around patient, and radiation detectors also rotate so that detectors remain opposite the x-ray source. Data from radiation detectors generate computer-reconstructed images of the patient's body at multiple levels.

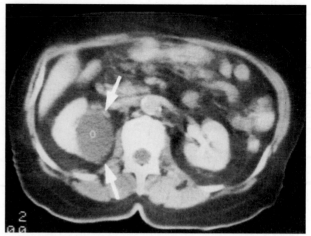

Figure 1–9 CT views of the abdomen at the level of kidneys, illustrating a fluid-filled cyst in the kidney (arrow). The cyst appears less dense than surrounding renal tissue. The opposite kidney (right side of photograph) appears normal.

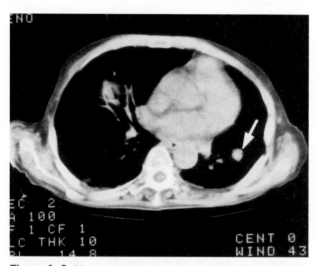

Figure 1–8 CT scan of chest. Mediastinum and heart appear white in the center of scan, with less dense lungs on either side. The arrow indicates a lung tumor, which appears as white nodule in lung.

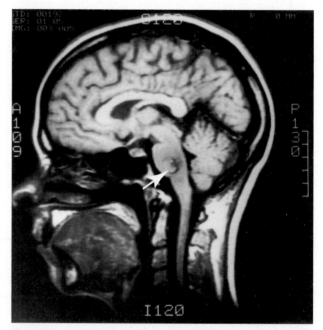

Figure 1–10 MRI view of brain, which is clearly visible because skull bones are not visualized by MRI. The white line surrounding the brain represents scalp tissue. The arrow indicates a malformation composed of blood vessels within the brain stem.

isotopes into the body. They are similar to radioisotope tests (see below). *Positrons* are defined as subatomic particles with the same mass as electrons but carrying a positive charge. PET scans provide information about organ or tissue metabolic activities, sites of metabolism of the injected compound, and blood flow to specific organs. Images that are generated are similar to those obtained from CT scans. PET scans are primarily used for brain function tests. Examples include brain tumors, strokes, Alzheimer's disease, Parkinson's disease, and certain nervous system disorders. They are also used for evaluation of the heart after a heart attack and to determine malignancy of

certain tumors. However, PET scans are currently very expensive because of the equipment and compounds that are needed.

10. Radioisotope (radionuclide) tests: Use **radioactive** materials to determine various body functions and states. Specially designed radiation detectors measure the radioisotope's uptake and excretion. These include conditions such as certain types of anemia, thyroid conditions, pulmonary conditions, skeletal conditions, cancers, and cardiovascular conditions. For example, when bone tumors are present, radioisotopes are concentrated around the tumor deposits and can be easily seen on a radioisotope bone scan (**Figure 1–11**).

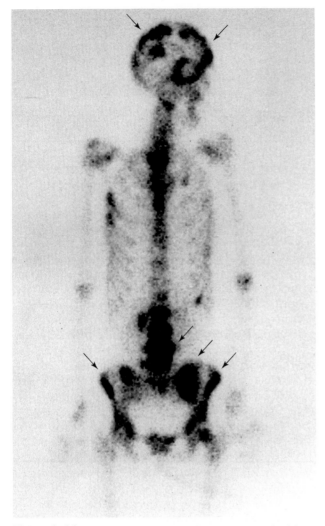

Figure 1–11 Radioisotope bone scan of head, chest, and pelvis. Dark areas (arrows) indicate the concentration of radioisotope around tumor deposits in bone.

11. Ultrasound procedures: These techniques map the sound vibrations that are produced by high-frequency sound waves transmitted into the body. Changes in tissue density cause echoes to reflect, from which images are produced. **Ultrasound** is used for a variety of procedures, including studies of the uterus and fetus during pregnancy (**Figure 1–12**), the heart valves and structures, for cardiovascular conditions, to detect gallstones, and for prostate abnormalities. Ultrasound is safer than radiologic studies because it does not use radiation.

Treatment

Once a diagnosis has been made, decisions are made as to the best treatment options. These options may be either specific or symptomatic. A *specific treatment* is based on the major cause of the disease. For example, a patient with diabetes may be treated with insulin. However, for many diseases there are no specific treatment regimens. A *symptomatic treatment* alleviates disease symptoms but may or may not affect the underlying course of the disease. For example, coughing is treated by antitussive medications, but these do not necessarily cure the cause of the coughing, which can be varied. Because many

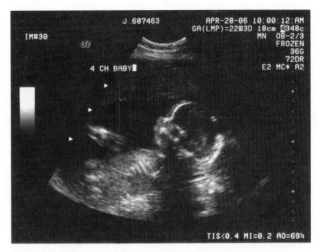

Figure 1–12 Ultrasound examination of a 22-week-old fetus.

diseases do not have specific treatments, the goal of symptomatic treatment is palliative: to reduce patient symptoms during the disease course. Also, a disease or condition may sometimes be caused by a medical treatment. When this occurs, the disease or condition is described as **iatrogenic**.

SUMMARY

Disease is defined as a deviation from normal physical, mental, and social well-being that causes a disruption or loss of homeostasis. Pathophysiology is the study of structural and functional changes that are related to disease. Disease effects depend on which organs or tissues are affected. Diseases may be classified as congenital, hereditary, degenerative, inflammatory, metabolic, or neoplastic. Today, various methods are used for the diagnosis of diseases and conditions. The procedures used may be invasive or noninvasive. Examples include clinical laboratory tests, cytology, histology, and diagnostic imaging. The prevention of disease depends on adequate early screening. Physical examination and patient history are also helpful. It is vital that health care practitioners be aware of the latest information about diseases and conditions, testing, and treatments.

REVIEW QUESTIONS

Select the best response to each question.

1. The term that means the body is in a state of equilibrium or balance is
   a. metabolism
   b. homeostasis
   c. physiology
   d. pathology
2. The time in early disease development when a patient is aware of a nonspecific change in the body is referred to as
   a. exacerbation
   b. epidemic
   c. occurrence
   d. prodromal

3. Outbreaks of a disease that occur over a given area with many cases of the disease are called
   a. endemics
   b. pandemics
   c. epidemics
   d. none of the above

4. The causative factors of a particular disease are called its
   a. idiopathy
   b. etiology
   c. pathology
   d. iatrogenicity

5. A disease that lasts for a short time but develops quickly is known as
   a. prodromal
   b. chronic
   c. latent
   d. acute

6. The development of a disease is referred to as
   a. pathology
   b. pathogenesis
   c. pathogen
   d. neoplasm

7. The study of changes to cells and tissues that is associated with a disease is referred to as
   a. cytology
   b. histology
   c. physiology
   d. pathology

8. Prevalence of disease is always a higher number than incidence and is called
   a. morbidity
   b. mortality
   c. prodromal
   d. occurrence

9. The probability or likelihood for recovery from a disease is called
   a. prognosis
   b. prevention
   c. syndrome
   d. convalescence

10. A technique used to study body functions that involves injecting glucose (or other compounds), labeled with isotopes, into the body is known as
    a. MRI
    b. CT scan
    c. PET scan
    d. Ultrasound

CASE STUDIES

Karen Coupe, PT, DPT, MSEd

Case 1

A PTA is performing a chart review for a 72-year-old woman admitted to the hospital for an elective total hip replacement. Two days after surgery the patient began to complain of shortness of breath and chest pain with a postsurgical complication of pulmonary embolism.

1. What do you suspect is the reason for the elective surgical procedure? Would this be classified as an acute or chronic issue? Would this be considered an inflammatory, degenerative or metabolic disorder?
2. What were the clinical manifestations of the pulmonary embolism?
3. The pulmonary embolism was a complication of the surgical procedure. Why is it important for the PTA to understand and be able to react to potential complications of any condition?
4. How could complications affect convalescence?
5. How could complications affect mortality rates?

Case 2

A 58-year-old man was admitted to the hospital complaining of shortness of breath, lightheadedness, and left-sided shoulder pain. Diagnostic testing included a blood workup and an electrocardiogram. Diagnosis: Myocardial infarction. Patient medical history: coronary artery bypass graft 2 years ago, hypertension controlled by medication, borderline type 2 diabetes. Social history: Sedentary lifestyle, smokes one pack of cigarettes a day, social drinker. Prior level of function: Independent in all activities of daily living. Patient was referred to physical therapy for cardiac phase I rehab.

1. What were the clinical manifestations of the myocardial infarction?
2. Explain the basic purpose of the diagnostic tests performed on this patient.
3. Why is it important that the PTA understand the patient medical history? What could be potential consequences of not understanding the patient medical history?
4. What role does the patient's social history have on physical therapy treatment?
5. Explain the rationale behind knowing the prior level of function before beginning physical therapy treatments.

WEBSITES

http://www.americanheart.org/presenter.jhtml?identifier=4720

http://www.cdc.gov/mmwr/

http://www.emedicinehealth.com/gangrene/article_em.htm

http://www.health-disease.org/

http://www.meddean.luc.edu/lumen/MedEd/orfpath/cellch.htm

http://www.medscape.com/viewarticle/421471

http://www.nd.gov/cte/programs/health-careers/ppt/pathophysiology.ppt

http://www.nlm.nih.gov/medlineplus/ency/article/003416.htm

http://www.nova.edu/healthcare/forms/patient_medical_history.pdf

http://www.pathguy.com/autopsy.htm

Mechanisms of Disease

LEARNING OBJECTIVES

After completion of the chapter the reader should be able to

1. Describe the effects of age and gender on various diseases.
2. Explain how socioeconomic status can affect development of disease.
3. Describe the effects of lifestyle on the progression of disease.
4. Define obesity and explain its effects on the body.
5. Define "body mass index."
6. Describe the effects of physical trauma on development of disease.
7. List the factors that are important to understand about culture diversity.
8. Explain how psychological factors impact the development and progression of disease.

KEY TERMS

Bariatrics: the branch of medicine that deals with the treatment of obesity and its complications.

Hydrostatic weighing: underwater weighing; a method to determine the mass density of a body.

Metabolic syndrome: a combination of medical disorders that increase the risk of developing cardiovascular disease and diabetes.

Ozone: a compound made up of three oxygen atoms that in the lower atmosphere is an air pollutant harmful to the respiratory system.

Pathogens: infectious agents that cause disease in their hosts.

Shaken baby syndrome: a form of physical child abuse occurring when a person violently shakes an infant or small child; it creates a whiplash-type motion that causes acceleration-deceleration injuries of the brain.

Somatoform: a mental disorder characterized by physical symptoms that suggest physical illness or injury.

X-ray absorptiometry: a means of measuring bone mineral density that uses two x-ray beams with different energy levels.

Overview

The mechanisms of disease have a connection with many different features that disrupt the normal state of an individual's health. Disruptions of internal equilibrium can result in degenerative changes in cells that can cause disease symptoms. The body's homeostasis is disrupted by fluid and electrolyte imbalances and conditions of acidosis or alkalosis. Predisposing (risk) factors for disease are those that determine an individual's susceptibility to pathogenic conditions. Other factors related to the mechanisms of disease include obesity, cultural diversity, and mental (psychological) states.

Predisposing Factors

Predisposing factors are also known as *risk factors*. Although they make people more vulnerable to diseases, they do not predict the development of a disease. However, in the absence of predisposing factors, this does not guarantee that a person will remain disease free. These factors frequently overlap or occur in numerous combinations with varying outcomes. Predisposing factors include age, gender, environment, heredity, lifestyle, physical activity, and socioeconomic status.

Age

Age is related to a variety of predisposing factors, and physiologic changes become more evident at approximately 30 years of age. Throughout a person's lifespan, certain risks are increased at certain ages and decreased at others. It may relate to long-term environmental and genetic factors as well. No one ages in the same exact way, although certain general steps in the process occur in basically the same order. As we age, cellular metabolism changes and cellular damage continually occurs.

The period from old age to death is called *senescence*. Average human lifespan is increasing, with women living longer, overall, than men. There are more elderly people alive today, proportionally, than at any other time in history. This is based on better nutrition, medical advances, and standards of living. Aging occurs as the body experiences reduced function at all levels and can no longer adapt to changing conditions. Each individual may be predisposed to certain pathologies that affect the rate at which aging occurs.

Aging is believed to occur either through genetic programming that predetermines the rate of cellular death (*apoptosis*), from the stressors of life upon the body, as a result of accumulating wastes and other substances, or because of degeneration of collagen and elastin. An additional opinion is that viruses or autoimmune reactions influence permanent damage to the body, intensifying the effects of aging. *Free radicals* (reactive chemicals produced during cell metabolism) damage nucleic acids and cells, which may lead to many types of diseases, influencing the rate of aging.

As we age, cells become less regular, elasticity is lost, and abnormal structures in tissues and organs increase. There is decreased tissue repair due to the slow down of mitosis (cellular reproduction). Function is reduced as neurons and muscle cells die, unable to be replaced. Prolonged exposure to factors such as chemicals, viruses, and radiation leads to increased risk of many diseases. **Table 2–1** lists significant changes that occur with aging.

> **RED FLAG**
> Osteoarthritis, the most common type of arthritis, impairs mobility in many older individuals. Physical therapy intervention can be of great help in combating the effects of osteoarthritis.

Gender

Gender affects the development of various diseases as well. Diseases affecting women more than men include multiple sclerosis, osteoporosis, breast cancer, and rheumatoid arthritis. Diseases affecting men more than women include gout, Parkinson's disease, and lung cancer. **Table 2–2** lists the seven most common diseases for males and females.

Environment

Environmental risk factors for disease include air and water pollution, noise, poor living conditions and sanitation, harsh geographic locations, and chronic psychological stress. Pollutants in the environment have been linked to asthma, cardiovascular problems, cancer, gastrointestinal problems, and

TABLE 2–1	**Age-Related Changes to Body Systems**	
Body System	**Changes**	**Comments**
Cardiovascular	Fatty tissue and collagen accumulation interfere with impulse conduction and cardiac muscle contraction. Heart valves thicken. Vascular degeneration causes a decrease in oxygen supply. Cardiac output and reserve are diminished. Arterial walls thicken, leading to arteriosclerosis and elevated blood pressure. Cholesterol and lipids accumulate in large arteries (atherosclerosis), obstructing blood flow and predisposing thrombus formation.	Cardiac muscle fibers cannot be replaced because they do not undergo mitosis. Adequate fluid intake is important to maintain cardiovascular function. Regular fitness programs combined with good diet are extremely helpful. Atherosclerosis leads to angina, heart attacks, peripheral vascular disease, and strokes.
Endocrine	As the number of tissue receptors to hormones decreases, the body has a reduced response to hormones. However, most endocrine glands remain relatively normal in their hormone production. Women during menopause experience lower levels of estrogen and progesterone and higher levels of follicle-stimulating hormone and luteinizing hormone.	Type 2 diabetes is an example of reduced response to hormones—enough insulin is produced but the body's reduced number of cell receptors means that glucose does not enter the cells. Hormone secretion in older men is lower, but the testes do not totally cease to function.

TABLE 2-1 Age-Related Changes to Body Systems (*Continued*)

Body System	Changes	Comments
Gastrointestinal	Decreased saliva and periodontal disease often influence dietary choices. Oral tissues are more prone to irritation and damage. With aging, lack of exercise and improper diet often lead to obesity. Complications of obesity include heart problems, gallstones, and osteoarthritis. Reduced digestive secretions are related to inadequate absorption of essential nutrients.	Older adults must maintain adequate nutrition. "Dry mouth" is common. Swallowing may become more difficult due to obstructions or neurologic causes. Peptic ulcers are more prevalent due to changes in mucosa and mucous production. Malignancies are more prevalent. Chronic constipation often leads to hemorrhoids.
Integumentary	Skin and mucous membranes become thin and fragile. Wounds heal more slowly and skin glands atrophy. Elastic and collagen fibers reduce in amount and flexibility. Skin lesions and spots proliferate. The hair turns gray because of reduced melanocytes and thins due to decreased amounts of hair follicles.	Skin bruising and ulcerations become more likely due to less moisture and other conditions.
Musculoskeletal	Bones lose calcium and overall bone mass, leading to osteoporosis. Fractures are more common. Spontaneous vertebral fractures result in decreased height and kyphosis. Cartilage degeneration results in osteoarthritis. Intervertebral discs may become herniated, resulting in severe back pain.	Ventilation and mobility are often impaired by degenerative changes in the spine. Joint pain is common, and serious conditions may result in joint replacement, the most common of which involves the hips or knees. Overall in flexibility occurs as a result of bone, cartilage, joint, and muscular changes. Regular exercise greatly improves mobility.
Neurologic	A natural reduction in brain mass occurs, varying with each individual. Lipids may accumulate in neurons, the myelin sheaths are lost, and neurofibrils or plaques develop on the cells. There is a decreased cell response to neurotransmitters in the brain. Tolerance to extreme temperatures is reduced. Neurologic changes lead to reduced sensory functions.	Maintaining high activity levels appears to maintain brain function. Aging leads to slower responses and reflexes, as well as lapses of short-term memory. Eyesight and hearing often become poorer. Night vision is usually greatly impaired. Also, taste and smell may be reduced because of neurologic changes.
Reproductive	The most significant change is menopause in women. Hormone reduction may lead to a variety of conditions. Breast tissue decreases in volume. "Hot flashes" are common, as well as headaches, irritability, and insomnia. In men testosterone decreases gradually, the testes shrink, and sperm or glandular secretion production reduces.	Declining hormones in women may lead to vaginal changes and potential pain during intercourse. Changes in pH may result in recurrent vaginal infections. In men benign prostatic hypertrophy may develop around the urethra, leading to surgery. Breast, prostate, and uterine cancers become more common with aging.
Respiratory	Inspiration and expiration become limited due to reduced elasticity of lung tissue, calcification of cartilage between ribs and the sternum, weakening of skeletal muscle, and reduced thoracic movement. Vascular degeneration occurs, leading to reduced oxygen levels.	Residual volume increases. As lung movements are restricted, there is decreased expansion for deep breathing and coughing. Coughing is less effective, causing secretions to accumulate and risk of pneumonia to increase. Regular physical exercise, breathing exercises, and oxygen therapy assist in maintaining respiratory function.
Urinary	The kidneys lose glomeruli and experience degeneration of tubules and blood vessels. This diminishes their ability to compensate for electrolyte and acid level changes. Bladder function cannot be controlled as readily due to weakened muscles. Incontinence may occur, resulting in incomplete bladder emptying.	Kidneys usually have reduced capacity to secrete drugs into urine. Common urinary changes include frequency, nocturia, and infections. Women, after childbirth, may experience decreased ability to restrict urinary outflow. Smooth muscle tone decreases.

many other diseases. Common air pollutants include **ozone**, particulate matter, carbon monoxide, nitrogen oxides, sulfur dioxide, and lead. Occupational diseases are higher in workers who are exposed to large amounts of dust or other particles in the air. These workers include miners and farmers. Common water pollutants include detergents, disinfectants, insecticides, petroleum hydrocarbons, industrial solvents, ammonia, fertilizers, and heavy metals.

RED FLAG

People living in countries with high rates of pollution (such as Peru, Pakistan, Kuwait, Saudi Arabia, Ethiopia, Russia, and Indonesia) are at much higher risk of disease.

TABLE 2-2 Diseases That Most Affect Males and Females

Males	Females
Heart disease	Heart disease
Cancer	Cancer
Stroke	Stroke
Chronic obstructive pulmonary disease	Chronic obstructive pulmonary disease
Type 2 diabetes	Alzheimer's disease
Influenza	Type 2 diabetes
Kidney disease	Influenza

Heredity

Genetic predisposition is also a major risk factor to the development of disease, as family history is a strong influence. Genetic risk factors may also be linked to environmental factors (for example, mental illness, hypertension, and diabetes). If a patient already has a family history of certain diseases, activities such as smoking, high-fat diets, and lack of exercise may greatly increase the likelihood of developing these diseases. The chance of developing a heredity-linked disease is decreased with adequate, regular self-examinations and improving lifestyle.

Lifestyle

Many components of a person's normal lifestyle can increase risk factors for disease. A dangerous or hazardous job, habit (such as cigarette smoking), or behavior may lead to serious illness or other conditions. Lifestyle choices that may lead to disease include smoking, excessive alcohol use, risky sexual behavior, use of illegal drugs, lack of exercise, poor nutrition, and psychological stressors. The most common diseases related to lifestyle include Alzheimer's disease, atherosclerosis, asthma, cancer, liver disease, chronic obstructive pulmonary disease, type 2 diabetes, heart disease, metabolic syndrome, Crohn's disease, kidney disease, osteoporosis, acne, stroke, depression, and obesity.

Physical Activity

Adequate physical activity is essential to prevent many different disease states. Regular exercise (20 minutes, three times per week) is important in preventing heart disease, stroke, type 2 diabetes, obesity, back pain, osteoporosis, and other conditions. Psychological states are also benefited by exercise. Combined with a healthy diet, physical activity is one of the best ways of preventing the development of many different illnesses. Unfortunately, more than 60 percent of men and women do not exercise daily. Simple methods of physical exercise include walking, using stairs instead of elevators, participating in sports, joining a gym or health club, aerobic exercises, stretching, and weight training.

Socioeconomic Status

Socioeconomic status plays a strong role as a risk factor for the development of disease. More people in low socioeconomic classes have a likelihood for developing certain diseases than any other classes. For example, people of lower income are more susceptible to developing chronic diseases, which are reported three times more often than in the highest income classes. Diagnosis and treatment may be delayed because of lack of health insurance or the ability to pay for medical assistance. The homeless population is usually much more likely to develop diseases that will go untreated or receive only limited treatment.

Cancer

Cancer is a term used to describe a disease process characterized by uncontrolled cell proliferation. This proliferation of cells leads to the development of *tumors* or *neoplasms*. Benign tumors are not considered life threatening in most cases, whereas malignant tumors usually are more dangerous. Benign tumors are usually slow to develop and are well differentiated, rarely recurring after surgical removal. Malignant tumors usually develop more quickly, with disorderly appearances, and often recur after surgical removal. Malignant tumors often invade surrounding tissue, the bloodstream, and/or lymphatic vessels. For a more detailed discussion of the various types of cancer, see Chapter 7.

Genetic Diseases

When a genetic or chromosomal abnormality has been identified, an individual may be tested for the presence of a mutation that caused a specific disease. Family history is vital in this regard. Common genetically linked diseases or conditions include cancer, coronary disease, various arthritic conditions, and kidney disease.

Genetic counseling is used to inform patients about the likelihood of their contracting a genetically linked disease or in passing it on to their offspring. Genetic counselors help families to understand disease diagnoses, disease courses, and available treatments. Available tests and their benefits are explained by these counselors. These professionals function on many different levels, preparing families for genetic testing outcomes, relieving feelings of guilt, helping to deal with insurance problems, and giving advice as to steps to take when a disease is not curable. As a result of the increased availability of genetic testing, most major hospitals now have genetic counselors available for their patients. For a more detailed discussion of genetic diseases, see Chapter 6.

> **RED FLAG**
> Screening programs are available to determine if a person is a carrier of a variety of genetic disorders. Ultrasonography and amniocentesis may detect certain developmental defects in fetuses.

Immune Disorders

Immune disorders are those resulting from the body's natural defense system breaking down. These occurrences may generate three types of conditions:

1. Hypersensitivity (allergy)
2. Autoimmune diseases
3. Immunodeficiency disorders

The immune system is made up of specialized cells and organs that defend the body against foreign microorganisms and substances. For a more detailed discussion of immune disorders, see Chapter 10.

Infection

Pathogens cause infections and their symptoms, such as redness, heat, pain, fever, swelling, pus, enlarged lymph glands, and red streaking of the skin. When an infection is widespread, symptoms include fever, body ache, headache, fatigue, loss of appetite, delirium, and weakness. Pathogens cause disease in two essential ways:

1. Invasion and localized destruction of tissue
2. Intoxication or production of substances that are poisonous

Infection results in tissue damage, and potential systemic involvement.

Infection may be from within the body (endogenous) or from outside the body (exogenous). Pathogenic agents include bacteria, viruses, fungi, and protozoa. Pathogenic microorganisms are transmitted in a variety of ways:

- Direct or indirect physical contact
- Inhalation or droplet nuclei
- Contaminated food or water
- Inoculation by an insect or an animal

Patients who do not have symptoms of a disease they carry are referred to as *asymptomatic*, and animals may also be carriers of certain diseases. A *communicable (contagious) disease* is one that can be directly transmitted from one person to another. For a more detailed discussion of infectious diseases, see Chapter 8.

> **RED FLAG**
> Infection may be eradicated without drug treatment when a microbial colony has only limited growth.

Inflammation and Repair

Inflammation, when acute, is a normal protective physiologic response to disease and tissue injury. Symptoms of inflammation include heat, redness, pain, swelling, and loss of function. When inflammation spreads to become systemic, it is accompanied by fever, loss of appetite, and malaise. At this stage blood tests will reveal an elevated erythrocyte sedimentation rate or elevated white blood cell count.

Repair and replacement of damaged tissue begin after these mechanisms of inflammation have removed the damaging microorganisms. However, the use of certain medications (such as steroids) can reduce the inflammatory response. Chronic illness and immune disorders can also slow the body's ability to use the inflammatory response to combat disease. For a more detailed discussion of inflammation and healing, see Chapter 9.

Nutrition and Obesity

Nutrition has direct yet controllable effects on chronic disease. Diet has both positive and negative effects on health and can both prevent and control morbidity and mortality. The most significant diseases related to diet are diabetes, cardiovascular disease, cancer, obesity, and osteoporosis. Diets high in fruits and vegetables are associated with lower risks for many chronic diseases and conditions.

Consuming a diet high in saturated fat and low in unprocessed carbohydrates is almost always a choice that will have serious consequences. Many countries, including all of North America, are well above the recommended average of fat-to-energy ratio. This is defined as the percent of energy that is derived from fat in the total number of calories supplied. It also concerns the recommended amount of saturated fat per total calories, which is 10 percent.

Malnutrition is a nutritional disorder that may be caused by deficient diet or diseases that cause the body to become unable to break down, absorb, or use food. Starvation due to famine results in a severe form of malnutrition known as *kwashiorkor*, a protein-calorie deficiency. Other examples of malnutrition are various anemias, hypervitaminosis, and obesity.

Obesity is defined by excessive fat accumulation, which contributes to many chronic diseases and early mortality and morbidity. The branch of medicine that deals with the treatment of obesity and its complications is called **bariatrics**.

Obesity is considered a pandemic that has begun to replace other causes of death, including undernutrition and infectious disease.

Diseases Related to Obesity

Obesity is defined as a body mass index (BMI) greater than or equal to 30 kilograms per square meter (kg/m^2). *BMI is a ratio of height to weight.* Any BMI greater than or equal to 25 is associated with increased risk for premature death and disability. *Morbid obesity* refers to a BMI greater than 40 kg/m^2. Some health care professionals still choose to define obesity as weight greater than 20 percent of desirable weight for a patient, based on gender, height, and body structure.

BMI is an accepted measurement for obesity worldwide. When fat distribution is in and around the abdomen, obesity is extremely risky for health and longevity. Because extremely muscular individuals may have a higher than desirable BMI, it is important to remember that health risks only occur if BMI is related to excess body fat.

> **RED FLAG**
> BMI varies with age and gender in children and adolescents. Special charts have been developed to gauge this for patients who are still growing, at various ages. One child of every five in the United States is obese, with a BMI that is at (or above) the 95th percentile.

In the United States obesity is second only to cigarette smoking as the leading cause of preventable death. Nearly 65 percent of adults in this country are overweight or obese. Approximately 500,000 deaths occur annually as a result of obesity. Unfortunately, the condition is on the rise across all age groups.

Obesity is usually caused by an imbalance between energy intake and energy expenditure. Inactivity and poor diet usually contribute to this situation. Medications such as antidepressants, corticosteroids, and antihypertensives may influence weight gain, as do hypoglycemia and water retention. Biochemical defects may also be responsible to a lesser degree, and it is becoming more widely believed that obesity is a central nervous system–mediated *neuroendocrine dysfunction*. It may be heavily related to hormonal dysfunction. Psychosocial and behavioral factors such as history of sexual abuse, eating disorders, cessation of smoking, and stressful lifestyle play a role in obesity.

Pathogenesis of obesity depends on evidence that the condition is a central nervous system–mediated neuroendocrine dysfunction. This is believed to be caused either by spontaneous genetic mutations or targeted gene deletions that affect food intake and body weight control. Hormonal dysfunction that affects the hypothalamic-pituitary-adrenal axis results in complicated events that occur in series. As regulated by stressors, this leads to poorly regulated secretion of cortisol, elevated blood pressure, resistance to insulin, and central obesity (the visceral accumulation of body fat). Obese patients use less energy and burn fewer calories than nonobese patients. Some patients have excessive fat cells of increased size. Obesity is also related to intestinal microorganisms, which can regulate energy intake, absorption, and storage.

The effects of obesity are not easy to define in earlier stages. It is, however, associated with the three leading overall causes of death: cardiovascular disease, cancer, and diabetes mellitus. Obesity is a known risk factor for hormone-related cancers (breast, cervical, endometrial, liver, prostate, colon, and rectal cancer).

Complications associated with obesity include **metabolic syndrome**, liver diseases, osteoarthritis, sleep apnea, atherosclerosis, hypertension, cardiovascular diseases, stroke, asthma, cancer, menstrual disorders, infertility, impaired mobility, gallbladder disease, psychological disturbances, premature death, and type 2 diabetes mellitus. It is a common cause of back and joint pain in multiple sites throughout the body.

Preventing obesity or slowing its progression is important in combating disease. This involves maintaining a healthy weight, weight loss, and preventing weight gain. Determining obesity involves measurements of height, weight, body circumference, and nutritional status. A waist circumference of more than 40 inches for men and 35 inches for women increases risks for premature death or disability and relates closely with BMI. Other methods of analysis include dual-energy **x-ray absorptiometry** and **hydrostatic weighing**.

To combat obesity it is important to combine physical activity with proper nutrition. A reduction of 10 percent of an individual's body weight has been shown to improve the quality of life for an obese patient. Treatments include moderate calorie intake, behavior modification, exercise, and social support. When these modifications and medications fail, surgical treatment (*bariatric surgery*) may be indicated. The most preferred surgery is *laparoscopic Roux-en-Y gastric bypass*. Benefits of bariatric surgery are improved serum lipids, weight loss, decreased blood pressure, improved or resolved diabetes mellitus, improved or resolved sleep apnea, reduced venous stasis, decreased joint pain, improved quality of life, and overall improved function.

> **RED FLAG**
>
> With obese patients the physical therapist assistant (PTA) should assist with reduction of back pain, arthritis symptoms, dysfunctions of the various parts of the lower limbs, preventing breakdown of the skin, and improving cardiopulmonary condition.

Working with obese patients is more difficult, requiring careful planning for transferring, using proper body mechanics, and asking for assistance when the patient needs lifting or hands-on therapy. The PTA may be involved in hypertension and obesity screening because regular exercise is important for physical and mental well-being as well as for prevention of conditions affecting morbidity that are associated with obesity. Graded exercise testing may be required before an exercise program can be prescribed. Treadmills are typically used to evaluate patients by slowly increasing the grade of the treadmill.

Physical Trauma and Chemical Agents

In children and young adults, physical trauma is the leading cause of death. Acute injuries commonly occur because of falls, motor vehicle accidents, penetrating injuries, physical abuse, burns, and drowning. When a person undergoes trauma, efforts must be made to minimize insult to body tissues, to offer precise assessment and management to prevent infection from developing, to restore homeostasis, and to treat shock and hemorrhage.

Potentially dangerous chemical agents (or irritants) include poisons, pollutants, drugs, preservatives, cosmetics, and dyes. The body may also be harmed by extreme heat or cold, electrical shock, insect or snake bites, and radiation.

Domestic Violence

Domestic violence includes intimate partner violence, child abuse, and elder abuse. PTAs may encounter individuals of all ages who have been victims of some form of domestic violence. Many state practice acts include wording that describes the PTA as being a *mandated reporter* of suspected domestic violence. Domestic violence occurs in all socioeconomic and racial-ethnic groups. The following list describes types of domestic violence:

- Physical abuse: Nonaccidental physical injuries such as bruises, welts, broken bones, burns, serious internal injuries, and death
- Emotional and psychological abuse: From acts or omissions potentially causing behavioral, cognitive, emotional, or mental disorders
- Sexual abuse: Includes exhibitionism, fondling, rape, molestation, or forced use of any age individual in the production of pornographic materials
- Neglect: Withholding of or failure to provide adequate food, shelter, clothing, hygiene, medical care, and/or supervision required for optimal health and well-being
- Stalking: Conduct directed at a specific person involving repeat visual or physical proximity, nonconsensual communication, threats, or any combination of these

Child Abuse

Child abuse may be physical or emotional in nature. It includes neglect and sexual abuse, with nearly 12 of every 1,000 children in the United States being victims. Nearly 1,500 children die every year from some form of abuse, many under 3 years of age. Health care professionals, at all levels, must be knowledgeable about determining signs of accidental injuries and child abuse. Similar to domestic violence, many states also consider the PTA to be a *mandated reporter* of suspected child abuse.

Explanation of injuries that are incompatible with a child's age, size, and developmental skills may signify child abuse. Common symptoms include a history of frequent illness related to the ears, throat, lungs, chest, and gastrointestinal tract. **Shaken baby syndrome** results in retinal hemorrhage and signs of traumatic brain injury. Often, subdural hematoma and skull fractures in infants result from this. If feedings are forced upon an infant, there may be upper lip and frenulum injuries. Behavioral manifestations of child abuse include neglect, which can result in head banging and rocking; failure to thrive; developmental delays; speech delays; and an aversion to being touched.

Elder Abuse

Elder abuse is defined as intentional or negligent acts by caretakers or others that cause harm or serious risk of harm to older patients over 60 or 65 years of age. Each state has its own clearly defined regulations concerning elder abuse. More than 1.8 million seniors may be victims of elder abuse in the United States. Unfortunately, many cases are never reported. Common types of elder abuse include physical abuse, emotional and/or psychological abuse, and financial exploitation.

Physical manifestations of elder abuse include soiled clothing or bedding, smell of fecal matter or urine, health or safety hazards, lack of hair or hemorrhaging below the scalp, dehydration or malnourishment or weight loss without illness, poor skin condition or hygiene, marks around the mouth that may indicate gagging attempts, rope burns or abrasions that indicate restraint attempts, and inadequate clothing, heat, or food. Behavioral manifestations of elder abuse include increased use of alcohol or other drugs and a caregiver always being present when a senior is questioned about treatment. When a caregiver answers all questions instead of the patient, this may be a realistic sign of elder abuse.

Cultural Diversity

It is important to understand cultural diversity when dealing with patients. The United States has more foreign-born residents than ever before in its history. This brings about differences in language, how health issues are viewed, religious beliefs, and general life experiences. Dietary preferences and traditions concerning birth and death must also be understood.

PTAs must be willing to learn about cultural issues, take the time needed to fully understand patients, and to overcome language barriers. PTAs should also show patience and be flexible about each patient's cultural background and how it affects the anticipations they may have concerning health care.

Mental Disorders

Mental disorders include dementia, grief response, mood disorders, and **somatoform** disorders. In general, they are clinically significant psychological or behavioral syndromes related to psychic pain, distress, or impairment of function. They may cause serious disability and deserve to be handled with the same medical professionalism as any other disease state. Specific patient behaviors that affect health and disease include coping with stressful situations. People react to a stressful event by using coping mechanisms.

Coping mechanisms are also called *relief behaviors*. They can resolve, reduce, or replace stress, depression, and anxiety. Stressors with multiple physiologic events may require physiologic coping mechanisms called *generalized adaptation responses*. When chronic, the body enters a stage of exhaustion, and damage to the involved systems occurs. Women and men respond differently to various stressors to protect themselves individually. Stress is linked to premature aging and death. Chronic depression is linked to heart disease and immune system dysfunction.

Stress includes social, psychological, and physiologic factors. Along with other emotional responses, stress is a component of complex interactions of genetic, behavioral, environmental, and physiologic factors. Stress is regulated by the endocrine, immune, and nervous systems. The stress response may be altered by early life events that are adverse or traumatic. Psychological stress and aging combine to impact the immune system, with interactive effects.

Stress causes different reactions in each person. Women often feel stress more than men at comparable life stages and circumstances. Women often are "stressed" longer after the experience than men. Stress is very strong, and its effects on the body and mind are wide reaching. Even slight physical or psychological stressors can harm immune function and delay healing.

> **RED FLAG**
> Severe prolonged stress or multiple stressors may have serious consequences such as development of peptic ulcer or acute renal failure.

Stress may be a neurophysiologic, hormonal, and behavioral event. Stress responses and symptoms are listed in **Table 2–3**.

Psychological Factors

Psychological factors can affect a person's health in many ways. A physical evaluation also includes an assessment of the patient's mental status. To evaluate psychological factors, all of the following are observed regarding the patient:

- Appearance
- Behavior
- Communication
- Judgment
- Mood
- Thought processes

TABLE 2–3 Stress

Stress Responses	Stress Symptoms
Changes in respiratory system	Allergic responses
Contraction of spleen	Chest pain
Decreased blood clotting time	Depression, anxiety, panic attacks
Decreased peristalsis and gut function	Discouragement, boredom
Decreased immune response (chronic stress)	Eating disorders
Dilation of pupils	Gastrointestinal symptoms
Increased heart rate, blood pressure	Headache
Increased sweat production	Hypertension
Redirection of blood supply (brain, muscles)	Myalgia, arthralgia, fibromyalgia
Release of adrenaline, glucose	Poor work or school performance with errors in judgment
	Prolonged fatigue (chronic fatigue syndrome)
	Sleep disturbances

Treatments must take into account the patient's physical as well as psychological needs to preserve self-esteem. Disease interrupts daily life and changes the patient's body image, emotions, and social outlook. Parental treatment of a patient's childhood illnesses may have a profound effect on how he or she handles illness later in life. Chronic diseases may affect a patient's behavior, causing feelings of fear, helplessness, and lack of control. As the patient adjusts to a serious disease, there will be stages of anxiety, shock, denial, anger, withdrawal, and depression. If long-term, or if the patient cannot accept the reality of the condition, psychological disturbances may manifest.

Role of the PTA in Patients with Stress

PTAs can assist with preparing a patient for a stress therapy program by using the following steps:

- Allowing self-regulation, self-efficacy perception, and outcome expectations to be described by the patient
- Assessing the patient's readiness to change before prescribing changes to exercise and lifestyle
- Promoting wellness and strategies that are correct for the patient's ability to change and his or her perception of self-efficacy
- Providing opportunities for improving self-efficacy, including feedback to his or her initial exercise attempts

When stress is major, illness is chronic, or the patient is psychologically disturbed, the PTA may need to develop personal coping mechanisms to provide the best care. If not anticipated, these factors may create obstacles to successful physical therapy. When the patient's ability to change is recognized, the resultant physical therapy program design is more likely to be correct and effective.

SUMMARY

Predisposing factors, also known as risk factors, make people more vulnerable to diseases. Predisposing factors include age, gender, environment, heredity, lifestyle, physical activity, and socioeconomic status. Neoplasms may become life-threatening malignancies. Genetic diseases are those caused by the presence of a mutation that may be related to genes or chromosomes. Immune disorders include hypersensitivity, autoimmune diseases, and immunodeficiency disorders. Pathogens cause infections by invasion and localized destruction of tissue and intoxication or production of poisonous substances.

Acute inflammation is a normal response to disease and tissue injury. Diet has both positive and negative effects on health. Obesity is second only to cigarette smoking as the leading cause of preventable death. To combat obesity it is important to combine physical activity with proper nutrition. In children and young adults physical trauma is the leading cause of death. Potentially dangerous chemical agents include poisons, pollutants, drugs, preservatives, cosmetics, and dyes. Domestic violence, including child and elder abuse, occurs in all socioeconomic and racial-ethnic groups. It is important for the PTA to understand cultural diversity when dealing with patients. Treatments must take into account a patient's physical as well as psychological (and mental) needs. PTAs must be able to deal with different levels of stress in their patients to avoid obstacles to successful physical therapy.

REVIEW QUESTIONS

Select the best response to each question.

1. Which of the following diseases is more common in men?
   a. osteoporosis
   b. Parkinson's disease
   c. rheumatoid arthritis
   d. multiple sclerosis

2. Pollutants in the environment have been linked to which of the following disorders?
   a. gastrointestinal problems
   b. asthma
   c. heart attack
   d. all of the above

3. All of the following are among the most common diseases related to lifestyle, except
   a. liver disease
   b. type 2 diabetes
   c. endocarditis
   d. obesity

4. Which of the following diets are associated with lower risks for many chronic diseases?
   a. diets high in carbohydrates
   b. diets high in fats
   c. diets low in proteins
   d. diets high in fruits and vegetables

5. Obesity is defined as a BMI greater than how many pounds per square inch?
   a. 30
   b. 45
   c. 60
   d. 90

6. A combination of medical disorders that increase the risk of developing cardiovascular disease and diabetes is referred to as
   a. nephrotic syndrome
   b. metabolic syndrome
   c. myxedema
   d. proliferative disease

7. The branch of medicine that deals with the treatment of obesity and its complications is called
   a. telomere
   b. orthopedics
   c. pediatrics
   d. bariatrics

8. All of the following medications may contribute to obesity, except
   a. fat-soluble vitamins
   b. corticosteroids
   c. antidepressants
   d. antihypertensives

9. Common types of elder abuse include
   a. financial exploitation
   b. emotional abuse
   c. physical abuse
   d. all of the above

10. Physiologic coping mechanisms are referred to as
    a. relief behaviors
    b. generalized adaptation response
    c. psychological disturbances
    d. self-efficacy perceptions

CASE STUDIES

Karen Coupe, PT, DPT, MSEd

Case 1

A 58-year-old woman was admitted to the hospital with nausea, vomiting, abdominal pain, and lethargy. Patient height 5′4″ weight 364, blood pressure 160/95, heart rate 88, respiration rate 17. Patient was at birthday party where she had consumed a large amount of cake and alcoholic beverages. Patient admits to overeating as well as consumption of four or more drinks on a daily basis. Diagnostic testing revealed type 2 diabetes with subsequent lower extremity (LE) peripheral vascular disease (PVD) and neuropathy.

1. What are some predisposing factors that put this patient at risk for type 2 diabetes?
2. What were the precipitating factors that caused the onset of a hyperglycemic episode? What were the clinical manifestations of this episode?
3. Is the subsequent LE PVD and neuropathy a separate diagnosis or a complication of diabetes?
4. Are the patient's vital signs normal? Does this put the patient at risk for any other pathology?
5. How might the patient change her lifestyle behavior to prevent future episodes as well as any further exacerbation of the disease?

Case 2

A 7-year-old is currently comatose in pediatric intensive care. The patient has a brain injury, a right humeral fracture, and multiple cigarette burns over her abdominal region, anterior thorax region, and multiple contusions throughout her body. Injuries were sustained through a beating from the mother's boyfriend. X-rays demonstrate a healed fracture of the right clavicle and right fifth and sixth ribs. Observation: Multiple healed cigarette burns on the back and inner thighs. Both the mother and the boyfriend are currently incarcerated. The boyfriend has previous arrests for assault and battery. Both the mother and the boyfriend have previous arrests for drug possession.

1. Are there any environmental and/or lifestyle factors that could have contributed to this child's abuse?
2. Are there any indications that this patient had suffered abuse before this incident?
3. What could be some signs and symptoms if a child were physically abused?
4. How might the signs and symptoms be different if the child is being sexually abused?
5. As a PTA you are required to follow the laws regarding the report of child abuse. What are the laws in your state?

WEBSITES

http://diversityhealthworks.blogspot.com/2009/05/diversity-disease-management-and.html

http://helpguide.org/mental/domestic_violence_abuse_types_signs_causes_effects.htm

http://www.amnh.org/nationalcenter/infection/03_inf/03_inf.html

http://www.cdc.gov/nccdphp/dnpao/index.html

http://www.drhoffman.com/page.cfm/193

http://www.mentalhealth.com/p20-grp.html

http://www.iom-world.org/research/mechanisms.php

http://www.ornl.gov/sci/techresources/Human_Genome/medicine/assist.shtml

http://www.pathguy.com/lectures/inflamma.htm

http://www.wrongdiagnosis.com/i/immune/intro.htm

Growth and Development of Children

LEARNING OBJECTIVES

After completion of the chapter the reader should be able to

1. Describe the major events that occur during prenatal growth and development.
2. Define the embryonic period.
3. Define the terms "low birth weight," "small for gestational age," and "large for gestational age."
4. Identify the reasons for abnormal intrauterine growth.
5. Describe the grasp and Babinski's reflexes.
6. List four methods of heat loss in the newborn.
7. Explain the major cardiovascular changes after birth.
8. Describe the immaturity of the urinary system after birth.

KEY TERMS

Achondroplasia: A type of dwarfism that is usually a sporadic mutation.

Amniotic fluid: A liquid produced by and contained within the fetal membranes during pregnancy.

Blastocyst: A thin-walled, hollow structure that contains the inner cell mass (embryoblast), from which the embryo arises.

Cleavage: The process of mitotic cell divisions that produces a blastula from a fertilized ovum.

Ductus arteriosus: The shunt that connects the pulmonary artery to the aortic arch in developing infants.

Embryo: The developing offspring, from the 2nd through the 8th week of pregnancy.

Embryoblast: The inner cell mass, from which the embryo arises.

Fertilization: The union of a male sperm and a female ovum; also called conception.

Fetus: The developing offspring, from the 8th week until birth.

Foramen ovale: The second shunt in a fetal heart; it allows blood to enter the left atrium from the right atrium.

Full term: A fetus that has reached 37 weeks of development and is essentially able to survive outside of the womb.

Grasp reflex: A pathologic reflex induced by stroking the palm, with the result that the fingers flex in a grasping motion. In newborns and young infants the tonic grasp reflex is normal.

Hyperplasia: An abnormal increase in cells that causes enlargement of a tissue or organ.

Hypokalemia: Lower than normal potassium in the blood.

Implantation: The process by which a fertilized egg implants in the uterine lining.

KEY TERMS CONTINUED

Morula: The round mass of blastomeres that results from cleavage of the fertilized ovum; it forms the blastula.

Polycythemia: Increased numbers of erythrocytes in the blood circulation.

Sepsis: A potentially serious systemic inflammatory response, affecting numerous parts of the body, commonly caused by septicemia (the presence of pathogenic microorganisms in the bloodstream).

Startle reflex: A reflex response to a sudden unexpected stimulus. The reaction may be accompanied by physiologic effects, including

increased heartbeat and respiration, closing of the eyes, and flexion of the trunk muscles.

Sucking reflex: Involuntary sucking movements of the circumoral area in newborns in response to stimulation.

Trophoblast: Also called the "trophoderm"; it is the outermost layer of cells of the blastocyst that attaches the fertilized ovum to the uterine wall, providing nutrition to the embryo.

Zygote: The cell formed by fertilization, before the occurrence of cleavage.

Overview

Growth and development influence which illnesses may affect children and their response to these illnesses. Today, infant mortality rates are lower than ever before because of great advances in the development of medications and other treatments. Mortality rates for infants are higher today in Black, non-Hispanic people than for other groups of people. The incidence of premature births continues to cause higher numbers of infant deaths because the bodies of these infants may not be mature enough to survive. Infants with very low birth weight (less than 3.3 pounds) are increasing in number, partially because of an increase of twin, triplet, and higher-order multiple births.

Growth and Development

Growth and development include changing from a fertilized ovum (**zygote**) to an **embryo**, fetus, infant, child, and adult. *Physical growth* consists of changes in the body or its individual parts. Changes in body function or psychosocial behaviors are termed *development*. Rapid growth occurs during the first year of life, continuing throughout childhood.

Middle to late childhood is the period from beginning school (approximately age 6) through adolescence (beginning approximately at age 12), and is the period when children begin to develop strong peer relationships. Adolescence is a transitional period, between childhood and adulthood, considered to be from ages 13 to 19. It begins with the development of secondary sex characteristics and continues until the end of somatic growth. At puberty, growth spurts cause rapid development of specific areas of the body at certain times.

Linear growth results from skeletal growth, and it stops when the skeleton is fully mature. Beginning at age 3 years a normal child grows between 5 and 6 centimeters for the next 9 years. Growth then slows down, and most organ systems reach maturity. To reach adult height, growth spurts occur during adolescence. Boys gain about 20 centimeters and girls 16 centimeters during adolescence.

Prenatal Growth and Development

Human growth and development begin when an ovum is fertilized by a sperm cell (**Figure 3–1**). Fertilization is also known as *conception*. When a developing offspring is implanted into the wall of the uterus, *pregnancy* begins. A pregnancy consists of three periods, called trimesters. At least several hundred sperm cells must be present to produce enough enzymes to allow one sperm cell to penetrate the ovum.

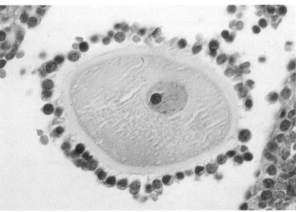

(A)   **(B)**

Figure 3–1 (A) Normal sperm in vaginal secretions. The darkly staining head containing the genetic material is covered by a lightly staining head-cap that contains the enzymes needed to penetrate the ovum during fertilization. The long narrow tail provides propulsion (original magnification 1,000). (B) Mature ovum with adherent granulosa cells. The nucleus is seen near the center of the cell. The homogeneous band surrounding the ovum is the zona pellucida (original magnification X 400).

In just 24 hours the one-celled organism divides into two cells. Within 72 hours it further divides into 16 cells and is called a **morula**. These mitotic divisions are referred to as **cleavage**. Peristaltic movements propel the morula down the oviduct to the uterus. About 4 days after **fertilization** the morula is divided into two parts by uterine fluids. The placenta (**trophoblast**) forms from the outer layer, and the embryo (**embryoblast**) forms from the inner layer. The structure that is now developed is called the **blastocyst**, which attaches to the endometrium of the uterus by the 6th day (**Figures 3–2** and **3–3**). This **implantation** period continues during the 2nd week of development.

There are two main periods of prenatal development. The *embryonic period* takes place from the 2nd week to the 8th week after fertilization, with main organ systems developing and functioning at minimal levels. The *fetal period*, beginning during the 9th week, involves growth and differentiation of the organ systems of the body until birth.

Embryonic Development

When the blastocyst is implanted and days go by, a tiny space appears in the embryoblast. This becomes the primordium of the amniotic cavity. A flat, semiround *embryonic disk* forms, which becomes all three germ layers of the embryo (ectoderm, mesoderm, and endoderm). Development increases during the 3rd week as the embryonic disk matures (*gastrulation*) (**Figure 3–4**). The ectoderm differentiates to become the epidermis and nervous system. The endoderm develops into the epithelial linings of the respiratory and digestive tracts as well as glandular cells of the liver, pancreas, and other organs. The mesoderm forms many structures, including the connective and smooth muscle tissues, skeletal tissue, striated muscle tissue, blood cells and vessels, bone marrow, and the reproductive and excretory organs.

The axial skeleton and neurologic system also begin to form during the 3rd week. Many neural-related structures form during the 4th week, and during this period

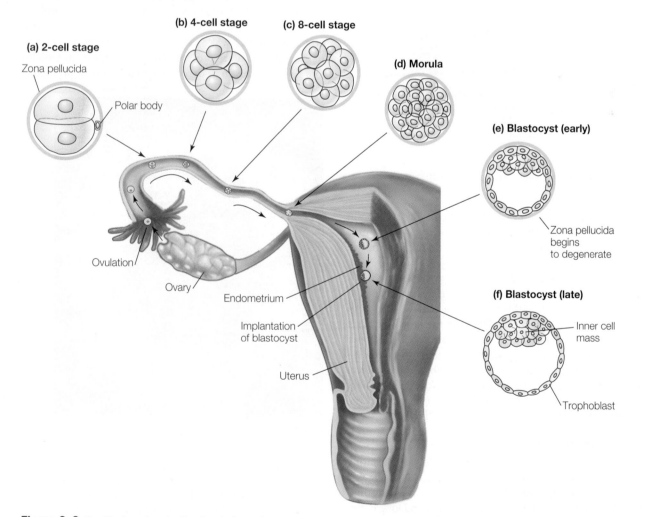

(a) 2-cell stage
Zona pellucida
Polar body

(b) 4-cell stage

(c) 8-cell stage

(d) Morula

(e) Blastocyst (early)
Zona pellucida begins to degenerate

(f) Blastocyst (late)
Inner cell mass
Trophoblast

Ovulation
Ovary
Endometrium
Implantation of blastocyst
Uterus

Figure 3–2 The blastocyst contacting the uterine wall.

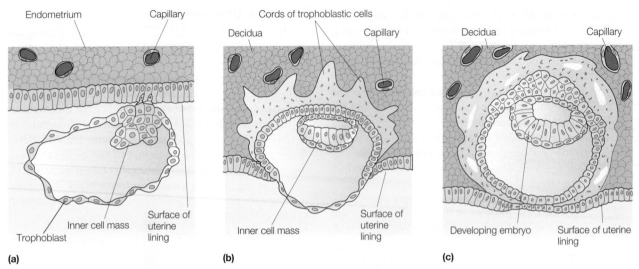

Figure 3–3 The blastocyst beginning to implant.

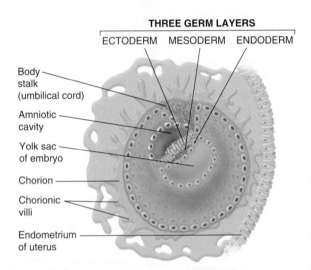

Figure 3–4 Formation of the three primary germ layers.

the 12th week. Most red blood cells are formed in the liver before this point, and this process (erythropoiesis) now transfers into the spleen. Urine begins to form between weeks 9 and 12 and is excreted into the amniotic fluid.

Between weeks 13 and 16 the skeleton greatly ossifies, the scalp shows signs of hair patterns, and, in females, the ovaries differentiate. Growth slows between weeks 17 and 20, and the skin of the fetus is covered with fine hair (*lanugo*) and a cheese-like white *vernix caseosa*. The eyebrows and hair on the head are present. The uterus forms in females and the testes begin to descend in males. Brown protective

disturbances to embryonic development may result in brain and spinal defects. The first functional organ system to develop is the cardiovascular system, including a primitive version of the heart.

Also during the 4th week the embryo curves and folds into a "C"-shaped structure, with small visible buds that form the limbs. Also visible at this time are the basic structures of the eyes and ears. During the 5th week the head and brain develop and grow rapidly. During the 6th week the upper limbs are formed, with the fingers beginning to form during week 7 (**Figure 3–5**). The intestines enter the umbilical cord during this time. By only the 8th week of development the embryo appears human-like. Its eyes are open, and the eyelids and auricles of the ears can be identified.

Fetal Development

Between week 9 and birth the embryo is called a **fetus**. During the 9th to 12th weeks the growth of the fetal body increases while growth of the head slows. By week 11 the chitestines have returned to the abdomen, and the skull and long bones begin ossification. The fetal external genitalia mature during

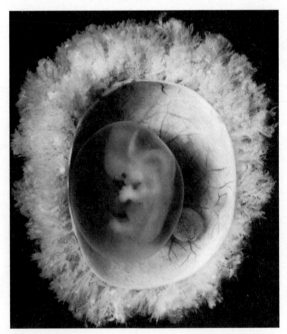

Figure 3–5 Relationship of the embryo to the amnionic sac, yolk sac, and chorionic cavity at about 7 weeks after conception. The chorionic sac has been bisected. At this stage, villi still arise from the entire periphery of the chorion, and the amnionic sac surrounding the embryo does not completely fill the chorionic cavity. The embryo is attached to the chorion by the umbilical cord (not shown in the photograph). The yolk sac is located to the right of the amnionic sac, between the amnionic sac and the chorion.

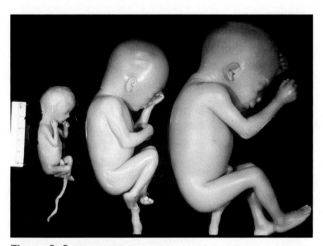

Figure 3–6 Progressive changes in size of the fetus at various stages of gestation. Left, Three and one-half months (32 grams). Center, Four and one-half months (230 grams). Right, Five and one-half months (420 grams).

fat forms near the heart and the blood vessels of the brain and kidneys.

The fetus gains significant amounts of weight during weeks 21 to 25. Rapid eye movements begin at week 21, and the fetus may become visibly startled beginning at weeks 22 to 23. **Figure 3–6** shows the development of a fetus between 3½ and 5½ months of gestation.

> **RED FLAG**
>
> The startle reflex includes an attempt to move away from the stimulus, contraction of the arms and legs, and blinking of the eyes. This protective reflex persists into adulthood but is usually not as pronounced as in childhood.

The alveolar lung cells begin to secrete surfactant, and the pulmonary system is able to support respiration starting at weeks 26 through 29. Breathing movements are present, and if the fetus is delivered prematurely at this stage it has a higher potential for survival.

During weeks 30 to 34 white body fat increases significantly. At week 35 the fetus can grasp and its pupils have a light reflex. If a normal-weight fetus is born at this time it is not premature in regards to weight but only to delivery date. Most infants are born at 266 days (38 weeks) after fertilization, or 40 weeks after the last menstrual period. All major systems are then developed well enough to ensure life outside of the womb.

Birth Weight and Gestational Age

Fetal weight gain is linear between 20 and 38 weeks of gestation. In the final half of the pregnancy the fetus gains 85 percent of its birth weight. Growth rates decline after 38 weeks of gestation because of reduced function of the placenta and the size of the uterus. Weight gain increases again after birth.

Most newborns average in weight between 6.6 and 8.8 pounds. Those weighing less than 5.5 pounds are classified as low-birth-weight infants; other subclassifications are very low birth weight, which is less than 3.3 pounds, and extremely low birth weight, which is less than 2.2 pounds. **Full-term** infants are born between weeks 38 and 41. Newborns with the highest survival rate weigh between 6.6 and 8.8 pounds at birth, which normally occurs between weeks 38 and 42.

Abnormal Intrauterine Growth

Normal intrauterine growth requires many different factors. When something goes wrong, abnormal growth can occur at any time, with immediate and long-term consequences. Classifications of newborns by birth weight and gestational age are shown in **Figure 3–7**. These classifications illustrate the standards with which gestational age can be assessed and normal or abnormal growth rates can be identified.

Small for Gestational Age

Smaller than normal fetal growth is described as *small for gestational age* (SGA). It is defined as being less than two standard deviations below the average for gestational age (which means below the 10th percentile). SGA is also described as *intrauterine growth retardation* (IUGR). Growth retardation can be symmetric, asymmetric, proportional, or disproportional. Symmetric growth retardation can be reversed after birth. Proportional growth retardation may be caused by chromosomal abnormalities, congenital infections, and environmental toxins. Asymmetric growth retardation may be corrected after birth with good nutrition. The most common form of disproportional growth retardation is **achondroplasia**, which is recognizable after the 24th week of gestation. It is signified by a slightly enlarged head, short limbs, underdevelopment of the middle of the face, and shortened fingers.

The maternal environment can drastically affect birth weight and size. Poor maternal nutrition, adolescent pregnancy, short intervals between pregnancies, heavy physical

> **RED FLAG**
>
> Among the common problems of the premature infant are variations in thermoregulation, chilling, apnea, respiratory distress, **sepsis**, and poor sucking or swallowing reflexes.

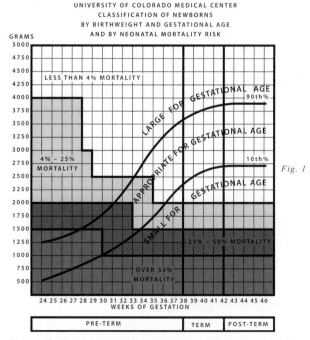

Figure 3–7 Classification of newborns by birth weight, gestational age, and neonatal mortality risk.

Source: Reprinted from Battaglia, C., Lubchenco, L. A Practical classification of newborn infants by weight and gestational age. *J Pediatr.* 1967 Aug;71(2):159–63.

labor while pregnant, and unusual dietary habits may all cause poor fetal growth. Diseases that may also contribute to SGA or IUGR include hypertension, diabetes mellitus, and chronic illnesses and infections. Drugs, including alcohol and tobacco, have numerous potential risks to the fetus. Mortality rates among infants with IUGR are 10 to 20 times higher than for normal infants and may be related to congenital anomalies, hypoxia, hyperbilirubinemia, hypoglycemia, and **polycythemia**.

Long-term effects of growth retardation may cause the individual to remain small throughout life, especially if the problem began earlier in development.

> **RED FLAG**
> Low birth weight is a significant criterion for identifying the high-risk infant with incomplete organ system development. It may result in significant long-term problems.

Large for Gestational Age

Fetal overgrowth and a birth weight above the 90th percentile are described as *large for gestational age* (LGA). Maternal causes include diabetes (if poorly controlled during pregnancy) and maternal body size, with heavy women tending to have LGA infants. Fetal causes include mostly chromosome and gene disorders.

> **RED FLAG**
> Important functions of the PTA are to involve the parents in the care of the infant (teaching handling techniques that enhance motor development), to explain therapeutic procedures, and to facilitate attachment between the infant and the family.

Complications of LGA include trauma and asphyxia during birth. This is often due to difficulties during labor, hypoglycemia, and polycythemia. Increased levels of glucose stimulate the pancreas of the fetus to increase secretion of insulin and undergo **hyperplasia**. Insulin increases fat deposits in the infant, and those with macrosomia have enlarged viscera and appear large and plump. Hyperinsulinemia in the fetus is related to fetal hypoxia and polycythemia (which puts them at direct risk for hyperbilirubinemia). They are also at risk for hypoglycemia.

Prenatal assessment of gestational age includes careful menstrual history, uterine size, detection of fetal heart rate and movements, ultrasonography, and **amniotic fluid** studies. *Postnatal assessment* of gestational age requires examination of external physical and neuromuscular characteristics and should be a part of every initial examination of newborns.

> **RED FLAG**
> LGA infants born of mothers with gestational diabetes are generally obese and plethoric, with very pink skin and red, shiny cheeks.

Growth of Organ Systems

Most full-term infants range in length between 18.9 and 20.9 inches, with height increasing by 1 inch per month over the first 6 months. The trunk of the infant's body grows more than other body areas, and at 1 year of age length is about 50 percent longer than at birth. Many organ systems are at

TABLE 3–1	Periods of Childhood Development	
Period	**Ages**	**Comments**
Newborn (neonatal period)	Birth to 4 weeks	Greatest risk of death at any time in life up to 65 years. Skeleton is not fully developed, and many bones are soft and pliable. Body systems are very immature.
Infancy	5 weeks to 12 months	Organ systems mature rapidly so that the infant develops immunity. The infant normally will begin rolling over, sitting up, standing, and eventually walking.
Early childhood	13 months to 5 years	Includes the toddler and preschool years. Growth slows, most organ systems have matured, and the child becomes independent and mobile.
Middle to late childhood	6 years to 12 years, ending in adolescence	Schooling begins, and the child begins to develop strong peer relationships. Growth is still slower than it will become during adolescence. Muscle mass increases while baby fat decreases. Motor skills are greatly increased.

minimal functioning levels at birth, potentially leading to a variety of infant health problems. A summary of the various periods of development from birth to adolescence is listed in **Table 3–1**.

Nervous System

During infancy the nervous system matures and grows rapidly. In fact, this system grows more rapidly (proportionally) before birth than after. The most rapid periods of nervous system growth are between weeks 15 and 20 of gestation and then again between 30 weeks, gestation up to 1 year of age. The nervous system is incompletely integrated at birth yet still able to sustain

> **RED FLAG**
> The grasp reflex involves the stimulation of the infant's palm or fingers, resulting in the infant grasping onto the stimulating object.

life outside of the uterus. Normal reflexes can be used to evaluate the level of the developing infant's central nervous system. These include the **startle reflex**, the **sucking reflex**, and the **grasp reflex** (**Figure 3–8**). Other reflexes, with their normal and abnormal states, are listed in **Table 3–2**.

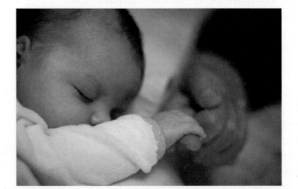

Figure 3–8 Newborn baby grasping a finger.

TABLE 3–2 Infant Reflexes

Reflex	Description	Comments
Asymmetric tonic neck reflex (ATNR)	When the infant's face is turned to one side, the arm and leg on that side of the body extend, and the arm and leg on the opposite side bend, resembling the position of a classically trained fencer. It is important in helping the infant to coordinate body movements on both sides of the body.	Normally lasts from birth until 6 months of age. Also known as the "fencing reflex." Beyond 6 months of age, this reflex may signify developmental delays. This reflex develops muscle tone and vestibular stimulation in utero. It also develops kicking movements and provides continuous motion, which stimulates the balance mechanism and increases neural connections.
Babinski's reflex	When the sole of the foot is firmly stroked, the big toe bends back and the other toes fan out.	This reflex disappears after the age of two years. After age two, this reflex signifies damage to the nerve paths connecting spinal cord and brain.
Rooting reflex	When the side of the infant's cheek is stroked with a finger, the baby will turn the head and open the mouth to follow the direction of the stroking. This is how the baby hunts for the mother's breast.	This reflex disappears after three to four months. If retained, there may be hypersensitivity around the lips or mouth. Speech or articulation problems may result, as well as difficulty chewing or swallowing, and there may be drooling or dribbling from the mouth.
Stepping reflex	If the baby is held upright with the feet on a hard surface, the feet will make a stepping action, even though actual walking may be many months away.	This reflex usually disappears after a few months, with no commonly associated abnormalities.
Symmetric tonic neck reflex (STNR)	When the infant's head and neck are extended, a "crawl" position is achieved by extending the arms and bending the knees.	Also called the "crawling reflex" it disappears when neurologic and muscular development allows independent limb movement for actual crawling. If it remains present in older children, it may result in poor posture, poorly developed muscle tone, poor hand-eye coordination, and inability to sit still and concentrate.
Tonic labyrinthine reflex (TLR)	Tilting the infant's head back while lying on the back causes the back to stiffen and/or arch backwards, the legs to straighten and push together, the toes to point, the arms to bend at the elbows and wrists, and the hands to become fisted or the fingers to curl.	After the newborn stage, the presence of this reflex is referred to as "abnormal extensor" tone or pattern. This may result in poor posture, tendency to walk on the toes, poor balance, motion sickness, spacial orientation difficulties, oculo-motor problems, visual-perceptual problems, and a dislike of physical activities such as sports.

Thermoregulation

Stable body temperature combines heat production, heat conservation, and heat loss. Heat may be produced in response to cold stress via voluntary and involuntary muscle activity (such as shivering) and non-shivering thermogenesis. This requires heat that is liberated from burning stores of brown fat. Heat is lost to the environment through the following four methods:

1. Radiation: transfer of heat from a warmer to cooler area that is not contacting the body
2. Convection: transfer of heat to surrounding environment via air currents
3. Conduction: transfer of heat to cooler surfaces in direct contact with the body
4. Evaporation: cooling that occurs secondary to water loss from the skin

Because preterm infants have a higher ratio of surface area to body mass, reduced subcutaneous tissue insulation, and immature skin with heightened water loss, their heat loss is accelerated.

Cardiovascular System

Major cardiovascular changes occur after birth. The circulation of blood changes as fetal shunts (the **foramen ovale** and **ductus arteriosus**) begin to close. The heart is large in relation to the chest cavity during birth, and it doubles in size and weight during the first year of life. At birth the right ventricle is stronger than the left ventricle, but this reverses during infancy. Systolic blood pressure rises as the heart rate gradually slows. Congenital disorders of the cardiovascular system are discussed in Chapter 6.

Respiratory System

The respiratory system makes major changes to allow the infant to breathe outside of the uterus. Respiration must begin at birth for the infant to survive, with the first breaths expanding the alveoli and initiating gas exchange. Infants breathe rapidly at first, usually from the abdomen, but this slows gradually. The respiratory system matures, increasing the amount of alveoli while the airways grow. Infants breathe through their noses until between 3 and 4 months of age. Therefore, upper airway obstructions can cause airway distress. Infectious agents can be easily transmitted through the lungs because the trachea is small and near to the branching structures of the bronchi. Normal infant respiration rates, as well as blood pressure and heart rates, with changes during development, are shown in **Table 3–3**. Middle ear infections are common in infants because their eustachian (auditory)

> **RED FLAG**
>
> For preterm infants the thermal environment must be carefully regulated. They should be kept in neutral environments to maintain stable core temperatures. These infants must be kept in incubators to maintain a controlled, regulated temperature. In general, neutral temperatures inside incubators for preterm infants (based on the weight of the newborn) should range between 32.6 and 35.5°C.

> **RED FLAG**
>
> Infants may be at risk for airway obstruction due to the small diameter and softness of the supporting trachea cartilage.

TABLE 3–3 Various Normal Rates from Infancy through Childhood

Age	Respiration Rate (Breaths per Minute)	Systolic Blood Pressure (mm Hg)	Heart Rate (Beats per Minute)
From birth to 1 year	30 to 40	70 to 90	110 to 160
From 1 to 2 years	25 to 35	80 to 95	100 to 150
From 2 to 5 years	25 to 30	80 to 100	95 to 140
From 5 to 12 years	20 to 25	90 to 110	80 to 120

tubes are short, straight, and in close communication with the ears.

Gastrointestinal System

Because of immaturity, most infants have poor digestive processes until about 3 months of age. Solid food may be incompletely digested and be actually visible in the stool. The first stool passed by an infant is called the *meconium*. It may contain amniotic fluid, intestinal secretions, shed mucosal cells, and blood. The meconium should occur within 24 to 48 hours after birth. However, because of lack of enteral nutrition due to illness or because of prematurity, the meconium may not occur for up to 7 days. The sucking reflex may be poor at birth, requiring days to be effective.

RED FLAG
Touching the roof of the infant's mouth with a finger, pacifier, or nipple stimulates the sucking reflex in newborns. It later becomes a conscious effort on behalf of the newborn.

The tongue thrust reflex is present, which helps in sucking, but it disappears at around 6 months of age. Infants require frequent feeding because of limited stomach capacity and rapid emptying. Stomach capacity increases quickly in the first months after birth.

Urinary System

The urinary system of infants is immature at birth. It is difficult for urine to be concentrated. The kidneys of infants are immature until 6 months of age. They may have limited ability to adjust to a restricted fluid intake. Infants should not be given water or very diluted formula, which can result in the retention of sodium ions and loss of potassium ions. This causes **hypokalemia** and arrhythmias, which are life threatening. Because their bladders are small, infants usually urinate frequently. When urinary tract system development is affected, this can be especially significant for girls, predisposing them to urinary tract infections as infants. Because the urethra in females is shorter than in males, they are more susceptible to urinary tract infections as newborns and infants.

PRECAUTION
Infant girls are more susceptible to urinary infections because bacteria such as *E. coli* from the feces may contaminate the urethra when the baby is cleaned.

SUMMARY

The growth and development of a child begin with the uniting of the ovum and sperm. Prenatal development consists of the periods of embryonic and fetal development. A zygote becomes an embryo, then a fetus, and, once born, must adjust to living outside of the womb. An infant is considered full term when born between the 38th and 41st weeks. Normal full-term birth weights are between 6.6 to 8.8 pounds.

The term *newborn* is defined as the period from birth to 4 weeks of age. Infancy is defined as the period from 5 weeks to 12 months of age. During this time the relative immaturity of many organ systems changes rapidly so they can become mature enough to protect against diseases and other conditions. Early childhood is the period from 13 months to 5 years of age and includes the toddler and preschool years. Growth slows down during this period, and most organ systems reach maturity.

Middle to late childhood is the period from beginning school through adolescence and is considered to be from age 6 to age 12. Children in this period begin to develop strong peer relationships. Adolescence is a transitional period, between childhood and adulthood. It generally is considered to cover from ages 13 to 19, beginning with the development of secondary sex characteristics and continuing until the end of somatic growth. Major growth spurts occur during this period, and major body changes are seen.

REVIEW QUESTIONS

Select the best response to each question.

1. During which period in a child's life is weight gain fastest in proportion to the child's total weight?
   a. the first 6 months
   b. from 6 months to 1 year of age
   c. preschool period
   d. adolescent period
2. The embryonic period takes place from the
   a. time of fertilization to the second week
   b. 1st week to 4th week after fertilization
   c. 2nd week to 8th week after fertilization
   d. 9 weeks to birth
3. The ectoderm differentiates to become
   a. smooth muscle tissues
   b. the nervous system
   c. the reproductive organs
   d. bone marrow
4. Proportional growth retardation may be caused by
   a. environmental toxins
   b. congenital infections
   c. chromosomal abnormalities
   d. all of the above
5. Most full-term infants increase in height how much per month, over the first 6 months?
   a. 1/8 inch
   b. 1/4 inch
   c. 1/2 inch
   d. 1 inch

6. What is the percentage of increase in length of an infant at 1 year of age, compared with his or her length at birth?
   a. 15
   b. 25
   c. 50
   d. 65

7. Which of the following fetal shunts begins to close after birth?
   a. foramen ovale
   b. foramen magnum
   c. ductus deferens
   d. foramen spinosum

8. Which of the following describes a newborn's action of flexing the fingers around an adult's finger?
   a. startle reflex
   b. sucking reflex
   c. grasping reflex
   d. none of the above

9. The round mass of blastomeres that results from cleavage of the fertilized ovum is called the
   a. zygote
   b. trophoblast
   c. blastula
   d. morula

10. The developing offspring from the 2nd through 8th week of pregnancy is called the
    a. embryoblast
    b. embryo
    c. fetus
    d. morula

CASE STUDIES

Karen Coupe, PT, DPT, MSEd

Case 1

A PTA is employed in a pediatric setting that treats a large population of infants who were born prematurely. Ninety percent of the preterm infants were born to parents with a variety of unhealthy behaviors. As part of a community service, the PTA is working in collaboration with the PT and a local physician to develop an educational workshop for parents-to-be. The focus of the workshop is to provide information on timelines, system development, and the promotion of healthy behaviors.

1. What are some important health behaviors the parent can do and/or avoid to help promote a healthy environment for the developing baby?

2. What are some of the potential negative effects of unhealthy health behaviors on the development of the baby?

3. Explain the prenatal timeline difference between the embryonic period and the fetal period of development.

4. During the embryonic period of development, explain in medical and then layman's terms which systems are developing.

5. During the fetal period of development, explain in medical and then layman's terms how the systems of the fetus are further developing. What is the critical timeline for survival if a fetus is born prematurely during this stage?

Case 2

A 6-month-old girl is referred to an early intervention program secondary to low muscle tone, difficulty feeding, and developmental delays. The PTA is reviewing the history and finds the following: premature birth at 28 weeks, birth weight 3 lb 2 oz.

1. The patient was born at 28 weeks. What is the normal gestation period?

2. Based on the time of birth, what systems were not yet fully developed?

3. Convert the birth weight into grams. What category of birth weight does this fall within?

4. Would you expect this infant to meet the same timeline for developmental milestones as a 6-month-old infant who went full term? Why or why not? How is the gestational age different from the chronological age?

5. Research the early intervention program in your city. What services are available?

WEBSITES

http://web.jjay.cuny.edu/~acarpi/NSC/14-anatomy.htm

http://www.aafp.org/afp/980800ap/peleg.html

http://www.benbest.com/science/anatmind/anatmd4.html

http://www.epigee.org/fetal.html

http://www.kidsgrowth.com/stages/guide/index.cfm

http://www.lpch.org/DiseaseHealthInfo/HealthLibrary/
   hrnewborn/sga.html

http://www.merck.com/mmhe/sec23/ch264/ch264f.html

http://www.unm.edu/~lkravitz/Article%20folder/
   thermoregulation.html

http://www.whattoexpect.com/pregnancy/your-baby/
   week-12/organ.aspx

http://www.visembryo.com/baby/

Health Problems in Children

LEARNING OBJECTIVES

After completion of the chapter the reader should be able to

1. Define the terms "hypotonia," "kernicterus," "macrosomia," and "retinopathy."
2. Discuss the common health problems of newborn infants.
3. Explain sudden infant death syndrome.
4. Describe respiratory distress syndrome in premature infants.
5. Identify the two most common causes of bacterial sepsis.
6. Identify the leading cause of death in children between 1 and 4 years of age.
7. Explain the most common health problems in middle to late childhood.
8. Identify the common reasons for obesity in children and adolescents.

KEY TERMS

Acidosis: A condition of excessive acid in the body fluids.

Acne: A skin condition characterized by inflammation of the oil-producing glands and ducts, commonly occurring during adolescence.

Antenatal: Occurring before birth.

Apnea: Absence or severe reduction in breathing.

Atelectasis: Lack of gas exchange within the alveoli.

Bilirubin: A pigment released into the blood after the destruction of old or damaged red blood cells.

Bradycardia: A slower than normal heart rate.

Bronchopulmonary dysplasia: A condition in premature infants wherein the lung tissue develops abnormally and is characterized by inflammation and scarring.

Colic: Painful spasms in the colon, usually affecting infants.

Egocentric: Concerned with the "self" rather than society.

Fontanels: Spaces covered by tough membranes between the bones of an infant's cranium, sometimes referred to as "soft spots."

Glucagon: A pancreatic hormone that increases blood sugar; it has the opposite effect of insulin.

Glucometer: Also called a "glucose meter"; a medical device that measures the approximate concentration of glucose in the blood.

Glycogen: A starch-like substance composed of linked glucose molecules that acts as an emergency supply of glucose.

KEY TERMS CONTINUED

Hyperbilirubinemia: Higher than normal amounts of bilirubin in the blood.

Hyperinsulinemia: A condition of abnormally high levels of insulin in the blood due to either excessive secretion from the pancreas or by decreased metabolism of insulin.

Hyperlipidemia: A condition of excessive levels of any specific fat or fats in the blood.

Hypoglycemia: Abnormally low blood sugar.

Hypotonia: A state of low muscle tone.

Hypoxemia: Low concentration of oxygen in the blood.

Klumpke's palsy: Atrophic paralysis of the forearm and hand that may be present at birth; it involves the seventh and eighth cervical nerves and the first thoracic nerve.

Lethargy: A state of drowsiness, sluggishness, or indifference.

Macrosomia: Also known as "big baby syndrome," it is sometimes referred to as "large for gestational age" (LGA). Macrosomia describes a fetus that weighs more than 8.8 pounds.

Morbidity: A state of illness or disease.

Mortality: Death, or the state of being subject to dying.

Myelinated: Covered with myelin, which is a substance composed of various fats, proteins, and cholesterol.

Precipitous delivery: Birth of an infant after less than 3 hours of labor; it usually involves intense contractions and pain for which there is not adequate time to relieve.

Retinopathy: Any degeneration of the blood vessels supplying the retina of the eye that is not caused by inflammation.

Scoliosis: A lateral or "side-to-side" curvature of the spine, often in the form of an "S" shape.

Surfactant: A lipoprotein-based substance secreted in the lungs that reduces the surface tension of fluids that coat the lung.

Transient tachypnea: Temporary, abnormally rapid breathing.

Unconjugated: Not commonly united with a compound or compounds.

Vertex: Cephalic; a type of presentation during childbirth wherein the infant's head comes through the pelvis of the mother before the rest of his or her body.

Overview

Childhood illnesses, and how children respond to them, are greatly influenced by physical and psychological maturation and development. Many diseases, while they may affect people of all ages, are more prevalent in children. A child's health care needs reflect his or her developmental stages.

A major factor concerning infant mortality is the incidence of preterm birth among women of all races and economic classes. The leading cause of death in African American infants is prematurity and the resulting low birth weight. The leading causes of death in White infants are congenital anomalies. Sudden infant death syndrome is the third leading cause of overall infant mortality in the United States, regardless of race.

In early childhood, major achievements include development and refinement of locomotion and language. These achievements take place as children progress from dependence to independence. Injuries are the leading cause of death in children between the ages of 1 and 4 years. The most common causes of death during this period include car accidents, drownings, fires, poisonings, playground injuries, and child abuse. During adolescence risks for morbidity and mortality include accidents, homicide, and suicide.

Neonatal Health Problems

As a neonate transfers from intrauterine to extrauterine life, many physiologic changes occur. After birth the *foramen ovale* and *ductus arteriosus* are functionally closed when the newborn takes the first breath and full circulation through the lungs begins. Blood circulation becomes entirely self-contained. Heat regulation is critical to the survival of the infant, with excessive heat loss potentially occurring because of the lack of subcutaneous fat. **Hypoglycemia** may occur because the fetal blood glucose concentration is about 15 mg/dL less than the maternal blood glucose concentration.

Birth Injuries

Birth injuries cause a significant amount of neonatal **morbidity** and **mortality**. They may be predisposed by **macrosomia**, forceps delivery, abnormal fetal presentation (position), cephalopelvic disproportion, prematurity, **precipitous delivery**, and prolonged labor. The major forms of birth injuries are cranial injuries, fractures, and peripheral nerve injuries.

Cranial Injuries

A newborn's head shape is able to change during birth (**Figure 4–1**). This is because the cranial bones have loose connections at the sutures and **fontanels**. When the infant is delivered head-first (vertex), the head is basically flattened at the forehead with the apex rising to form a plane at the end of the parietal bones. The posterior skull (occipital area) drops abruptly. Within just 1 to 2 days after birth, the head assumes an oval shape. Infants born by breech presentation (foot-first) or by cesarean section do not experience such molding of the skull bones.

The scalp may experience edema due to sustained pressure against the mother's cervix. This condition usually resolves itself during the 1st week after birth. *Cephalohematoma* describes a collection of blood below the periosteum due to ruptured blood vessels. Subperiosteal

> **RED FLAG**
> Large cephalohematomas may cause significant blood loss, anemia, hyperbilirubinemia, subdural or subarachnoid hemorrhage, calcium deposits, and swelling that can last for up to 1 year.

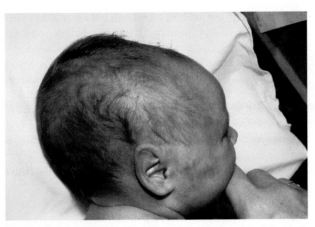

Figure 4–1 Molding (changing) of the posterior portion of the skull in a newborn infant.

bleeding may be very slow and not cause any signs or symptoms until 24 to 48 hours after birth. Although the overlying skin is normal in color, skull fractures may still be present. In most cases these fractures do not require treatment, but monitoring for hyperbilirubinemia is indicated. The condition usually resolves itself in 2 weeks to 3 months.

Fractures

Skull fractures, although uncommon due to the skull's ability to mold into various shapes, may follow forceps delivery or severe, prolonged pelvic contractions. Uncomplicated linear skull fractures usually do not require treatment. Depressed skull fractures are visible as indentations of the infant's head and require surgery if the brain tissue is compressed. Simple linear skull fractures usually heal within a few months.

During birth, the clavicle (collar bone) is the bone that is most fractured, though overall this is not a very common occurrence. This occurs more often in lower than normal gestational age infants when delivery is difficult due to various reasons. The infant will show signs of pain, discoloration, and physical deformity in the area, and there may be a crackling sound (crepitus) due to bones rubbing together. If the fracture is complete, it is treated by immobilizing the arm and shoulder and with pain medications.

Peripheral Nerve Injuries

Sometimes, during **vertex** deliveries, peripheral nerve injuries may occur because of excessive stretching of the head and neck away from the shoulders. During breech deliveries, excessive lateral traction on the trunk of the body before the head is delivered can tear the cervical cord, causing Erb's palsy. This condition is a paralysis that occurs because of traumatic injury to the upper brachial plexus. It occurs most commonly as a result of forcible traction during childbirth, with injury to one or more cervical nerve roots. Signs of Erb's palsy include loss of sensation in the arms as well as paralysis and atrophy of the deltoid, biceps, and brachialis muscles. Erb's palsy is also called Erb-Duchenne paralysis. Brachial plexus injuries affect the nerves of the upper arm, lower arm, or entire arm. The upper arm is most commonly injured, and this occurs mostly in small-for-gestational-age infants or because of difficult or traumatic deliveries. Signs and symptoms include the infant holding the affected arm so

that the shoulder is rotated internally, the elbow is extended, the forearm pronated, and the wrist and fingers flexed. The arm will appear very limp whenever the infant is lifted. Treatment of various peripheral nerve injuries initially requires immobilization, exercise, and appropriate positioning, with most infants recovering in 3 to 6 months. Physical therapy and splinting may be required to improve muscle function and to prevent flexion contracture of the elbow. If paralysis continues, surgery may be indicated.

Hypoglycemia

The immediate postnatal period sees changes in glucose concentration levels, with levels below 40 to 45 mg/dL indicating hypoglycemia. Usually, within 3 hours after birth glucose stabilizes between 50 and 80 mg/dL. Any concentrations below 40 to 45 mg/dL should at this point be considered abnormal. Hypoglycemia in the newborn may not be correlated with the standard manifestations of the condition in other age groups. In the newborn, signs and symptoms of hypoglycemia include apnea, cyanosis, hypothermia, **hypotonia, lethargy**, poor feeding, and seizures. Symptoms may even be very mild. **Hypoxemia** and ischemia can lead to permanent brain damage. Infants at highest risk of hypoglycemia are those born to diabetic mothers, premature infants, and those who are small for gestational age. Blood glucose is commonly measured by using a **glucometer** and the heel stick technique. All infants should be screened for indications of hypoglycemia.

Infants of diabetic mothers are exposed to elevated blood glucose levels, because glucose readily crosses the placenta. These infants also have a lower than normal **glucagon** response to hypoglycemic stimuli. Those who have **hyperinsulinemia** are often larger than normal gestational age. When a diabetic mother adequately controls her diabetes, the newborn is usually of nearly normal size and usually does not experience neonatal hypoglycemia.

Premature and small-for-gestational-age infants are vulnerable to hypoglycemia because they have inadequate stores of liver **glycogen**, muscle protein, and body fat, all of which are needed to maintain energy needs. Their enzyme systems are not fully developed. Also, the presence of transient hyperinsulinemia promotes hypoglycemia. The physical therapist assistant (PTA) should discuss reasons for hypoglycemic episodes with the families of infants. Together, they should explore ways to prevent this from recurring.

> **RED FLAG**
>
> There are several familial forms of hyperinsulinemic hypoglycemia with an inheritance pattern. One form has been linked to a mutation in the human insulin receptor gene.

Jaundice

Jaundice is a yellow-orange discoloration of the skin and sclera (**Figure 4–2**). It affects more than 50 percent of full-term infants and nearly all preterm infants. The discoloration is usually due to excessive circulating **bilirubin**, as the newborn's system adjusts to normal metabolizing levels. Bilirubin is formed from the breakdown of hemoglobin in the red blood cells. Usually, nearly two-thirds of **unconjugated** bilirubin in a newborn can be cleared by the liver. However, because newborn red blood cells have shorter life spans, the infant may be predisposed to **hyperbilirubinemia**. The liver usually adjusts

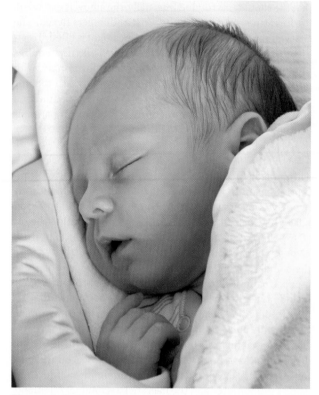

Figure 4–2 Jaundiced infant.

to normal clearance rates as sufficient nutrition, regular bowel movements, and normal fluid volume are developed.

Physiologic jaundice commonly develops in newborns and disappears after a few days. Normally, bilirubin in the umbilical cord blood is 1 to 3 mg/dL, which rises to just under 5 mg/dL within 24 hours. It peaks between the 2nd and 4th days after birth and then decreases to below 2 mg/dL between the 5th and 7th days. If the time that jaundice occurs is outside these parameters, it is considered pathologic. The most serious resulting condition is *kernicterus* (bilirubin encephalopathy). This neurologic syndrome results from bilirubin deposits in the basal ganglia and brainstem. To prevent kernicterus, the aim of treatment is to prevent bilirubin blood levels from becoming neurotoxic.

Useful diagnostic procedures include a clinical evaluation of the signs and symptoms, tests of liver function, and blood and urine tests. Treatment includes frequent breastfeeding (to prevent dehydration), phototherapy, and, sometimes, blood transfusions. Phototherapy involves the use of a special blue light that alters bilirubin for better excretion via the urine and stool. Exchange transfusion is indicated only when bilirubin levels reach 25 to 30 mg/dL or to correct anemia. A less common form is *breast milk jaundice*, which occurs 7 days after birth. Maximal concentrations may be between 10 and 12 mg/dL, and cessation of breastfeeding, substituted by formula, usually causes a rapid decline in serum bilirubin.

Erythroblastosis Fetalis

Erythroblastosis fetalis is also known as *hemolytic disease of the newborn*. It is a type of hemolytic anemia that results from sensitization of the mother to a "foreign" blood group antigen

that is present in the fetal red blood cells but not in the maternal cells. It is usually caused by Rh incompatibility when the mother is Rh negative but the fetus is Rh positive, although it may also be caused by incompatibility involving other blood group systems. The term *erythroblastosis fetalis* is based on large numbers of nucleated erythroblasts (red blood cells) in the blood of severely affected infants. These infants appear with severe edema, and this level of the condition is termed *hydrops fetalis* (**Figure 4–3**). The edema occurs because of heart failure and impaired plasma-protein synthesis in the liver, both of which are caused by the severe anemia. If the infant is born alive, he or she will be moderately or severely anemic. Sometimes, those with a mild form of the disease may at first appear normal but become anemic and jaundiced as time progresses.

> **RED FLAG**
> Before birth, treatment options for erythroblastosis fetalis include blood transfusion, early induction of labor in specific circumstances, and plasma exchange of the mother's blood.

Premature Infants

Infants are considered to be premature when they are born before 37 weeks of gestation. Their birth weight is usually very low, often between 3.3 and 5.5 pounds. Mortality and morbidity rates are much higher for premature infants. Premature infants less than 3.3 pounds at birth are on the increase, which may be associated with an increase in the amount of multiple births (twins, triplets, etc.).

The organ systems of premature infants are immature and may not be able to sustain life. All body systems are underdeveloped. Complications of premature births include pulmonary hemorrhage, respiratory distress syndrome, congenital pneumonia, **transient tachypnea**, **bronchopulmonary dysplasia**, pulmonary air leaks, glucose instability, recurrent **apnea**, hyperbilirubinemia, hypocalcemia, anemia, intraventricular hemorrhage, circulatory instability, necrotizing enterocolitis, bacterial infections, hypothermia, viral infections, disseminated intravascular coagulopathies, and **retinopathy**.

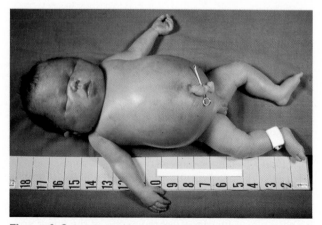

Figure 4–3 A stillborn infant with fetal hydrops. Because the fetus was head down in the uterus, the edema is more marked in the face than in the legs and feet. The abdomen is swollen because the liver and spleen are enlarged, and fluid has also accumulated in the peritoneal cavity.

Respiratory Problems

The most common complication of premature births is *respiratory distress syndrome*. It is usually caused by a lack of **surfactant** in the lungs. Respiratory distress syndrome is also called *hyaline membrane disease*. If an infant is born at approximately week 24 of development, he or she will probably die because there is only partial development of pulmonary vascularity. By 26 to 28 weeks there is usually enough surfactant and development of the lungs to allow the infant to survive. When surfactant is deficient, lung compliance is decreased, alveolar ventilation is reduced, and **atelectasis** usually develops. Signs and symptoms include grunting on expiration, nasal flaring, cyanosis, intercostal and subcostal retractions, and peripheral edema. The respiration rate is greater than 60 breaths per minute.

Exogenous surfactant replacement therapy is now available, which has greatly helped in treating respiratory distress syndrome. Corticosteroids, when given to women in preterm labor, can accelerate lung maturation in the developing infant. **Antenatal** steroids are regularly used for women in preterm labor of up to 34 weeks. However, other complications are on the increase, including air leak syndromes, bronchopulmonary dysplasia, and intracranial hemorrhage.

The disease is self-limited. The infant dies in 3 to 5 days or completely recovers with no aftereffects. Treatment measures include correcting shock, **acidosis**, and hypoxemia. To prevent alveolar collapse, continuous positive airway pressure is used.

Other common respiratory problems affecting premature infants are *apnea* and *periodic breathing*. Apnea is cessation of breathing for 20 seconds or more, often accompanied by bradycardia or cyanosis. Periodic breathing is an intermittent failure to breathe for 10- to 15-second periods and commonly occurs in infants weighing less than 4 pounds. Underdeveloped respiratory centers in the medulla oblongata of premature infants often impair sustained ventilatory drive. When hypoxemia occurs, infants usually respond with a brief period of increased ventilation followed by apnea or hypoventilation.

Medications and ventilatory support may be required to manage apnea and periodic breathing until the infant's central nervous system is developed enough to sustain ventilatory drive. If accompanying **bradycardia** during apnea is profound, more aggressive therapies, including the use of methylxanthines, may be indicated. These drugs, which include caffeine and theophylline, stimulate the brainstem respiratory neurons to decrease the frequency and severity of apnea.

> **RED FLAG**
> About 50% of infants weighing less than 3.3 pounds require intervention for apnea.

Torticollis

Torticollis is an abnormal condition in which the head is usually rotated and laterally flexed. It is a result of the contraction of muscles on that specific side of the neck. Torticollis may be congenital or acquired and is also known as *wry-neck*. Treatments include surgery, heat, support, immobilization, and physical therapy. The treatments of choice depend on the cause and severity of the condition. Spasmodic torticollis may result from spasms in the neck muscle and is often transient. Examination usually does not reveal a physical cause. In certain cases torticollis may be brought on by severe stress.

Infection and Sepsis

Sepsis in neonates causes higher rates of mortality and morbidity. Preterm infants are 3 to 10 times more likely to experience infection and sepsis. Causative factors include maternal genitourinary tract infections, lack of infant immunity, infant surgical procedures, asphyxia, congenital abnormalities, invasive procedures, and administration of medications that may alter normal microbial flora.

Bacterial sepsis (bacteremia) is characterized by bacteria in the bloodstream and affects nearly 30 percent of infants admitted to neonatal intensive care units. As a precautionary measure, preterm infants are often treated for sepsis even if a positive blood culture is not obtained. Despite the use of antibacterial agents and other supportive treatments, the mortality rate due to neonatal bacterial sepsis is about 25 percent.

Group B streptococcus and *Escherichia coli* cause between 70 and 80 percent of positive blood cultures in neonates. The microorganisms responsible for bacterial sepsis in infants have changed significantly over the years. *Early-onset infections* are those acquired before or during delivery. They are usually severe and progress rapidly.

Late-onset infections are those acquired after delivery in the nursery, neonatal intensive care unit, or outside of the medical treatment facility. They often have neurologic involvement and are of slower progression. Meningitis is an example of a condition seen with late-onset infections. Other causative microorganisms for these types of infections include *Staphylococcus aureus*, *Staphylococcus epidermidis*, and other enterobacteria.

The signs of bacterial sepsis are not easy to distinguish from other conditions. Usually, when an infant appears to be even slightly abnormal in health status, bacterial sepsis should be suspected and investigated. Early diagnosis and treatment are vital.

> **RED FLAG**
> Group B streptococcus is the most common causative bacterium of sepsis in preterm infants.

Administration of antimicrobial agents may save the life of the infant. Group B streptococcus disease threatens newborns throughout the world, with preterm newborns being at highest risk.

Infants

Infants may be prone to numerous health problems because of the immaturity of their organs and systems. They are prone to feeding difficulties, nutritional disturbances, colic, injuries of many types, aspiration of foreign objects, suffocation, falls, poisoning, and motor vehicle accidents. Adequate and timely childhood immunizations are recommended.

Nutrition

Infants grow rapidly and require good nutrition, beginning with either breast milk or commercial infant formulas. Breastfeeding is recommended by the American Academy of Pediatrics for the first year after birth. Fluoride is recommended for infants who are breastfed and for those receiving infant formulas that contain unfluorinated water. At about 6 months of age dietary or supplemental iron should be added.

Commercial infant formulas are designed to match the nutritional values of human breast milk. If an infant is lactose intolerant, consuming either breast milk or infant formulas may be problematic. Lactose is a simple sugar contained in human breast milk or cow's milk. A specific enzyme (*lactase*) is required to break down lactose. If an infant lacks this enzyme, he or she is termed *lactose intolerant.* Therefore, infant formula made from soybeans should be used. Newborns and infants often regurgitate formula, regardless of its mixture. Usually, cow milk–based formulas are preferred over soybean-based formulas. Therefore, soybean-based formulas should only be used when an infant cannot tolerate a cow milk–based formula. Thorough investigation of intolerances is required.

Although breastfeeding is recommended for the first year of life, in most cases solid foods may be introduced at 6 months of age. These usually involve bland infant cereals, slowly progressing to individual vegetables, fruits, and, finally, meats. Infants are usually able to drink from a cup rather than a bottle during this time. Between 9 and 12 months of age intake of solid foods and formula increases so that weaning from the breast or bottle can occur. This should be done very gradually because it can cause anxiety in the infant.

Colic

Colic is also known as *irritable infant syndrome*. It usually causes signs and symptoms such as abdominal pain or cramping, loud crying, extreme irritability, and "drawing up" of the legs to the abdomen. Episodes may last from several minutes to several hours each day, with efforts to calm the infant usually being unsuccessful. Colic is most common in infants younger than 3 months of age, although it can occur up to 9 months of age. Colic usually is referred to by the *rule of three* (3 hours a day, or more, of crying; continuing for more than 3 days a week; continuing for longer than 3 weeks) in well-fed, healthy infants.

Apnea, cyanosis, or difficulty breathing may indicate undiagnosed cardiac or pulmonary conditions. If the infant has gastroesophageal reflux, he or she may tilt the head and arch the back.

RED FLAG

Health care providers should determine if colic is an underlying organic cause, involving a careful history and thorough physical examination.

Treatment of colic is not precise because there is no specific cause. Breastfeeding, in general, seems to be better for infants and results in less "colicky" infants. Non-pharmacologic interventions should always be attempted before using drugs to treat the condition. Parents need to be educated about the condition to alleviate their own fears. Frustration is normal, and parents should be counseled about effective methods and treatments used for colic.

Sudden Infant Death Syndrome

Sudden infant death syndrome (SIDS) has its highest incidence during months 2 and 3 of life. SIDS is defined as infant death that remains unexplained after autopsy, investigation, and review of history. It accounts for more infant deaths beyond the prenatal period than any other cause. Infants should be put to sleep on their backs to reduce the risk of SIDS. Other factors that increase risks for this condition include prematurity, low birth weight, exposure to cigarette smoke, and African American or Native American race.

Infants sleeping on their stomachs (the prone position) have significantly higher risk of SIDS. Sleep surfaces should not be too soft, and comforters and pillows should be avoided. Also, adults should not sleep with their infants due to risk of smothering. Though the exact cause of SIDS is unknown, immature cardiorespiratory control from the brainstem is suspected. Features of the condition may include sleep apnea, pauses during inspiration, excessive periodic breathing, and impaired response to higher levels of carbon dioxide or lower levels of oxygen. If autopsy confirms no other causes, SIDS may be diagnosed. Child abuse must be investigated and ruled out.

When an infant dies of SIDS, support of family members is essential. Feelings of guilt or inadequacy may be overwhelming. Parents and other family members must receive information about SIDS so they can fully understand the situation.

Infectious Disease

Widespread immunization for children has greatly decreased the incidence of childhood infectious disease. Recommended immunizations are for diphtheria, pertussis, polio, tetanus, measles, mumps, rubella, hepatitis B, and *Haemophilus influenzae* type B infection. These immunizations are given at specific times during development. Parental concerns about these immunizations must be handled effectively, with complete education about the dangers of avoiding proper scheduling. Many children, unfortunately, still do not routinely receive immunizations or do not receive all of them.

Injuries

Injuries are the major cause of death in infants between 6 and 12 months of age. Injuries can be from aspiration of foreign objects, falls, poisonings, drowning, burns, suffocation, and other bodily damage. It is vital to "childproof" the house and other environments. Close supervision of children is required at all times. Another significant factor is motor vehicle accidents, which become the number one cause of accidental infant death after 1 year of age. Approved infant safety restraints are required now by most states when they ride in a car or other vehicle. The safest place for infants to ride is considered to be the middle of the back seat of a vehicle. Often, a hospital will verify that the vehicle transporting a newborn home has the proper safety equipment before the infant is discharged. Health care providers must educate parents about the dangers of carrying infants and children in vehicles without proper protective measures.

Early Childhood

Early childhood is the period of 18 months to 5 years of age. This period is broken up into the following:

- Toddler: a child between 18 months and 3 years of age
- Preschooler: a child between 3 and 5 years of age

Major changes occur during early childhood, including those that relate to language, locomotion, and a sense of independence. However, physical growth during early childhood is not as dramatic as during infancy. Most children between 2 and 5 years of age gain about 4.4 pounds in weight and 2.8 inches in height. Their bodies become leaner, they have more energy, and they need to sleep between 11 and 13 hours per day, which includes a nap. By age 4 years normal children will have all 20 of their primary teeth and also have 20/20 vision.

The respiratory systems of those in early childhood are still immature, and respiratory infections and otitis media (middle ear infections) are common. Respiratory rates average only 20 to 30 breaths per minute, and respirations remain abdominal until age 7. The brain is about 90 percent of adult size by 2 years of age, and by this time the spinal cord is usually completely **myelinated**. Control of urination and defecation becomes possible at age 2, although not all children become "potty-trained" by that age.

During this period the skeletal system ossifies, with leg growth and changes in muscle and fat proportions becoming apparent. After 1 year of life nearly two-thirds of increase in height of the child is due to leg growth. Gross and fine motor abilities improve greatly, and learning now includes interactions with others. Children learn appropriate social behaviors and sex roles. Toddlers overcome senses of doubt and shame while acquiring a sense of autonomy. Preschoolers acquire a sense of initiative and also develop a conscience.

Common Health Problems

Injuries are also the leading cause of death in children between 1 and 4 years of age. Because toddlers and preschoolers have increased abilities for locomotion and lack an awareness of danger, they have an increased risk for injuries. As their immune systems are immature, infectious diseases are a significant problem. Entering day care facilities or preschools also increases the risk of exposure to infectious disease. Common communicable diseases during this period are the common cold, influenza, chickenpox (varicella), otitis media, and gastrointestinal tract infections.

Child abuse is another significant factor. Approximately 1.4 million children in the United States undergo some form of abuse annually. This may include physical or emotional neglect, physical abuse, and sexual abuse. Neglect is the most common form and is often attributed to poor parenting. Physical abuse is described as the deliberate infliction of injury. Sexual abuse is unfortunately on the rise and is usually committed by males. Children often do not report abuse because they are afraid of not being believed.

Middle to Late Childhood

Middle to late childhood is defined as the period when a child begins school, at about 5 or 6 years of age, until the beginning of adolescence, which is approximately age 12. This period of childhood has an important, well-remembered effect on future physical, psychosocial, and cognitive development. The future adult life of a child is greatly determined by this period.

Physical growth is slower during this period than during other times. In late childhood, children usually gain up to 7.7 pounds in weight per year and average 2.4 inches of growth (in height) per year. Growth "spurts" occur about three to six times per year. The legs increase in length, posture improves, and the center of gravity descends to a lower area. Children become more graceful and better prepared for increased physical activity. Body fat decreases and lean muscle mass increases. By age 12 the body has doubled its strength and physical capabilities. However, muscles are still immature and can be injured from strenuous activities such as sporting events. Facial proportions change as facial areas grow more quickly than cranial areas. Primary teeth are lost and permanent teeth replace them.

During middle to late childhood caloric requirements are lower, cardiac growth is slow, blood pressure slowly rises, and heart and respiratory rates decrease. Frequent eye checkups should occur during this period to assess the need for glasses because vision is continually developing. Bones continue to strengthen but are not at adult strength. Children should be checked for posture problems that may indicate spinal conditions such as scoliosis, and proper footwear and workspaces should be provided.

Near age 12, physical differences between girls and boys become apparent. Girls usually enter puberty about 2 years before boys and are often taller. Differences in the development of sex characteristics between all children as well as genders are great.

Psychosocial development is strongly impacted by the entry into school. Peers outside of the family unit become very important to children. The basic temperament and approach to life become apparent as the child's personality develops. Basic personality elements may change in adulthood but never disappear completely.

Common Health Problems

Immunity has, by the time of late childhood, greatly increased. However, respiratory infections and gastrointestinal disorders are still common. During this period the chief cause of mortality is accidents, with motor vehicle accidents ranking highest. The addition of fluoride to most U.S. water systems has decreased the incidence of dental caries (tooth cavities). However, in this age group dental caries may be of higher incidence because of inadequate dental care and higher amounts of dietary sugar being consumed. Often, children resist adult assistance in tooth brushing and flossing and perform these functions inadequately themselves.

Bacterial or fungal infections are also common, usually affecting the respiratory, gastrointestinal, and integumentary systems. Skin infections are at their highest peak of incidence during this time of development. Acute or chronic health problems may appear for the first time, including asthma, epilepsy, childhood cancers, and developmental or learning disabilities.

Weight Problems and Obesity

Weight problems, including overweight or obesity, are more common today in children during middle to late childhood. A standard body mass index is used to determine normal weight ranges for children of specific ages and heights (**Figure 4–4**). The following information is of concern for these specific ages of children:

OVERWEIGHT AND OBESE: WHAT DO THEY MEAN?

Body weight status can be categorized as underweight, healthy weight, overweight, or obese. Body mass index (BMI) is a useful tool that can be used to estimate an individual's body weight status. BMI is a measure of weight in kilograms (kg) relative to height in meters (m) squared. The terms overweight and obese describe ranges of weight that are greater than what is considered healthy for a given height, while underweight describes a weight that is lower than what is considered healthy for a given height. These categories are a guide, and some people at a healthy weight also may have weight-responsive health conditions. Because children and adolescents are growing, their BMI is plotted on growth charts[25] for sex and age. The percentile indicates the relative position of the child's BMI among children of the same sex and age.

Category	Children and Adolescents (BMI for Age Percentile Range)	Adults (BMI)
Underweight	Less than the 5th percentile	Less than 18.5 kg/m²
Healthy weight	5th percentile to less than the 85th percentile	18.5 to 24.9 kg/m²
Overweight	85th percentile to less than the 95th percentile	25.0 to 29.9 kg/m²
Obese	Equal to or greater than the 95th percentile	30.0 kg/m² or greater

Adult BMI can be calculated at http://www.nhlbisupport.com/bmi/. A child and adolescent BMI calculator is available at http://apps.nccd.cdc.gov/dnpabmi/.

25. Growth charts are available at http://www.cdc.gov/growthcharts.

Figure 4–4 Body mass index.
Source: Courtesy of U.S. Department of Agriculture and U.S. Department of Health and Human Services. Dietary Guidelines for Americans, 2010. 7th Edition, Washington, DC: U.S. Government Printing Office, December 2010.

- Children aged 6 to 11 years: 18.8% are now considered overweight
- Children aged 12 to 19 years: 17.4% are now considered overweight

African American and Mexican American children and adolescents are affected more than other ethnic groups.

Common reasons for children or adolescents to become overweight or obese include the obvious ones, such as over-consumption of calories and lack of adequate physical activity, but there are other factors as well. Excessively large portion sizes, consuming meals away from home (where control of balanced food quality is less likely), frequent snacking, and high-calorie beverages all contribute to excessive calorie intake. Watching television and spending too much time working or playing on computers makes people more sedentary and less physically active. Genetic factors concerning weight gain may also be contributory.

Pediatric obesity harms health as well as psychological states. It may also influence the remainder of their lives, carrying through into adulthood. Nearly 60 percent of overweight children have a higher risk factor for cardiovascular disorders such as **hyperlipidemia**, hyperinsulinemia, or *hypertension*. Obesity may also contribute to heart attack, stroke, and joint problems (especially in the knees and lower extremities) later in life. More than 25 percent have risk factors for two or more related conditions. They are also more likely to be predisposed to type 2 diabetes mellitus.

Adolescence

Adolescence describes the period of transition between childhood and adulthood, signified by much emotional, cognitive, and physical growth. Changes occur at varying times in each individual. Adolescence begins as secondary sex characteristics develop (usually at ages 11 or 12) and ends with the completion of somatic growth (usually at ages 18–20). Adolescence begins and ends earlier for girls than for boys. The adolescent period may be referred to as the *teenaged years* (from 13–19). Adolescents commonly achieve independence from their parents, have strong peer support, make their own personal choices about lifestyles, work on their body images, and establish **egocentric**, moral, sexual, and vocational identities.

As the body matures sexually, hormonal activity also influences physical growth. The greatest gains in height are seen during this period. Growth spurts usually occur in girls between ages 10 and 14, with most girls gaining between 5 and 7.9 inches in height and 15.4 to 55.1 pounds in weight. In boys, growth spurts are more pronounced, with increases in height of 4 to 11.9 inches and increases in weight of 15.4 to 66.1 pounds commonly seen. Boys often gain in height until ages 18 to 20, though increases are possible until age 25.

Growth occurs first in arms, legs, hands, feet, and neck, followed by growth in hips, chest, shoulder, and trunk. Growth spurts may cause clothing and shoe sizes to change several times over only a few months. Often, muscle growth is not aligned with skeletal growth, making adolescents less coordinated than during other periods of growth. Boys experience a widening of the chest while the pelvis remains narrow, with girls experiencing the opposite.

Heart rate during adolescence increases to that of adults, as does blood pressure. Blood volume and hemoglobin also increase. The skin thickens and hair growth increases, especially in boys. Sebaceous and sweat gland activity increases, influencing the development of **acne**, increased perspiration, and body odor. Voice changes occur, with boys experiencing greater degrees of voice deepening. Due to continued eruption of permanent teeth while facial bones are growing, there may be a need for orthodontic appliances such as braces.

Hormonal activity increases, affecting levels of growth hormone, adrenal hormones, thyroid hormones, insulin, and gonadotropic hormones. The thyroid gland enlarges, as do the pancreatic islets of Langerhans. The anterior pituitary gland produces follicle-stimulating hormone and luteinizing hormone, influencing the secretion of sex hormones.

The ovaries and testes release hormones that influence the maturation of primary sex characteristics. The internal and external genitalia mature, and secondary sex characteristics such as the growth of pubic and axillary hair occur.

Because psychosocial development also occurs in uneven "spurts," adolescents often experience irregular periods of emotional upset. The majority (80 percent) of adolescents mature without any permanent disability, although at the time many parents believe they have become "out of control." Adolescents need to be reassured their feelings are not abnormal but are due to continued growth and hormonal release. They may have conflicts with parents, siblings, authority figures, and peers as their personal identity is continually developing.

Physical symptoms of maturation include headaches, insomnia, and stomachaches, though occasionally these symptoms may be psychosomatic. Anxiety and mild depression are commonly seen, and health care workers should monitor adolescents if these conditions worsen. Adolescents are often rebellious, lazy, moody, and likely to take dangerous risks in behavior. They may be easily influenced to experiment with drugs or sexual activity. Often, problems at school occur due to these various behavioral states. Open communication is advised to help the adolescent make the transition to adulthood as easy as possible.

Common Health Problems

Although adolescence usually contains fewer health problems than other periods, there is a greater risk of morbidity and mortality from accidents, homicides, and suicides. The fourth leading cause of death in adolescents is cancer, including lymphomas and bone or genital tumors. Overall, accidents are most prevalent, often because of a lack of maturity, which places the adolescent into situations where harm is more likely to occur. They often believe they are impervious to harm even though their behaviors may be quite risky.

Motor vehicle accidents are of primary concern, often due to reckless driving habits or the use of alcohol and other substances. Attempts at suicide maintain nearly constant levels in adolescents of every generation. Cigarette smoking and risky sexual behavior also may be risk factors for adolescents. Adolescent pregnancy, sexually transmitted infections, and the transmission of HIV are of major concern. Health care providers should attempt to discuss all these behaviors openly and honestly with adolescents and educate them while remaining nonjudgmental, factual, and open to their comments.

Nearly 1 million adolescents in the United States become pregnant each year, with 4 of every 10 female teenagers becoming pregnant before age 20. Of this 1 million, 47 percent gave birth, 40 percent had therapeutic abortions, and 13 percent spontaneously abort. Adolescent pregnancies pose great risks to the fetus or newborn as well as the mother. Lack of maturity often causes poor parenting or other behaviors that may harm the offspring.

Substance abuse among adolescents is still of major concern, and health care workers must be knowledgeable about its symptoms. Peer pressure often plays a strong part in convincing an adolescent to "try" various substances, because they want to "fit in." Education is the best way to explain the dangers of the use of tobacco, alcohol, and both legal and illegal drugs.

SUMMARY

Infancy is described as the period from 5 weeks to 12 months of age. During this period growth and development are ongoing. Infants are at risk for a variety of illnesses because many of their organ systems are relatively immature. Birth begins a series of changes in an infant's organ systems as the body adjusts to postnatal life.

During the birth process maladjustments or injuries may cause disability or death. Premature delivery is a significant health problem in the United States. Premature infants are at risk for many health problems due to the interruption of intrauterine growth and immaturity of organ systems.

Significant health risks during early childhood include infectious diseases and injuries, with injuries being the main cause of death during this period. Child abuse is also increasing as a major health problem. During middle to late childhood respiratory diseases are a major cause of illness, whereas motor vehicle accidents are the major cause of death. Chronic health problems during this period include asthma, childhood cancers, and epilepsy. Being overweight or obese is an increasingly common problem during this period. During adolescence, health risks include substance abuse, risky sexual behavior, and accidents. Homicide and suicide are also more likely to occur in this age group than in other times of early life.

REVIEW QUESTIONS

Select the best response to each question.

1. Hypoxemia in newborns can lead to permanent damage to the
   a. bone marrow
   b. spleen
   c. brain
   d. liver

2. Kernicterus is also known as
   a. bilirubin encephalopathy
   b. viral encephalitis
   c. physiologic jaundice
   d. cephalohematomas

3. The most common bone fracture during birth is fracture of the
   a. scapula
   b. clavicle
   c. humerus
   d. ulna

4. The most common complication of premature birth is
   a. retinopathy
   b. intraventricular hemorrhage
   c. intracranial hemorrhage
   d. respiratory distress

5. Which entry is *not* true about the causes of sepsis in newborns?
   a. Lack of infant immunity
   b. A mother with diabetes

c. Asphyxia and congenital abnormalities

d. Infant surgical procedures

6. At which age should dietary or supplemental iron be added to the diet?

   a. 2 months
   b. 4 months
   c. 6 months
   d. 10 months

7. Lactose intolerance may occur in infants when they lack

   a. a specific enzyme
   b. vitamin B_{12}
   c. iron
   d. bile

8. Sudden infant death syndrome has its highest incidence during months

   a. 1 to 2
   b. 2 to 3
   c. 5 to 7
   d. 8 to 10

9. The leading causes of death in children between ages 1 and 4 years are

   a. otitis media and encephalitis
   b. osteomyelitis and osteopathy
   c. testicular cancers
   d. injuries

10. A greater risk of morbidity and mortality in adolescents is due to

    a. homicides and suicides
    b. pneumonia
    c. obesity and diabetes
    d. sexually transmitted infections

CASE STUDIES

Karen Coupe, PT, DPT, MSEd

Case 1

A 3-month-old infant sustained a right upper extremity injury during a difficult birthing process. Magnetic resonance imaging (MRI) results confirm a diagnosis of Erb-Duchenne palsy. The parents were taught early movement and positioning techniques. Subsequent electromyography testing results were positive for nerve activity, and the patient was referred to physical therapy for progressive strengthening activities.

1. Explain the difference between an MRI and electromyography.

2. What are the clinical manifestations of Erb-Duchenne palsy? Position your arm in a manner to replicate the arm position you might observe with this patient.

3. This patient was referred for progressive strengthening activities. Based on the level of injury with Erb-Duchenne palsy, which muscles require strengthening?

4. Although this infant isn't old enough to have all of his developmental reflexes, which developmental reflexes would be affected by this condition?

5. Compare and contrast Erb-Duchenne palsy with **Klumpke's palsy** and whole arm palsy.

Case 2

A 10-year-old boy was referred to outpatient physical therapy secondary to greenstick fracture of the right tibial shaft. The patient was in a full knee/ankle cast for 6 weeks and has been non-weight bearing (NWB) using axillary crutches. Prior level of function: independent in all activities of daily living, active in soccer, basketball, and baseball. The PT evaluation reveals decreased right lower extremity range of motion, strength, and observes that the patient is still using an NWB status regardless of the PT order to begin weight bearing as tolerated (WBAT). Plan of care includes range of motion/stretching, strengthening, and gait training WBAT beginning with axillary crutches and progressing to gait training without an assistive device.

1. What is a greenstick fracture, and why is it more common in children?

2. The fracture was at the tibial shaft. Based on bone development and the patient's age, what could have been damaged if the patient had suffered a fracture at the proximal or the distal tibia?

3. When the patient was NWB with axillary crutches, what type of gait pattern was most likely used? Why do you suspect the patient is still using an NWB status?

4. The plan of care includes range of motion and strengthening. Based on the length of the cast, which joints would be affected? What muscles would most likely require strengthening?

5. The plan of care includes gait training WBAT beginning with axillary crutches. What type of gait pattern would you use? How would you progress this patient to independent ambulation without an assistive device?

WEBSITES

http://kidshealth.org/parent/medical/

http://www.mayoclinic.com/health/colic/DS00058

http://www.merck.com/mmhe/sec23/ch264/ch264a.html

http://www.merck.com/mmpe/sec19/ch272/ch272c.html

http://www.nlm.nih.gov/medlineplus/ency/article/007306
.htm

http://www.nlm.nih.gov/medlineplus/toddlerhealth.html

http://www.oregon.gov/DHS/ph/ah/docs/Middle_
childhood_population.pdf?ga=t

http://www.premature-infant.com/

http://www.sids.org/nprevent.htm

http://www.who.int/child_adolescent_health/topics/
prevention_care/adolescent/dev/en/index.html

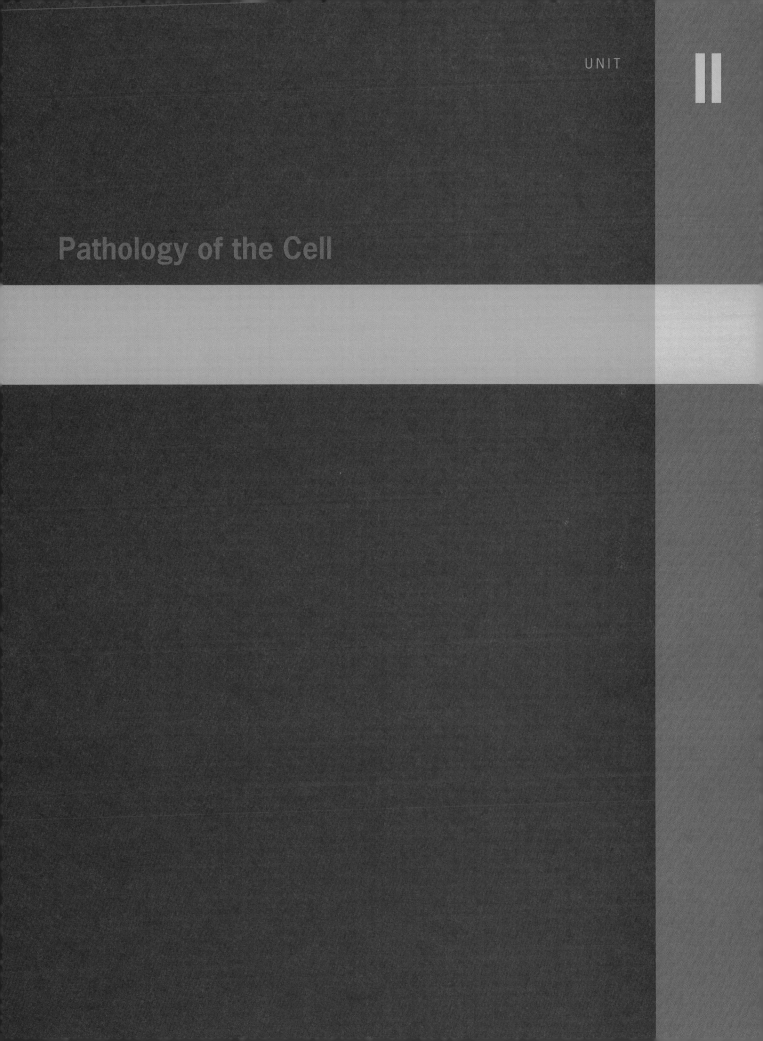

Pathology of the Cell

Cell Injury and Cell Death

LEARNING OBJECTIVES

After completion of the chapter the reader should be able to

1. Explain cellular changes.
2. Describe tissue necrosis.
3. Discuss cellular adaptation.
4. Explain the mechanisms of cell injury.
5. List various types of asphyxial injuries.
6. Describe accidental injuries and list six examples.
7. Define hypertrophy, metaplasia, and hyperplasia.
8. Explain the mechanisms of chemical injury.

KEY TERMS

Abrasion: Scraping away of the skin.
Anaerobic: Without air; lacking oxygen.
Anoxia: A total lack of oxygen.
Apoptosis: The process of programmed cell death.
Asphyxial injuries: Harmful events caused by lack of oxygen for breathing.
Atrophy: Wasting away of tissue due to disease, poor nutrition, or disuse.
Contusion: A bruise; an injury with no break in the skin, characterized by discoloration, pain, and swelling.
Dysplasia: The development of abnormal cells.
Endogenous: Occurring within the body.
Exogenous: Occurring outside the body.
Gangrene: A condition involving a large amount of necrosis (body tissue death).
Hematoma: Blood loss into a tissue, organ, or other confined space.
Hyperplasia: An increase in the amount of normal cells in a tissue or organ.
Hypertrophy: Enlargement or overgrowth of an organ or body part due to hyperplasia.
Hypoxia: Low concentration of oxygen in a tissue, or lack of an adequate supply of oxygen.
Inflammation: Redness, pain, and swelling due to infection or other causes.
Ischemia: A temporary reduction of blood supply to an organ or tissue because of an obstruction of a blood vessel.
Karyolysis: Complete dissolution of a cell's chromatin as a result of the actions of deoxyribonuclease (DNase).
Laceration: A torn wound with ragged edges.
Lysis: The breaking down of cells.
Metaplasia: A reversible replacement of one differentiated cell type with another mature differentiated cell type.

KEY TERMS CONTINUED

Necrosis: The premature death of living cells and tissue.
Neoplasia: The abnormal proliferation of body cells.
Strangulation: Compression of the throat that leads to unconsciousness via lack of oxygen; it

may lead to cerebral ischemia, asphyxia, and death.
Suffocation: The process of being asphyxiated.

Overview

When a body cell encounters any type of stressor that may be harmful to its normal structure and functions, it undergoes adaptive changes that allow it to survive and maintain its functions. When the stress is overwhelming or the adaptation is ineffective, cell injury and death occur. Various types of cellular injury may cause cell damage or cell death.

Cellular Changes

Body cells react to altered body conditions by adapting their differentiation and growth. Some alterations are minor. Environmental irritants and hormonal stimulation often modify tissues. Changes are usually reversible once the stimulus is removed. When cell structure and function change, a disease may develop. The structure of deoxyribonucleic acid (DNA) in the cells may be significantly and irreversibly changed in certain conditions. Though cancer or permanent tissue damage may not occur, the cause of abnormalities must be determined in early stages. Changes in metabolic processes may damage or destroy cells. Other causes of cell damage or destruction include altered cell pH, cell membrane damage, and reduced levels of adenosine triphosphate (ATP).

Cellular Adaptation

Cellular adaptation helps cells to protect themselves; however, an *adapted* cell is not the same as a normal cell yet is not an injured cell either. Cellular adaptation is part of many different diseases, and many cells actually show increased function during the early stages of an adaptive response. The most important cellular adaptive responses to understand are atrophy, dysplasia, hypertrophy, hyperplasia, metaplasia, and neoplasia (**Figure 5–1** and **Table 5–1**).

Atrophy

Atrophy is defined as a decrease (or shrinkage) in cellular size and can occur in enough cells of a specific organ to cause the entire organ to become atrophic. Atrophy is most common in the skeletal muscle, heart, brain, and secondary sex organs. It may be classified as *pathologic* or *physiologic. Pathologic atrophy* is caused by decreases in pressure, workload, blood supply, use, hormonal stimulation, nutrition, and nervous stimulation, such as when a bedridden patient experiences *disuse atrophy* in his or her skeletal

> **RED FLAG**
> **Dysplasia**, defined as "deranged cellular growth," is considered an atypical type of hyperplasia.

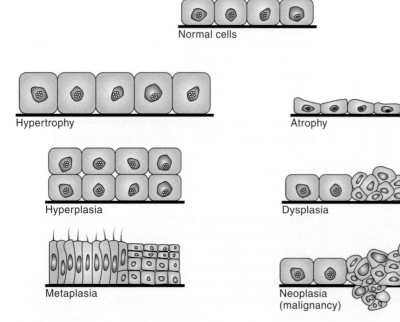

Figure 5–1 Normal and abnormal cellular growth.

TABLE 5-1 Cellular Adaptation Vocabulary

Term	Definition	Comments
Anaplasia	Loss of differentiation in a cell, usually associated with cancer	Associated with cancer or malignancy; used in the grading of tumors
Atrophy	A decrease in the size of cells, resulting in a reduced tissue mass	Causes of atrophy include insufficient nutrition, reduced tissue use, aging, and decreased hormonal or neurologic stimulation Example: shrinkage of skeletal muscle due to limb immobilization in a cast because of previous injury
Dysplasia	Describes tissue in which cells vary in size and shape, often have very large nuclei, and have an increased rate of mitosis	Dysplasia may be due to chronic infection or irritation or may be precancerous; detection of dysplasia is influential in tests such as the Pap smear
Hyperplasia	An increased number of cells resulting in an enlarged tissue mass	May occur simultaneously with hypertrophy; there may be an increased risk of cancer with developing hyperplasia
Hypertrophy	An increase in the size of individual cells, resulting in an enlarged tissue mass	Example: consistent exercise resulting in enlarged skeletal muscle mass
Metaplasia	An acquired condition in which a fully developed adult tissue changes abnormally into a different kind of tissue	May be caused by lack of vitamin A or as a result of certain activities (such as smoking)
Neoplasia (neoplasms)	New growth; a tumor, either benign or malignant	Malignant neoplasms are referred to as cancer; benign tumors are usually not life threatening unless in the brain or certain other areas

muscles. *Physiologic atrophy* occurs in early development, such as when the thymus gland undergoes physiologic atrophy during childhood. Whether pathologic or physiologic, atrophic cells show the same basic changes.

Normal muscle cells have more endoplasmic reticulum, mitochondria, and myofilaments than atrophic muscle cells. When nerve loss causes muscle atrophy, amino acid uptake and oxygen consumption are reduced immediately. When chronic malnutrition causes muscle atrophy, it is often accompanied by *autophagic vacuoles* in greater numbers than normal. These are vesicles that are membrane-bound inside cells and contain hydrolytic enzymes and cellular debris. These enzyme levels rise rapidly when atrophy occurs.

The vacuoles form to protect uninjured organelles from those that are injured. Some contents of the vacuoles resist destruction by lysosomal enzymes. These contents may include granules containing *lipofuscin*, an age pigment that is yellowish-brown in color. Lipofuscin primarily accumulates in atrophic cells, liver cells, and myocardial cells.

Diagnosis of muscular atrophy involves a complete blood count to evaluate health status. Blood serum chemistries, such as creatine kinase, may be performed to measure muscle enzymes. *Electromyography*, wherein needle electrodes are inserted into the muscle to measure its action potential or ability to respond to stimuli, may also be helpful. A muscle needle *biopsy* may be performed under local anesthesia if *polymyositis* (polymyalgia-rheumatica) is suspected. Because so many different issues surround muscle abnormalities (myopathies), *magnetic resonance imaging* (MRI) studies are often used because they provide more detailed images of tissue.

Regular exercise may be helpful in cases of muscular atrophy. Treatments include strength training for certain types of muscular atrophy, although strength training is not useful for atrophy from diseases such as muscular dystrophy. Physical therapy is tailored to each individual patient to strengthen muscles and restore as much normal function as possible.

Electrical stimulation may be used in conjunction with exercises to stimulate the muscle and promote strength gains. If atrophy was caused by a systemic illness (known as *neurogenic atrophy*), intramuscular injections of anabolic steroids may be indicated. If atrophy is severe, and joints are likely to become involved, orthotics may be used to minimize the risk of contracture development.

Dysplasia

The abnormal development and maturation of body cells is called dysplasia. These cells may exhibit abnormal size, shape, and relationship to other cells (**Figure 5–2**). When epithelial cells experience dysplasia, it may be due to chronic inflammation or irritation. Sometimes, dysplasia may progress and cause the formation of a tumor, which is known as **neoplasia**. An example of a common site of dysplasia is the epithelium that covers the cervix of the uterus, progressing to cervical cancer. Another common site where dysplasia occurs is the respiratory tract.

Dysplasia is related to hyperplasia (often called *atypical hyperplasia*). Dysplastic changes are often found close to cancerous cells. Dysplasia may range from mild to severe and is often referred to as "low grade" or "high grade." Atypical hyperplasia appears to be related to breast cancer development. The development of malignant tumors is referred to as *neoplasia*. Dysplastic changes may be reversible if the causative stimulus is removed.

Hypertrophy

Hypertrophy is defined as an increase in cellular size and, as a result, the size of the affected organ. It mostly affects the cells of the kidneys and heart. Protein accumulates in the cellular components of these organs, helping to increase cellular size. Hypertrophy, like atrophy, can be pathologic or physiologic and is caused by increased functional demand or specific hormonal stimulation.

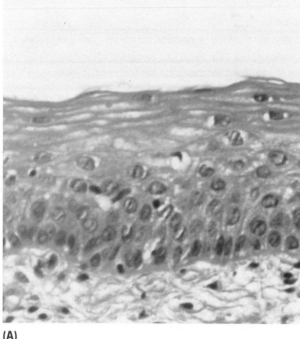

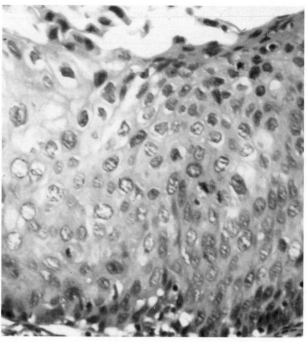

(A)

(B)

Figure 5–2 Comparison of normal, nonkeratinized stratified squamous epithelium (A) with dysplastic epithelium. (B) Note the variation in nuclear size, polarity, and staining reaction (original magnification X 400).

Hypertrophy may be triggered by mechanical signals or trophic signals (such as growth factors, hormones, and vasoactive agents). For example, when a diseased kidney is removed, the other kidney adapts to the increased workload, causing it to increase in number of cells and overall size. A pathologic example is when pathophysiologic hypertrophy of the heart occurs secondary to hypertension or problem valves.

Hyperplasia

Hyperplasia is defined as an increase in the number of cells due to an increased rate of cellular division. In response to injury, hyperplasia occurs when an injury has been severe and prolonged and caused cell death. Increased cell growth involves production of growth factors that stimulate remaining cells to synthesize new cell components and eventually divide. Both hyperplasia and hypertrophy often occur at the same time, taking place if the cells can synthesize DNA. In nondividing cells such as myocardial fibers, only hypertrophy occurs.

There are two types of normal (physiologic) hyperplasia:

- Compensatory: Enables certain organs (such as the liver) to regenerate
- Hormonal: Usually occurs in estrogen-dependent organs such as the breast or uterus

Nerve cells, skeletal muscle cells, myocardial cells, and cells of the lens of the eye do not, however, regenerate. Myoblasts can fuse to create additional skeletal muscle cells. Compensatory hyperplasia commonly occurs in epidermal and intestinal epithelia, bone marrow cells, fibroblasts, and hepatocytes. Some hyperplasia occurs in bone, cartilage, and smooth muscle cells. Another example is when the skin thickens to form a callus, as a result of hyperplasia of epidermal cells, which is caused by a mechanical stimulus.

Pathologic hyperplasia is the abnormal proliferation of normal cells. This usually occurs in response to excessive hormonal stimulation or growth factors on target cells. Pathologic hyperplasia of the endometrium is the most common example, caused by an imbalance between estrogen and progesterone secretion, with oversecretion of estrogen. Excessive menstrual bleeding may be caused by pathologic endometrial hyperplasia. When regular growth-inhibition controls fail, hyperplastic endometrial cells may undergo malignant transformation.

Diagnosis of hyperplasia differs based on which organs are involved, but for confirmation needle biopsy is essential. When hyperplasia involves the prostate or breast, for example, treatment often involves surgery. For hyperplasia that results in skin lesions, treatments such as *diathermy* may be used. This involves the application of heat by using high-frequency electromagnetic currents.

Metaplasia

Metaplasia is defined as the reversible replacement of a single mature cell type by another (sometimes less differentiated) cell type. It is believed to occur due to stem cell "reprogramming" in epithelial or connective tissue. Signals generated by cytokines and cell growth factors cause these precursor cells to mature. An example of metaplasia is the replacement of normal columnary ciliated epithelial cells in the bronchial lining by stratified squamous epithelial cells. Because these new cells neither have cilia nor secrete mucus, the condition causes a loss of vital protection. If the inducing stimulus (usually cigarette smoking) ceases, the bronchial metaplasia may be reversed. However, prolonged exposure to an inducing stimulus may result in dysplasia and cancerous transformation.

In cases of myelofibrosis with myeloid metaplasia, bone marrow biopsy is the most accurate method of diagnosis. Although there is no curative treatment, bone marrow transplant can potentially cure some patients. However, the treatment does carry significant risks.

Cellular Injury

Cellular injury occurs when a cell cannot maintain homeostasis because of harmful stimuli. Most diseases result from cellular injury. A *reversible injury* is one in which injured cells may recover. An *irreversible injury* is one in which injured cells die. Cellular injury may result from chemical agents, hypoxia (lack of sufficient oxygen), free radicals, infectious agents, immunologic reactions, physical and mechanical factors, genetic factors, and nutritional imbalances.

The type, state, and adaptive processes of a cell, along with the type, severity, and duration of the injurious stimulus, determine the extent of cellular injury. The extent of injury can be greatly influenced by modifying factors such as nutritional status. It is not fully understood at which point cellular death is not preventable.

Mechanisms of Cell Injury

There are four common mechanisms of cell injury:

- ATP depletion: Loss of mitochondrial ATP and decreased ATP synthesis.
- Oxygen and oxygen-derived free radicals: Lack of oxygen is vital in progression of cell injury in ischemia.
- Intracellular calcium and loss of calcium steady rate: Normally, intracellular cytosolic calcium concentrations are very low, but changes can damage membranes and cells.
- Defects in membrane permeability: Early loss of selective membrane permeability is found in all forms of cell injury.

There are three common forms of cell injury:

- Hypoxic injury, from lack of oxygen
- Free radicals and reactive oxygen species injury, from oxygen ions and peroxides
- Chemical injury, from toxic substances

Hypoxic Injury

Hypoxia, defined as the lack of sufficient oxygen to the tissue, is the single most common cause of cellular injury. Hypoxia may result from loss of hemoglobin or hemoglobin function, a decreased amount of oxygen in the air, diseases of the respiratory and cardiovascular systems, decreased production of red blood cells, and poisoning of the cytochromes (oxidative enzymes) inside the cells. Hypoxia is usually caused by **ischemia** (reduced blood supply).

Ischemia often results from gradual narrowing or complete blockage of arteries. Gradual arterial obstruction that causes progressive hypoxia is better tolerated than sudden, acute **anoxia** (total lack of oxygen) caused by a sudden obstruction (usually from a blood clot). An acute coronary artery obstruction can cause myocardial cell death (infarction) in only a few minutes if blood supply is not restored.

Stroke and myocardial infarction usually result from atherosclerosis and resultant ischemic injury.

The process of cellular response to hypoxic injury occurs within 1 minute after myocardial blood supply is interrupted. The heart loses color and cannot contract normally. Between 3 and 5 minutes after this begins, the heart ceases to contract because of a rapid decrease in mitochondrial phosphorylation and lack of ATP. This leads to increased anaerobic metabolism, generating ATP from glycogen because of insufficient oxygen. Once the supply of oxygen is depleted, anaerobic metabolism also ceases.

Lack of ATP causes failure of the plasma membrane's sodium-potassium pump and sodium-calcium exchange. Sodium and calcium accumulate as potassium diffuses out of the cells. At this point water and sodium enter cells freely, causing cellular swelling and dilation of the endoplasmic reticulum. Ribosomes detach from the endoplasmic reticulum, and protein synthesis is reduced. As hypoxia continues, each entire cell swells greatly. However, if oxygen is restored, these disruptions may be reversed. If not, vacuolation (formation of vacuoles) inside the cytoplasm occurs and the mitochondria swell, damaging the membrane.

At this time the cells are irreversibly damaged, and extracellular calcium moves into the cells to accumulate in the mitochondria. If oxygen is restored at this time, *reperfusion injury* may occur. This results from the generation of high reactive oxygen intermediates such as hydroxyl radical, superoxide, and hydrogen peroxide. Antioxidants such as superoxide dismutase, beta-carotene, and vitamin E can decrease the amount of damage.

> **RED FLAG**
> Vitamin C, vitamin E, and beta-carotene are natural antioxidants.

The cells of the body are bathed in a calcium-rich fluid. Muscle cells must have calcium to activate actin and myosin. When the plasma membrane is damaged, calcium easily enters and accumulates in the mitochondria, causing swelling and rapid cell death. When atherosclerosis causes hypoxic injury, lack of ATP production increasingly deprives the myocardium of energy required for contraction.

Mechanisms of Chemical Injury

When a toxic substance interacts with a cell's plasma membrane, chemical injury to the cell begins. The following are the two general mechanisms of chemical injury:

- Direct toxicity: Due to a chemical combining with a cell's membrane or organelles
- Formation of reactive free radicals and lipid peroxidation

An example of chemical injury is when carbon tetrachloride is converted by enzymes in the smooth endoplasmic reticulum of liver cells into chloromethyl (CCl), which is a highly toxic free radical. CCl rapidly destroys the liver cells' endoplasmic reticula by lipid peroxidation, breaking down the lipid component of the reticula.

Lipid molecules accumulate inside the cytoplasm, beginning inside the cisternae of the endoplasmic reticulum. The liver becomes fatty as the CCl blocks the synthesis of *lipid-acceptor proteins (apoproteins)*. Blockage of lipoprotein (triglyceride) secretion begins 10 to 15 minutes after CCl exposure. Fat droplets combine to form larger droplets and fill vacuoles and, eventually, the entire cytoplasm. About 10 to 12 hours later the liver is greatly enlarged and pale due to fat accumulation. This condition is reversible if the toxicity is removed, with cellular changes the same as in hypoxic injury.

Accidental Injuries

In the United States both unintentional and intentional injuries cause over 148,000 deaths every year. Black males are most often affected by various types of injuries, and men of all groups are affected by injuries more than twice as often as women. Injury-related deaths are highest in young adults and the elderly. Unintentional injuries are the leading cause of death for people between the ages of 1 and 34 years. In this age group suicide ranks as the second greatest cause of death. Nonfatal injuries are a significant cause of morbidity and disability. Classifications of injury include blunt force injuries, contusion, abrasion, laceration, fractures, sharp force injuries, gunshot wounds, and asphyxial injuries. The most common of these are discussed following.

Contusion

A **contusion** is a bruise, defined as bleeding into the skin and/or underlying tissues due to trauma that crushes the soft tissues and ruptures blood vessels but does not break the skin. Often, a contusion is not seen until several hours after injury. Colors of contusions include reddish-purple, bluish-black, yellowish-brown, and/or green. Contusions change color as tissue damage and healing progress. The area of the injury helps to determine the pattern of bruising. Contusions can heal in days or weeks. Deeper bleeding may cause discoloration in areas that were not actually directly injured.

A **hematoma** refers to a collection of blood in soft tissues or an enclosed space. A *subdural hematoma* describes a collection of blood between the inner surface of the dura mater and the brain surface. This results in a shearing of small veins bridging the subdural space. Subdural hematoma may be due to blows, falls, or sudden acceleration/deceleration of the head. An *epidural hematoma* describes a collection of blood between the inner skull surface and the dura and is caused by a torn artery (usually due to a skull fracture).

Brain contusions may result from blows, falls, or other impact. A blow to the skull causes a cerebral contusion that is grouped in a *coup* pattern. In falls or impacts when the head strikes the ground or another object, the cerebral contusion is seen in a portion of the brain opposing the external injury site, known as a *contrecoup* pattern of injury. A contrecoup injury occurs when the head accelerates in motion while the brain "lags behind," causing it to press against the opposite side of the skull from the direction of motion. As the head suddenly stops, the portion of the brain pressing into the skull is injured.

For example, for subdural hematoma diagnosis is confirmed by computed tomography, MRI, x-rays, and angiogram. Subdural hematoma requires emergency hospitalization and surgery. For recovery, various types of physical therapy may be indicated, as well as aquatic therapy and speech therapy.

Abrasion

An **abrasion** is a scrape that is caused by removal of the superficial skin layers, due to friction between an object and the skin. Abrasions range greatly in size. Nonperpendicular abrasions may result in tags of tissue being heaped up at the trailing (downstream) edges. At first, abrasions usually have a pale, moist, yellow-brown appearance that darkens to brown (or black) as the injury dries. Tissue fluid may ooze from the injury for 1 to 2 days until completely covered over by a crust or scab, which eventually flakes off of the underlying new skin.

> **RED FLAG**
> Another example of the importance of patterned injury is a bite mark, which may actually identify the assailant.

Often, both abrasions and contusions may result in a patterned appearance based on the shape and features of the injuring object. When an assault, automobile accident, or homicide occurs, these patterned injuries may be important for documentation of the case.

Laceration

A **laceration** is a tear or rip in skin or tissue. It is different from an incision, wherein the skin or tissue is cleanly divided using an extremely sharp edge. Lacerations are more jagged and irregular, with abraded edges to the wound. Depths of lacerations may be highly irregular, with stretched but unbroken vessels or nerves crossing the wound area. Surrounding tissue may be crushed, abraded, and contused if force is applied in a perpendicular motion to the skin. Tangential force causes undermining of the wound, and the trailing edge will be lifted away to create a pocket in the opposite direction from where the blow occurred. An *avulsion* is an extreme example of this, wherein a large tissue area is pulled away to create a large flap.

Blunt impact to the abdomen often causes lacerations of internal organs such as the liver, kidneys, intestines, and spleen. The thoracic aorta is often lacerated as a result of automobile accidents. Severe blows to the chest may also lacerate the aorta or ventricles, causing rupturing of the heart.

Fractures

Fractures and shattering of bones may occur because of blunt force blows or impacts. See Chapter 16 for a discussion of fractures in detail.

Asphyxial Injuries

Asphyxial injuries occur when the cells fail to receive or use oxygen. Oxygen deprivation may be total (*anoxia*) or partial (*hypoxia*) and includes suffocation, strangulation, chemical asphyxiation, and drowning.

Suffocation

Suffocation occurs when oxygen fails to reach the blood and can be due to a lack of environmental oxygen or blockage of the external airways. Common examples of suffocation include suicide by tying a plastic bag over the head or a child stuck inside an unused refrigerator. If the oxygen level drops below 5%, death can occur within only a few minutes. *Choking asphyxiation* is based on obstruction of the internal airways and depends on locating and removing material that obstructs them. Disease or injury may also cause the soft airway tissues to swell, obstructing them and blocking respiration. Also, suffocation may be due to compression of the chest or abdomen. Symptoms of suffocation include petechiae (pinpoint hemorrhages) of the eyes and face and florid facial congestion. Diagnosis is based on the patient history and signs and symptoms.

Strangulation

Strangulation may be caused by compression and closure of the air passages and blood vessels due to external pressure on the neck. Cerebral hypoxia or anoxia secondary to cessation or alteration of blood flow to and from the brain may result. Most strangulation deaths and injuries occur from alteration of cerebral blood flow, not from lack of airflow. Complete blockage of the carotid arteries can cause unconsciousness within only 10 to 15 seconds.

Attempts at suicide often involve *hanging strangulations*, wherein a noose around the neck, combined with the hanging weight of the body, constricts the noose to compress the neck. Only partial suspension of the body is sufficient to cause injury or death.

Contusions and abrasions on the outside of the neck are common. Usually, internal damage is severe, including deep bruising and fractures of the hyoid bone and throat cartilages, as well as petechiae.

Chemical Asphyxiants

Chemical asphyxiants either block utilization of oxygen or prevent its delivery to the tissues. The most common chemical asphyxiant is *carbon monoxide*, followed by *cyanide* and *hydrogen sulfide* (sewer gas). Carbon monoxide is odorless, colorless, and undetectable unless mixed with a pollutant that can be seen or smelled. It causes a cherry-red appearance because it prevents oxygen molecules from binding with hemoglobin. Cyanide blocks intracellular utilization of oxygen, causing a similar cherry-red appearance in the victim. However, cyanide also causes an odor of bitter almonds that can be detected by certain individuals when they get close to a cyanide-poisoning victim. Hydrogen sulfide may cause the symptom of brown-tinged blood as well as other nonspecific signs of asphyxiation.

Drowning

Drowning causes alteration of oxygen delivery to tissues from breathing in water or other fluids. The major mechanism of injury is low blood oxygen levels (hypoxemia). Though large amounts of fluids can pass through the alveolar–capillary interface, airway obstruction by the fluids is the usual cause of damage or death. It is possible to drown in small amounts of water or other fluids (*dry-lung drowning*) due to vagal nerve–mediated laryngospasms that result.

Cerebral hypoxia after the breathing in of fluids leads to unconsciousness in a few minutes. Irreversible injury occurs much more quickly in warm water than in cold water. Complete submersion is not required for the person to drown. When water enters the lungs, a common symptom is large amounts of foam coming out of the nose and mouth.

Cellular Death and Necrosis

Cellular death eventually leads to **necrosis** (cellular dissolution), which results after localized cell death and *autolysis* (cellular self-digestion) have occurred. Stages of necrosis, including normal cell condition, *pyknosis*, and **karyolysis**, are shown in **Figure 5–3**.

Irreversible cell injury is signified by dense clumping, progressive disruption of genetic material, and disruption of the plasma and organelle membranes. Fragmentation of the nucleus of a cell into smaller particles is known as *karyorrhexis*. There are five major types of necrosis:

- Coagulative necrosis: Usually results from hypoxia caused by severe ischemia or hypoxia due to chemical injury
- Liquefactive necrosis: Usually results from ischemic injury to neurons and glial cells in the brain, sometimes caused by bacterial infection
- Caseous necrosis: Usually results from tuberculous pulmonary infection, with tissues resembling soft, clumped cheese
- Fat necrosis: Usually results from powerful lipase enzymes that break down triglycerides to release free fatty acids; the tissue appears opaque and chalk white
- Gangrenous necrosis (**gangrene**): Usually results from severe hypoxic injury due to arteriosclerosis of major arteries; may lead to dry or wet gangrene (**Figure 5–4**)

When cell development is abnormal, cell numbers are excessive or cells are injured or aged. **Apoptosis** is a normal occurrence and is defined as *programmed cell death*. In apoptosis cells appear to "digest" themselves via enzymatic action. This self-destruction allows them to disintegrate into fragments. The following are examples of various types of cell injury:

- Ischemia: Oxygen deficit in cells due to circulatory obstruction or respiratory problems
- Mechanical damage: Pressure or tearing of tissue
- Physical agents: Radiation exposure or excessive heat or cold
- Microorganisms: Bacteria, viruses, or parasites
- Chemical toxins: Including foreign substances
- Nutritional deficits
- Abnormal metabolites that accumulate in cells
- Fluid or electrolyte imbalance

Ischemia may occur locally due to a blocked artery or may occur systemically due to respiratory problems. Brain, heart, and kidney cells, which have a high oxygen demand, are affected very quickly by hypoxia. This may interfere with the production of ATP in the cells, causing a sodium pump loss in the cell membranes, and loss of cellular function. When sodium ions increase inside the cell, it swells and eventually ruptures its membrane. When oxygen is lacking, **anaerobic** metabolism leads to a pH decrease and continued impairment of metabolism.

Both **exogenous** and **endogenous** chemicals may damage cells by altering the membrane's permeability or by

> **RED FLAG**
> Ischemia is the most common cause of cell damage and tissue necrosis.

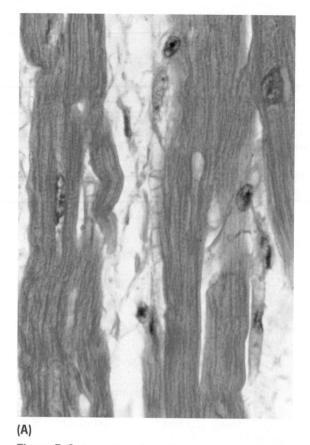
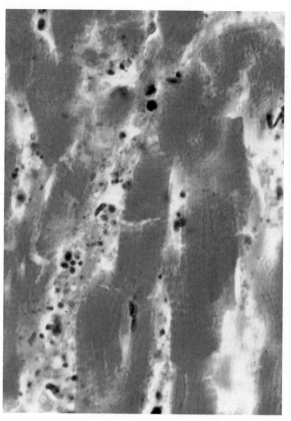

(A)   **(B)**

Figure 5–3 Comparison of normal cardiac muscle fibers (A) with necrotic fibers. (B) Note the fragmentation of fibers, the loss of nuclear staining, and the fragmented bits of nuclear debris (original magnification X 400).

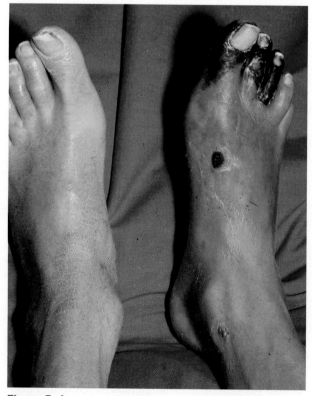

Figure 5–4 Gangrene of right foot as a result of arterial obstruction.

producing free radicals. Infectious diseases, via the actions of *microorganisms*, may also cause cell injury. Cell damage by various sources occurs with either *initial* metabolic changes or *loss of cellular function*. Cells may recover from damage if the causative factor is quickly removed. If the noxious factor remains, damage becomes irreversible and kills the cell. Increased damage is shown by detectable *morphologic* or structural cell changes.

When the cell dies, the nucleus disintegrates. **Lysis** (dissolution) releases *lysosomal* enzymes into tissues, causing **inflammation**. Large amounts of dead cells can cause this to be extensive, potentially killing more cells. Dead cells release enzymes into the bloodstream, helping to identify the types of cells that are damaged.

An *infarction* describes an area of dead cells that were harmed by a lack of oxygen. Functional loss may be significant when large amounts of cells die, as when the heart fails because the heart muscle is infarcted or dies. Connective or scar tissue may form to fill the gap left by the dead tissue. Heart muscle cells do not reproduce because they do not undergo mitosis.

Each type of cell dies at a different rate from other cells. When deprived of oxygen brain cells die in only 4 to 5 minutes, whereas heart cells can survive for up to 30 minutes. Because cardiac and respiratory function can be artificially maintained, it is harder to determine actual *somatic death* of the body. Usually, *brain death* is sufficient in determining somatic death. It is based on lack of any electrical brain activity, measured by absence of responses and electroencephalography.

Aging and Altered Cellular and/or Tissue Biology

Aging, as it relates to alterations in cellular and tissue biology, may cause injuries due to ultraviolet light exposure, mechanical injuries, and metabolic reactions. The connection between aging and disease is not clear. Certain levels of atrophy of tissues are normal with aging until they reach a clinically significant disease state. Atherosclerosis usually progresses with age; however, it may not significantly affect one individual but lead to the death of another. Aging may be the result of the accumulation of multiple random injuries and other events. It also may be the result of self-destructive processes unique to each individual or because of a genetically predetermined developmental "schedule."

SUMMARY

Cells adapt to increased work demands or threats to their survival. They do this by changing their size (hypertrophy and atrophy), number (hyperplasia), and form (metaplasia). Normal cellular adaptation occurs as a reaction to an appropriate stimulus. It stops once the need to adapt has ceased. Cells can be damaged by physical trauma, temperature extremes, electrical injuries and exposure to chemicals or radiation, biologic agents, and because of lack of nutrition. Most damaging effects of injurious agents come from the uncontrolled production of free radicals or because of impaired delivery or utilization of oxygen. Cell injury is either reversible, which allows cells to recover, or irreversible, in which the cells become necrotic and die.

REVIEW QUESTIONS

Select the best response to each question.

1. An area of dead cells, due to a lack of oxygen, is called
   a. ischemia
   b. an infarction
   c. atresia
   d. gangrene

2. The breaking down of cells is called
   a. lysis
   b. gangrene
   c. autopsy
   d. biopsy

3. The premature death of living cells and tissue is called
   a. metaplasia
   b. karyolysis
   c. necrosis
   d. contusion

4. A condition that describes tissue cells that vary in size and shape is referred to as
   a. dysplasia
   b. hyperplasia
   c. metaplasia
   d. hypertrophy

5. The four common mechanisms of cell injury include all the following *except*
   a. lack of oxygen and ischemia
   b. decreased ATP formation in the cells
   c. decreased intracellular potassium
   d. defects in membrane permeability

6. An increase in the size of individual cells is called
   a. dysplasia
   b. hyperplasia
   c. metaplasia
   d. hypertrophy

7. A contusion is called
   a. a bruise
   b. gangrene
   c. atrophy
   d. anoxia

8. A collection of blood between the inner surface of the dura mater and the brain surface is called
   a. an epidural hematoma
   b. a subdural hematoma
   c. a brain concussion
   d. a brain contusion

9. The most common chemical asphyxiant is
   a. cyanide
   b. hydrogen sulfide
   c. nitrous oxide
   d. carbon monoxide

10. A torn wound with ragged edges is called
    a. a laceration
    b. gangrene
    c. an abrasion
    d. a contusion

CASE STUDIES

Karen Coupe, PT, DPT, MSEd

Case 1

A 24-year-old woman is hospitalized due to multiple injuries sustained in a motorcycle accident 2 days ago. The patient underwent an *open reduction internal fixation* (ORIF) secondary to a left trimalleolar ankle fracture, presents with multiple abrasions on the lateral aspect of the right upper and lower extremities, a 6-inch laceration on the right lateral forearm, as well as multiple contusions. Patient medical history: Unremarkable. Prior level of function: Independent in all activities of daily living, marathon runner. The physical therapist evaluation reveals bed mobility with mod X 1 assist for right lower extremity; transfers sit to stand with min x 1 secondary to loss of balance, ambulation with axillary crutches non–weight-bearing on right lower extremity x 25 ft with multiple verbal cues for correct crutch placement, maintaining a non–weight-bearing status and instruction to refrain from leaning on the axillary pads. Plan of care includes bed mobility, transfers and gait training with axillary crutches and therapeutic exercise.

1. Explain the difference in what you would observe with an abrasion versus a contusion versus a laceration.

2. Would each of the above undergo an inflammatory process? If so, how would this contribute to what you would observe?

3. What is an ORIF? Why do you suspect the physician did an ORIF rather than just a simple casting of the ankle?

4. Because this patient is casted and non–weight-bearing on the right, what will occur to the musculature on the right lower extremity? Why?

5. Why is it important that the patient refrain from leaning on the axillary crutch pads?

Case 2

A 16-year-old boy suffered brain damage from hypoxia and secondary cerebral edema from a near-drowning accident 3 days ago. Magnetic resonance imaging (MRI) revealed a frontal lobe subdural hematoma. Secondary complication of acute renal tubular necrosis. According to a friend the patient was diving into the ocean, hit his head, was found unconscious, and required cardiopulmonary resuscitation (CPR). The patient is comatose, and the physical therapist plan of care is for tone reduction, *passive range-of-motion* (PROM), and positioning.

1. What type of cellular injury occurred in the brain tissue with the hypoxia? Is this reversible or irreversible?

2. What is a subdural hematoma? Could this be a contributing factor in the brain damage?

3. The frontal lobe of the brain contains many important areas that allow us to function both physically and cognitively. List some specific functions controlled by the frontal lobe.

4. The patient has renal tubular necrosis. What has happened to the renal tubules? Depending on the severity, how could this affect the patient?

5. Why would PROM and positioning be important for this patient?

WEBSITES

http://geography.about.com/od/populationgeography/a/lifeexpectancy.htm

http://library.thinkquest.org/04oct/00206/ta_cause_of_death.htm

http://ocw.tufts.edu/data/51/551831.pdf

http://publications.nigms.nih.gov/insidethecell/chapter5.html

http://www.humpath.com/Atrophy

http://www.uvm.edu/~jkessler/PATH301/301celli.htm

http://www.wakeems.com/ICE/Hypothermia/pediatric%20brain%20injury%20from%20ca.pdf

http://www.wrongdiagnosis.com/a/accidents/intro.htm

http://www.wrongdiagnosis.com/sym/necrosis.htm

http://www.wrongdiagnosis.com/sym/suffocation.htm

Genetic and Congenital Disorders

LEARNING OBJECTIVES

After completion of the chapter the reader should be able to

1. Define the terms congenital, gene mutation, genotype, phenotype, and karyotype.
2. Describe three types of single-gene disorders.
3. Compare disorders due to multifactorial inheritance with those caused by single-gene inheritance.
4. Describe the meaning of autosomal recessive disorders and list three disorders in this group.
5. Define X-linked recessive disorders.
6. Explain the diagnostic tools used to determine certain abnormalities during pregnancy.
7. Describe gene therapy.
8. Relate maternal age and occurrence of Down syndrome.

KEY TERMS

Alleles: Alternative forms of a gene that occupy a corresponding position on homologous chromosomes.

Amniocentesis: An obstetric procedure in which small amounts of amniotic fluid are removed for laboratory analysis. It is usually performed between the 16th and 20th weeks of gestation to aid in the diagnosis of fetal abnormalities.

Anomaly: A congenital malformation, such as the absence of a limb.

Autosomes: Chromosomes that are not sex chromosomes and appear as a homologous pair in a somatic cell.

Brainstem: The lower extension of the brain, where it connects with the spinal cord.

Cranium: The part of the skull that encloses the brain.

Expression: The indication of a physical or emotional state through facial appearance or vocal intonation.

Genotype: The complete genetic constitution of an organism or group, as determined by the specific combination and location of the genes on the chromosomes.

Heterozygous: An organism whose somatic cells have two different allomorphic genes on the same location of each pair of chromosomes.

Homozygous: Having two identical alleles at corresponding locations on homologous chromosomes.

Karyotype: A diagrammatic representation of the chromosome complement of an individual or species, in which the chromosomes are arranged in pairs in descending order of size and according to the position of the centromere.

KEY TERMS CONTINUED

Meiosis: The division of a sex cell as it matures into two and then four haploid cells. The nucleus of each receives one half of the number of chromosomes present in the somatic cells of the species.

Melanin: The natural pigment that gives color to the hair, skin, and irises of the eyes.

Mitosis: The separation of chromosomes in a cell nucleus into two identical sets in two cell nuclei.

Mutation: An unusual change in a gene or a gene sequence.

Neonates: Infants between birth and 28 days of age.

Organogenesis: The formation and differentiation of organs and organ systems during embryonic development.

Penetration: A stage in which genetic material enters a host cell.

Phenotype: The complete observable characteristics of an organism or group, including anatomic, physiologic, biochemical, and behavior traits.

Polygenic: Pertaining to or dominated by several different genes.

Spina bifida occulta: The type of spina bifida that does not involve herniation of the meninges or the contents of the spinal cord.

Teratogenic: Capable of causing the formation of one or more developmental abnormalities in the fetus.

Trisomy: The presence of a third chromosome of one type in a cell that would normally have two of the same chromosomes.

Overview

Genetic and congenital disorders are important factors in health care. These disorders affect every age group, involving nearly all body tissues and organs. Congenital defects are also known as *birth defects* and can develop prenatally or at birth. The term *congenital* does not indicate or exclude genetic disorders, which are usually hereditarily linked.

Genetic disorders may occur from chromosomal disorders, multifactorial disorders, or single-gene disorders. Single-gene disorders are due to one defective gene that is passed on the chromosome to younger generations along the specific inheritance gene pattern. Sometimes, the **expression** or **phenotype** (effect) of an altered gene causes clinical signs that may vary in severity. This may depend on the activity or **penetration** of the gene.

Genetic Control

Each human cell contains 23 pairs of chromosomes. The genetic information for each cell is stored on these chromosomes. Of the 23 pairs, 22 of them are called **autosomes**, which are numbered by size and shape in a **karyotype** (**Figure 6–1**). The final pair consists of the sex chromosomes (XY for males and XX for females). If the child receives an X chromosome from the mother and a Y chromosome from the father, sex is defined as male. If the child receives X chromosomes from both parents, sex is defined as female.

Each sperm and each ovum receive only 23 chromosomes during **meiosis**. Once the ovum is fertilized by the sperm, the zygote that forms has a combined total of 46 chromosomes (23 pairs). The genetic information from both parents they contain may differ widely because there are so many possible combinations of genes. It is almost completely unlikely that any two people can have the same genes and deoxyribonucleic acid (DNA) sequence. Each individual therefore has a unique identifying characteristic—their DNA (**Figure 6–2**).

Genes matched for a certain function are called **alleles**. They are located at specific locations on the paired chromosomes. Each gene uses DNA to determine the protein synthesis of the cells. A **genotype** describes the same chromosomes

and genetic content contained in each person's body. However, not all genes are active in every cell. *Gene expression* is defined as this limited activity. Each cell's specific function is usually controlled only by a small group of genes.

DNA strands, which determine cell functions, compose genes. A communication link with DNA is known as ribonucleic acid (RNA). RNA communicates with DNA when protein synthesis is occurring, helping to control cellular activities. When cells are undergoing **mitosis** during embryonic and fetal development, chromosomes replicate, with each daughter cell receiving identical DNA to the DNA that

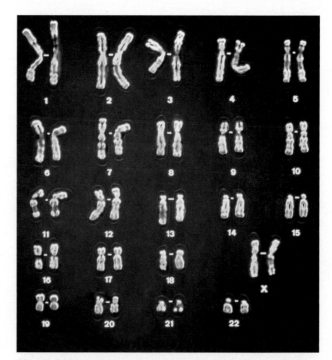

Figure 6–1 Karyotype. Chromosomes from a normal human female arranged in order of decreasing size. Note that there are 46 chromosomes—or 23 pairs—in somatic cells. Each pair is similar in size, banding pattern, and location of the centromere.

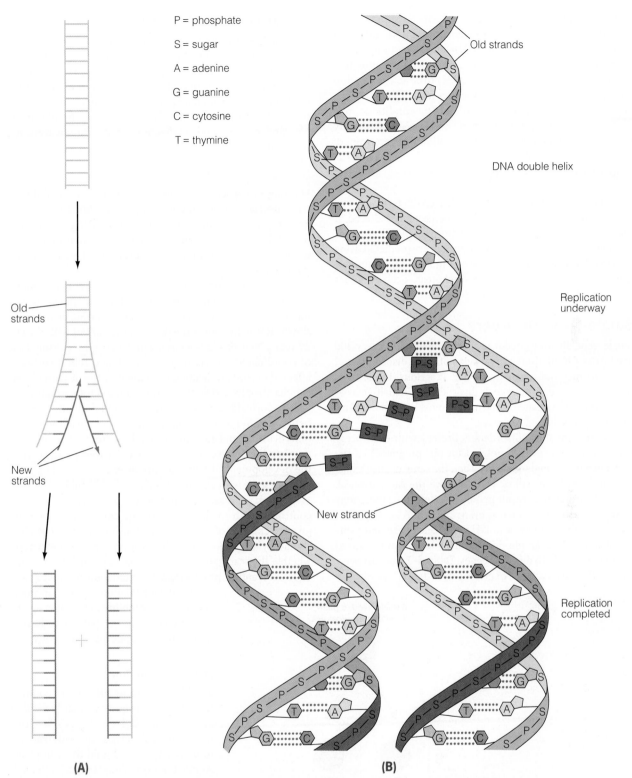

P = phosphate

S = sugar

A = adenine

G = guanine

C = cytosine

T = thymine

Old strands

DNA double helix

Replication underway

Old strands

New strands

New strands

Replication completed

(A)   **(B)**

Figure 6–2 DNA replication. DNA replication is semiconservative. (A) Each double helix unwinds, and each half of the helix serves as a template for the production of a new strand of DNA. When replication is complete, each new helix contains one old and one new strand. (B) Nucleotides attach to the template one at a time and are joined together with the aid of enzymes.

exists in the parent cell. Unless an error occurs during meiosis or mitosis, the same genetic information is replicated. A **mutation** (alteration) in genetic material can be caused by radiation, exposure to harmful drugs, or spontaneously.

Genes may differ in location on chromosomes, and research known as *gene mapping* continues to progress as scientists identify the roles of each human gene. The *International Human Genome Project* is attempting to identify and map every gene on every human chromosome. Millions of different pairings have already been listed. Approximately 25,000 protein-coding genes are believed to exist in human chromosomes.

DNA sequences regulate gene activity in some capacity, although there are DNA sequences that have unknown functions. Information about DNA and its actions grows every year. When a specific gene is identified in relation to a pathologic condition, we are more likely to be able to develop blood tests that can screen for the presence of that particular gene. Increased knowledge of genetic conditions may lead to improved cures, preventions, and treatment. Already there have been hundreds of genetic conditions determined. Congenital disorders present at birth are also referred to as *congenital defects*. They include genetic (inherited) disorders and developmental disorders.

Genes control every type of physical characteristic. They also control metabolic processes. When a gene is altered, it often causes a disease to develop. Patterns of inherited genes include dominant and recessive traits that are predicted using a system known as *Punnett squares* (**Figure 6–3**). Dominant genes are shown in capital letters, whereas recessive genes are shown in lowercase letters.

Single-Gene Disorders

Single-gene disorders occur in approximately 1 of every 200 live births. Often, there are no signs of these disorders, and diagnosis may not occur until later. If serious, the fetus is often miscarried. Single-gene disorders are usually classified by their inheritance pattern, with most being dominant, recessive, or X-linked recessive.

The risk for these disorders is present with each pregnancy in a family at risk, not just for one pregnancy. If the first-born has a single-gene disorder, the same chance exists that the next-born will or will not have the same disease. These disorders may result in only one defect, or there may be widespread effects such as cystic fibrosis. Also, a specific physical symptom may be linked to not one but to many different genes. For example, deafness in children may be caused by approximately 16 different genes. **Table 6–1** gives an overview of the various types of genetic disorders.

Autosomal Dominant Disorders

Some autosomal dominant disorders do not become clinically evident until mid-life, and by this time the defective gene may have already been passed on. In these disorders a defect present in only one allele produces clinical expression of the disease. An affected parent has a 50 percent chance of passing the disorder on to each child, irrespective of gender. No carriers exist, and unaffected parents do not transmit these disorders.

Huntington's Disease

Huntington's disease is an example of an autosomal dominant disorder for which screening is available. Its causative gene results in brain degeneration developing in mid-life. Sometimes, two dominant genes are expressed in a single individual. Type AB blood is an example of such *codominant* genes.

Huntington's disease is characterized by progressive mental deterioration and abnormal writhing or "jerky" movements. It usually occurs between ages 30 and 50, progressing slowly. It usually causes the death of the patient within 15 to 20 years. Neurons in the basal ganglia atrophy, causing lack of coordinated muscle movements. The cerebral cortex is affected eventually, leading to dementia. Cortical and basal ganglia atrophy is diagnosed by computed tomography.

The normal *HD* gene on chromosome 4 normally contains between 6 and 35 repeating groups of the nucleotides adenine, cytosine, and guanine. When these "repeats" increase in number, the disease develops—the more *repeats*, the earlier the development of Huntington's disease. The male parent passes a gene with expanded repeats to the child.

Though the disease cannot be stopped, it can be partially controlled with medication. Genetic counseling should be given to children of persons with Huntington's disease. They should be told about available testing that can determine whether they carry the abnormal gene. Physiotherapy focuses on fall prevention, promoting safe ambulation, improving balance and coordination, wheelchair management and mobility in the later stages, and encouraging the patient to have a good attitude about his or her body.

Marfan's Syndrome

Marfan's syndrome affects the connective tissue of the body, primarily *fibrillin I* in the extracellular matrix. Connective tissues normally give shape and structure to body tissues and hold them in place. About 1 of every 5,000 births is affected, primarily occurring within families. The clinical features of Marfan's syndrome include eye problems, skeletal (including vertebral) deformities, longer than normal arms, cardiovascular abnormalities, and hypermobility of the joints. The skeletal deformities are most obvious, with the body appearing long and thin, including the extremities and fingers (**Figure 6–4**). Chest deformities may require

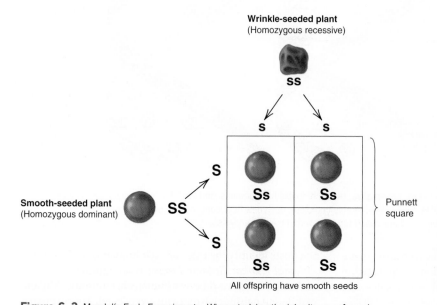

Wrinkle-seeded plant
(Homozygous recessive)

SS

S   S

Smooth-seeded plant
(Homozygous dominant)

SS

S

S

Ss	Ss
Ss	Ss

Punnett square

All offspring have smooth seeds

Figure 6–3 Mendel's Early Experiments. When studying the inheritance of seed conformation, Mendel first crossed homozygous-recessive (ss) and homozygous-dominant (SS) plants. The offspring were all heterozygotes (Ss).

TABLE 6-1 Genetic Disorders and Inheritance

Single-Gene Disorders	Multifactorial Disorders	Chromosomal Disorders
Autosomal Dominant	Anencephaly	Cri du chat syndrome
Adult polycystic kidney disease	Cleft lip and palate	Down syndrome
Familial hypercholesterolemia	Clubfoot	Monosomy X (Turner's syndrome)
Huntington's disease	Congenital heart disease	
Marfan's syndrome	Myelomeningocele	Polysomy X (Klinefelter's syndrome)
	Schizophrenia	
Autosomal Recessive		Trisomy 18 (Edwards' syndrome
Albinism		
Color blindness		
Cystic fibrosis		
Phenylketonuria		
Sickle cell anemia		
Tay-Sachs disease		
X-linked Recessive		
Duchenne muscular dystrophy		
Hemophilia A		

surgery. The associated eye conditions predispose patients to retinal detachment.

The most dangerous effects of the condition involve the cardiovascular system, including mitral valve prolapse, aortic valve ring dilation, and weakness of the aorta and other arteries. The condition cannot be cured, but low to moderate activities are recommended. Surgery may be required in cases of acute aortic dissection or progressive aortic dilation. The physical therapist assistant (PTA) should explain to the patient with Marfan's syndrome that strenuous activities should be avoided as much as possible. These include contact sports, high-impact aerobics, scuba diving, and weight training. The patient should be advised that the cardiovascular components of Marfan's syndrome might result in surgery to treat progressive aortic dilation or acute aortic dissection.

Autosomal Recessive Disorders

Autosomal recessive disorders include albinism, phenylketonuria (PKU), and Tay-Sachs disease. For these disorders to develop both parents must pass on the defective gene. This

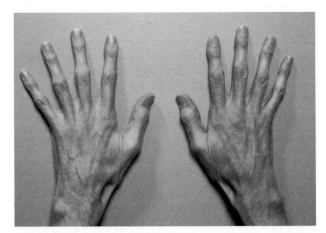

Figure 6-4 Marfan's syndrome.

produces an affected (**homozygous**) child, with males and females being equally affected. A child who is **heterozygous** has received one normal gene and one defective gene, meaning that he or she is a carrier with no clinical signs of the disorder.

The genotypes of each parent determine the risk of transmitting an autosomal recessive disorder to a child. In each pregnancy the probability of inheriting a defective recessive gene is as follows:

- 50% from one carrier parent, resulting in a carrier child
- 25% from two carrier parents, resulting in an affected child
- 25% that no defective gene will be passed, and the child will be normal

Some defective genes for one disorder may cause additional resistance to other disorders. Sickle cell gene carriers may have increased resistance to malaria, for example.

Recessive gene disorders are often related to an enzyme defect causing toxic metabolites to accumulate. This interferes with cell function and may even cause death. PKU is an example of one of these *storage diseases* or *inborn errors of metabolism*. In PKU, toxic levels of phenylalanine may result in brain damage.

Certain genes are not entirely recessive or dominant. An *incomplete dominant* gene, such as the gene for sickle cell disease, may cause different effects. A heterozygous child may display sickle cell trait, whereas a homozygous child may have the full range of sickle cell anemia.

Albinism

Albinism is a very common genetic defect, occurring in 1 of every 38,000 White births and 1 of every 22,000 African American births. When two recessive genes are inherited, they result in a metabolic pathway deficiency related to the production of **melanin**. This brown pigment is responsible for coloration in the eyes, hair, and skin. Individuals with albinism have reduced levels of melanin, or absolutely none. An albino's skin appears pale, his or her hair is white, and the irises of the eyes are pink (**Figure 6-5**). The lack of protective melanin makes these individuals more susceptible to sunburn and skin cancer because ultraviolet light is able to cause more damage. Their eyes also must be protected from ultraviolet light to prevent blindness. The PTA should inform patients with albinism about reducing risks of cancer by protecting themselves from ultraviolet radiation and to have any suspicious lesions screened for malignancy immediately. Information may be given about using glasses and any visual aids such as large print books to minimize eyestrain.

Cystic Fibrosis

Cystic fibrosis (CF) is an autosomal recessive disease that often causes death early in life. CF changes how the sweat glands in the skin function and alters the effects of the respiratory system's mucous glands and the pancreatic ducts. When the sweat glands are defective, excessive salt is released from the body. However, the most serious symptoms affect the lungs and pancreas. Pancreatic digestive enzymes do not normally drain into the small intestine because of clogging of the ducts. Digestion is impaired, and the buildup of enzymes

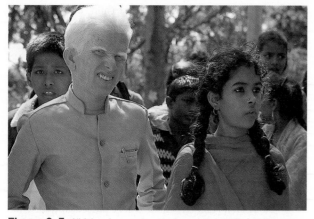

Figure 6–5 Albinism is an autosomal-recessive trait. An albino man with his wife in India.

results in cyst formation. The pancreas slowly degenerates, with fibrous tissue replacing glandular tissue.

Malnutrition is a symptom of CF because of the pancreatic effects. Patients must eat granular or powdered extracts of animal pancreases that contain digestive enzymes. Nutrients and vitamins must also be taken in large quantities to offset malnutrition caused by the digestive symptoms.

In the lungs, CF causes large amounts of mucus to be produced, blocking the respiratory passages and making breathing difficult. Several times a day patients must be treated to remove the mucus and prevent infections from trapped bacteria (**Figure 6–6**).

Unfortunately, most patients with CF only live into their late teens or early twenties. CF is a very common genetic disease, with 1 of every 22 Whites carrying a gene for CF. About 1 of every 2,000 Whites in the United States suffers from CF. However, only about 1 in 100,000 to 150,000 individuals carries the gene for the disease.

RED FLAG
It is important to make sure that early diagnosis and effective treatment for CF occur.

Treatment is focused on instructing patients, their parents, or their caregivers about slowing the progression of

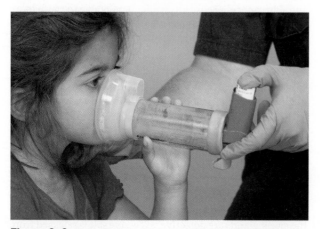

Figure 6–6 Cystic Fibrosis. Inhalants, antibiotics, and physical therapy are used to treat patients with cystic fibrosis. To remove mucus from the lungs, parents or physical therapists must treat the patient two or three times a day. Pounding on the rib cage with a cupped hand (clopping) loosens the mucus.

secondary organ dysfunction and sequelae (including chronic lung infection and pancreatic insufficiency). Treatments include antibiotics, chest percussion, postural drainage (chest physiotherapy includes the mechanical and positioning part of postural drainage), mucolytic agents, pancreatic enzyme replacement, and nutritional therapy. Patients, parents, or caregivers should be made aware of the need for routine laboratory evaluations to assess pulmonary function as well as response to therapeutic interventions.

Phenylketonuria

Phenylketonuria (PKU) is a rare metabolic disorder. It is caused by a deficiency of the liver enzyme phenylalanine hydroxylase. As toxic levels of phenylalanine accumulate, the disorder can result in mental retardation, delayed speech, microcephaly, and other symptoms of impaired neurologic development. Because symptoms develop gradually, mental retardation is often present before it is detected. Today, newborns are routinely screened for abnormal levels of serum phenylalanine.

Infants with PKU are treated with special dietary therapy. This must be started early in neonatal life (by days 7–10) to prevent brain damage. Infants with PKU should be tested weekly during the first year of life, then twice per month between ages 1 and 12, and monthly after 12 years of age. Women with PKU of childbearing age must carefully control their diet to regulate phenylalanine levels. Parents of infants with PKU should be instructed how vital diet control is to the health of these infants. Also, women with PKU must be instructed about controlling their own diet before they conceive a child and during pregnancy to protect the health of the infant.

Tay-Sachs Disease

Tay-Sachs disease is defined as a failure to break down components of cell membranes known as gangliosides. It is usually a disorder of Eastern European Jews, with about 1 of 30 being carriers. With this condition the gangliosides accumulate in the lysosomes of the brain, retina, and other organs. Over time the neurons are destroyed, affecting the cerebellum, basal ganglia, brainstem, spinal cord, and autonomic nervous system. Infants with the disease may appear normal initially but then develop muscle flaccidity, weakness, and decreased attentiveness. This usually develops between months 6 and 10 and is followed by rapid deterioration of mental and motor functions, with resultant seizures. Visual impairment and blindness often occur. Unfortunately, death usually occurs before age 5. There is no cure for Tay-Sachs disease, but tests are available to identify genetic carriers of the disease. There is no way for the PTA to assist patients with this condition, although people in the affected population should be instructed about the tests available to identify its carriers.

X-Linked Disorders

Most often, sex-linked disorders are carried by the female (X) sex chromosome. These are recessive yet manifest in heterozygous males who lack the blocking (or matching) normal gene on the Y chromosome. Females with a heterozygous pair are carriers, with no clinical signs. X-linked recessive disorders include Duchenne muscular dystrophy and hemophilia A.

Female carriers have a 50 percent chance of producing a male child who is affected with an X-linked recessive disorder. They also have a 50 percent chance of producing a female child who is a carrier. An affected male parent will transmit the defect to any female children (who become carriers), although his sons will not be affected or become carriers.

Duchenne Muscular Dystrophy

There are several types of *muscular dystrophy* (MD), which is a progressive weakening and degeneration of skeletal muscle. All types of MD are relatively rare, but the most common type is Duchenne MD, which develops soon after birth or in childhood before age 5. MD usually first attacks the shoulder, hip, thigh, and calf muscles. It may also result in various spinal deformities. The condition makes normal activities such as standing, running, or climbing stairs extremely difficult. Eventually, MD involves all skeletal muscles, resulting in immobility (**Figure 6–7**).

MD makes the patient more susceptible to pneumonia and other serious pulmonary infections, and mental impairment may occur. Duchenne MD only affects males and is caused by a genetic defect that is usually carried by the mother of the affected patient. The disease may be caused by a newly acquired mutation, as there may be no family history. There is no known successful treatment for MD, and more severe cases may cause cardiac or respiratory complications that result in death within 15 years after diagnosis.

Physical therapy is designed to provide regular range-of-motion exercises to keep joints as flexible as possible. Adequate physical therapy also helps to prevent contractures from developing, and reduces or delays the curvature of the spine. Aquatic therapy may also be helpful in maintaining range of motion in joints. Parents and caregivers must be educated about the importance of physical therapy. Occupational therapy may also be used and can include the use of wheelchairs.

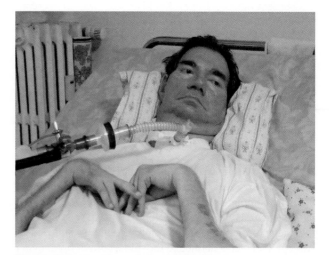

Figure 6–7 The effects of muscular dystrophy.

Areas in which bleeding usually occurs include the gastrointestinal tract and joints of the ankle, elbow, hip, or knee. In the joints this is often seen around the time the child begins to walk. Acute pain and inflammation may accompany the bleeding, and if untreated, chronic bleeding and inflammation lead to joint contractures and fibrosis. About one-third of patients experience muscle hematomas. Intracranial hemorrhage is also a rare, yet deadly, symptom.

Factor VIII replacement therapy may be helpful in reducing musculoskeletal damage. In 2003, the U.S. Food and Drug Administration approved a new recombinant factor VIII replacement product called *Advate*, which helps to keep cells viable so they can produce the factor VIII protein.

Gene replacement therapy is making advances in curing hemophilia A. Carriers can now be identified, and the condition is easier to diagnose during the prenatal stages. Amniocentesis or chorionic villus sampling is used to predict outcomes of the condition and to determine gene therapy.

Patients with hemophilia A can exercise regularly, which helps to build muscles and prevent joint problems. However, they should be instructed to avoid contact sports. Physical therapy for the hemophiliac patient should include stretching, movement exercises, and resistance training (including weight lifting). Regular exercise routines can help to prevent severe bleeding.

> **RED FLAG**
>
> The beginning physical symptoms of Duchenne MD include excessive tripping, increasing difficulty climbing stairs, and difficulty in standing. The condition can be confirmed via muscle biopsy, electromyography, or elevated serum creatine kinase levels in the blood.

Hemophilia A

Hemophilia A is one of the most common inherited bleeding disorders. It affects about 1 of every 5,000 male live births. It only rarely affects females. Hemophilia A is caused by a deficiency of *factor VIII*, encoded by the *F8 gene*, which is essential for normal blood clotting. Though usually hereditarily linked, 30 percent of new cases have no familial history, meaning this condition can arise because of a new gene mutation. When the disease is mild to moderate, bleeding usually does not occur unless a lesion or trauma is present, as seen during surgery or dental procedures. This is not usually detected during childhood. However, when the disease is severe, bleeding usually occurs in childhood spontaneously, several times a month.

Multifactorial Inheritance Disorders

Multifactorial inheritance disorders affect nearly 10 percent of the population. They may be **polygenic** in nature or because of an inherited tendency to develop a disorder after exposure to environmental factors. A combination of different factors is required, regardless of the time of occurrence (at birth or later in life). Often, family members have an increased risk of developing a certain disorder, although not every family member will contract it.

Common examples of these disorders include congenital hip dislocation, cleft palate, type 2 diabetes mellitus, congenital heart disease, hydrocephalus, and anencephaly. Multifactorial disorders are usually limited to a single, localized area of the body, with the same defect likely to recur in siblings. If the genetic tendency is determined, avoidance of causative environmental factors may minimize the risk of development of these disorders. Familial tendency for breast cancer or colon cancer are examples. Familial tendency can be determined via a family pedigree through several generations (**Figure 6–8**).

Neural Tube Defects

Neural tube defects are one of the most common birth defects. They occur in approximately 1 of 1,000 live births in the United States. A neural tube defect is defined as an opening in the spinal cord or brain that occurs very early in the development of the fetus. When the neural tube does not close completely during the third or fourth week of pregnancy, a neural tube defect develops. The two types of neural tube defects are open (which is more common) and closed. An "open" defect is defined as the spinal cord or brain being exposed outside of the body. A "closed" defect is when the opening is covered by skin.

A reduction in *neural tube defects* has been shown when folic acid is taken before conception and continued through the first trimester of pregnancy. Folic acid deficiency is related to open defects such as anencephaly and spina bifida. Anencephaly is a congenital absence of major portions of the brain and malformation of the **brainstem** (**Figure 6–9**). In this condition the **cranium** does not close and the vertebral canal remains a groove. Anencephaly can be detected early during gestation by amniocentesis or by ultrasonography.

Spina bifida is another congenital open neural tube defect in which a developmental anomaly exists in the posterior vertebral arch. This condition is relatively common. It occurs in 7 of every 10,000 live births. If the separation is wide enough, the contents of the spinal canal protrude posteriorly. A *meningomyelocele* will be evident (**Figure 6–10**), which is the most serious type of spina bifida. In this type the meninges and a portion of the spinal cord protrude through the opening in the vertebral column. This causes neurologic symptoms. Physical therapy for meningomyelocele is based on the patient's level of muscle function, joint alignments, posture, contractures,

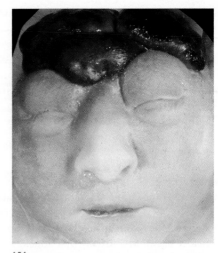

(A)

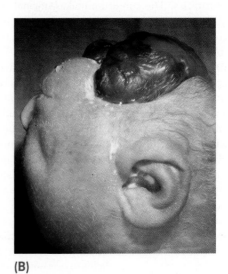

(B)

Figure 6–9 Characteristic appearance of anencephalic infant. Most of brain, top of skull, and scalp are absent. Maldevelopment of skull causes protrusion of eyes. (A) Frontal view. (B) Lateral view.

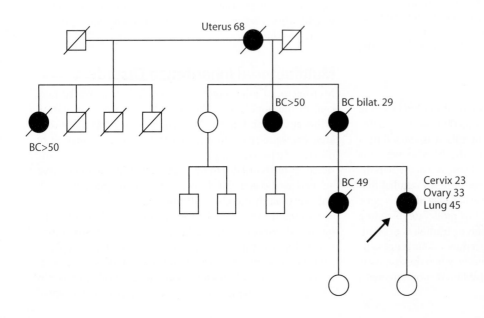

Figure 6–8 A family pedigree for an X-linked recessive trait.

Source: Reprinted from Boettger et al. BRCA1/2 mutation screening and LOH analysis of lung adenocarcinoma tissue in a multiple-cancer patient with a strong family history of breast cancer Journal of Carcinogenesis 2003 2:5.

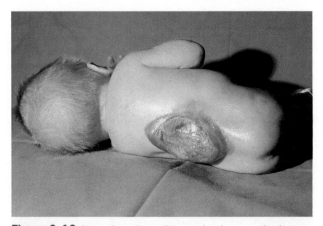

Figure 6–10 Large thoracic meningomyelocele covered only by a thin membrane. This condition is associated with neurologic disturbances resulting from incorporation of neural tissue into the wall of the sac.

and signs of progressive neurologic dysfunction. Parents of these patients should be instructed about handling and positioning techniques and the use of orthotics. Infants with the condition should be provided with activities to promote normal motor development.

Spina bifida occulta is a type of spina bifida that does not involve herniation of the meninges or the contents of the spinal canal and rarely requires treatment (**Figure 6–11**). Another type of spina bifida, *spina bifida cystica*, is a defect of the central nervous system involving a hernial cyst containing meninges (meningocele), the spinal cord (myelocele), or both (myelomeningocele). Neurologic deficits do not usually accompany the anomalies that only involve bone deformities. In spina bifida direct signs and symptoms are rarely noted

unless there is an obvious visible cyst. In adults the condition may be diagnosed accidentally during radiographic examinations given for other reasons, such as to diagnose the cause of back pain. This is generally not true in children because x-rays are commonly not done.

Folic acid plays an important role in spina bifida conditions. It is recommended that all women of childbearing age take 400 micrograms of folic acid daily, especially if they have had a previously affected pregnancy, have a close (first-family) relative with a related disorder, have diabetes mellitus, or are taking anticonvulsants. Folic acid is now added to all enriched cereal grain products. Folate-rich foods include dark, leafy green vegetables, legumes, and orange juice.

Cleft Lip and Cleft Palate

Cleft lip and cleft palate are very common birth defects, resulting in an abnormal facial appearance and speech impediments. In the United States this condition affects between 0.3 to 3.6 infants of every 1,000 live births, with Native Americans as the highest risk group. Cleft lip, with or without cleft palate, is more common among boys, whereas isolated cleft palate is twice as common in girls (**Figure 6–12**).

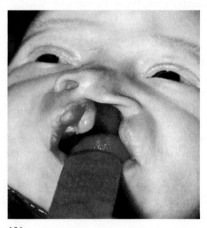

(A)

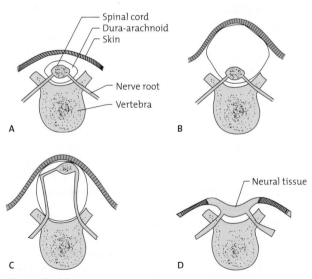

Figure 6–11 Various types of spina bifida. (A) Occult spina bifida. Failure of formation of vertebral arches. No protrusion of meninges. (B) Meningocele. Meninges protrude through defect in the vertebral arches. Cord and nerve trunks are not present in the sac. (C) Meningomyelocele. Protrusion of both meninges and nerve tissue. The spinal cord and nerve trunks are frequently incorporated into the wall of the sac. (D) Failure of the neural tube to form and separate from the surface ectoderm. The neural tissue is continuous with the adjacent skin.

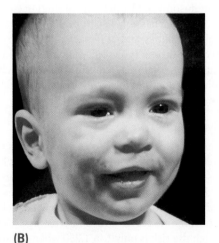

(B)

Figure 6–12 (A) Widely cleft lip and palate in a 2-week-old infant. (B) The same child at 14 months of age after surgical correction of the defect.

The defect originates around the 35th day of gestation, controlled by environmental or hereditarily linked gene disturbances. It also may be caused by teratogens and chromosomal abnormalities. These defects may be only small notches in the upper lip or may be much more severe, involving complete separation of the palate that extends to the floor of the nose. The teeth may also be deformed, missing, or excessive in number.

These conditions may take years, with many surgeries, to correct. Infants with cleft palate may require specialized feeding equipment so they can correctly suckle for feeding. With surgery, closure of the lip is usually performed by 3 months of age. Surgical closure of the palate is usually done before 1 year of age. Additional surgery, based on the severity of the condition, may be indicated later. Also, dental or orthodontic procedures may be required to correct tooth problems that have resulted.

Cleft lip and palate may cause speech defects due to the "open" malformation, which causes lack of normal control of airflow through the area. When speaking, it is usually difficult for the patient to create many consonant sounds due to the lack of sufficient pressure in the mouth. Speech therapy is usually required, which, in combination with surgery, greatly assists patients in achieving normal speech.

Chromosomal Disorders

Chromosomal disorders often occur due to an error during meiosis as DNA fragments are displaced or lost. They occur during the process of spindle formation ("crossover"). Chromosomal disorders are more common when a mother is over age 35 and may result in a chromosomal translocation, deletion, or an abnormal number of chromosomes. Down syndrome is an example of a **trisomy**, meaning there are three chromosomes instead of two at the "21" position (called *trisomy 21*). In most cases an infant with Down syndrome has 47 instead of 46 chromosomes. The disorder may be caused spontaneously or because of a specific substance.

Chromosomal disorders occur during the first trimester of pregnancy, occurring in about 7 of every 1,000 births. When only one sex chromosome (the X chromosome) is present, monosomy X (Turner's syndrome) occurs. In this syndrome the infant has only 45 chromosomes, causing many physical abnormalities and, if female, a lack of ovaries. In Klinefelter's syndrome (polysome X) an extra X chromosome results in a total of 47 chromosomes in each cell. In males with this condition the testes are usually small and no sperm are produced.

Down Syndrome

Down syndrome, also referred to as *trisomy 21*, is the most common chromosomal disorder. It occurs in about 1 of every 900 births. Nearly all cases of Down syndrome are caused by a cell division error during meiosis, which results in a trisomy of chromosome 21. The risk of having a child with Down syndrome increases with maternal age. For example, although the risk is only 1 in 1,250 when the mother is age 25, it is 1 in 100 if she is 45. A female's oocytes are of a finite amount and appear to change with the aging process.

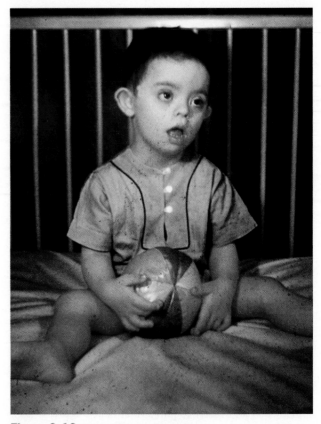

Figure 6–13 Child with Down Syndrome.

Environmental agents appear to play a part in changing or damaging oocytes.

The physical features of a child with Down syndrome are distinctive (**Figure 6–13**) and include reductions in normal body growth, a head that is smaller and "squared" in appearance, a flatter than normal facial profile, a small and depressed nose, slanted eyes, malformed ears, fatty deposits at the back of the neck, a tendency for the mouth to be opened, and the tongue to appear large and protruding. Also, the hands are usually short and stubby, with inwardly curled fingers. The space between the large and second toes is increased. In infants and young children hypotonia and joint looseness (laxity) appear. There may be gastrointestinal and heart defects. There is a 10 to 20 percent greater risk of developing leukemia in children with Down syndrome. If a patient with Down syndrome lives to senescence, there is a higher risk of developing Alzheimer's disease.

Prenatal screening tests are available to diagnose the condition. Usually, maternal serum levels of alpha-fetoprotein, human chorionic gonadotropin, unconjugated estriol, inhibin A, and pregnancy-associated plasma protein A are measured. The mother's age, along with the results of three or four tests, determine the probability of the infant having Down syndrome. Other tests may be conducted between 10 and 13 weeks gestation to verify whether the infant has the syndrome. The condition is confirmed through amniocentesis, chorionic villus sampling, or percutaneous umbilical blood sampling.

The goal of physical therapy for the child with Down syndrome is to minimize the development of compensatory movements a child is prone to develop. It is important to use physical therapy to instruct about proper posture for standing while the child is still very young. This helps the child to avoid abnormal mobility patterns. The child should also be taught the proper posture for sitting, because most children with Down syndrome naturally assume a sitting position with the trunk rounded and the head resting back on the shoulders.

Turner's Syndrome

Turner's syndrome is caused by an absence of all or part of the X chromosome. It affects about 1 of every 2,500 live births, although nearly all fetuses with the causative karyotype are spontaneously aborted. The syndrome only affects females, causing short stature (but with normal body proportions), poor breast development, infertility, lymphedema of extremities, neck "webbing," bone age retardation, heart problems, and other symptoms (**Figure 6–14**).

The syndrome may also cause kidney problems, changes in normal nail growth, lack of coordination of visual-oriented tasks, poor psychomotor skills, and attention deficit disorders. Diagnosis is often delayed until late childhood or early adolescence. Early diagnosis, however, is important so the more severe symptoms can be screened. Basically, any female with unexplained short stature, webbed neck, peripheral lymph edema, delayed puberty, or coarctation of the aorta should undergo chromosomal studies.

The syndrome is usually treated beginning in early childhood with growth hormone therapy to correct height problems. Around the normal age of puberty, estrogen may be used to promote normal development of secondary sex characteristics. For adult women with the syndrome it is important to continue to monitor their cardiovascular and other affected systems for normal health.

Klinefelter's Syndrome

Klinefelter's syndrome affects males and is described as testicular dysgenesis with the presence of one or more extra X chromosomes. Usually, there is only one extra X chromosome, although in rare cases there may be several. Additional X chromosomes are of maternal origin in two-thirds of cases, and advanced maternal age increases the risk of this syndrome developing.

Klinefelter's syndrome is one of the most common genetic abnormalities, occurring in 1 of every 500 to 1,000 live births. In many cases one additional X chromosome is undetected, whereas additional X chromosomes make the condition more detectable. Signs and symptoms include enlarged breasts, less than normal body hair, small testes, and infertility (due to lack of sperm production) (**Figure 6–15**).

This syndrome is usually not detected at birth, although at puberty the testes do not respond to normal hormonal stimulation and begin to degenerate. The lower part of the body appears longer than the upper part. As aging occurs the body may become more heavily built than normal, with a female-like distribution of subcutaneous fat and breast enlargement. The voice may not sound masculine, and facial and pubic hair growth may be sparse. There may be varying degrees of language impairment and difficulty reading and writing.

Treatment involves early detection in infancy and childhood and may include physical and speech therapy programs. Androgen therapy is often initiated when testosterone deficits are discovered, as early as 12 to 14 years of age. Men with Klinefelter's syndrome should conduct breast self-examinations regularly, because gynecomastia predisposes males to breast cancer. If the patient has a low but existent sperm count, cryopreservation of sperm should be undertaken if a future family is desired. Genetic counseling is indicated because of increased risk of autosomal and sex chromosomal abnormalities.

Physical therapy for Klinefelter's syndrome is designed to increase muscle strength and improve motor coordination. Physical therapy techniques include various exercises, stretching, electric stimulation, and massage. For infants with the condition, parents may be instructed in how to exercise the infant's muscles.

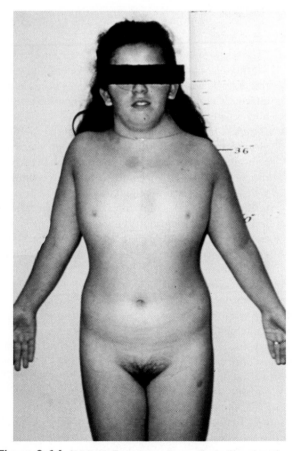

Figure 6–14 Child with Turner's syndrome, illustrating a broad neck resulting from prominent lateral skin folds, a broad chest with widely spaced nipples, and a short stature.

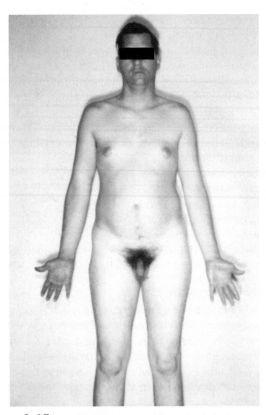

Figure 6–15 Klinefelter's syndrome. The patient's body configuration is male, although there is slight breast hypertrophy.

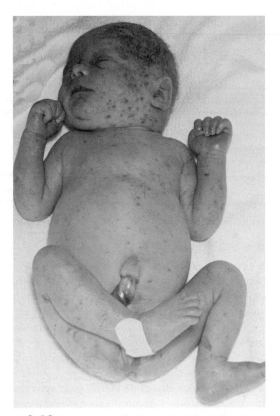

Figure 6–16 Severe systemic disease in newborn infant caused by an inapparent infection of the mother during pregnancy.

Developmental Disorders

Developmental disorders may be caused by difficult labor or delivery, premature birth, or exposure to harmful agents. They may affect many organs or only one. These disorders may be spontaneous or due to environmental factors. During the first few months of fetal development, the DNA of embryonic cells may be easily altered because of rapid mitosis and differentiation. Maternal nutrition may also play a part, such as when low folic acid levels are linked to the development of spina bifida.

Radiation, alcohol, cigarette smoking, drugs, and maternal infections may all play roles in developmental disorders. A systemic infection of the fetus that results from an unapparent infection of the mother during pregnancy illustrates the clinical features, as shown in **Figure 6–16**. Routine prenatal screening tests for high-risk maternal infections are signified by the acronym *TORCH*:

- *Toxoplasmosis*: An infectious disease caused by the one-celled protozoan parasite *Toxoplasma gondii*: This common disease is asymptomatic, with 25 percent of women in their reproductive years having antibodies to this organism. However, intrauterine *Toxoplasma* infection affects only 0.1 percent of all pregnancies.
- *Other* (hepatitis B, mumps, rubeola, gonorrhea, syphilis, varicella).
- *Rubella*: Although of high risk to the fetus during pregnancy, routine vaccination against rubella has nearly eliminated congenital rubella in the United States, with only 10 cases reported each year.

- *Cytomegalovirus*: About two-thirds of women of childbearing age in the United States have antibodies to this disease, with nearly 2 percent of newborns being affected. Cytomegalovirus is usually diagnosed by antibodies detected in urine cultures.
- *Herpes*: Intrauterine infection with the herpes simplex virus is uncommon, but neonatal infection is usually acquired as the fetus passes through the birth canal if the mother has active genital herpes. The condition is diagnosed by examination of the mother, serologic testing and culture, and the appearance of typical skin lesions in the newborn. If the mother with herpes is treated with antiviral drugs or a cesarean section delivery is performed, the newborn will not show signs of the disease.

In most cases embryonic damage occurs before the pregnancy is suspected, with most malformations being of unknown cause. The embryo dies within the first 2 weeks of embryonic life. However, the most critical time is during the first 2 months of development because the cells divide rapidly and differentiate. **Organogenesis** is also taking place, and basic body structures are forming. Damage to basic cells may have long-term effects, depending on the stage of development at the precise exposure time.

An **anomaly** is a developmental abnormality. In addition, substances such as cocaine may cause premature birth,

> **RED FLAG**
> It is recommended that women, during childbearing years, avoid exposure to all drugs, chemicals, or radiation not prescribed by their physicians.

higher risk of other illnesses, and increased likelihood of sudden infant death syndrome. An example is cerebral palsy, a type of brain damage that can occur at various times before, during, or just after birth. It may be caused by insufficient oxygen, excessive bilirubin in the blood, or trauma. Effects may be localized or in several areas of the brain.

Musculoskeletal Conditions

Musculoskeletal conditions are some of the more familiar genetic and developmental disorders. Diseases range quite widely in severity. Congenital hip dysplasia, clubfoot, spinal muscular atrophy, Legg-Calvé-Perthes disease, osteogenesis imperfecta, and arthrogryposis multiplex congenita are discussed further.

Congenital Hip Dysplasia

Congenital hip dysplasia is defined as an abnormality of the acetabulum (inner surface of the hip joint) that results in the ball (femoral head) slipping out of the normal position. It is more common in females, usually appearing during the first months of life. It usually occurs because of either improper fetal position in the uterus or the effects of maternal hormones that relax the mother's pelvic ligaments in labor. This relaxes the joint ligaments in the infant.

The condition is diagnosed because of asymmetric skin folds on the affected thigh, limited abduction (positive Ortolani's sign), and a difference in leg length. Diagnosis is confirmed by hip joint x-ray studies and physical examination (**Figure 6–17**). Treatment involves placing the femoral head in the proper position (closed reduction), maintained with a splint or cast for 2 to 3 months. Outcome is often successful, especially if treatment is done early. An older child may require surgery.

To diagnose hip dysplasia, determining the infant's position in the womb is required. During early life, hip dysplasia may be aggravated by wrapping the infant's body too tightly in a blanket or forcing the infant's legs into a closed, straight position. This places excessive stress on the hip joints.

Clubfoot

Clubfoot (talipes equinovarus) is a common congenital foot deformity. It is believed to be caused by either genetic factors or fetal position inside the uterus. Although a true clubfoot deformity cannot be corrected with manipulation, some positional deformities can be straightened by special procedures. In this condition the affected foot (or both feet) turn inward with the toes pointed downward and the heel(s) drawn upward (**Figure 6–18**). Clubfoot is diagnosed with physical examination, and x-rays are used to determine the severity of the condition.

Treatment is better if begun during infancy. A cast or splint may be applied to straighten the foot gradually, changed frequently over time until the desired position is achieved (serial casting). Surgery is indicated if these efforts fail. The PTA should instruct parents that attention must be paid to the position of the child's foot or feet throughout childhood to ensure normal positioning. There are no known preventive measures for clubfoot.

Spinal Muscular Atrophy

Spinal muscular atrophy is defined as degeneration of motor neurons that leads to wasting away of spinal muscles and weakness. The severity of this condition may be quite varied. Many types of medical care may be required, including pulmonology, neurology, orthopedic surgery, orthosis, nutritional supplementation, respiratory therapy, medications, and physical therapy or rehabilitation. Diagnosis is confirmed by genetic testing or tests conducted after birth. Physical therapy interventions may include exercise and massage. It may involve stretching, strengthening, braces, walkers, standing frames, hand splints, and wheelchairs.

Legg-Calvé-Perthes Disease

Legg-Calvé-Perthes disease is also called *coxa plana*. It is defined as ischemic necrosis that leads to flattening of the head of the femur because of vascular interruption (**Figure 6–19**). This disease mostly affects boys between ages 4 and

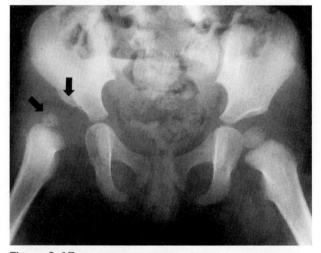

Figure 6–17 A congenital dislocation of the right hip in an 18-month-old child. Radiograph shows that right hip socket (left) is shallow, and its upper end (upper arrow) is less well developed than normal, permitting the head of the femur (lower arrow) to be displaced upward out of the hip-joint socket. The dislocated head is also less well developed than normal.

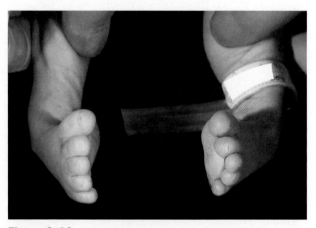

Figure 6–18 Common type of congenital clubfoot (talipes equinovarus) in newborn infant.

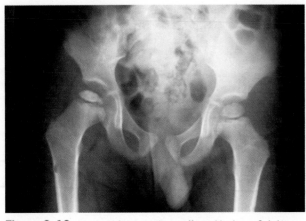

Figure 6–19 A normal femur and one affected by Legg-Calvé-Perthes disease.

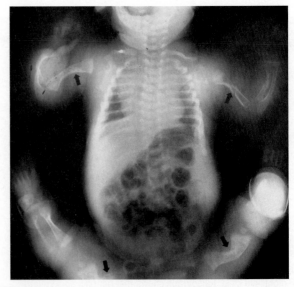

Figure 6–20 Hip spica cast.

Bilateral long leg hip spica cast

One and one-half hip spica cast

10 years and has a familial link. It is usually unilateral but may be bilateral in 20 percent of patients. Although it usually only persists for 3 to 4 years, it may lead to premature osteoarthritis due to misalignment of the acetabulum.

Legg-Calvé-Perthes disease is believed to occur due to venous obstruction with secondary intraepiphyseal thrombosis, retinacular vessel trauma, vascular irregularities, vascular occlusion due to increased intracapsular pressure, or increased blood viscosity. The disease occurs in four stages: synovitis, necrosis of the ossification center of the femoral head, revascularization, and then healing and regeneration. Residual deformity may occur based on the amount of necrosis that occurred in stage two.

The first indication of the disease is usually persistent thigh or knee pain. It is diagnosed by physical examination, recurrent x-rays every 3 to 4 months, and magnetic resonance imaging. Treatment involves several weeks of bed rest, traction, a hip splint or cast, or a leg brace. Physical therapy with passive and active range-of-motion exercises after cast removal helps to restore motion. If surgery is required, the patient must usually wear a hip spica cast for approximately 2 months. This cast immobilizes part of the entire trunk of the body and, in this case, the legs, which must remain extended (**Figure 6–20**).

Osteogenesis Imperfecta

Osteogenesis imperfecta is also called *brittle bone disease*. It is defined as thin, poorly developed bones that fracture easily. It occurs in about 1 in 30,000 people and, if inherited, is an autosomal recessive disorder. The homozygous child usually dies very near the time of birth due to multiple fractures sustained in the uterus or during delivery (**Figure 6–21**). Most forms of the disease appear related to gene mutations causing abnormal collagen structures. Signs and

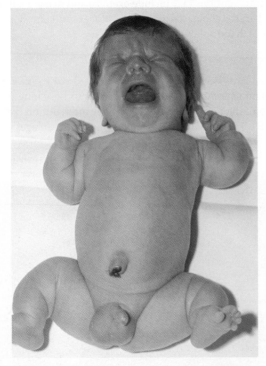

(A)

(B)

Figure 6–21 Severe form of osteogenesis imperfecta. (A) Shortening and bowing of the limbs resulting from multiple intrauterine fractures that have healed in poor alignment. (B) X-ray film showing multiple fractures of ribs and limb bones, some showing poor alignment and evidence of healing. Arrows indicate the location of four fractures.

symptoms include frequent fractures, poor healing, short stature, deformed cranial structure and limbs, thin skin, bluish-colored sclera, a visible choroid layer, abnormal tooth and enamel development, and middle ear deafness due to bone deformity.

Diagnosis involves the above signs and symptoms, elevated serum alkaline phosphatase levels, skin culture showing low quantities of fibroblasts, x-rays, and echocardiography, showing mitral insufficiency or floppy mitral valves. Treatment includes prevention of fractures with splints and supports and internal fixation of fractures, ensuring stabilization to prevent deformities.

Arthrogryposis Multiplex Congenita

Arthrogryposis multiplex congenita is a rare congenital disorder characterized by multiple joint contractures. It may also involve muscle weakness and fibrosis. The condition is non-progressive. In its most common form arthrogryposis affects the hands, wrists, elbows, shoulders, hips, feet, and knees (**Figure 6–22**). Contractures are often accompanied by muscle weakness. Quality of life can be greatly improved by physical therapy, including stretching, casting or splinting of affected joints, strengthening, and mobility training. Orthopedic correction may also be indicated. Surgery may be indicated in certain circumstances, but contractures usually recur.

Teratogenic Agents

Often, no signs that a genetic disorder is present occur at birth. They often occur months or years later. **Teratogenic** agents, which can cause embryonic or fetal damage, are usually difficult to define. Women are always advised to avoid using drugs or chemicals during their childbearing years to avoid teratogenic effects. If the risk of genetic disorders is known, parents often choose not to conceive children.

Radiation

Although diagnostic levels of radiation do not cause congenital abnormalities, heavy doses of ionizing radiation have been linked to microcephaly, mental retardation, and skeletal malformations. For safety, a woman's last day of menstruation should be recorded on all radiologic requisition forms. Some facilities require pregnancy tests before any extensive x-ray studies are conducted.

> **RED FLAG**
> Radiation is teratogenic and mutagenic (able to cause gene mutations).

Radiation can cause inheritable changes in genes and genetic materials. For example, during the 13th week of gestation administration of therapeutic radioactive iodine can interfere with thyroid development in the fetus.

Chemicals and Drugs

Although only 2 to 3 percent of developmental defects are related to drug or environmental causes, environmental chemicals and drugs can cross the placenta to damage the embryo or fetus. Documented harm has been caused by organic mercurials (substances containing mercury), often resulting in blindness or neurologic deficits. Effects of

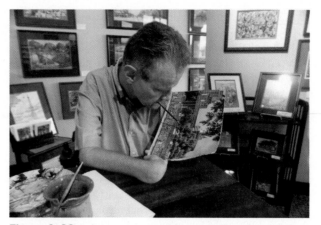

Figure 6–22 Arthrogryposis multiplex congenita.

exposure to chemicals and drugs may depend on the time of and length of exposure.

Lipid-soluble drugs usually cross the placenta more readily, entering the fetal circulation. A drug's molecular weight also plays a part, with lower molecular weight drugs crossing the placenta more easily. Proven teratogens include thalidomide, antimetabolites used to treat cancer, warfarin, certain anticonvulsants, ethyl alcohol, and cocaine. Other agents such as vitamin A have been shown to cause fetal harm. The classic example is thalidomide, which was widely used in Europe in the 1960s to treat nausea and vomiting associated with pregnancy (morning sickness) but was never marketed in the United States. The drug caused some malformation in the bones of the extremities, which were much reduced or absent. In severe cases the hands or feet arose directly from the trunk (**Figure 6–23**).

> **RED FLAG**
> The drug isotretinoin (Accutane), used to treat acne, has been proven to cause cleft palate, heart defects, eye defects, and central nervous system abnormalities.

The U.S. Food and Drug Administration created five categories of teratogenic drugs:

- Class A: Adequate human studies show no risk: *ascorbic acid, thyroid hormone, pyridoxine, liotrix, niacin, many vitamins*
- Class B: Animal studies may or may not show a risk, human studies show no risk, or there have not been adequate human studies: *acetaminophen-paracetamol, amoxicillin, cefotaxime, loperamide*

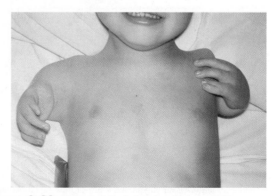

Figure 6–23 Characteristic limb deformities caused by thalidomide.

- Class C: Animal studies show a risk, and there are no adequate human studies: *diclofenac, rifampicin, theophylline, topical triamcinolone*
- Class D: Human studies have shown a risk, but there still may be a potential benefit that outweighs the risk: *paroxetine, phenytoin, tetracycline*
- Class X: All studies show a definite risk, with no outweighing potential benefits: *isotretinoin, leflunomide, thalidomide*

Fetal Alcohol Syndrome

Fetal alcohol syndrome (FAS) consists of a variety of signs and symptoms caused by maternal alcohol consumption. Between 1,000 and 6,000 infants, of 4 million born each year, will have FAS. Alcohol passes across the placental barrier, meaning the alcohol concentration is nearly the same in the fetus as in the mother.

Abnormalities caused by alcohol during pregnancy include growth retardation, neurologic abnormalities, developmental delays, behavioral dysfunction, intellectual impairment, and malformations of the skull, brain, and facial features. FAS infants often have small eye openings, a thin upper lip with a central groove, and a flattened midfacial area.

> **RED FLAG**
> The harmful effects of alcohol extend throughout an entire pregnancy.

The criteria for diagnosis of FAS include three facial abnormalities, growth deficits, and central nervous system abnormalities (including a small head circumference, a small jaw, cognitive or intellectual deficits, motor function delays, and attention problems or hyperactivity). Even small amounts of alcohol during pregnancy may be teratogenic. If used during organogenesis, many skeletal and organ defects may result. If used later in pregnancy, the defects may be only behavioral or cognitive in nature. Chronic alcohol consumption during pregnancy causes a variety of effects, usually more severe. Therefore, it is recommended that women avoid *all alcohol consumption* during conception and pregnancy.

Prenatal Screening and Diagnosis

There are diagnostic tests available to determine certain abnormalities during various times in life, but particularly in the prenatal period. When a family history of a specific disease exists, testing is recommended. Testing is also indicated for those who have given birth to a child with an abnormality and for pregnant women over age 35.

Examples of commonly screened disorders include Tay-Sachs disease and sickle cell disease. Prenatal diagnosis may play a part in deciding on the abortion of the infant or in the preparation for a lifelong dedication to specialized care. Minor or severe birth defects occur in 1 of every 28 births.

Diagnostic tools include ultrasonography, maternal blood tests, **amniocentesis (Figure 6–24)**, and chorionic villus sampling. The growing of fetal cells, along with their harvesting and examination of chromosomes or karyotype, can detect chromosomal abnormalities. Additional testing includes DNA tests, enzyme deficits, and verification of the presence of abnormal constituents. Extraction of uterine arterial blood can help to diagnose blood and metabolic disorders. A drawback to some prenatal tests is they may not show conclusive results until between 16 and 18 weeks into the pregnancy.

Neonates are often tested about 48 hours after birth via the pricking of their heels to sample capillary blood. Most

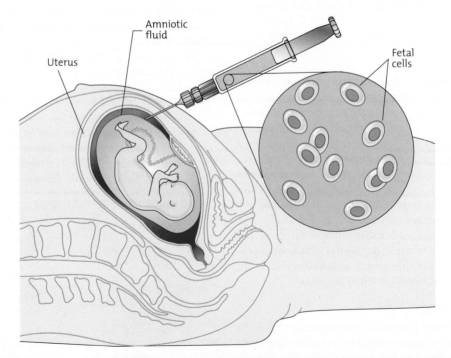

Figure 6–24 Amniocentesis. Amnionic fluid containing some free cells derived from the fetus is withdrawn. The fetal cells can be grown in tissue culture so that their karyotype and many of their metabolic functions can be determined. Studies of fetal DNA can also be performed in selected cases.

areas of the world require neonates to be tested for congenital metabolic disorders because prompt treatment can prevent mental retardation. A variety of conditions may be detected, including sickle cell anemia, congenital adrenal hyperplasia, and congenital toxoplasmosis. CF and hearing function are also commonly tested.

Gene Technology

Gene technology includes gene testing, DNA testing, genetic engineering, and gene therapy. It is a relatively new area of health care, with significant advances occurring every year.

Gene and DNA Testing

Gene testing identifies genetic disorders in both embryos and newborns. It is used via in vitro fertilization to ensure the birth of a child who will have compatible tissue to those of an older sibling who is ill with a disease such as leukemia. Stem cells from the younger sibling can then be used to save the life of the older sibling. Embryo testing has also been used to avoid serious defects in a future offspring (known as *preimplantation genetic diagnosis*).

Gene testing has also been used to identify genes that may be causes of serious future disease, including cancer. Much controversy exists regarding the ethical use of gene and DNA testing. Questions about the use of genetic information, and who has access to it, are ongoing. DNA testing is important in identifying individuals because DNA is unique to every person. Forensic scientists commonly use genetic markers in blood and other body fluids to identify suspects in criminal cases. DNA from a crime scene can tell investigators a lot about a perpetrator, including whether the individual is male or female.

Genetic Engineering and Gene Therapy

Genetic engineering describes methods of manipulating genes, which can be altered by changing a DNA sequence or even replacing a section of the sequence. Gene manipulation focuses on removing a defective gene to supply a normal one, with the goal of eliminating genetic defects. Recombinant DNA technology was an early achievement in this field. Altered DNA can produce identical molecules or *clones*. When human genes that code for hormones are transferred into bacterial cells, larger quantities of hormones can be generated (**Figure 6–25**). Other important factors that can be produced include blood-clotting factors. As a result of these techniques, there are now larger than ever supplies of hormones such as growth hormone, insulin, and oxytocin.

Genetic engineering is also used to mass produce vaccines at a lower cost. Two types of genetically engineered vaccines are produced: proteins or polypeptides that are identical to those found in the capsids of viruses and genetically modified (but inactive) viruses. There are many concerns that genetic changes that may occur during these processes could have unpredictable effects when the vaccines are administered to humans. Genetically altered viruses could exchange genetic material with live viruses, with uncertain outcomes.

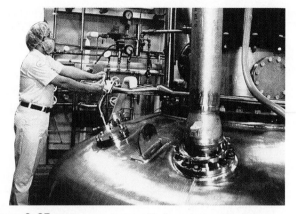

Figure 6–25 Mass producing genetically engineered bacterial products. Large vats like this one contain hundreds, sometimes thousands of gallons of culture medium and genetically modified bacteria that produce valuable proteins such as human growth hormone for treating human diseases.

The technique of inserting normal human genes into genetically defective cells to obtain a cure for a disease is known as *gene therapy*. Gene therapy promises future cures for certain diseases, including CF, Huntington's disease, and polycystic kidney. By introducing normal genes into living target cells, cell activity can be changed and missing genes can be replaced. Inserting a gene to supply a missing enzyme can help children with severe combined immunodeficiency disease.

> **RED FLAG**
> Genetic-based treatments may soon be available for cancer, mental illnesses, criminal behaviors, and substance abuse.

The major difficulty in gene therapy is getting genes into the DNA of body cells in which they are missing. A promising method is the use of bone marrow transplants. Already, tests with animals are proving highly successful. Also, the use of liposomes allows genes that are coated with antibodies for specific target cells to be delivered to the correct cells. Many other techniques are being perfected, and the future of genetic engineering and gene therapy is bright.

SUMMARY

Genetic and congenital disorders may affect single or multiple genes. Single-gene disorders may be expressed as dominant or recessive traits. In autosomal dominant disorders a single mutant allele is transmitted from one parent to the offspring regardless of sex. Autosomal recessive disorders occur only when both members of a gene pair are affected. Sex-linked disorders are associated with the X chromosome, and an unaffected mother carries one normal and one mutant allele on the X chromosome. Chromosomal disorders result from a change in the number or structure of chromosomes and include Turner's syndrome, Klinefelter's syndrome, and Down syndrome.

Developmental disorders may be caused by difficult labor or delivery, exposure to harmful agents, or premature birth. Alcohol, cigarette smoking, drugs, radiation, and maternal infections may all play roles in developmental disorders. Congenital hip dysplasia, clubfoot, spinal muscular atrophy,

Legg-Calvé-Perthes disease, osteogenesis imperfecta, and arthrogryposis multiplex congenita are examples of musculoskeletal conditions.

Teratogenic agents are those that produce abnormalities during embryonic or fetal life. They are more likely to affect the embryo in the early part of a pregnancy. Women of childbearing age should avoid taking any nonprescription or recreational drug, smoking tobacco products, or drinking alcohol. When pregnant, it is extremely dangerous to use any of these substances.

REVIEW QUESTIONS

Select the best response to each question.

1. The reason that each individual has unique identifying characteristics is that
   a. two people cannot have the same genes and DNA sequence
   b. two people may have different numbers of chromosomes
   c. two people may have abnormal genes
   d. two people may have abnormal chromosomes

2. A mutation in genetic material can be caused by
   a. certain drugs
   b. exposure to radiation
   c. spontaneous occurrences
   d. all of the above

3. Clubfoot is an example of
   a. single-gene disorders
   b. multifactorial disorders
   c. autosomal recessive disorders
   d. autosomal dominant disorders

4. Which of the following is *not* a chromosomal disorder?
   a. Cri du chat syndrome
   b. Klinefelter's syndrome
   c. Marfan's syndrome
   d. Turner's syndrome

5. A disease characterized by progressive mental deterioration and abnormal writing or "jerky" movements is called
   a. Huntington's disease
   b. Cystic fibrosis
   c. Edwards' syndrome
   d. Tay-Sachs disease

6. The most dangerous effects of Marfan's syndrome involve which of the following body systems?
   a. nervous
   b. cardiovascular
   c. urinary
   d. respiratory

7. Deficiency related to the production of melanin may result in
   a. phenylketonuria
   b. hemophilia A
   c. anencephaly
   d. albinism

8. Down syndrome is also referred to as

   a. trisomy 18
   b. trisomy 21
   c. trisomy 5
   d. none of the above

9. Enlarged breasts, small testes, infertility, and less than normal amounts of body hair are manifestations of
   a. Klinefelter's syndrome
   b. Turner's syndrome
   c. Marfan's syndrome
   d. Edwards' syndrome

10. Hemophilia A is caused by a deficiency of clotting factor number
    a. II
    b. IV
    c. V
    d. VIII

CASE STUDIES

Karen Coupe, PT, DPT, MSEd

Case 1

A 2-year-old boy was diagnosed at birth with L5 myelomeningocele. Patient medical history: developmental hip dysplasia reduced with a Pavlik harness, chiari type II malformation, and subsequent insertion of a ventriculoperitoneal shunt. This patient was referred for home physical therapy secondary to developmental delays. The parents report the primary method of mobility is through creeping. Bilateral hinged ankle-foot orthoses (AFOs) have been custom-made for ambulation activities, but the patient is not currently ambulatory. The physical therapist evaluation reveals lower extremity (LE) weakness, hypotonia, bilateral flexible calcaneovalgus. Plan of care includes static and dynamic standing activities, ambulation with bilateral hinged AFOs, and family education.

1. What is the difference between spina bifida occulta, meningocele, and myelomeningocele?

2. Why would a patient with myelomeningocele have a ventriculoperitoneal shunt?

3. At approximately what age would the sutures of the cranium fuse together? Once the cranium is fused, what signs and symptoms should alert the PTA of a shunt malfunction?

4. What would be considered a normal developmental age range for ambulation?

5. This patient has custom AFOs. Why would this patient require this orthotic?

Case 2

A 10-year-old boy with Down syndrome qualified for physical therapy and other services under Part B of the Individuals with Disabilities Education Act (IDEA). The patient underwent a spinal fusion with subsequent application of a halo vest secondary to significant atlantoaxial instability with neurologic signs and symptoms. During hospitalization the patient developed an infection that extended his stay by 1 week. Prior level of function: Independent in ambulation, transfers and bed mobility. Current level of function: Ambulation with a front-wheeled rolling walker x 6 feet secondary to fatigue and loss of balance x 3 with modx1 to recover. Individualized education program (IEP) goals include arriving to class on time with independent ambulation.

1. Explain the etiology and clinical manifestations of Down syndrome.

2. Where is the atlantoaxial joint? Was the instability a primary diagnosis or a complication of Down syndrome? Why?

3. This patient was previously independent in ambulation. What are some of the contributory factors for the current level of function with ambulation?

4. What is Part B of the IDEA? What types of services are available for eligible individuals?

5. What is an IEP? What is the PTA's role in the IEP? Do parents have a voice in the IEP?

WEBSITES

http://www.biology-online.org/3/1_genetic_control.htm

http://www.cdc.gov/ncbddd/fasd/index.html

http://www.cdc.gov/ncbddd/single_gene/x-link.htm

http://www.columbia.edu/itc/hs/medical/humandev/2004/Chpt23-Teratogens.pdf

http://www.genengnews.com/

http://www.gpnotebook.co.uk/simplepage.cfm?ID=-1818623966

http://www.marchofdimes.com/Baby/birthdefects_chromosomal.html

http://www.merck.com/mmhe/sec01/ch002/ch002d.html

http://www.nature.com/scitable/topicpage/multifactorial-inheritance-and-genetic-disease-919

http://www.ndss.org/

http://www.ninds.nih.gov/disorders/pdd/pdd.htm

http://www.reproductivegenetics.com/single_gene.html

Oncology

LEARNING OBJECTIVES

After completion of the chapter the reader should be able to

1. Contrast benign and malignant tumors.
2. List the warning signs of cancer.
3. Describe the local and systemic effects of cancer.
4. Explain common diagnostic tests.
5. Discuss metastasis and spread of malignancy.
6. Describe cancer staging.
7. List common risk factors for cancer.
8. Discuss possible treatments for malignant tumors.

KEY TERMS

Anemia: A decrease in the normal number of red blood cells or less than the normal quantity of hemoglobin.

Angiogenesis: The growth of new blood vessels from preexisting vessels.

Antineoplastic: Inhibiting or combating the development of cancer.

Atypical: Not common in form, as in the symptoms of a disease.

Biopsies: Medical tests that involve the removal of cells or tissues for examination.

Cachexia: Wasting syndrome, which includes loss of weight, muscle atrophy, fatigue, weakness, and significant loss of appetite.

Chromosomes: Organized structures of DNA and proteins found in cells.

Deoxyribonucleic acid (DNA): A nucleic acid that contains genetic instructions needed for development and normal functioning of living organisms.

Differentiation: The process by which a less specialized cell becomes a more specialized cell type.

Hematopoietic: Related to hematopoiesis, the formation of blood cellular components.

Leukemia: A cancer of the blood or bone marrow characterized by an abnormal increase of white blood cells.

Metastasis: The spread of a disease from one organ or body part to another that is not adjacent.

Micrometastases: Multiple metastases too small in size to be detected.

Mutations: Sudden changes in the nature of genes as opposed to gradual genetic changes that develop over the course of generations.

Oncology: The medical specialty that deals with tumors and cancers.

Palliative: Improving patient comfort but not treating the underlying condition.

Prognosis: A prediction of the course and outcome of a disease.

Prophylactic: Used to prevent rather than to treat or to cure.

Recurrence: The returning of a disease state.

Remission: The state of absence of disease activity in patients with a chronic illness.

Seeding: A final cancer process, wherein the disease spreads via body fluids or membranes.

Overview

Cancer is the second leading cause of death in the United States. It affects all age groups, but the risk of developing cancer increases greatly with age. Cancer is actually a collection of many different diseases, all caused by an accumulation of genetic alterations. It can originate in almost any organ, with skin cancers being the most common site in persons in the United States. Excluding skin cancers, the prostate is the most common site in men, and the breast is the most common site in women (**Table 7–1**). Environment and heredity interact, modifying the risk of developing cancer as well as the response to treatment. Increased understanding of the basic pathophysiology of cancer has contributed to the many effective therapies available today.

Benign and Malignant Tumors

A *neoplasm* is an abnormal tissue that grows by cellular proliferation more rapidly than normal. It continues to grow after the stimuli that initiated the new growth cease. A neoplasm is also called a *tumor*. This unneeded cellular growth deprives other cells of needed nutrients. Neoplasms usually have no useful function and consist of immature or **atypical** (abnormal) cells. Tumor growth depends on the cells from which the tumor develops, each with unique growth patterns and appearances. Surrounding structures are affected by pressure as a tumor expands in size.

Names of Tumors

Oncology is the study of malignant tumors, also referred to as the study of cancer. Tumors are named according to their related body system. **Table 7–2** shows tumor classifications and lists roots, suffixes, and examples of tumors. The root word specifies the cell of origin, with the suffix indicating whether it is benign or malignant and the type of tissue involved. Numerous specialized names have arisen as well, such as *leukemia*, *Hodgkin's disease*, and *Wilms' tumor*.

Characteristics of Tumors

Depending on the cell of origin, tumor characteristics differ. **Table 7–3** summarizes benign and malignant tumors.

TABLE 7–2 Tumor Classifications

Root	Suffix	Example
Adeno- (glandular tissue)	-carcinoma (malignant epithelial tissue)	Adenocarcinoma: Malignant tumor of the epithelial lining of a gland
Fibro- (fibrous tissue)	-sarcoma (malignant connective tissue)	Fibrosarcoma: Malignant tumor of the fibrous tissue
Lip- (fatty tissue)	-oma (benign)	Lipoma: Benign tumor of the fatty tissue

TABLE 7–3 Benign and Malignant Tumors

Focus Area	Benign Tumors	Malignant Tumors
Cells	Differentiated, fairly normal mitosis, similar to normal cells	Many undifferentiated, increased and atypical mitosis, varied sizes and shapes with large nuclei
Growth	Expanding mass, often encapsulated, relatively slow-growing	Cells infiltrate tissue and are not adhesive, with no capsule and rapid growth
Life-threatening potential	Only in the brain and other certain locations	Yes, due to tissue destruction and spread of tumors
Spread	Localized	Invades nearby tissues, or metastasizes to distant sites via the lymph vessels and blood
Systemic effects	Rare	Commonly present

Benign, or *nonmalignant*, tumors are often encapsulated. They expand without spreading and usually consist of differentiated cells that reproduce more quickly than normal cells (**Figure 7–1**). These tumors may damage tissues because of compression of adjacent structures. They are not considered life threatening unless in an area where increased pressure

TABLE 7–1 Common Sites of Cancer in Males and Females

Males		Females	
New Cases	**Deaths**	**New Cases**	**Deaths**
Prostate (29%)	Lung/bronchus (31%)	Breast (26%)	Lung/bronchus (26%)
Lung/bronchus (15%)	Prostate (9%)	Lung/bronchus (15%)	Breast (15%)
Colon/rectum (10%)	Colon/rectum (9%)	Colon/rectum (11%)	Colon/rectum (10%)
Urinary bladder (7%)	Pancreas (6%)	Uterine corpus (6%)	Pancreas (6%)
Non-Hodgkin's lymphoma (4%)	Leukemia (4%)	Non-Hodgkin's lymphoma (4%)	Ovary (6%)
Melanoma of the skin (4%)	Liver/intrahepatic bile duct (4%)	Melanoma of the skin (4%)	Leukemia (4%)
Kidney and renal pelvis (4%)	Esophagus (4%)	Thyroid (4%)	Non-Hodgkin's lymphoma (3%)
Leukemia (3%)	Urinary bladder (3%)	Ovary (3%)	Uterine corpus (3%)
Oral cavity/pharynx (3%)	Non-Hodgkin's lymphoma (3%)	Kidney/renal pelvis (3%)	Brain/other nervous system (2%)
Pancreas (2%)	Kidney/renal pelvis (3%)	Leukemia (3%)	Liver/intrahepatic bile duct (2%)
All other sites (19%)	All other sites (24%)	All other sites (21%)	All other sites (23%)

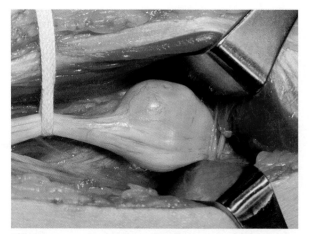

(A)

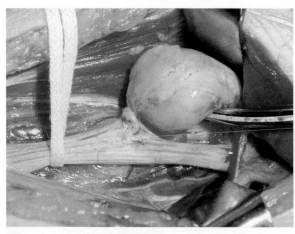

(B)

Figure 7–1 (A) Benign tumor (neuroma) arising from the sciatic nerve. (B) Tumor dissected from surrounding nerve. The cleavage plane is easily established, indicating that the tumor is sharply circumscribed and does not infiltrate the adjacent nerve.

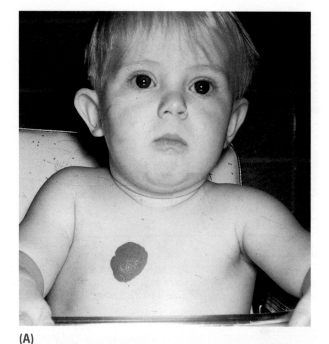

(A)

(B)

Figure 7–2 Benign blood vessel tumor (angioma) of skin. (A) Clinical appearance. (B) Histologic appearance revealing well-formed mature blood vessels (original magnification X 400).

may have serious effects, such as in the brain. A benign tumor of the blood vessels is referred to as an *angioma* (**Figure 7–2**).

Malignant tumors usually consist of nonfunctioning, undifferentiated cells that reproduce quickly. Tumor cells penetrate into surrounding tissue. They can easily break away and spread to other tissues and organs (**Figure 7–3**). This process is known as *metastasis*.

Cancer

Malignant neoplasms are commonly called cancers. Cancer affects all ages of people, but overall risk increases with age.

Pathophysiology

Tumors are usually composed of more primitive cells than other body structures. They proliferate because growth, inhibition, and cell-to-cell communications are no longer occurring normally. Expansion of a tumor compresses blood vessels, causing inflammation, increased pressure, and tissue necrosis. Tumor cells often secrete enzymes that break down proteins and normal cells. As inflammation and growth increase, organ function progressively becomes reduced.

Enlargement of a tumor deprives its inner cells of blood and nutrients, resulting in continued necrosis, inflammation, and localized infection. Certain tumor cells secrete growth factors that stimulate **angiogenesis**, promoting tumor development. Tumor cells may prevent normal cells from receiving nutrients so they cannot regenerate normal tissues.

Tumors vary widely in the speed of their growth and development. The term *in situ* refers to neoplasms that exist in a preinvasive stage of cancer that can last for months or years. When neoplasms are in situ, the possibility of early diagnosis is increased, as seen in some oral cancers and cervical cancer. Tumors are *graded* based on the amount of **differentiation** of malignant cells (G1 is well-differentiated and G4 is undifferentiated and highly malignant).

> **RED FLAG**
>
> Progression of cancer involves the mutated cell's exposure to factors that affect its growth. Promoters may be hormones (such as estrogen), food additives (such as nitrates), or drugs (such as nicotine).

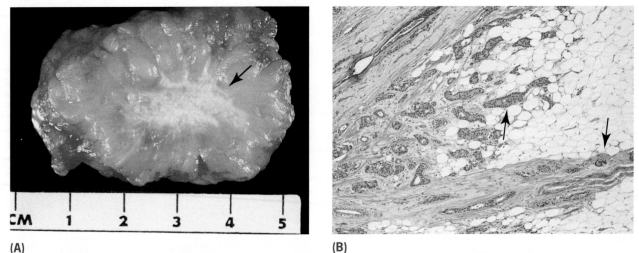

(A)   **(B)**

Figure 7–3A Breast carcinoma. (A) Breast biopsy illustrating breast carcinoma (arrow) infiltrating adjacent fatty tissue of breast. There is no distinct demarcation between tumor and normal tissue. (B) Low-magnification photograph illustrating the margin of infiltrating breast carcinoma. Small clusters of tumor cells (arrows) infiltrate adipose tissues of breast (original magnification X 20).

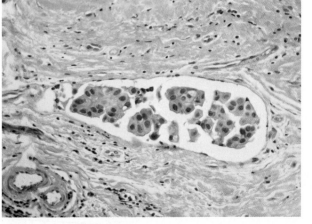
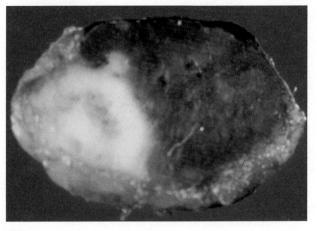

(A)   **(B)**

Figure 7–3B Lymphatic spread of carcinoma. (A) Cluster of tumor cells in lymphatic vessel (original magnification X 400). (B) Deposit of metastatic carcinoma (white mass within node) that has spread via lymphatic channels into a small regional lymph node.

Tumor grade should not be confused with the stage of a cancer. Cancer *stage* refers to the extent or severity of the cancer, based on factors such as the location of the primary tumor, tumor size, number of tumors, and lymph node involvement (spread of cancer into lymph nodes) (**Table 7–4**). It is

important to remember that staging of different types of cancers varies widely in prognoses.

Warning Signs of Cancer

It is important, as a health care professional, to understand all early indicators and warning signs of possible malignancies. It is possible to save a patient's life by critically observing and reporting warning signs of cancer. The following are nine important warning signs of cancer:

- Unusual bleeding or discharge from any area
- Changes in bowel or bladder function, such as discomfort or diarrhea
- Changes in the color, size, and shape of moles or warts
- Sores that do not heal, in any body area
- Unexplained weight loss
- Anemia or low hemoglobin

TABLE 7–4 **General Cancer Staging**

Stage	Comments
0	Precancerous state
I	Confined to the organ where it originated
II	Has invaded nearby tissues or organs
III	Has spread to lymph nodes or other tissues
IV	Has metastasized to distant locations

- Persistent fatigue
- Persistent cough or hoarseness without a real reason
- A solid, often painless lump, in any body area

These are just a few, as there are other warning signs of cancer as well. In oncology, *evidence-based practice* is used to identify, appraise, and use evidence to solve clinical problems.

Localized Effects of Tumors

Tumors have many localized effects, including pain, obstruction, tissue necrosis, and ulcerations. There is often no pain when a tumor is in its early stages. Although not always present, pain often occurs when a tumor has developed to an advanced stage. Pain may occur due to direct pressure upon sensory nerves, such as in bone cancer. If pain is dull and aching, it may be because of the stretching of a visceral capsule, such as with kidney or liver cancer. Pain may also be caused by inflammation, irritation of nerve endings by chemical mediators, infection, ischemia, and bleeding. In some malignant tumors there may be marked enlargement of the cervical lymph nodes, such as with malignant lymphoma.

When tumors compress ducts or passageways or grow inside or around body structures, *obstruction* may result. For example, an obstruction of the digestive tract leads to ulceration or edema. Obstructions often cause serious complications in all stages of their development.

If tissue necrosis or ulceration occurs, an infection may develop around the tumor. This often occurs in areas when the normal body flora can become *opportunistic*, such as in the oral cavity. Cancer often causes the host to have reduced resistance to microbial invasion.

Systemic Effects of Tumors

When malignant tumors have metastasized, systemic (general) effects may appear. These include weight loss, pain, **cachexia**, anemia, infections, bleeding, and paraneoplastic syndromes.

Weight loss and severe tissue wasting (*cachexia*) are commonly caused by many malignancies. Factors that contribute to these symptoms include anorexia, fatigue, pain, trapping of nutrients from normal cell use, stress, and altered metabolism of carbohydrates and proteins. Macrophages may produce cachetic factors in response to tumors. Cachexia leads to added fatigue, weakness, and tissue breakdown.

In the early stages of cancer pain is usually absent or mild. As cancer progresses, however, the severity of pain usually increases. It results most often from pressure or compression, obstruction, inflammation, and visceral surface stretching.

Anemia commonly results from anorexia and decreased food intake, bone marrow depression, and chronic bleeding with iron loss. It decreases the oxygen that is available to cells. This leads to poor tissue regeneration and fatigue. As host resistance declines, infections occur frequently. The immune system becomes less effective as tissue breakdown develops. Immobility contributes to lung infections because of the stoppage of normal movement of lung secretions and a reduced cough effort.

When tumor cells erode blood vessels or cause tissue ulceration, bleeding may occur. Poor clotting may be caused by bone marrow depression and hypoproteinemia. Often, chronic bleeding is seen in the digestive tract due to the slow regeneration of the mucosa, leading to iron deficiency anemia. *Paraneoplastic syndromes* are related to conditions such as *bronchogenic carcinoma* in the lungs. Hormonal-type effects may occur from substances released by tumor cells that affect blood clotting or neurologic functions. In bronchogenic carcinoma, *adrenocorticotropic hormone* may be produced, causing Cushing's syndrome, which can confuse diagnosis and complicate monitoring of the patient.

Infection is common in the patient with advanced cancer. This is particularly true with myelosuppression from treatment, direct invasion of bone marrow, the development of fistulas, or immunosuppression from hormone release in response to chronic stress.

Diagnostic Tests

Diagnostic tests, when conducted regularly and early enough in the development of cancer, can save a patient's life. Self-examination programs and routine screening tests can never be promoted enough. During treatment for cancer, as well as during follow-up treatment, frequent monitoring is required to assess treatment effectiveness and provide warnings about possible **recurrence**. Although the only 100 percent accurate test for malignant tumors is examination of tumor cells, diagnostic tests are still greatly helpful in discovering warning signs. Diagnostic tests for cancer are as follows:

> **RED FLAG**
>
> Several important characteristics of the host affect tumor growth. These include age, gender, overall health status, and immune system function.

- Blood tests: Low hemoglobin and erythrocytes are a general sign of cancer.
- Tumor marker tests: Examination of various body fluids may indicate enzymes, antigens, hormones, or other substances produced by malignant cells; these tests are commonly used to diagnose colon cancer, testicular cancer, liver cancer, ovarian cancer, prostate cancer, and certain types of leukemia. When tumor markers are found in abnormal amounts in blood, urine, or tissues, they are often (but not always) indications of the presence of cancer. They cannot be used alone to diagnose cancer but must be combined with other tests. Research about tumors is ongoing, because these tumor marker tests are not currently consistently reliable indicators of cancer.
- Radiographic and imaging tests: These include x-rays, ultrasound, magnetic resonance imaging (MRI), and computed tomography (CT) scans; these tests look for changes in tissues or organs. In some tests *radioisotopes* may be incorporated to trace metabolic pathways and functions.
- Histologic and cytologic tests: Bone marrow examination confirms certain types of cancer (such as leukemia); these tests evaluate **biopsies** of tissues, cells, and

tumors and are the most accurate methods of diagnosing cancers such as cervical and bone cancers.

Spread of Malignancy

Tumors spread in a variety of ways, producing *secondary* tumors that are identical to the parent (*primary*) tumor. Unfortunately, many cancers have already spread before being diagnosed. **Metastasis** must be diagnosed before beginning treatment. There are three basic mechanisms for the spread of malignancy:

- *Invasion*: The localized spread of tumor cells into adjacent tissue, which destroys normal cells. Tumor cells are attached loosely to other cells, secreting enzymes that break down tissue. Tumor cells often have a "crablike" image, and the origin of the word *cancer* comes from the Latin word for "crablike" (**Figure 7–4**).

- *Metastasis*: The spread of cancer from the primary tumor (**Figure 7–5**) to distant sites via the lymph or blood; tumor cells erode into a vein or lymphatic vessel, eventually traveling and lodging in another body area that is hospitable to their growth. Only a few tumor cells are required for this to occur, with regional lymph nodes often being the first site of metastasis.

  Often, lymph nodes may be removed or treated to eradicate any **micrometastases** of early-stage–metastasizing cancers such as breast cancer. Because many cancers spread via venous and lymphatic flow, the lungs and liver are common secondary tumor sites.

- **Seeding**: This final process refers to cancer that spreads via body fluids or membranes (usually in body cavities). Tumor cells break off to travel easily with fluid and tissue movements (as in ovarian cancer). Diagnostic procedures or surgery are more dangerous with this type of cancer spread because they can increase the spread of the tumor cells.

> **RED FLAG**
> Most commonly, metastasis occurs through the blood vessels and lymphatic system.

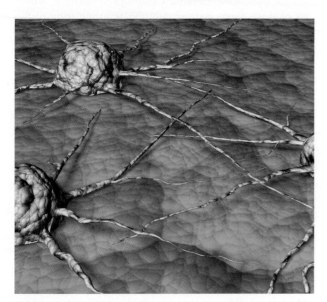

Figure 7–4 "Crablike" shape of invading tumor cells.

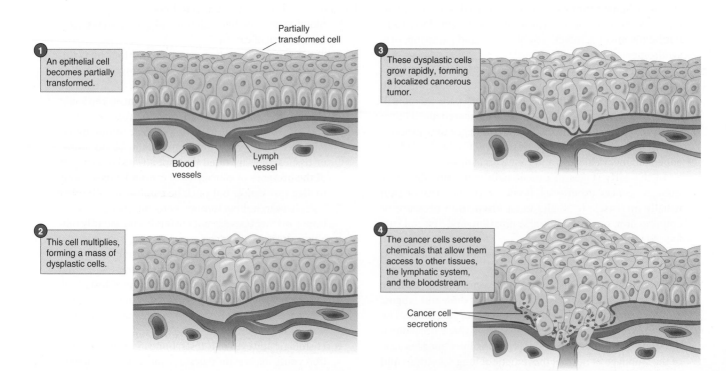

① An epithelial cell becomes partially transformed.

Partially transformed cell

Blood vessels

Lymph vessel

② This cell multiplies, forming a mass of dysplastic cells.

③ These dysplastic cells grow rapidly, forming a localized cancerous tumor.

④ The cancer cells secrete chemicals that allow them access to other tissues, the lymphatic system, and the bloodstream.

Cancer cell secretions

Figure 7–5 Cancer growth and metastasis. Cancers grow by cell division. Cells can break free from the tumor and spread in the blood and lymphatic systems to other parts of the body where they establish secondary tumors. Secondary tumors often develop in the liver, lungs, and lymph nodes.

Cancer Staging

Cancer staging is used to describe the extent of the disease and provides a basis for treatment and **prognosis**. It is applied to a specific malignant tumor when it is diagnosed and may be repeated at critical points in the disease progress. The components of cancer staging are size of the primary tumor (T), extent of regional lymph node involvement (N), and invasion or metastasis of the tumor (M). **Table 7–5** clearly explains cancer staging as it relates to breast caner. More complex subgroups for each cancer stage have been established for a wide variety of cancers.

Etiology

The etiology of cancer is based on carcinogenesis, risks and prevention methods, and host defenses. Various genes may be responsible for cell growth and replication. Those that cause cancer are called *oncogenes*. Changes in cell **deoxyribonucleic acid (DNA)** are a base cause of malignant transformation.

Viruses are capable of producing many different types of tumors, including certain types of leukemias and lymphomas. HIV can produce Kaposi's sarcoma, as seen in AIDS patients. Certain papilloma viruses may cause genital condylomas, predispose certain women to cervical carcinoma, and may cause various squamous cell carcinomas. Chronic viral hepatitis may lead to primary carcinoma in the liver. The Epstein-Barr virus, which causes mononucleosis, may lead to certain types of carcinomas and lymphomas.

Other etiologic factors include gene and chromosomal abnormalities. When genes mutate they may function differently, and altered function plays a part in the formation of tumors. *Proto-oncogenes* are normal genes that regulate some normal cellular growth but may mutate or translocate and develop derangements in functions. *Tumor suppressor genes* may mutate or become disrupted, causing unrestrained cellular growth to occur. *DNA repair genes* may become altered in structure, which increases the likelihood of DNA **mutations** in body cells.

Chromosomal abnormalities play a part in the development of certain cancers, such as leukemias. When certain components of **chromosomes** become translocated, they may fuse with different genes and form composite genes that allow for uncontrolled cellular growth.

When immunologic defenses fail, mutations and cellular growth may become uncontrolled. Evidence shows that patients with congenital immunologic deficiencies have a higher than normal incidence of tumors. This is because the body cannot identify and destroy abnormal cells as readily as when the immune system is functioning normally. Heredity also plays a role in some common tumors, including those of the breasts, colon, ovaries, or lungs.

Risk Factors

One of the most significant risk factors for cancer is advancing age, though predisposing factors influence susceptibility to the disease. Risk factors for cancer include previous cancer, lifestyle or personal behaviors such as smoking, exposure to certain viruses, exposure to certain hormones, geographic location and related environment, previous cancer treatments, gender, ethnicity, socioeconomic status, type of occupation, family history, presence of precancerous lesions or polyps, stress, and inflammatory bowel disease. More than one-third of cancer deaths in the world are related to one or more of nine modifiable risk factors: tobacco use, excessive alcohol use, inactivity, diet and nutrition, obesity, unsafe sex, urban air pollution, household fuels that cause indoor smoke, and contaminated injections.

Signs and Symptoms

Although signs and symptoms differ based on the type of cancer and its staging, there are general manifestations of the disease. These are listed in **Table 7–6**.

> **RED FLAG**
> Some cancers and precancerous lesions may result directly or indirectly from genetic predisposition.

TABLE 7-6 General Signs and Symptoms of Cancer

- Abnormal bleeding
- Anemia
- Anorexia
- Cachexia
- Coagulation disorders
- Decreased immunity
- Fever
- Gastrointestinal obstruction
- Growing lumps or masses
- Hoarseness
- Muscle wasting
- Nausea
- Pain
- Paraneoplastic syndromes
- Pulmonary obstruction
- Retching
- Secondary infections
- Stroke-like symptoms
- Tissue damage, necrosis, ulceration
- Vascular obstruction
- Visible changes in lesions
- Vomiting
- Weight loss

TABLE 7–5 Breast Cancer Staging

Stage	Size	Lymph Node Involvement	Metastasis
I	T1: tumor 2 cm or less in diameter	N0: no lymph nodes involved	M0: no metastasis
II	T0 to T2: tumor less than 5 cm in diameter	N1: nodes involved	M0: no metastasis
III	T3: tumor larger than 5 cm in diameter	N1 or N2: nodes involved, tumor may be fixed	M0: no metastasis
IV	T4: tumor any size, but fixed to chest wall or skin	N3: clavicular nodes involved (spread)	M1: metastasis present

Carcinogenesis

Carcinogenesis is the process wherein normal cells are transformed into cancer cells, developing from sequenced changes over a fairly long period of time. Either a combined group of risk factors or repeated exposure to a single risk factor may be causative. Although some cancers, such as lung cancer, have direct risk factors (such as smoking), many are less defined. Oncogenic viruses may play a role, such as the *human papillomavirus* triggering cervical cancer. Radiation exposure is linked to **leukemia**, whereas ultraviolet radiation is linked to skin cancer. There are three stages of carcinogenesis:

- Initiating factors (procarcinogens): Those that cause the first irreversible cell DNA changes, including genetic changes or exposure to environmental risks (**Figure 7–6**).
- Exposure to "promoters" (including hormones or chemicals): Causes later DNA changes, less differentiation, and increased mitosis, with possible changes in cell development. This process leads to tumor development, and promoters and prolonged time intervals complicate the establishment of cancer risk factors.
- Continued exposure and DNA changes: Result in malignant tumors.

Risks and Prevention Methods

Risks for cancer include geographic areas, ethnic background and genetics, environment, and diet. Risk factors are described in **Table 7–7**. Prevention methods for cancer include regular medical examinations, regular dental examinations, limiting sun exposure, and eating a healthy diet. High fiber intake, regular consumption of fresh fruits and vegetables, and eating foods that contain antioxidants are all recommended.

Host Defenses

Neoplastic growth is inhibited in the body by *cancer suppressor genes*. The immune system reacts to changes in tumor cell membranes, which it determines are "foreign" to the body. Cell-mediated and humoral immunity are used in the immune response. The immune surveillance and destruction of foreign or abnormal cells involves cytotoxic T lymphocytes, natural killer cells, and macrophages. Cancer risk is increased when the body is immunodeficient. Therefore, conditions that reduce immunity, such as HIV and AIDS, often lead to the development of cancers such as Kaposi's sarcoma and lymphomas. This is due to the decreased number of T lymphocytes because of the immunodeficient state.

> **RED FLAG**
>
> Research suggests that cancer cells develop continually but that the immune system recognizes these cells as foreign and destroys them.

Diagnosis

Diagnosis of cancer, as early as possible, greatly improves prognosis. Any early changes in appearance of a body structure, its function, and the way it feels may all be indicative of cancer. Examples of changes that may signify cancer include "lumps," ulcers, changes in warts or moles, bleeding, sudden changes in bowel habits, and so on. A physician should be consulted, who will first take a complete medical history and

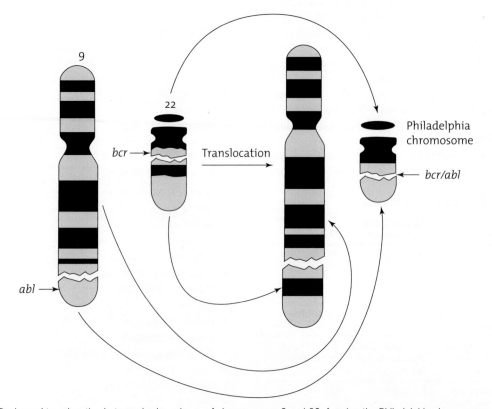

Figure 7–6   Reciprocal translocation between broken pieces of chromosomes 9 and 22, forming the Philadelphia chromosome containing the composite gene that disrupts normal cell functions.

TABLE 7–7 Risk Factors for Cancer

Risk Factors	Descriptions	Examples
Genetic factors	Oncogenes that regulate all growth	Breast cancer: high family incidence Retinoblastoma: inherited Leukemia: chromosomal abnormalities
Viruses	Oncogenic viruses alter host cell DNA	Cervical cancer: papilloma virus (HPV) or herpes simplex II Kaposi's sarcoma: HIV Hepatic cancer: hepatitis virus
Radiation	Ultraviolet rays from the sun, x-rays, gamma rays, and radioactive chemicals cause cumulative chromosomal damage in cells	Leukemia: radiation exposure Skin cancer: sun exposure
Chemicals	Exposure to both natural and synthetic products in excess may be hazardous: the effects of carcinogens depend on amount and duration of exposure	Bladder cancer: aniline dyes and rubber Leukemia: solvents such as benzene Lung cancer: asbestos, nickel
Biologic factors	Chronic irritation and inflammation with increased mitosis	Colon cancer: ulcerative colitis Oral cancer: leukoplakia
Age	Increasing	Many cancers are more common in the elderly
Diet	Natural substances, additives, or processing methods	Colon cancer: high-fat diet Gastric cancer: smoked foods
Hormones	Various	Endometrial cancer: estrogen

conduct a physical examination. This may include localized examinations based on the signs and symptoms. Common studies include rectal and colon exams, vaginal exams, Pap smears, gastrointestinal exams, and various types of x-ray studies. If a tumor is found, a biopsy or complete removal may be indicated. Histology will provide an exact diagnosis. If the tumor is malignant, additional surgery and other treatments may be needed.

As cells are shed from tumor cells, they may be seen in the blood and other body fluids. The widespread use of procedures that examine surface cells, such as the Pap smear, has allowed for much earlier detection of various cancers than ever before in history. Another procedure used for cytologic diagnosis is fine-needle aspiration. A very fine needle, attached to a syringe, is used to aspirate material from organs or tissues. Most commonly, this method is used for breast or thyroid cancer screening. Other organs for which fine-needle aspiration may be used include the lungs, liver, kidneys, and pancreas.

Sometimes, *frozen sections* of resected neoplasms are used, wherein a portion is examined after being frozen solid at subzero temperatures. Only a thin section of the frozen tissue is cut and used for the preparation of microscope slides. This method is very quick and extremely accurate. *Tumor-associated antigen tests* are another method of cancer diagnosis. Some cancers secrete *tumor-associated antigens* such as *carcinoembryonic antigen*. Other substances that may be secreted by tumor cells include *alpha-fetoprotein* and *human chorionic gonadotropin*. While these two substances are normally released in the body at various times, when they are released by tumor cells it is in much higher quantities.

> **RED FLAG**
> Because lymphangiography is invasive and may be difficult, utilizing x-rays, CT scans, and MRI have largely replaced this method.

> **RED FLAG**
> Ultrasound helps differentiate cysts from solid tumors and is commonly used to provide information about abdominal and pelvic cancer.

Treatment

Treatment for cancer includes chemotherapy, radiation, and surgery. Each type of cancer is treated with its own specified treatment regimen. For example, leukemia is treated by chemotherapy because the cancer cells are dispersed in the blood and are **hematopoietic**. Solid tumors often are removed surgically, and the patient is then treated with chemotherapy, radiation, or both depending on the sensitivity of these cells to each type of therapy.

If a tumor is small and localized, treatments often cure the condition. However, if the cancer is advanced, treatments may only be **palliative**. This type of treatment is focused on reducing the manifestations and complications of the cancer to prolong life. Patients may be made more comfortable and less symptomatic with palliative care. Types of palliative care for cancer include the following:

- Physical: Common problems include pain, nausea, fatigue, loss of appetite, shortness of breath, vomiting, and insomnia. Physical symptoms may be treated with medications, nutrition therapy, physical therapy, deep breathing techniques, chemotherapy, radiation therapy, or surgery.
- Emotional: Depression, anxiety, and fear are treated with coping methods that include counseling, support groups, family meetings, and referrals to mental health professionals.
- Practical: Concerns about finances, legalities, insurance, employment, and advance directives are handled by professionals in each of these areas for the best benefit of the patient and his or her family.
- Spiritual: Palliative care experts can discuss concerns about the disease, outcomes, reasoning, and other issues and contact spiritual and religious authorities to ease the patient and family.

Adjuvant therapy is additional **prophylactic** treatment used when a cancer is known to metastasize early. For example, after a localized breast tumor that has not spread is removed, chemotherapy and radiation are often administered to kill any cancer cells that may have broken away and traveled to a lymph node or nearby tissue. Additional treatments for cancer include nutritional counseling, physiotherapy, psychotherapy, and other methods that may last for the lifetime of the patient.

Surgery may involve removal of a tumor as well as surrounding tissue and lymph nodes. Tumor cells and their boundaries must be verified to ensure complete removal. Occasionally, removal of enough surrounding tissue can affect function of organs or other body structures. Complete tumor removal may not be possible in certain situations, although reduction in its size may help to reduce symptoms and prevent complications.

Radiation and chemotherapy are usually administered repeatedly at specific intervals to kill tumor cells but not greatly harm normal cells. Usually, not all tumor cells are destroyed in just one treatment. Therefore, tumors may grow slightly in between treatments, requiring long-term, repeated treatments.

Radiation

Radiation is used alone or in combination with other therapies. It often causes DNA alterations or mutations that kill cancer cells while not harming normal cells. Radiation also damages blood vessels that carry blood supply to tumor cells. This type of treatment is most effective on cells that are undergoing DNA mitosis or synthesis. However, some cancers are unresponsive to radiation. Also, radiation may be used before tumor surgery or 6 weeks after surgery to help ensure reduction of any remaining tumor cells.

The most serious negative effect of radiation is *bone marrow depression*. The blood cell counts of the patient must be continually monitored, with decreased leukocytes increasing the risk of infection. Because platelets are also decreased, there may be excessive bleeding. Fatigue and tissue breakdown occur because erythrocytes become reduced by radiation as well. Blood transfusions may be required, and treatment may need to be postponed until these conditions are resolved. Potentially life-threatening complications include septicemia and pneumonia.

Radiation also damages epithelial cells in the blood vessels, causing *vasculitis*, and in the skin. When the skin is damaged in this manner, it resembles the effects of a sunburn, with alopecia (hair loss) occurring. In the digestive tract the mucosa is damaged, causing nausea, vomiting, diarrhea, and possible malnutrition and dehydration. Potential inflammation and ulcerations in this tract may cause bleeding. Radiation to the head or neck may cause oral mucosa ulceration, dry mouth (xerostomia), difficulty swallowing, tooth damage, and respiration problems. When radiation is directed at the abdomen, there may be ovary or testis damage, leading to sterility or increasing the risk of teratogenesis.

Overall, radiation usually causes fatigue, lethargy, and mental depression. Long-term effects include inflammation, necrosis, and localized scar tissue. It is possible for scar tissue to cause adhesions, obstructions, and other "secondary" problems.

Chemotherapy

Different cancer cells respond uniquely to **antineoplastic** drugs. Therefore, chemotherapy is sometimes combined with surgery or radiation to treat specific tumors. Small tumors and those that reproduce most quickly are best treated with antineoplastic drugs. Most commonly, 6 weeks after tumor removal surgery, antineoplastics are begun. Often, two to four different types of antineoplastics are used at periodic intervals.

Classifications of antineoplastic drugs include antimetabolites, antimitotics, antibiotics, and alkylating agents, which interfere with DNA replication and protein synthesis. These agents work best when used at the proper times in the tumor cell cycles. Each type of cancer is matched to specific drugs so the maximum number of tumor cells is destroyed.

Bone marrow depression is the most significant adverse effect of chemotherapy because very low blood counts may require transfusions or the stopping of the treatment until the bone marrow can recover. Blood tests are taken before each treatment. Each drug causes a specific *nadir* (point of lowest cell count, referred to as *neutropenia* or *leukopenia*) at different points in the cycle. If *thrombocytopenia* occurs, hemorrhaging is a major risk. Neutropenia commonly causes infections, whereas septicemia causes gastrointestinal tract tumors. Lung cancers often cause pneumonia.

Nausea and vomiting may occur around the time of each chemotherapy treatment because these agents stimulate the emetic (vomiting) center in the brain. Vomiting may continue after treatment because the digestive tract and mucosa are often irritated by the agents that are used.

Ongoing mitosis easily damages epithelial cells, with hair loss and breakdowns of mucosa and skin being common. Oral stomatitis and diarrhea often lead to malnutrition. Oral candidal infections are often seen. Some antineoplastic drugs have very specific damaging effects such as lung fibrosis.

Other Treatments

Additional treatments for various cancers include hormones such as prednisone, which decreases mitosis and increases erythrocyte counts. Hormones usually improve appetite and the attitude of the patient while decreasing tumor-related swelling and inflammation. If tumor growth depends on hormone levels, sex hormones may be administered. For example, prostate cancer may be treated with estrogens. Hormone-blocking agents such as tamoxifen may help to reduce tumors and prevent recurrences. Newer drugs such as exemestane block the conversion of androgens to estrogens and have been used to treat postmenopausal, hormone-dependent breast cancer.

Nutrition

Advanced stages of cancer usually result in malnutrition. This may be caused by anorexia, vomiting, tooth loss, soreness in the mouth, fatigue, pain, malabsorption, altered metabolism, and nutrient trapping by tumor cells. Both the cancer itself and the effects of chemotherapy and radiation can cause malnutrition.

To treat mouth discomfort, ice and mouthwashes may be used. Smaller meals with nonirritating foods are generally preferred. They should be adequate in vitamin and protein levels. Appetite may increase when pain is controlled and antiemetic drugs are used. Total parenteral nutrition may be required, wherein nutrients are injected directly into a peripheral vein.

Prognosis

Cancer is usually considered to be "cured" when a patient has survived for 5 years without recurrence after diagnosis and treatment. **Remission** is defined as having no clinical signs of a disease. It has been documented that several periods of remission may occur before a disease becomes terminal.

Early diagnosis and treatment may be beneficial, although certain cancers involve prolonged illness with very acute episodes occurring intermittently. The prognosis for various types of cancer differs widely. Lung cancer treatment has not improved prognosis even with aggressive treatment plans. Survival rates, however, have been greatly improved for specific childhood leukemias, as well as for Hodgkin's lymphoma. Prognosis for any type of cancer depends on many different factors and the overall health of the patient before the development of the disease. **Table 7–8** lists the prognoses for various types of cancers, according to the American Cancer Society.

Screening

To help detect cancer early in its development, regular cancer *screening* is recommended. This can be performed in a variety of ways:

- Observation: External genitalia, mouth, skin
- Palpation: Breast, lymph nodes, prostate, rectum and anus, thyroid
- Laboratory tests and procedures: Pap smear, colonoscopy, mammography

Cancer screening is designed to detect early cancers or premalignancies. Ideally, it is cost effective and improves therapeutic outcomes. Most cancers are more readily curable when detected in their early stages. When a tumor is small and has not metastasized, the chance of a successful treatment is heightened. However, in certain types of cancer even a small primary tumor will metastasize early.

The unfortunate aspect of cancer screening is that for some cancers no screening methods are available (for example, pancreatic cancer). Development of screening for these types of cancer using tumor markers is ongoing. Screening or early detection is usually relatively successful for breast, cervical, colorectal, prostate, and malignant melanoma skin cancers. Screening is advised during periodic health examinations for thyroid, testicular, ovarian, lymph node, and mouth cancers.

SUMMARY

Tissue growth and repair involves cell proliferation and differentiation. Cell proliferation is the process wherein tissue acquires new or replacement cells through cell division. A new growth or neoplasm is called a tumor. Benign neoplasms are well-differentiated tumors that resemble the tissue of origin but have lost the ability to control cell proliferation. They grow by expansion and are enclosed in a fibrous capsule. Malignant neoplasms are less well-differentiated tumors that have lost the ability to control both cell proliferation and differentiation. They travel to distant sites to form metastases.

Various diagnostic tests for cancer include blood tests, tumor marker tests, radiographic and imaging tests (including CT scan and MRI), and tissue biopsy. The prognosis of cancer depends on cancer staging. Various carcinogens, genes, and viruses may be risk factors for the development of cancer. Cancer treatments include chemotherapy, radiation, and surgery. Each type of cancer requires its own specific treatment regimen. Adjuvant therapy is additional prophylactic treatment that is used when a cancer is known to metastasize early.

TABLE 7–8 Cancer Prognoses

Cancer Type	Prognosis (percentage of patients who will survive for 5 years or more)	Comments
Lung	Varies widely: 1–67%	Kills more Americans than any other type, more than 130,000 annually
Colorectal	63–70%	Kills more than 55,000 Americans annually but produces about 150,000 new cases per year
Breast	Varies widely: 14–99%	The most common type affecting women; nearly 150,000 women develop breast cancer in the United States annually, with 35% dying from the disease
Stomach	Varies widely: 15–65%	One of the more frequently diagnosed types of cancer, with nearly 10 of every 100,000 Americans dying from the disease; men are more than twice as likely than women to have stomach cancer
Prostate	Varies widely: 33–99%	The most common type of cancer in men, and second only to lung cancer in male deaths from cancer; about 30,000 American men die from it annually
Bladder	53–84%	Associated with industrial growth; new cases number 40,000 per year, with 15,000 Americans dying from this disease annually
Oral	55–90%	25,000 Americans contract oral cancers annually, and 9,000 die from the disease
Skin	Varies widely: 15–99%	The largest source of malignancy in the United States; new cases of skin cancers number 500,000 annually, with about 6,000 Americans dying from these every year
Uterine	61–86%	The most common type of reproductive system cancer
Ovarian	39–44%	The fifth most common type of cancer in women, with 21,000 new cases per year

REVIEW QUESTIONS

Select the best response to each question.

1. A sudden change in the nature of a gene as opposed to a gradual genetic change that develops over the course of generations is referred to as
   a. oncology
   b. metastasis
   c. differentiation
   d. mutation

2. A benign tumor of the fatty tissue is known as a
   a. liposarcoma
   b. lipoma
   c. lipoatrophy
   d. lipoid

3. The growth of new blood vessels from preexisting vessels is called an
   a. angioma
   b. angioid
   c. angiogenesis
   d. angioglioma

4. A cellular growth that no longer responds to normal body controls is called a
   a. papule
   b. osteoblast
   c. cytotoxin
   d. neoplasm

5. Exposure to radiation may be linked to
   a. leukemia
   b. cervical cancer
   c. breast cancer
   d. hepatic cancer

6. Tumors are graded based on the amount of
   a. risk factors related to age
   b. cell-to-cell communication
   c. differentiation of malignant cells
   d. pain they cause

7. If a malignant tumor is advanced, treatment may only be
   a. prophylactic
   b. palliative
   c. radiation
   d. surgery

8. The most serious adverse effect of radiation is
   a. oral mucosa ulceration
   b. xerostomia
   c. bone marrow depression
   d. lethargy

9. How long after a malignant tumor is removed by surgery should antineoplastic drugs be started?
   a. 2 days
   b. 2 weeks
   c. 4 weeks
   d. 6 weeks

10. Prostate cancer may be treated with which of the following hormones?
    a. estrogen
    b. growth hormone
    c. testosterone
    d. progesterone

CASE STUDIES

Karen Coupe, PT, DPT, MSEd

Case 1

A 58-year-old woman was admitted to the hospital secondary to shortness of breath and coughing up blood. Chest x-ray, bronchoscopy, mediastinoscopy, and positron emission tomography scan indicate stage IV non–small-cell lung cancer with metastasis to the brain. Patient medical history: Chronic bronchitis, chronic fatigue, 30-lb weight loss, coughing up blood, which she attributed to the bronchitis. Social history: Three pack a day smoker, employed as a desk clerk. Prior level of function: Independent in ambulation short distances (10–20 ft), patient required frequent assistance with other activities of daily living secondary to fatigue. Physical therapist evaluation reveals generalized weakness, shortness of breath, and mod assist of one w/ bed mobility, transfers, and ambulation x 5 ft. Frequent rests secondary to low O_2 saturation rates.

1. This patient is in stage IV lung cancer. What does this mean? Is it common to find lung cancer in the early stages?

2. Are there any indications in the patient's medical history that she may have had cancer? Did this patient have any contributing factors in her lifestyle?

3. What are other general indications, for anyone, to watch for that may indicate cancer?

4. Briefly describe the purpose of the diagnostic testing used to confirm the diagnosis in this case.

5. Based on lung physiology, what effects will lung cancer have on the physical therapy plan of care? How could the metastasis to the brain affect the plan of care?

Case 2

A 46-year-old man was diagnosed with a brainstem glioma, underwent radiation therapy, and is currently in remission in an inpatient rehabilitation setting. Prior level of function: Independent in all activities of daily living, mechanical engineer. Physical therapist evaluation reveals a nonambulatory patient secondary to severe ataxia, dysphagia, and generalized weakness.

1. What is a brainstem glioma? Is a patient in remission considered to be cured?

2. List all functions and/or pathways controlled by the brainstem. Based on those functions, what are some other clinical manifestations that could be possible with a brainstem lesion?

3. What are the effects of radiation on the glioma? Does the radiation have any effect on the surrounding areas?

4. Why would this patient be nonambulatory secondary to severe ataxia? What other activities of daily living would be difficult for a patient with ataxia?

5. Many patients with neurologic pathology present with dysphagia. What would be some important precautions during treatment for any patient with dysphagia?

WEBSITES

http://www.cancer.gov/cancertopics/types/alphalist/a-d

http://www.cancer.org/

http://www.newsweek.com/2009/07/22/a-death-sentence-reexamined.html

http://www.oncolink.org/treatment/

http://www.oncologystat.com/index.html

http://www.scienceclarified.com/Ti-Vi/Tumor.html

Infection, Inflammation, and Repair

Infectious Disease

LEARNING OBJECTIVES

After completion of the chapter the reader should be able to

1. Describe the basic characteristics of bacteria, viruses, chlamydiae, rickettsiae, mycoplasmas, and fungi.
2. Describe pathogens and resident (normal) flora.
3. Explain the factors contributing to pathogenicity and virulence of microbes.
4. Describe the methods of transmitting microbes.
5. Describe the stages in the development and course of an infection.
6. Explain the common diagnostic tests for infection and the purpose of each.
7. Differentiate between septicemia and bacteremia.
8. Explain the basic guidelines for the use of antimicrobial drugs.

KEY TERMS

Antiseptics: Agents that can be applied to the skin to destroy pathogens.
Autoclaving: Process of using an "autoclave," a device that combines intense pressure and high temperatures to sterilize equipment and other items.
Bacteria: Single-celled microorganisms that do not need living tissue to survive.
Culture: A substance (medium) used to grow microorganisms (usually bacteria or viruses) for the purpose of further examination or study.
Disinfectants: Agents used to destroy microorganisms or their toxins.
Endemic: Occurring only in a specific area or population of the world.
Fungi: Single-celled or multiple-celled microorganisms that can change shape and grow well in warmth or moisture.
Leukocytosis: An increase in white blood cells in the blood.
Leukopenia: A decrease in white blood cells in the blood.
Lymphadenopathy: Any disease of the lymph nodes.
Microorganisms: Organisms visible only under a microscope, including bacteria, fungi, protozoa, and viruses.
Monocytosis: Increase in the number of monocytes circulating in the blood; monocytes are important for immunity.
Mutate: Change of a microorganism, either spontaneous or because of environmental conditions or medications.

KEY TERMS CONTINUED

Neutropenia: An abnormally low number of neutrophils in the blood; neutrophils are the most important type of white blood cells.

Nosocomial: Occurring as a result of hospital (or other institutionalized) medical treatment; nosocomial infections are often caused by microorganisms becoming resistant to commonly used antimicrobial agents.

Pathogenicity: The capacity of microorganisms to cause disease.

Pathogens: Disease-causing microbes commonly called "germs" and "bugs."

Protozoa: Single-celled microorganisms that may live independently, on dead matter, or inside (or upon) living hosts.

Resident flora: Indigenous or "normal" microorganisms that live on the skin and inside most areas of the body; also called "resident microbiota."

Seizures: Symptoms of brain abnormalities that often cause convulsions; they occur because of sudden, abnormal electrical activity in the brain.

Sepsis: Presence of various pus-forming (and other) pathogenic organisms, or their toxins, in the blood or tissue.

Septicemia: An overwhelming systemic infection that may occur when pathogens circulate and reproduce in the blood; septicemia is a common type of sepsis.

Staining: Process of using a dye (e.g., Gram stain) to color cells and subcellular structures to facilitate microscopic examination.

Sterilization: Process of completely eradicating pathogens from equipment, surfaces, and so on.

Toxins: Poisonous substances (often proteins) produced by living cells or organisms; toxins are capable of causing diseases and other harm to the body.

Unicellular: Having or consisting of one cell.

Virulence: Degree of pathogenicity of a specific microorganism.

Viruses: The smallest type of microorganism; viruses must have living hosts to replicate.

Overview

Many people afflicted with a chronic or critical illness die as a result of infection. Very young and very old patients are more susceptible to infections. When sufficient quantities of microorganisms exist, the general signs and symptoms of infection become apparent.

Different types of microorganisms occur in various environments, such as the food supply, water, hospitals, and human (or animal) vectors. Hospitalized patients are often at risk for **sepsis**, which is an overwhelming infection that can become fatal. The transmission of infection may be affected by preserving the food supply, by specific areas of the world, population density, and societal waste management practices. Worldwide spread of infection has changed with the improvements in air travel, allowing for quicker transmission of infections between people of different countries.

Today, some microorganisms have been used as biological *weapons of mass destruction*, along with nuclear and chemical weapons, as tools of war and terrorism. Examples include the spreading of anthrax spores or the smallpox virus. The prevention, detection, and management of infections are the vital roles of healthcare professionals. The physical therapist assistant (PTA) must be cautious of the potential spread of infection.

Causative Infectious Diseases

Microorganisms are visible only under a microscope and include bacteria, viruses, fungi, parasites, mycoplasmas, rickettsiae, and chlamydiae. Some microorganisms are pathogenic, whereas others are either beneficial or neutral in relationship to human beings.

Pathogens are disease-causing microbes that are commonly called "germs" and "bugs." When the body is invaded by microorganisms and microbes and they multiply, infectious disease occurs. Microorganisms have different needs in order to grow, including oxygen, carbohydrates, specific temperatures, specific pH, or a living host. Each type of organism seeks its own hospitable environment.

Classes of Infectious Microorganisms

Microorganisms can be separated into eukaryotes (fungi and parasites) and prokaryotes (bacteria). Eukaryotes are organisms containing a membrane-bound nucleus, and prokaryotes are organisms in which the nucleus is not separated. Viruses, which are the smallest pathogens, have no organized cellular structure. Viruses consist of a protein coat surrounding a nucleic acid core of deoxyribonucleic acid (DNA) or ribonucleic acid (RNA).

Parasites (protozoa, helminthes, and arthropods) are members of the animal kingdom. They cause infections and disease in other animals, which then transmit them to humans. Many types of microorganisms can be grown in the laboratory by using the correct environment and a suitable **culture** medium in a test tube or Petri dish (**Figure 8–1A and B**).

> **RED FLAG**
> Unlike eukaryotes and prokaryotes, viruses are incapable of replication outside of a living cell.

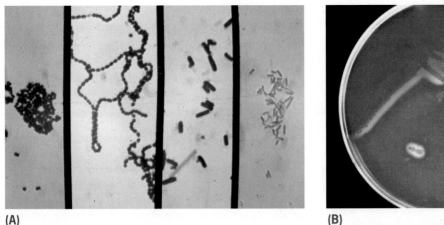

(A)   **(B)**

Figure 8–1 (A) Appearance of bacteria as seen in Gram stains. From left to right: gram-positive cocci in clusters (staphylococci), gram-positive cocci in chains (streptococci), gram-positive bacilli, gram-negative bacilli (original magnification X 1,000). (B) Bacteriologic culture plate (blood agar) containing colonies of hemolytic staphylococci. Enzymes produced by the bacteria break down (hemolyze) the blood cells in the culture medium, which causes the clear zones surrounding the colonies.

Bacteria

Bacteria are **unicellular** (single-cell) organisms. They do not need living tissue to survive. Bacteria are classified and named based on their size and shape (**Figure 8–2**). The major groups of bacteria are listed in **Table 8–1**.

Bacteria are classified as either *gram positive* or *gram negative*. Once classified, the appropriate antimicrobial medication can be chosen. Penicillin is an example of a drug that affects the cell wall of gram-positive bacteria. Because human cells do not have cell walls, but bacteria do, penicillin is able to target just the bacterial cells. Certain bacteria secrete **toxins** and enzymes. *Exotoxins* are usually produced by gram-positive bacteria and often interfere with nerve conduction (*neurotoxins*) or stimulate vomiting (*enterotoxins*).

Endotoxins are found in gram-negative organisms and are released after the bacterium dies. They may cause fever, weakness, circulatory effects, increased capillary permeability, vascular fluid loss, and endotoxic shock. *Enzymes* from bacteria may damage host tissues and cells. Other enzymes help the bacteria to invade tissue by breaking down various components.

TABLE 8–1	Major Groups of Bacteria	
Group	**Shape**	**Example**
Bacilli	Rod	*Clostridium tetani*, which causes tetanus ("lockjaw"); it survives as a spore in soil and contaminates puncture wounds, with its toxin causing seizures, muscle spasms, and respiratory failure
Spirilli	Spiral	Includes spirochetes and vibrios; *Treponema pallidum* causes syphilis and *Borrelia burgdorferi* causes Lyme disease (affecting the brain, heart, and joints)
Cocci	Spherical	*Diplococci:* pairs of bacteria (including pneumococcus, which causes pneumonia)
		Streptococci: chains of bacteria (often causing respiratory infections)
		Staphylococci: grape-like clusters of bacteria (such as *Staphylococcus aureus*, which causes skin infections)

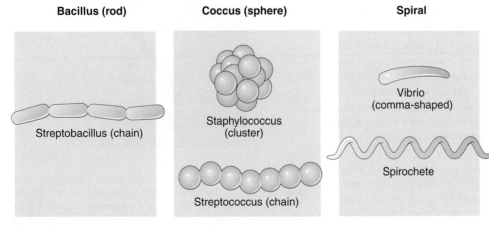

Bacillus (rod)   **Coccus (sphere)**   **Spiral**

Streptobacillus (chain)

Staphylococcus (cluster)

Streptococcus (chain)

Vibrio (comma-shaped)

Spirochete

Figure 8–2 Variations in bacterial shape and cell arrangements.

Certain bacteria form *spores* (*endospores*) that are very resistant to heat and adverse conditions. Spores can survive for a long time but must resume a bacterial vegetative state to reproduce. Examples of infections caused by bacterial spores are tetanus and botulism. Bacteria duplicate via *binary fission*, wherein two daughter cells are produced by division of the parent bacterium. These daughter cells are identical to the original bacterium. Binary fission may occur over only a few minutes or over many hours. Bacterial colonies may be damaged and destroyed by lack of nutrients or oxygen, high metabolic wastes, pH changes, and temperature changes.

Rickettsiae

Rickettsiae are gram-negative, bacteria-like organisms that can cause life-threatening illnesses. They may be coccoid, rod shaped, or irregularly shaped. Rickettsiae are similar to viruses in that they require a host cell for replication. They have no cell walls and weak cell membranes that easily leak. Therefore, they must live inside another cell that has better protection. Rickettsiae are transmitted by the bites of arthropods such as fleas, lice, and ticks or through exposure to the waste products of these organisms. These organisms are sensitive to some antibiotics, including tetracycline and chloramphenicol.

> **RED FLAG**
> Rocky Mountain spotted fever, Q fever, and typhus are examples of rickettsial infections.

Mycoplasmas

Mycoplasmas are bacteria-like organisms and the smallest of the cellular microbes that can live outside of a host cell. Some mycoplasmas may be parasitic. Lacking cell walls, they may assume a variety of shapes, ranging from coccoid to filamentous. Because they have no cell wall, mycoplasmas are resistant to penicillin and other antibiotics that work by inhibiting cell wall synthesis. Mycoplasmas can cause primary atypical pneumonia and many secondary infections. They respond to the antibiotics tetracycline and erythromycin.

Chlamydiae

Chlamydiae are smaller than rickettsiae and bacteria but larger than viruses. They require host cells for replication and are susceptible to antibiotics. Chlamydiae are transmitted by direct contact, such as during sexual activity. Chlamydia is called a "silent disease" because of the lack of symptoms. Chlamydiae are a common cause of infections of the bladder, urethra, fallopian tubes, and prostate gland. Chlamydiae are inhibited by antibiotics that inhibit protein synthesis (for example, erythromycin and tetracycline) as well as certain sulfonamide drugs.

> **RED FLAG**
> Annually, there are more than 40 million patients diagnosed with chlamydia in the United States, making it the most common sexually transmitted disease.

Several different types of diseases are caused by chlamydiae. Most commonly, chlamydial disease affects the genital tract. The disease may be spread by a pregnant mother to her fetus, causing *inclusion conjunctivitis*. Other resultant conditions include pulmonary infections and lymphatic-related inflammatory conditions of the groin and rectum.

Viruses

Viruses are very different from the other microbial groups. They are so small that most viruses can be seen only with an electron microscope. Viruses are acellular (not cellular). They are intracellular parasites that must have living hosts to replicate. Structurally, viruses are very simple. A virus particle contains a core made of only one type of nucleic acid, either DNA or RNA. This core is surrounded by a protein coat (**Figure 8–3A, B, and C**). Viruses exist in many types and subtypes, as shown in **Table 8–2**.

Viruses cause infection by attaching to host cells and using their genetic material to enter and take over the cells. The host cell's metabolism is used to synthesize protein and begin producing new components of viral cells. A *bacteriophage* is any one of a number of viruses that infect bacteria.

Viruses that cause the common cold and influenza frequently *mutate* (change slightly during replication), making it difficult for the host's immune system to develop adequate immunity against them. This is why both the common cold and seasonal influenza are not curable. Because viruses lack their own metabolic processes, drugs are generally less effective against them than bacteria. When an intracellular virus alters a

> **RED FLAG**
> Cervical cancer is directly linked to four different types of the human papillomavirus (HPV).

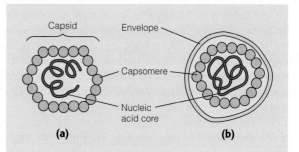

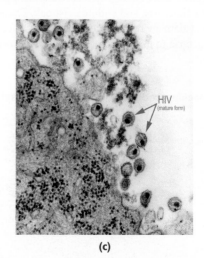

Figure 8–3 General structure of a virus. (A) The virus consists of a nucleic acid core of either RNA or DNA. Surrounding the viral core is a layer of protein known as the capsid. Each protein molecule in the capsid is known as a capsomere. (B) Some viruses have an additional protective coat known as the envelope. (C) Electron micrograph of the human immunodeficiency virus (HIV).

TABLE 8–2 Viruses and Disease

Virus	Disease	RNA or DNA
Flaviviruses	RNA	West Nile virus, encephalitis
Hepadnaviruses	DNA	Hepatitis B virus
Herpesvirus	DNA	Herpes simplex, infectious mono-nucleosis, varicella (chickenpox)
Orthomyxoviruses	RNA	Influenza A, B, C
Papovaviruses	DNA	Warts, cancer (human papillomavirus [HPV])
Paramyxoviruses	RNA	Mumps, measles
Picornaviruses	RNA	Poliovirus, hepatitis A virus
Retrovirus	RNA	Human immunodeficiency viruses
Togavirus	RNA	Rubella virus (German measles), hepatitis C virus

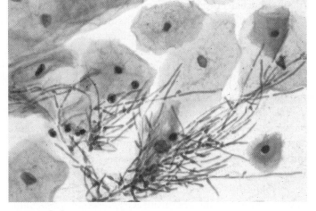

Figure 8–5 A cluster of hyphae in a vaginal smear from a patient with a vaginal infection caused by *Candida albicans* (original magnification X 400).

host cell's chromosomes, malignant cells (cancer) may develop.

Fungi

Fungi are found on almost every type of living organism as well as on dead organic material. There are five basic classes of fungi, based on how they reproduce and their structural appearance. These five classes include: chytridiomycota, zygomycota, glomeromycota, ascomycota, and basidiomycota. Infections result from single-celled yeasts or multicellular molds (similar to mycotic infections). Fungi are made up of either single cells or chains of cells that can assume different structural shapes (**Figure 8–4**). Fungi grow well in warmth and moisture, and "good" fungi are important in yogurt, beer, other foods, and as antibiotic sources.

Fungi have long filaments or strands called *hyphae* (**Figure 8–5**). These intertwine to form a visible mass (*mycelium*). Fungi reproduce either by budding, by extension of their hyphae, or by producing spores that spread easily through the air. Most fungi are not pathogenic. Examples of superficial fungal infections include *tinea pedis* (athlete's foot) and various *Candida* infections (thrush, vaginal infections; **Figure 8–6A and B**). Acute pulmonary infections caused by fungi commonly subside spontaneously and do not require treatment. Chronic systemic fungal infections must be treated with various antifungal medications.

Histoplasma capsulatum is the organism that causes *histoplasmosis* via the inhalation of dust that contains spores of the

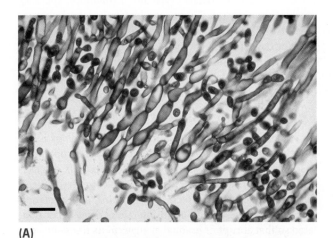

(A)

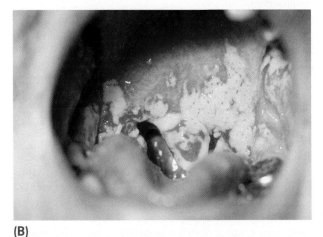

(B)

Figure 8–6 The agent of oral thrush. (A) A photomicrograph of stained *Candida albicans* cells (bar 40 μm). (B) Oral thrush.

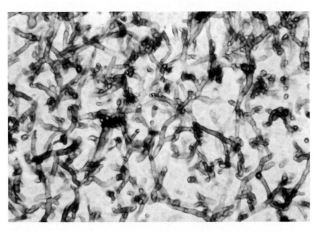

Figure 8–4 A low-magnification photomicrograph illustrating cluster of fungus hyphae (original magnification X 160).

fungus. It usually produces an acute respiratory infection but may cause a chronic infection that is similar to tuberculosis. Also, a related fatal form of histoplasmosis may develop. The disease *coccidioidomycosis* is caused by another fungus, *Coccidioides immitis*, found in the southwestern United States. This condition is also spread by inhalation of dust containing fungus spores and has similar symptoms.

The disease *blastomycosis* is caused by *Blastomyces dermatitidis*. It is similar to the above conditions, usually acute and self-limited, but may become a more chronic pulmonary infection or widespread systemic disease. Another important fungal condition, *cryptococcosis*, is caused by *Cryptococcus neoformans*. It is also found in soil and caused by inhalation of dust containing the organisms. *Cryptococcus neoformans* is yeast-like, with a large mucoid capsule, and can be transported in the bloodstream to the meninges of the brain, leading to chronic meningitis. Identification of the organisms is via spinal fluid smears and cultures.

Protozoa

Protozoa are more complex organisms than fungi and may live in a variety of ways. These unicellular organisms may live independently, on dead organic matter, or inside (or upon) living hosts. There are also a number of subcategories of protozoa. Primarily parasitic, protozoans may cause infections such as malaria (via the *Plasmodium* species), amebic dysentery (via *Entamoeba histolytica*), or trichomoniasis (via *Trichomonas vaginalis*). Some protozoans move by using flagellum or portions of their cytoplasm. The active, reproducing form of a protozoan (the *trophozoite*) adheres to intestinal mucosa and uses enzymes to spread and invade blood vessels and tissues.

Epidemiology of Infectious Diseases

As related to infection and immunity, *epidemiology* is the study of circumstances that influence how infectious diseases are transmitted among humans. Infectious diseases are classified based on incidence, portal of entry, source, disease course, site of infection, symptoms, and virulence. The expected frequency of an infectious disease is calculated so that abrupt or gradual changes in its frequency can be observed.

Infections have the potential to spread from a single infected individual to become a worldwide pandemic. Some areas of the world experience **endemic** infections (those that occur only in that specific area). Prevention and control of infections depends on knowledge of how they are transmitted, the microorganisms involved, and how they may be controlled and reduced in number.

Resident Flora

Indigenous, or "normal," flora is also known as *resident microbiota* or **resident flora**. This consists of microorganisms (primarily bacteria) that live on the skin and inside most areas of the body. For example, in the upper respiratory tract *streptococci*, *Hemophilus*, and *staphylococci* are commonly found. In most cases resident flora is completely harmless and usually helps the body to maintain its normal states. The areas of the body that are normally sterile (free from microorganisms)

are the blood, cerebrospinal fluid, lungs, stomach, uterus, fallopian tubes, ovaries, bladder, and kidneys.

In the intestinal tract resident flora is important for the synthesis of vitamin K and for normal digestion. However, resident flora from these areas may cause infections if it is transferred to other areas of the body. An *opportunistic infection* may occur when the body's defenses are impaired or the balance among species of resident flora is disrupted. Sometimes, antibacterial drugs intended to treat a specific infection will destroy some of the normal flora in another area, causing a different infection to occur.

Transmission

When an infection is transmitted, a *chain of events* occurs (**Figure 8–7**). These events are collectively called the "chain of infection." The source of infection (reservoir) may be either a person with an obvious, acute infection or one with no signs or symptoms. A person may be incubating an early stage of infection or be a lifetime carrier who never actually develops symptoms but still may transmit the infection to others. Often, hepatitis B is transmitted in this manner. Other sources of infection may also be animals or contaminated equipment, food, soil, or water. The mode of transmission from the reservoir to the new host is explained in **Table 8–3**.

The hands are a major route of transmission of many infections. Improper or inadequate hand washing spreads infections from many sources, in all environments. In healthcare facilities **nosocomial** infections may occur. These infections are due to the presence of many microorganisms because of sick patients in these settings. It is not uncommon for a patient undergoing a simple hospital or outpatient surgery to develop a serious systemic infection due to infected equipment, droplet transmission, food trays, or improper procedures. Common nosocomial infections include urinary tract infections, diarrhea, pneumonia, and surgical wound infection. *Clostridium difficile* is an example of a common nosocomial infection in intensive care units that is flourishing because of the use of antimicrobial drugs (which disrupt the body's normal flora).

Resistance

A host's resistance level is important in keeping infections from developing, especially with infections such as tuberculosis. Host resistance is maintained through the following measures:

- Intact skin and mucous membranes
- Body secretions such as tears and stomach acid
- Nonspecific phagocytosis
- Effective inflammatory response
- Lack of disease
- Effective immune system
- Production of interferons against viruses

Resistance may be lowered by increased microbial virulence, which includes production of exotoxins, endotoxins, and destructive enzymes. Other factors include the formation of spores, entry of many microorganisms into the body, and the presence of bacterial capsules and pili. *Interferons* are proteins made by human host cells when viruses invade.

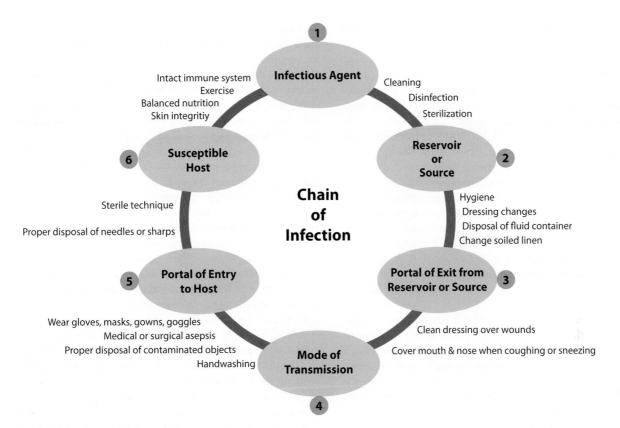

Figure 8–7 Transmission of infectious agents (chain of infection).

TABLE 8-3 Mode of Transmission

Contact	Mode	Example
Direct	Touching an infectious lesion, sexual intercourse, contact with body fluids, crossing the placental barrier to the fetus	*Treponema pallidum*, which causes syphilis and fetal defects or death; *Toxoplasma gondii*, which causes toxoplasmosis and neurologic deficits
Indirect	Via contaminated body part, contaminated food, or a fomite (inanimate object such as bed linens, which carry organisms)	Food poisoning, *Salmonella*, *E. coli*, *Giardia*, roundworm, *Enterovirus*
Droplet	Oral or respiratory; pathogens are expelled from the body and inhaled into or contacted by others	Legionnaire's disease, various skin infections, tuberculosis
Vector-borne	When an insect or animal transmits an infection	Malaria, Lyme disease, encephalitis, West Nile virus

They increase the resistance of nearby host cells to the viral invasion and interfere with viral replication, stimulating the immune system. Factors that decrease host resistance are as follows:

- Age, usually affecting the very young and very old
- Genetic predisposition
- Any type of immunodeficiency
- Malnutrition
- Chronic diseases such as cardiovascular disease, diabetes, and cancer
- Severe emotional or physical stress
- Damage to the skin or mucosa, invasive procedures
- Poor inflammatory response, often due to long-term use of glucocorticoids

In lower socioeconomic classes host resistance is commonly lowered because of open lesions, poor nutrition, fatigue, inadequate hygiene, lack of medical care, and drug or alcohol abuse. Antimicrobial medications may be indicated in patients with poor host resistance before any invasive procedures being performed.

Pathogenicity

Pathogenicity is defined as the capacity of microorganisms to cause disease. Even nonpathogens can become pathogens, such as when resident flora invades another part of the body in which it is not normally found. **Virulence** is defined as the degree of pathogenicity of a specific microorganism. This is based on its ability to invade and damage host cells and tissues; its ability to produce toxins; its ability to adhere to tissue via pili, fimbriae, or specific membrane receptor sites; and its ability to avoid host defenses. The latter may occur because organisms regularly **mutate**. These mutations may occur spontaneously or because of environmental conditions or medications. Once mutated, these organisms may not be susceptible to treatments that did affect them in their original form. Host resistance and the ability of a microorganism to cause a disease are delicately balanced.

Current Trends

There are many cases of "new" diseases and causative microorganisms that do not appear to respond to existing medications. As the world gets "smaller" because of the ease of international travel, the ability of the populace to carry and spread diseases from one area of the globe to another increases. Current trends in disease development are monitored and reported on by the Centers for Disease Control and Prevention, the World Health Organization, and even the United Nations. Recent outbreaks have included *severe acute respiratory syndrome*, or *SARS*, the *Ebola* virus, certain strains of *Escherichia coli*, "flesh-eating bacteria," and H_1N_1 *influenza* (previously called *Swine flu*). Today, common nosocomial infections also include *methicillin-resistant* Staphylococcus aureus *(MRSA)*, *vancomycin-resistant enterococcus*, and *Clostridium difficile*.

Many of these infections are highly virulent, causing relatively rapid morbidity and mortality, and appear to be on the increase. No apparent reason for this has been ascertained. It also appears that some vaccines are losing their effectiveness over time. For example, *whooping cough*, nearly eradicated, is on the rise once again. Multidrug-resistant microorganisms include strains of *Mycobacterium tuberculosis, Hemophilus influenzae, Streptococcus pneumoniae, Neisseria gonorrheae*, and *Staphylococcus aureus*. Health monitoring organizations emphasize that the use of antibacterial drugs for minor infections or as prophylactics should be reduced to lower multidrug resistance.

Development of Infection

Breaking the chain of infection is more important than ever in controlling its development. The development of infection may be slowed by using *universal precautions*, wherein all blood, body fluids, and wastes are considered "infected." Gloves and appropriate personal protective equipment (PPE) must be used to avoid contact with pathogens and infected materials.

> **RED FLAG**
>
> Disposal of needles, tissues, equipment, and wastes must follow the guidelines of federal and state regulatory agencies.

The development of infection may be minimized by locating and removing the reservoir or sources of infection. This can be accomplished by identifying contaminated food or water or food handlers who may be carriers. Also, infected travelers should postpone their travel to avoid spreading infections. The portal of exit of microorganisms must be blocked. This means that secretions such as blood, saliva, and urine must be kept from reaching uninfected persons. For each type of infection it is important to understand the modes of transmission to correctly block them. Surroundings and clothing should be regularly cleaned, and **sterilization** such as **autoclaving** should be used. **Disinfectants** should be used to destroy microorganisms or their toxins, and **antiseptics** may be applied to the skin to destroy pathogens without causing harm.

Before any clinical signs become apparent, microorganisms must enter the body, find a site to establish a colony, and begin reproduction. The infection becomes established if the host defenses are insufficient to combat the pathogenic microorganisms. The *incubation period* is the time between entry into the body and the appearance of clinical signs of infection. For most infections this period may last for as little time as a few days up to several months.

The next period is the *prodromal period*, wherein the patient feels fatigued, loses the appetite, and experiences other signs of illness. The *acute period* is when the infection is fully developed and symptoms are at their worst. *Onset* of a specific infection may be prolonged and subtle (referred to as *insidious*) or sudden and acute. The length of the acute period is based on the pathogen's virulence and the host's resistance. The acute period begins to subside either when the immune response becomes effective or if the pathogens are weakened by lack of nutrients or other factors.

Some infections can become *chronic* when microorganisms remain in the body, causing recurrent periodic acute episodes. Follow-up tests should be undertaken to ensure that all microorganisms have been eradicated. Chronic infections can cause serious damage to body tissues. An overwhelming systemic infection (**septicemia**) may occur when pathogens circulate and reproduce in the blood. When all body systems experience infection, the patient's life may be threatened. *Bacteremia* occurs when pathogens enter and circulate in the blood in smaller numbers for a short time. Occasionally, these circulating pathogens may lodge in an organ and cause a more serious infection. An example is when pathogens attack the heart's valves when they have been damaged previously by rheumatic fever or another condition. A serious infection within the heart may then occur.

Standard Precautions

Methods that may be implemented to minimize risk of exposure to employees, patients, and other individuals are referred to as *standard precautions*:

- Hand hygiene
- Standards for the handling of *sharps*
- Standards for cleaning up spills
- Standards for disinfection and disposal of equipment
- Standards for handling soiled linens
- Standards for cleaning up the facility
- Use of *personal protective equipment*

It is the role of the PTA to ensure that all universal and standard precautions are followed to minimize the chances of disease transmission.

Personal Protective Equipment

PPE is used for the protection of the skin and mucous membranes. It creates a barrier between blood or bodily fluids and employees of a healthcare facility. To minimize risk of exposure, *barrier precautions* such as gloves are used. Ideally, PPE protects workers from all pathogenic microorganisms. PPE includes gloves, laboratory coats, face shields, goggles, gowns, and masks (**Figure 8–8**).

After use, soiled PPE should be left in special storage areas at the work site (often inside or close to a patient's room). To

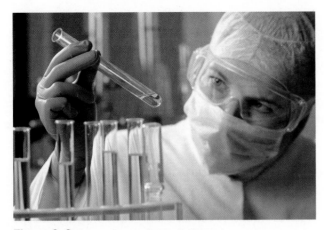

Figure 8–8 Personal protective equipment.

protect against contact with blood, bodily fluids, or chemical substances, specially designed face shields, goggles, and masks are used. Because of the potential of splashing or splattering with these various fluid substances, eyewash stations are required by law for all facilities wherein this may accidentally occur (**Figure 8–9**).

Employees can use eyewash stations to flush out their eyes or mucous membranes with water as soon as possible after

RED FLAG
After eye washing the employee should (usually) be taken to the emergency room at a local hospital. This depends on the policy of the facility involved.

exposure occurs. A minimum of 15 minutes is recommended for rinsing of eyes and mucous membranes. After contact with a potentially harmful substance, contact lenses should be removed before eye washing.
The employee should not rub the eyes, which may cause further irritation and absorption of the harmful substance.

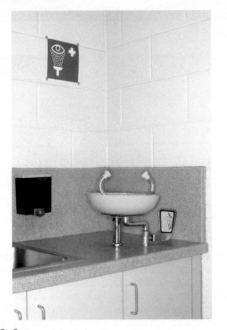

Figure 8–9 Eye wash station.

Airborne Precautions

Airborne precautions are used when a patient has, or may have, an infectious disease that may be spread by the airborne route. Airborne precautions are used in addition to standard precautions. They require a *negative pressure room* in addition to a private room. This prevents airflow from the patient's room into corridors and other areas where people may be exposed to the infectious disease. Special fans, vents, and HEPA filters are used to maintain negative pressure in the patient's room. The following diseases are characterized as requiring airborne precautions:

- Tuberculosis
- Varicella (chickenpox): also requires contact precautions
- Herpes zoster (shingles): also requires contact precautions
- Rubeola (measles)

Droplet Precautions

Droplet precautions are designed to reduce the risk of droplet transmission of infectious agents. Droplet transmission involves contact with large particle droplets that likely contain pathogenic microorganisms from an infected patient. These droplets usually are emitted from the nose, mouth, or conjunctivae. They may be generated because of talking, sneezing, coughing, suctioning, and bronchoscopy. Droplet transmission requires contact between a susceptible individual and the infected patient within a distance of 3 feet. Because of the size of these droplets, they do not remain airborne (hence the difference between droplet and airborne transmission). To avoid exposure via droplet transmission, it is advisable to wear a mask when entering the patient's vicinity. The following diseases are commonly transmitted via droplet transmission:

- The common cold
- Diphtheria: also by contact transmission
- Influenza
- Meningitis
- Mycoplasma
- Mumps
- Pertussis (whooping cough)
- Plague
- Rubella
- Strep (including strep throat, scarlet fever, pneumonia)

Contact Precautions

Contact precautions are "barriers" that stop the transmission of infection by physical contact. Contact transmission requires physical touching to transmit an infection. Contact can be between two people or between a person and an animal. An object that becomes contaminated by touch is referred to as a *fomite*. Although most microorganisms have to enter the mouth, nose, or eyes to cause an infection, others can be spread simply by skin-to-skin contact. *Skin-to-skin transmission* occurs when bacteria, viruses, or parasites on the skin are transferred to the skin of another. Breaks in the skin make transmission more likely. Diseases commonly transmitted by physical contact include the following:

- Abscesses
- Athlete's foot

- Cold sores
- Conjunctivitis ("pink eye")
- Croup
- Infectious diarrhea
- Cutaneous diphtheria
- Ebola
- Herpes zoster (shingles)
- Impetigo
- Lice
- Respiratory syncytial virus
- Ringworm
- Scabies
- Varicella (chickenpox)

Because physical therapy usually involves direct contact with patients, the PTA must use proper PPE at all times to reduce the likelihood of disease transmission. For example, if the PTA has a cold, equipment must be worn to prevent droplet as well as contact transmission, because accidentally coughing, sneezing, or touching the patient has the potential to transmit the infection.

> **RED FLAG**
> Hand washing is the most important step in preventing infectious disease.

Signs and Symptoms

When an infection develops, local signs and symptoms usually include inflammation, pain or tenderness, redness, swelling, and warmth. If an infection is caused by bacteria, *pus* (purulent exudate) is often present (**Table 8–4**). Additionally, there may be tissue necrosis and **lymphadenopathy** at the site of infection. Viral infections usually cause serous exudates (fluids that have escaped from blood vessels and leaked into tissues or their surfaces). The color and characteristics of pus or serous exudates help to identify the causative microorganism.

When an infection is systemic, signs and symptoms as listed above in Table 8–4 may affect any part of the body. Body temperature may be very high and also accompanied by chills or may only show a slight elevation. It may even be below normal.

> **RED FLAG**
> The nervous system may be affected by a systemic infection, resulting in **seizures**, confusion, disorientation, and loss of consciousness.

Diagnostic Tests

Diagnostic tests used to identify the type of infection include *culture* and **staining** techniques. Samples may be taken of sputum, blood, and other body fluids. Certain organisms can be grown on culture media in the laboratory, whereas others require a living host. A drug sensitivity test is one in which the growth of

microorganisms on a culture plate is measured in the presence of a variety of different drugs (**Figure 8–10A and B**).

Regardless of the type of infection, it is important to establish the most effective medical treatment as soon as possible, because any test requiring a culture takes several days to complete. Blood tests are mostly used to check for variations in the amounts of leukocytes. Bacterial infections usually cause **leukocytosis** (an increase in white blood cells in the blood). Viral infections usually cause **leukopenia** (a decrease in white blood cells in the blood). Changes in amounts of different types of leukocytes occur based on the causative microorganism, for example, **monocytosis** or **neutropenia**.

Acute infections usually cause neutrophils to increase, whereas chronic infections usually cause lymphocytes and monocytes to increase. Blood tests can also reveal antibodies to confirm diagnosis of different types of infections (mostly viral infections). *Radiologic* examinations may be used to identify the infection site and the causative microorganisms. The role of the PTA includes knowledge of how to review diagnostic tests and how to determine treatments that are based on test results.

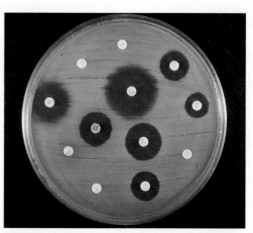

(A)

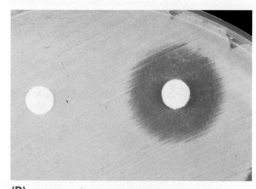

(B)

Figure 8–10 (A) Sensitivity test, illustrating antibiotic-impregnated filter paper disks on surface of culture plate. The clear zone around disk indicates that the antibiotic in the disk has inhibited bacterial growth. (B) Closer view of two disks on plate. The antibiotic contained in the disk on the left fails to inhibit growth of organism, which is resistant to antibiotic. The clear zone around antibiotic on the right indicates that the antibiotic in the disk inhibits the growth of the organism, which is sensitive to the antibiotic.

TABLE 8–4 Signs of Bacterial Infection	
Local	**Systemic**
Erythema (redness)	Elevated erythrocyte sedimentation rate
Lymphadenopathy	Fatigue, weakness, anorexia
Pain and tenderness	Fever
Purulent exudate (pus)	Headache, arthralgia
Swelling	Leukocytosis

Treatments

Because the human body can often combat many infections without needing antimicrobial drugs, and because many infections use up nutrients and create wastes that limit their development naturally, it is hoped that the use of antimicrobial drugs can be reduced. The increased use of these drugs has resulted in resistance and reduced the opportunities for infected patients to develop antibodies. *Drug resistance* due to bacteria adapting their metabolism to block drug action has developed. Bacteria can block drug action by producing certain enzymes, altering their cell membranes, and changing in other ways.

Antimicrobials may also be administered as prophylactics in immunosuppressed patients before invasive procedures. For acute infections they may be administered in a *loading dose* (a larger dose administered initially to achieve effective blood levels more quickly). **Table 8–5** explains the guidelines for effective antimicrobial therapy.

Antiviral agents do not destroy viruses. They inhibit viral reproduction and provide an opportunity for host defenses to remove the virus. Antibiotics are effective against bacteria but not against viruses. These agents block synthesis of bacterial cells walls or interfere with bacterial metabolism. Because viruses do not have cell walls or metabolism, antibiotics do not work against them. However, in certain viral infections antibiotics may be given to reduce risk of secondary bacterial infections. **Table 8–6** details the classifications of antimicrobial agents.

Most antibacterial agents work in one of these four ways:

- Interfering with bacterial cell wall synthesis (e.g., penicillin)
- Increasing permeability of the bacterial cell membrane to allow leakage of cell contents (e.g., polymyxin)
- Interfering with protein synthesis and reproduction (e.g., tetracycline)
- Interfering with synthesis of essential metabolites (e.g., sulfonamides)

TABLE 8–6 Classifications of Antimicrobial Agents

Type	Definition
Antibiotic	An older term meaning a drug derived from an organism (such as penicillin, which is derived from a mold); many antimicrobial drugs today are synthetic instead
Antibacterial	The current term used to describe a drug that attacks bacterial growth
Antiviral	A drug that inhibits the replication of a virus so the body's immune response can combat it
Antifungal	A drug that kills fungi by interfering with mitosis or increasing fungal membrane permeability
Bactericidal	A drug that destroys bacterial organisms
Bacteriostatic	A drug that decreases the rate of bacterial reproduction, allowing the host's defenses to destroy the organisms
Broad spectrum	An antibacterial agent that is effective against both gram-negative and gram-positive organisms
Narrow spectrum	An antibacterial agent that acts against either gram-negative or gram-positive organisms but not both
First generation	An antimicrobial agent that is from an original drug class
Second generation	An antimicrobial agent that is from a later, improved version of an original drug class

Common adverse reactions of antimicrobial agents include digestive tract discomfort and allergic reactions. Antiviral drugs often have significant adverse effects because they alter viral interaction inside host cells. Antifungal agents are mostly administered topically to skin or mucous membranes.

Immunotherapy

Immunotherapy involves the supplementation or stimulation of a host's immune response to limit or reverse the spread of a pathogen. Substances used for immunotherapy include cytokines and intravenous immune globulin. Cytokines are produced by human white blood cells to stimulate white cell replication, antibody production, and phagocytosis. Intravenous immune globulin uses antibodies obtained from normal, healthy immune donors that are infused as an intravenous solution.

The basic principle of immunotherapy is using pathogen-specific antibodies to neutralize, phagocytize, and remove infectious agents. It is predicted that therapies based on regulating the human inflammatory response will become more widely used in the coming years. Proper, timely immunizations also are important in immunotherapy and have greatly reduced the spread of disease such as measles, mumps, pertussis, and rubella. It is believed that in the not too distant future immunizations will become available to effectively treat HIV, hepatitis C, malaria, and many other serious diseases.

TABLE 8–5 Antimicrobial Drug Therapy

Action	Effect
The drug should be taken at regular, evenly spaced intervals over 24 h.	To maintain blood levels that are adequate to control and destroy microorganisms
It should be taken until completely used (usually 5–10 days) even if symptoms have subsided.	To ensure the infection is completely eradicated and to prevent development of resistant microorganisms
Directions should be followed with respect to administration along with food or fluid intake.	To ensure the drug is not inactivated or impaired regarding its absorption
The specific causative microorganism must be identified.	To ensure the most effective antibiotic can be chosen that has the least effect on resident flora and body tissues
A complete drug history must be obtained.	To ensure the patient doesn't receive a drug that may potentially cause a serious allergic reaction

Surgical Intervention

Surgical intervention, before the development of antimicrobial agents, was sometimes the only option to save the lives of patients with serious infections. Today, when pathogens are resistant to antimicrobial agents, surgery is still used. Examples of surgical procedures related to infections include the draining of abscesses, debridement (cleaning infected sites), and removal of infected organs (such as the appendix). Sometimes, an infected part of an organ (such as one of the heart valves) is indicated. In endocarditis, an infected heart valve may be removed and replaced by an artificial or transplanted valve. For cases of gas gangrene, surgical amputations may be required to stop the spread of disease and save the life of the patient.

SUMMARY

Pathogenic microorganisms cause infections. Bacteria are single-cell organisms enclosed inside cell walls and sometimes having an outer capsule. Viruses are intracellular parasites requiring living host cells for reproduction. Fungi may cause infection in lower numbers than bacteria or viruses because only a few fungi are pathogenic. Resident or normal flora refers to nonpathogenic microbes normally present in and on the body. The degree of a specific pathogen's virulence determines the severity of the resulting infection.

Pathogens may be transmitted by direct or indirect contact. The infection cycle may be broken by reducing the reservoir, blocking transmission, or increasing host resistance. Universal precautions must be taken with all individuals to reduce transmission of infection. Signs of infection are not apparent until sufficient amounts of microorganisms are established and reproduced in the body. Infection may be eradicated without drug treatment. Antibacterial drugs are classified by their activity and mechanism.

REVIEW QUESTIONS

Select the best response to each question.

1. Bacteria that are permanent and beneficial residents in the human body are called
   a. parasites
   b. pathogens
   c. hosts
   d. normal flora
2. The smallest organisms of all are known as
   a. chlamydiae
   b. viruses
   c. rickettsiae
   d. bacteria
3. Which of the following microorganisms appear in grape-like clusters?
   a. Staphylococci
   b. Spirochetes
   c. Streptococci
   d. *Neisseria gonorrheae*
4. If a virus has a bacterial host, it is called
   a. an obligate anaerobe
   b. a bacteriophage
   c. bacteriostatic
   d. bactericidal
5. Spiral-shaped bacteria are called
   a. cocci
   b. diplococci
   c. spirilla
   d. bacilli
6. A substance that inhibits the growth of bacteria is said to be
   a. sterile
   b. anaerobic
   c. bactericidal
   d. bacteriostatic
7. The degree to which an organism is pathogenic is known as
   a. resistance
   b. virulence
   c. pathogenicity
   d. toxicity
8. Which of the following is the reason that drugs are generally less effective against viruses than bacteria?
   a. Viruses lack their own metabolic processes
   b. Viruses are smaller
   c. Viruses are unable to reproduce
   d. Viruses are anaerobic
9. Bacterial infections usually cause
   a. leukopenia
   b. leukopia
   c. leukocytosis
   d. leukemia
10. A larger dose of antibiotics administered initially to achieve effective blood levels more quickly is called a
    a. maintenance dose
    b. ceiling dose
    c. starting dose
    d. loading dose

CASE STUDIES

Karen Coupe, PT, DPT, MSEd

Case 1

A PTA is working in a skilled nursing facility. The facility treats a wide variety of geriatric patients whose diagnoses range from cerebrovascular accident to total hip replacement. In addition, many of these patient's have multiple system disorders such as chronic obstructive pulmonary disease, congestive heart failure, diabetes, thyroid issues, hypertension, and PVD. Over the past 2 weeks over one-half of the patients have demonstrated signs and symptoms of *C. difficile*.

1. What is *C. difficile*? What is the transmission method?
2. Why would some of the patients in this facility have a lower resistance to any potential infection?
3. Which of the following terms could be used in relation to this outbreak: endemic, epidemic, nosocomial, iatrogenic, or idiopathic?
4. Although there are many ways to prevent transmission of disease, what is the most important method that all healthcare workers should use before, sometimes during, and after patient contact? Research the Centers for Disease Control and Prevention website and explain the preferred method for this procedure.

5. When working with patients with *C. difficile*, what other precautions would the PTA use to prevent transmission?

Case 2

A PTA is working in an outpatient department and is going to treat a 42-year-old man with a diagnosis of chronic right adhesive capsulitis. Patient medical history: Active integumentary MRSA with numerous boils on the right upper extremity, some with drainage. The patient does not have any protective covering over the boils, although he admits the physician instructed him to do so. The patient's wife is present and expresses her fear of getting MRSA. The PT plan of care includes joint mobilization by the PT followed by the PTA stretching and strengthening the right shoulder.

1. What is MRSA? What is the method of transmission?
2. What should the PTA have the patient do before working with the patient?
3. When working with this patient what precautions would the PTA use to prevent transmission?
4. Based on how the patient presents with open areas, what educational material could the PTA provide for this patient?

5. What educational material could the PTA provide for the patient's wife?

WEBSITES

http://library.thinkquest.org/CR0212089/micr.htm

http://microbiology.suite101.com/article.cfm/
    normal_flora_and_opportunistic_pathogens

http://www.cdc.gov/ncidod/EID/vol11no10/05-1014.htm

http://www.healthhype.com/microorganisms-types
    -harmful-effects-on-human-body-pictures.html

http://www.hhs.gov/pandemicflu/plan/sup4.html

http://www.medterms.com/script/main/art
    .asp?articlekey=12321

http://www.merck.com/mmhe/sec17/ch188/ch188c.html

http://www.symptom-diagnosis.com/infection-symptoms

http://www.uptodate.com/patients/content/topic
    .do?topicKey=~IZjIr4TcdeiLv/

http://www.who.int/whr/2007/07_chap3_en.pdf

Inflammation and Healing

LEARNING OBJECTIVES

After completion of the chapter the reader should be able to

1. Describe the purpose of inflammation.
2. List the five main signs of acute inflammation and describe the physiologic mechanisms involved in their production.
3. Differentiate between acute and chronic inflammation.
4. List four types of inflammatory mediators and state their function.
5. Name and describe the five types of inflammatory exudates.
6. Explain the components of "RICE" therapy for inflammation.
7. Describe tissue repair.
8. Describe the phases of wound healing.

KEY TERMS

Abscess: A localized pocket of pus in a solid tissue.
Acute: Of rapid onset and relatively short duration.
Adhesions: Bands of scar tissue that join two surfaces that are normally separated.

Anorexia: Lack or loss of appetite for food.
Blister: A small pocket of fluid within the upper skin layers.
Chemical mediators: Substances released as part of the inflammatory response that bring about vascular and cellular changes (e.g., histamine).
Chemotaxis: Movement based on specific chemical factors affecting a cell or organism.
Chronic: Of slow onset and relatively long duration.
Collagen: The protein portion of the white, shiny, nonelastic fibers of the skin, tendons, bone, cartilage, and all other types of connective tissue.
Contractures: Shortenings of specific structures.
Diapedesis: Outward passage of red or white blood cells through the intact walls of the capillaries.
Erythrocyte sedimentation rate (ESR): Rate at which red blood cells precipitate within 1 hour; an ESR test provides a nonspecific measurement of inflammation.
Exudate: Fluid, cells, or other substances that slowly escape from blood vessels and are deposited on tissues or tissue surfaces.
Fibrinogen: A soluble plasma glycoprotein formed in the liver that is converted (by thrombin) into fibrin during blood coagulation.
Fibrinous: Inflammation resulting in a large increase in vascular permeability that allows fibrin to pass through the blood vessels.
Fibroblasts: Cells that synthesize the extracellular matrix and collagen and play an important role in wound healing.
Fracture callus: A temporary formation of fibroblasts and chondroblasts at the site of a bone fracture as the bone attempts to heal itself.
Granulation tissue: Perfused, fibrous connective tissue that replaces the fibrin clot in wounds that are healing.

KEY TERMS CONTINUED

Granuloma: A roughly spherical mass of immune cells that forms when the immune system perceives substances that are foreign and not able to be eliminated.

Hemorrhagic: Related to bleeding, or bloody in appearance.

Hyperemia: Increase of blood flow to different body tissues.

Infection: Colonization of a host organism by a foreign microorganism.

Inflammation: A normal body defense mechanism that localizes and removes harmful agents signified by swelling, redness, heat, pain, and occasional loss of function.

Interferons: Blood proteins that have antiviral effects.

Isoenzymes: Enzymes that differ in amino acid sequence but catalyze the same chemical reaction.

Leukocytes: White blood cells; they defend the body against infectious disease and foreign materials and include five types: neutrophils, eosinophils, basophils, lymphocytes, and monocytes.

Macrophages: Large phagocytic cells produced in the bone marrow that are initially released from the marrow as monocytes. Macrophages are widely distributed throughout the body and may lodge in the walls of blood vessels or in connective tissue.

Malaise: A feeling of general discomfort or uneasiness.

Neutrophils: The most abundant type of leukocytes;

after trauma, they move quickly to the area as part of the acute inflammatory response.

Parenchymal cells: A type of cells that are functional elements of organs, such as the hepatocytes.

Perforation: A complete penetration of the wall of a hollow organ.

Permeability: The capacity of a blood vessel to allow ions, water, nutrients, or cells to move in and out of the vessel.

Phagocytosis: Cell eating; the engulfing of solid particles by a cellular membrane.

Purulent: Containing pus, which is a white, yellow, green, or brown exudate produced by dead and/or living cells that travel into intercellular spaces around infected cells.

Pyrexia: Fever, which may be mild or severe.

Pyrogens: Substances that induce a fever.

Regeneration: The regrowth of tissue so that normal function returns.

Scar: An area of fibrous tissue that replaces normal skin or other tissue after injury or disease.

Serous: Watery in appearance; resembling or producing serum.

Stenosis: Narrowing of structures such as tubes or ducts.

Ulcers: Sores or lesions that result from erosion to areas of organs or tissues.

Vasodilation: Widening of blood vessels.

Overview

Inflammation is a natural response on the part of the body to injury or infection. In the inflammatory process the body attempts to isolate an affected area to prevent injury or infection from spreading to other locations. The process of inflammation allows the body to repair damaged tissues and the immune response to heal the wound. Inflammation is a protective response that attempts to eliminate initial causes of cell injury and necrotic cells and tissues that result from that injury. This process occurs in tissues with blood vessels from biochemical and cellular involvement.

Most components of the inflammatory process are found in the circulatory system. Most early mediators (facilitators) of inflammation increase the movement of plasma and blood cells from the circulation into the tissues surrounding an injury. The collective term for such fluids is **exudate**. These fluids defend the host against infection and facilitate tissue repair and healing.

Physiologic Mechanisms of Inflammation

The body protects itself against injury in either specific or nonspecific ways, which include the skin, mucous membranes,

body secretions, cellular activities, and immune defenses. The first line of defense is the mechanical barrier created by the skin and mucous membranes, which block bacteria and harmful substances from entering the body tissues. Also, body secretions such as saliva and tears containing enzymes and other chemicals help to destroy foreign materials.

The second line of defense includes **phagocytosis** and **inflammation**. Phagocytosis involves **neutrophils** (one of the **leukocytes**) and **macrophages**, which engulf and destroy bacteria, cell debris, and foreign matter. Inflammation involves events that limit the effects of injury or foreign agents. Nonspecific agents that protect uninfected cells against viruses are known as **interferons**. The third line of defense is the immune system, which stimulates production of unique antibodies or sensitized lymphocytes after exposure to specific foreign substances.

Classifications of Inflammation

Inflammation is the reaction of vascularized tissue to local injury. It is a normal body defense mechanism that localizes and removes agents that are harmful to the body. Signs and symptoms of

RED FLAG

Localized infections produce a rapid inflammatory response with obvious signs and symptoms.

inflammation are actually warning signs of a problem in or on the body and should not be confused with **infection**. Inflammation can be caused by microorganisms that cause infection but also by cuts, allergic reactions, insect bites, sprains, ischemia, cell necrosis, infarction, caustic agents, splinters, dirt, and burns. It is signified by redness, heat, swelling, pain, and, sometimes, loss of function. Swelling occurs because of the leakage of plasma from the dilated and more permeable vessels. This causes the volume of fluid in the inflamed tissue to increase (**Figure 9–1**).

Acute Inflammation

Inflammation can develop immediately and last for a short time or have a delayed onset and last for a more severe, prolonged time. Tissue injury causes the damaged mast cells and platelets to release **chemical mediators** (histamine, serotonin, prostaglandins, leukotrienes, and others) into the interstitial fluid and blood (**Table 9–1**). It is nonspecific and may result from any injury.

> **RED FLAG**
> Serotonin is a vasoconstrictor mediator of inflammation released from platelets.

Histamine and certain other chemical mediators are released immediately from granules in mast cells for immediate effect. Others must be synthesized from arachidonic in mast cells before release. Many anti-inflammatory drugs and antihistamines reduce these chemical mediators' effects.

> **RED FLAG**
> Prostaglandin is a complex derivative of a fatty acid (prostanoic acid) that has widespread physiologic effects.

The rapid release of chemical mediators results in local **vasodilation**, which causes **hyperemia**. Capillary membrane **permeability** increases to allow plasma proteins to shift into the interstitial spaces along with more fluid. This fluid dilutes toxic materials, whereas globulins act as antibodies, and fibrinogen forms a fibrin mesh to localize the harmful agent. Vasodilation and increased capillary permeability constitute the "vascular response" to injury.

During the "cellular response" leukocytes are attracted via **chemotaxis** to the area of inflammation, acting like magnets

TABLE 9–1 Chemical Mediators and Inflammation

Chemical	Major Action	Source
Chemotactic factors	Attract neutrophils to site	Mast cell granules
Complement system	Vasodilation and increased capillary permeability, chemotaxis, increased histamine release	Activation of plasma protein cascade
Cytokines (interleukins, lymphokines)	Increasing of plasma proteins and erythrocyte sedimentation rate, induction of fever, chemotaxis, and leukocytosis	T lymphocytes and macrophages
Histamine	Immediate vasodilation and increased capillary permeability to form exudate	Mast cell granules
Kinins (such as bradykinin)	Vasodilation and increased capillary permeability, pain, and chemotaxis	Activation of plasma protein (kinogen)
Leukotrienes	Later response: vasodilation, increased capillary permeability, and chemotaxis	Synthesis from arachidonic acid in mast cells
Platelet-activating factor	Activation of neutrophils and platelet aggregation	Cell membranes of platelets
Prostaglandins	Vasodilation, increased capillary permeability, pain, fever, and potentiation of histamine effect	Synthesis from arachidonic acid in mast cells

for damaged cells. Neutrophils and then monocytes and macrophages collect along capillary walls to move through wider separations in the walls to the interstitial areas (**diapedesis**). **Figure 9–2** illustrates leukocytes adherent to capillary

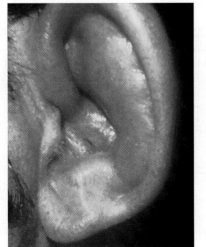

Figure 9–1 Marked swelling of ear caused by acute inflammation.

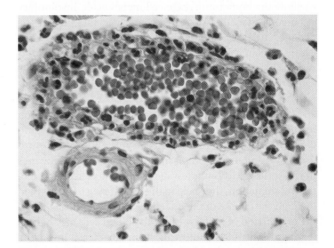

Figure 9–2 Photomicrograph illustrating leukocytes adherent to capillary endothelium and migrating through wall to site of tissue injury (original magnification X 160).

endothelium that migrate through vessel walls to sites of tissue injury. They destroy and remove foreign material, cell debris, and microorganisms via phagocytosis.

The functions of cellular elements in the inflammatory response are explained in **Table 9–2**.

When excessive fluid and protein collects in the interstitial compartment, blood flow in the area decreases. The fluid shifting out of the capillaries is reduced. Naturally occurring defense or control mechanisms in the body inactivate chemical mediators to prevent spreading or prolonging of inflammation. Redness and warmth are caused by increased blood flow to the damaged area. Swelling (edema) is caused by the shift of protein and fluid into the interstitial space. Pain is caused by the increased pressure of the fluid on the nerves as well as irritation by chemical mediators. Loss of function is caused when the cells lack nutrients or the swelling interferes with an action (such as joint movement).

A collection of interstitial fluid formed in the inflamed area is called *exudate*. Characteristics of exudate are as follows:

- **Fibrinous** exudates: Thick, sticky, with high cell and fibrin contents; this type increases the risk of **scar** tissue in the area (**Figure 9–3**).
- **Hemorrhagic** (bloody) exudates: Present if blood vessels have been damaged.
- **Purulent** exudates: Thick, yellowish green in color, with higher amounts of leukocytes and cell debris along with microorganisms; indicate bacterial infection; commonly called "pus." An **abscess** is a localized pocket of pus in a solid tissue (such as around a tooth).
- **Serous** (watery) exudates: Consist mostly of fluid and small amounts of protein and white blood cells; often caused by allergic reactions or burns. For example, after a severe burn of the skin, a **blister** may form (**Figure 9–4**).

General manifestations of inflammation may also include **malaise**, mild fever (**pyrexia**), fatigue, headache, and **anorexia**. Fever can be severe if infection has caused the inflammation, depending on the causative microorganism. High fever may impair the growth and the reproduction of the pathogen. Fever is caused by the release of **pyrogens** from white blood cells or macrophages. Shivering may occur to allow the body to increase cell metabolism. Involuntary cutaneous vasoconstriction reduces heat loss, and if the patient "curls up" voluntarily, the body will conserve heat. These mechanisms continue until the body temperature is reset to its new, higher level by the hypothalamus. Once the cause of the fever is removed, body temperature is normalized by reversing these mechanisms.

Diagnostic tests used to determine the type of infection include those that check for leukocytosis, elevated serum C-reactive protein (CRP), elevated **erythrocyte sedimentation rate**, and increased plasma proteins and cell enzymes in the serum. Although not indicating the cause or site of the inflammation, they help in the monitoring of the patient through the course of the infection. A *differential count* (of the proportion of each type of white blood cell) may help in distinguishing a viral infection from a bacterial infection. Examining a peripheral blood smear may disclose abnormal cells in high numbers. Increased circulating plasma proteins (**fibrinogen**, prothrombin, and alpha-antitrypsin)

TABLE 9–2	Cellular Element Functions in the Inflammatory Response
Type of Leukocyte	**Function**
Basophils	Release of histamine, leading to inflammation
B lymphocytes	Production of antibodies
Eosinophils	Increase in number for allergic responses
Macrophages	Active in phagocytosis (macrophages are mature monocytes that have migrated from the blood into the tissues)
Monocytes	Active in phagocytosis
Neutrophils	Active in phagocytosis
T lymphocytes	Active in the cell-mediated immune response

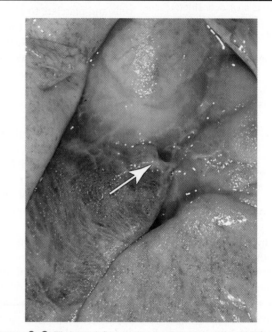

Figure 9–3 Fibrinous inflammation involving the surface of the heart (epicardium) and pericardium. The pericardial sac has been opened to expose the surface of the heart, which appears rough because fibrin has accumulated on the epicardium. The arrow indicates a large aggregate of fibrin adjacent to the right atrial appendage.

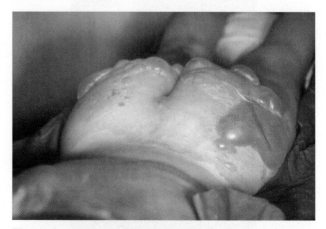

Figure 9–4 Extensive burn with marked leakage (extravasation) of fluid into the burned area leading to formation of large blisters.

may result from a liver response that increases protein synthesis.

When there is severe inflammation and necrosis, tissue is destroyed to some extent and must be repaired (**Figure 9–5**). This results in *cell enzymes* and **isoenzymes** becoming elevated in the blood. This event helps these substances to locate the site of the necrotic cells that have released enzymes into the blood and tissue fluids. Certain enzymes are not specific to certain tissues.

The amount of tissue necrosis that occurs is related to the specific type of trauma and other factors related to the inflammatory response. If necrosis is extensive, it may lead to **ulcers**, tissue erosion, or tissue death. Infection may develop in inflamed tissues because microorganisms can penetrate them more easily once they are damaged and blood supply is impaired. Inflammatory exudate is an excellent medium for microorganisms to use for reproduction and colonization.

> **RED FLAG**
> Inflammation caused by brief exposure to a substance usually subsides within 48 hours.

Deep ulcers that result from prolonged, severe inflammation may lead to complications such as **perforation** of the viscera or the development of scar tissue in large amounts. Inflammation can also cause strong muscle contractions or *skeletal muscle spasms*, which can force joints out of alignment.

> **RED FLAG**
> Joint inflammation often decreases its range of movement.

Chronic Inflammation

Chronic inflammation differs from **acute** inflammation in that it may last for weeks, months, or even years. Acute inflammation is usually self-limited and of short duration. Chronic inflammation may develop as the result of a recurrent or progressive active inflammatory process. Rheumatoid arthritis involves chronic inflammation with acute exacerbatory periods. Chronic inflammation may develop from **chronic** irritation due to bacteria, long-term immune abnormalities, and smoking. Chronic inflammation causes less swelling and exudate than acute inflammation. However, it increases the amounts of lymphocytes, *macrophages*, and **fibroblasts** and usually causes more tissue destruction. Increased scar tissue may form because of higher amounts of collagen being produced. Sometimes a **granuloma** develops around a foreign object such as a splinter or as a result of an immune response.

> **RED FLAG**
> Disseminated infections have a slow inflammatory response and take longer to identify and treat, thereby increasing morbidity and mortality.

Treatment of Inflammation

Inflammatory agents include such medications as acetylsalicylic acid (ASA), acetaminophen, nonsteroidal anti-inflammatory drugs (NSAIDs), and prednisone. A mnemonic used to remember the treatment for inflammation is "RICE": Rest, Ice, Compression, and Elevation.

Application of ice packs constricts blood vessels and decreases edema and pain. Chronic rheumatoid arthritis responds well to application of heat, but heat should be

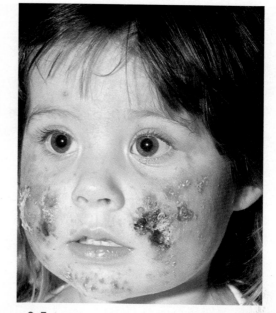

Figure 9–5 Acute inflammation of face with superficial necrosis of skin. Crusts of dried exudate (scabs) have formed on skin surface.

avoided in acute exacerbations of the condition. Elevation usually improves fluid flow away from the damaged area. Compression garments help the muscle pump to reduce accumulation of fluid. Mild-to-moderate exercise is useful for many chronic inflammatory conditions to improve blood and fluid flow. Orthotics help to prevent **contractures** and are often used along with rest, adequate nutrition, and good hydration.

Healing and Tissue Repair

Tissue repair overlaps the inflammatory process. It is a response to tissue injury and represents an attempt to maintain normal body structure and function. Tissue repair may take the form of **regeneration** of **parenchymal cells**, in which injured cells are replaced with cells of the same type. Sometimes there is no residual trace of previous injury, although it may take the form of replacement by connective tissue, leaving a permanent scar. There are several methods of wound healing:

- *Resolution*: Occurs after minimal tissue damage; cells recover and tissue returns to normal in a short period of time (e.g., mild sunburn).
- *Regeneration*: Occurs in damaged tissue in which cells are capable of mitosis; damaged tissue is replaced by identical tissue from proliferation of nearby cells (e.g., hepatocytes in the liver can undergo mitosis when needed to regenerate).
- *Replacement*: Connective tissue (scar or fibrous tissue) forms after extensive damage or when cells are incapable of mitosis (e.g., chronic inflammation in the brain or heart results in normal tissue being replaced by fibrous tissue).

Healing by *first intention* means that a wound is free of foreign material and necrotic tissue, with edges close together. Healing by *second intention* refers to a large break in tissue, increased inflammation, a longer healing period, and more scar tissue formation (**Figure 9–6**).

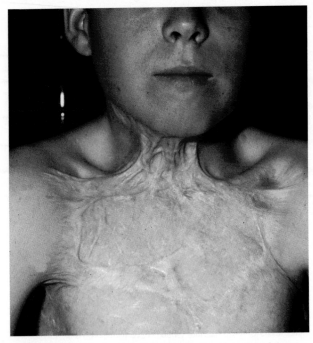

Figure 9–6 Marked scarring after the healing of a severe burn, which has restricted motion of neck and arms. Skin grafting was required to improve function.

Tissue repair begins after injury with a blood clot forming, inflammation developing, and phagocytosis beginning. After 3 to 4 days foreign material and cell debris have been phagocytized. **Granulation tissue** from nearby connective tissue grows into the gap caused by the injury. Granulation tissue is highly vascular. It appears moist and is pink or red, containing many new capillary buds. Nearby *epithelial cells* undergo mitosis, extending across the wound from the outside edges inward. **Collagen** is produced by fibroblasts, which strengthens the repairing tissue. Cross-linking and shortening of the collagen fibers form a strong, tight scar. The scar gradually fades from red to white. It is not as strong as normal, uninjured skin tissue.

The phases of healing are as follows:

- Inflammation: Beginning immediately and lasting for 2 to 5 days, the inflammatory phase involves both hemostasis and inflammation.
  - Hemostasis is divided into the processes of vasoconstriction, platelet aggregation, and the formation of a clot via the actions of thromboplastin.
  - Inflammation involves the processes of vasodilation and phagocytosis.
- Proliferation: Lasting from day 2 until 3 weeks after injury, the proliferative phase includes the processes known as granulation, contraction, and epithelialization.
  - Granulation occurs as fibroblasts lay a bed of collagen, filling defects and producing new capillaries.
  - Contraction is the process of wound edges pulling together to reduce defects.
  - Epithelialization involves a moist surface to cross the area, with cells traveling about 3 centimeters from the point of origin, in all directions.

- Maturation: Also known as the "remodeling phase," this lasts from 3 weeks to 2 years.
  - New collagen forms, which increases tensile strength to wounds, but scar tissue is only 80 percent as strong as the original tissue.

The *picture frame theory* of tissue healing describes the process of mitotically active cells migrating inward from the margin of a wound. This pulls the material within the margins of the defect. This is related to the *pull theory*, wherein the material within a healing wound contracts and pulls the margins of the wound together.

Factors Affecting Healing

Small gaps in tissue are healed quickly, with minimal scar tissue formation. Large or deep gaps take much longer and result in large scars. Healing is promoted by younger age, good nutrition, adequate hemoglobin, effective circulation, a clean and undisturbed wound, and no complications. Healing may be delayed by advanced age, poor nutrition, dehydration, low hemoglobin, circulatory problems, other disease states, irritation, bleeding, excessive mobility, infection, foreign materials, radiation, lack of insulin, chemotherapy, and prolonged use of glucocorticoids.

When scars are formed, there are often complications to the wound area. Loss of function may result from loss of normal cells and lack of specialized structures such as hair follicles, glands, and sensory nerve endings. Scar tissue tends to shrink over time, restricting range of joint movement, fixation, and joint deformity. Scar shrinkage can also cause shortening or narrowing (**stenosis**) of structures such as tubes or ducts. **Adhesions** are bands of scar tissue that join two surfaces that are normally separated, such as between loops of the intestine or between the pleural membranes. Hard ridges of scar tissue or the formation of keloids may occur due to excessive collagen deposits.

> **RED FLAG**
> Blood supply may be impaired around a scar, resulting in further tissue breakdown and ulceration.

Contact inhibition is defined as cessation of replication of dividing cells that come into contact, as in the center of a healing wound. When it occurs, a monolayer is formed. *Epibole* is defined as growth of epithelium that surrounds underlying mesenchymal tissue. This is to keep premature closure of wound edges from occurring, and both of these processes can cause poor, insufficient wound healing.

> **RED FLAG**
> It is important to avoid both contact inhibition and epibole during the healing process.

Regarding bone healing, there are three primary (yet overlapping) stages:

- Inflammatory stage (2–4 weeks after fracture): A hematoma forms within the fracture site during the first few hours and days. Inflammatory cells infiltrate the bone. Granulation tissue, vascular tissue, and immature tissue are formed.
- Repair stage (1–2 months after fracture): The bone ends become joined and stabilized. New bone tissue (**fracture callus**) forms, but it is weak and requires protection. Cartilage hardens near the end of the fracture and sweeps toward the center. New blood vessels

(for new growth) develop. Smokers should stop their habit during this phase because nicotine greatly slows down these processes.

- Late modeling (remodeling) stage (months to years after fracture): The body changes weak bone material into strong bone material. The body remodels the fracture callus down to normal sized bone. In general, the bone is restored to its original shape, structure, and mechanical strength. Mechanical stress (weight bearing) actually helps during this stage as the bone must endure the weight placed upon it, strengthening its structure.

SUMMARY

The ability of the body to repair damaged tissues is variable. The inflammatory response is a nonspecific defense mechanism. Other defenses include the barriers (skin, mucous membranes, and secretions) and phagocytosis. The five signs of acute inflammation include redness, warmth, pain, swelling, and loss of function. There are two types of inflammation: acute and chronic. Injured tissues are repaired by regeneration of parenchymal cells or by connective tissue repair, in which scar tissue replaces the parenchymal cells of the injured tissue. Chronic inflammation results in formation of fibrotic or scar tissue. Anti-inflammatory drugs include aspirin (acetylsalicylic acid) and nonsteroidal anti-inflammatory drugs. Healing in a small area of damage often occurs because of regeneration where cells are capable of mitosis. Extensive damage often causes formation of fibrotic or scar tissue. Factors promoting healing include youth, good nutrition, good circulation, and lack of infection or disease. Other factors include contract inhibition, epibole, and three stages of bone healing. These stages are the inflammatory stage, the repair stage, and the late modeling (remodeling) stage.

The phases of healing include inflammation, proliferation, and maturation. Inflammation is subdivided into hemostasis and the processes of vasodilation and phagocytosis. Proliferation is made up of the processes of granulation, contraction, and epithelialization. The final phase, maturation, is also known as the "remodeling phase," as new collagen forms and scar tissue develops.

REVIEW QUESTIONS

Select the best response to each question.

1. The following are signs and symptoms of inflammation *except*
   a. pain
   b. cyanosis
   c. warmth
   d. loss of function
2. Mast cell granules produce and release
   a. interleukins
   b. lymphokines
   c. histamine
   d. leukotrienes
3. Basophils release which of the following substances that cause inflammation?
   a. histamine
   b. antibodies
   c. interleukins
   d. lymphokines
4. Thick, yellowish-green exudate that contains higher amounts of leukocytes and microorganisms is what type of exudate?
   a. serous
   b. hemorrhagic
   c. fibrinous
   d. purulent
5. A differential count of leukocytes may help in distinguishing a viral infection from which type of infection?
   a. bacterial
   b. fungal
   c. protozoal
   d. rickettsial
6. Which of the following is an example of chronic inflammation?
   a. second-degree burn
   b. myocardial infarction
   c. rheumatoid arthritis
   d. allergic reaction
7. Which of the following suffixes means "inflammation"?
   a. -itis
   b. -iasis
   c. -iatric
   d. -ist
8. The sudden onset of a disease marked by intensity of symptoms is described as
   a. critical
   b. chronic
   c. morbid
   d. acute
9. An area of dead cells or tissue due to lack of oxygen is called
   a. ischemia
   b. an infarction
   c. atresia
   d. gangrene
10. Examples of corticosteroids include each the following *except*
    a. prednisone
    b. dexamethasone
    c. prostaglandin
    d. beclomethasone

CASE STUDIES

Karen Coupe, PT, DPT, MSEd

Case 1

An 18-year-old was referred to physical therapy with a right ankle sprain. The patient injured himself playing basketball. Patient is non–weight bearing and is using axillary crutches. Patient medical history: Unremarkable. Prior level of function: Independent in all activities of daily living, active in basketball and soccer. Physical therapist evaluation reveals an inversion grade II sprain with significant edema from the distal metatarsal heads to the mid-crural region, ecchymosis, decreased ankle range of motion (ROM) in all planes and c/o pain. Plan of care is for modalities, passive ROM, and patient education.

1. Is this patient's ankle injury acute, subacute, or chronic?
2. This patient has significant edema. What are the other cardinal signs of inflammation?
3. What is ecchymosis and why would the patient present with this?
4. Considering the stage of the patient's injury, would the physical therapist assistant want to use cold modalities or heat modalities? Explain the reasoning behind your choice.
5. Passive ROM is generally considered a ROM that is within the available ROM, whereas stretching is pushing beyond the available ROM. Why would the PT want passive ROM rather than stretching?

Case 2

A 22-year-old man is currently being seen in an outpatient physical therapy clinic secondary to a left femoral shaft fracture. The patient initially underwent an intramedullary nailing with nonunion resulting in two additional surgical stabilizations. The patient is now 8 months post initial fracture. Patient is currently ambulating, weight bearing as tolerated, with bilateral axillary crutches. PT evaluation reveals postsurgical scar is healed with adhesions on the distal one-third, antalgic gait pattern with decreased step length on the right, decreased hip ROM and strength. Plan of care is for scar mobilization, gait training, ROM, and strengthening.

1. This patient suffered a nonunion fracture that required three surgeries. What does this mean?
2. Explain the basic stages of bone healing. What would happen if the bone had not yet healed and orders were for physical therapy stretching and strengthening?
3. Why would a patient develop adhesions on a scar? Why is it important to mobilize the tissue?
4. How would the appearance of the scar differ if it developed keloids?
5. Define antalgic gait. Why would the patient have a decreased step length on the right uninvolved leg?

WEBSITES

http://courses.washington.edu/conj/inflammation/acute inflam.htm

http://emedicine.medscape.com/article/1298129-overview

http://www.britannica.com/EBchecked/topic/287677/inflammation/214905/Chemical-mediators-of-inflammation

http://www.medterms.com/script/main/art.asp?articlekey=3979

http://www.merck.com/mmhe/sec01/ch007/ch007b.html

http://www.mnwelldir.org/docs/terrain/chronic_inflammation.htm

http://www.wrongdiagnosis.com/medical/inflammation.htm

CHAPTER 10

Immune Response, Hypersensitivity, and Autoimmune Disorders

LEARNING OBJECTIVES

After completion of the chapter the reader should be able to

1. Describe the basic features of humoral and cell-mediated immunity.
2. Explain the role of lymphocytes in the immune response.
3. Compare hypersensitivity and immunity.
4. Explain the classification of antibodies and how they differ from one another.
5. Describe hypersensitivity reactions and the various types.
6. List the major autoimmune disorders.
7. Explain the methods of diagnosis for systemic lupus erythematosus.
8. Describe the pathophysiology of AIDS.

KEY TERMS

Anaphylaxis: A severe and acute type I hypersensitivity reaction, with potentially life-threatening symptoms.

Antigen: Any substance that stimulates the production of antibodies.

Antimicrobial: Preventing or inhibiting microbial infection.

Autoantibodies: Antibodies that attack the body's own tissue.

Bronchoconstriction: Narrowing of the breathing tubes of the lungs.

Complement: A protein that helps antibodies clear pathogens from the body.

Cytotoxic: Destructive or toxic to cells.

Erythema: Redness of the skin, often caused by inflammation.

Glycoproteins: Molecules made up of sugars and amino acids.

Humoral: Pertaining to or derived from a body fluid.

Hypogammaglobulinemia: An immune disorder characterized by a reduction of gamma globulins.

Hypoproteinemia: An abnormally low level of protein in the blood.

Interleukins: Proteins called lymphokines that help regulate the immune system.

Mast cells: Cells in connective tissue that contain histamine and heparin, which are released during allergic reactions or in response to inflammation or tissue injury.

KEY TERMS CONTINUED

Memory cells: Those that protect the body if an invading antigen returns by "remembering" the previous occurrence.

Monocytes: Large leukocytes that have only single nuclei.

Monokines: Cytokines (cell-signaling protein molecules) produced by monocytes and macrophages.

Mutate: To produce a change in the base pair sequences of chromosomal molecules.

Opportunistic: Able to take effect due to a lack of immune function.

Plasmapheresis: The removal, treatment, and return of components of blood plasma from the blood circulation.

Prophylactic: Preventing the spread of disease.

Pruritic: Itchy.

Retrovirus: Any virus containing RNA that replicates in targeted host cells.

Secondary: Not primary; a condition that develops as the result of a primary condition.

Splenectomy: Removal of the spleen.

Stem cells: Undifferentiated cells that can grow into any type of body cells.

Thymus: The lymphoid gland located near the sternum that is essential in the development of immunity before puberty.

Titer: The concentration of a substance in a solution as determined by titration (the process of adding amounts of different solutions to create a specific chemical reaction).

Vesicles: Small, raised skin lesions that usually contain fluid.

Overview

The immune system is a major part of the body's defense system. Immunity is the second major function of the lymphatic system. Lymphatic cells and biochemicals attack microorganisms to destroy infectious particles. Immunity against disease also protects against toxins and cancer cells. When an immune response is abnormal, the results may include persistent infections, allergies, autoimmune disorders, and cancer.

Immune System

The immune system responds to certain substances, cells, toxins, proteins, and other entities perceived as foreign to the body. The immune response is intended to recognize and remove unwanted materials. Unique antigens on the cell surfaces can distinguish "self" from "non-self" (foreign). The immune system recognizes a specific invading **antigen** as foreign and develops a specific response to that particular antigen. It stores the response in its **memory cells** to protect the body again if the invading antigen returns. A person must have been exposed to a specific foreign material and have developed immunity to it before this defense is effective. Defense mechanisms include phagocytosis (cell-eating) and the inflammatory response.

Cancer is also fought by the body in a similar fashion—it is identified as foreign. Cancer, therefore, often develops after the immune system has become compromised or depressed. Unfortunately, not all cancer cells are identifiable as foreign. Tolerance to self antigens prevents improper responses.

The immune system consists of the lymphoid structures, immune cells, and tissues concerned with immune cell development. The immune cells (lymphocytes) and macrophages provide the mechanism that identifies and removes "alien" material. They originate in bone marrow, which, along with the thymus, plays an important role in the maturation of the cells. The blood and circulatory system provide transportation and communication networks for the immune system.

Antigens (immunogens) can be foreign substances or human cell surface antigens unique to each patient. The *macrophage* is essential for the immune response to occur. They develop from *monocytes*, occurring throughout the body in the liver, lungs, lymph nodes, and other tissues. Macrophages intercept and engulf foreign material and present the antigens from the foreign material to the lymphocytes, initiating the immune response. They also secrete chemicals that activate additional lymphocytes and the inflammatory response. **Figure 10–1** shows the development of immunity.

The lymphocyte is the primary cell in the immune response. The two groups (T and B lymphocytes) determine which type of immunity will be initiated (either cell-mediated or humoral immunity). T lymphocytes (T cells) arise from **stem cells** in the bone marrow and then travel to the *thymus* for further differentiation and development. *Cell-mediated immunity* develops as T lymphocytes with protein receptors on the cell surface recognize antigens on the surface of target cells. They then directly destroy the invading antigens and reproduce to create many more cells that can battle the invaders. T cells are mostly effective against cells infected with viruses, fungal or protozoal infections, cancer cells, and foreign cells (such as transplanted tissue).

B lymphocytes (B cells) are responsible for **humoral** immunity by producing antibodies or immunoglobulins. Antibodies or immunoglobulins are proteins. They are found in the general blood circulation, forming the globulin portion of plasma proteins. Immunoglobulins are divided into five classes, shown in **Table 10–1**.

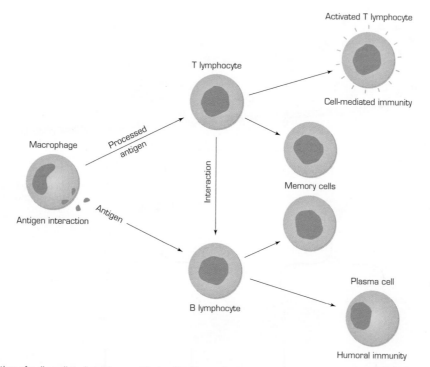

Figure 10–1 Interaction of cell-mediated and humoral immunity. Macrophage processes and presents processed antigen fragments to T lymphocyte; B lymphocyte processes intact antigen and displays fragments of the same antigen on its cell membrane. T lymphocyte, which has responded to the same antigen, stimulates the B lymphocyte to proliferate, mature into plasma cells, and make antibodies.

TABLE 10–1 Immunoglobulins		
Immunoglobulin (Ig)	**Function**	**Comments**
IgG	Activates complement; includes antibacterial, antiviral, and antitoxin antibodies; crosses placenta and creates passive immunity in newborn	Most common antibody in the blood, produced in both primary and secondary immune responses
IgM	Usually the first to increase in the immune response; activates complement; forms natural antibodies; involved in blood ABO type incompatibility reaction	Bound to B lymphocytes in circulation
IgA	From the colostrum, it provides protection for the newborn child	Found in secretions such as tears and saliva, in mucous membranes, and in colostrum
IgE	When linked to allergen, it causes release of histamine and other chemicals, resulting in inflammation	Binds to mast cells in skin and mucous membranes
IgD	Activates B cells	Attached to B cells

Process of Acquiring Immunity

The immune response consists of two steps:

■ A *primary response* occurs during initial exposure to an antigen (see **Figure 10–2**). The antigen is recognized and processed. Initiation of the development of antibodies or sensitized T lymphocytes begins. This can take up to several weeks and can be monitored by using the serum antibody **titer** (measure).

■ A *secondary response* results when a repeat exposure to the same antigen occurs. Memory cells produce large numbers of matching antibodies or T cells quickly and can continue to do so for years (see **Figure 10–3**).

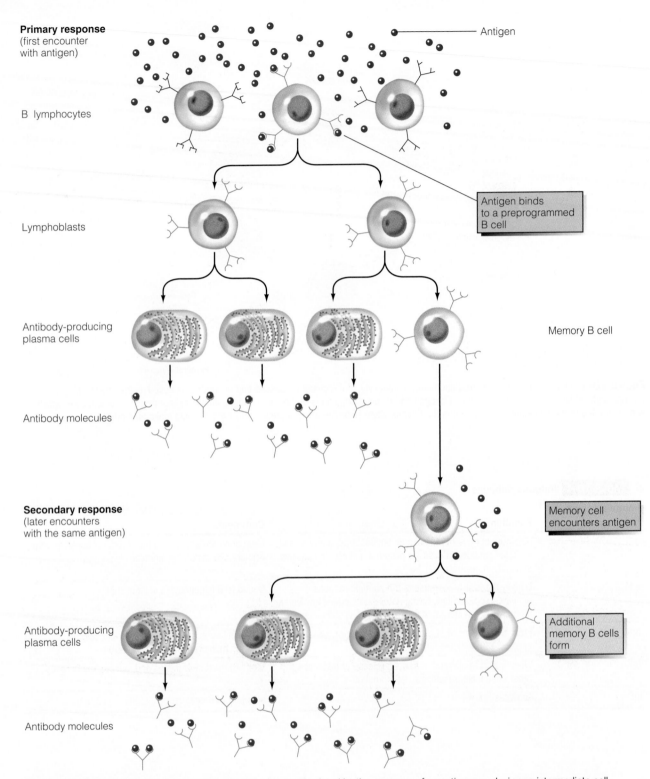

Figure 10–2 B-cell activation. Immunocompetent B cells are stimulated by the presence of an antigen, producing an intermediate cell, the lymphoblast. The lymphoblasts divide, producing plasma cells and some memory cells. Memory cells respond to subsequent antigen encroachment, yielding a rapid, secondary response.

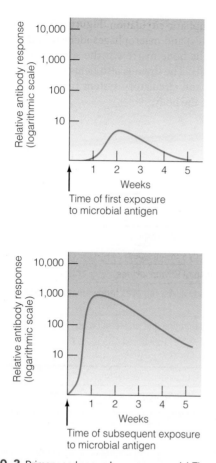

Figure 10–3 Primary and secondary responses. (a) The primary (initial) immune response is slow. It takes about 10 days for antibody levels to peak. Almost no antibody is produced during the first week as plasma cells are being formed. (b) The secondary response is much more rapid. Antibody levels rise almost immediately after the antigen invades. T cells show a similar response pattern.

Immunity is acquired in four ways (**Table 10–2**). *Active immunity* develops when the body develops antibodies or T cells in response to a specific antigen introduced into it. *Active natural immunity* is acquired by direct exposure to an antigen. *Active artificial immunity* develops when a specific antigen is introduced into the body stimulating the production of antibodies. *Passive immunity* occurs when antibodies are transferred from one person to another. *Passive natural immunity* occurs when IgG is transferred from mother to fetus. *Passive artificial immunity* results from the injection of antibodies from a person or animal into a second person.

The occurrence of infectious diseases such as polio and measles has declined where vaccines have been widely used. Smallpox has been virtually eradicated throughout the world. Those who are not immunized against recommended illnesses are still very susceptible to contracting them. A *toxoid* is an altered or weakened bacterial toxin that acts as an antigen. A *booster* is an additional immunization given 5 or 10 years after initial immunization that "reminds" the immune system about a particular antigen and promotes a better secondary response.

TABLE 10–2 Forms of Acquired Immunity

Form	Example	Description
Natural active	A patient who has chickenpox one time	Has memory; pathogens enter the body and cause illness, forming antibodies in the host
Artificial active	A patient who has the measles vaccine and gains immunity	Has memory; a live or attenuated vaccine is injected into the patient, forming antibodies but not forming illness
Natural passive	Passage of antibodies through the placenta during pregnancy or via the ingestion of breast milk	Does not have memory; antibodies are passed directly from mother to child to provide temporary protection
Artificial passive	Via gammaglobulin, if recently exposed to a microbe	Does not have memory; antibodies (antiserum) are injected into a patient to provide temporary protection to minimize severity of infection

Immune Response

Unique antigens (usually proteins) on individual cell surfaces help the immune system to distinguish foreign cells from normal cells. These are sometimes referred to as non-self (foreign) and self (normal). The immune system usually ignores the self cells, tolerating them while recognizing specific invader antigens as "non-self." It develops a specific response to that particular antigen and stores the response in *memory cells*, allowing them to "remember" the antigen if it returns.

A patient must have been exposed to a certain foreign material and developed immunity to it before it can defend against it. The immune system is assisted in destroying foreign material by general defense mechanisms such as phagocytosis and the inflammatory response. The removal of foreign material also helps in preparing injured tissue for the healing process.

A malignant neoplasm may have an abnormal cell membrane, allowing the immune system to identify it as "foreign" and remove it. Therefore, a normal immune system plays an important role in fighting off cancer. Often, a depressed immune system results in the development of various types of cancer. Unfortunately, not all cancer cells can be removed by the immune system because they are not able to be identified as foreign.

The immune system has specific controls to prevent excessive responses to antigens. If the causative antigen is removed, the response is also reduced. Many chemical messengers also have a short life span. Improper responses are prevented by tolerance to self antigens.

Immune System Components

The components of the immune system include the lymphoid structures, immune cells, and tissues that deal with immune cell development (**Table 10–3**). Chemical mediators also play essential roles. Lymphoid structures include the lymph nodes, spleen, tonsils, intestinal lymphoid tissue, and the lymphatic circulation (**Figure 10–4**). Immune cells (lymphocytes) and macrophages identify and remove alien material. The bone marrow is the site of origination of all immune cells. The thymus also helps these cells to mature. The blood and circulatory system transport immune cells throughout the body.

TABLE 10–3 Immune System Components

Components	Definition	Function
Organs		
Antibodies	Specific proteins produced in humoral response	Bind with antigens
Antigens	Foreign substances or cell components	Stimulate immune response
Autoantibodies	Antibodies against self antigens	Attack body's own tissues
Bone marrow	Source of stem cells and leukocytes	Maturation of B lymphocytes
Lymphatic tissue	Contains many lymphocytes	Filters body fluids, removes foreign matter, used in immune response
Thymus	Located in the mediastinum; larger in children but decreases in size in adults	Site of maturation and proliferation of T lymphocytes
Cells		
Basophils	White blood cells that bind IgE	Release histamine in anaphylaxis
B lymphocytes	Humoral immunity-activated cells	Become antibody-producing plasma cells or B-memory cells
Cytotoxic (killer T) cells	Large, differentiated T cells	Destroy antigens, cancer cells, and virus-infected cells
Eosinophils	Granulocytes important in allergic reactions	Participate in allergic responses
Helper T cells	T cells that conduct surveillance and secrete cytokines	Activate B and T cells to control or limit specific immune response
Macrophages	Phagocytic white blood cells	Process and present antigens to lymphocytes for the immune response
Mast cells	Connective tissue cells with allergic functions	Release chemical mediators in connective tissue
Memory T cells	T cells that help to remember foreign invaders	Remember antigens; quickly stimulate immune response upon reexposure
Monocytes	White blood cells with single nuclei	Migrate from blood into tissues to become macrophages
Neutrophils	Phagocytic white blood cells	Used in nonspecific defense, active in inflammatory process
NK lymphocytes	Natural killer cells	Destroy foreign cells, virus-infected cells, and cancer cells
Plasma cells	Develop from B lymphocytes	Secrete specific antibodies
T lymphocytes	White blood cells critical in immunity	Used in cell-mediated immunity
Chemical Mediators		
Chemotactic factors	Substances that respond to chemical stimulation	Attract phagocytes to area of inflammation
Complement	Group of inactive circulatory proteins	When activated, they stimulate release of other chemical mediators
Cytokines (messengers)	Lymphokines, monokines, interferons, and interleukins	Stimulate activation and proliferation of B and T cells, communication between cells
Histamine	Released from mast cells and basophils	Causes vasodilation and increased vascular permeability or edema
Kinins (such as bradykinin)	Polypeptides	Cause vasodilation, edema, and pain
Leukotrienes	Group of lipids derived from mast cells and basophils	Cause contraction of bronchiolar smooth muscle and develop inflammation
Prostaglandins	Group of lipids with varying effects	Some cause inflammation, vasodilation, edema, and pain
Tumor necrosis factor	A cytokine active in the immune response	Stimulates fever, chemotaxis, mediator of tissue wasting, stimulation of T cells and necrosis in some tumors, mediator in septic shock

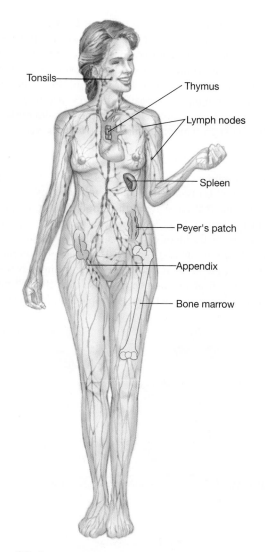

Figure 10–4 The lymphatic system and its pathways.

Tonsils

Thymus

Lymph nodes

Spleen

Peyer's patch

Appendix

Bone marrow

Functions of Monocytes and Lymphocytes

Monocytes play a big role in immunity. *Macrophages* develop from **monocytes**, occurring throughout the body. Macrophages are large phagocytic cells that engulf foreign material, processing and presenting antigens from the material to lymphocytes, which initiates the immune response. Macrophages secrete **monokines** and **interleukins**, which play a part in the activation of more lymphocytes and in the inflammatory response. This accompanies a **secondary** immune response.

The lymphocyte is the primary cell used in the immune response. It is produced in the bone marrow. When mature, lymphocytes are known as *immunocompetent* cells, which recognize and react to antigens (**Figure 10–5**). The two groups of lymphocytes, T lymphocytes and B lymphocytes, determine which type of immunity must be initiated (cell-mediated or humoral immunity).

T lymphocytes are also called T cells. They arise from *stem cells* in the bone marrow, traveling to the **thymus** for additional differentiation and to develop cell membrane receptors. When T lymphocytes that have protein receptors on their surfaces recognize antigens on surface target cells, *cell-mediated immunity* has developed. T cells, therefore, directly destroy invading antigens. These T cells reproduce and also activate other T lymphocytes and B lymphocytes. T cells are primarily effective against virus-infected cells, cancer cells, foreign cells, and fungal or protozoal infections.

There are many specialized subgroups of T cells. **Cytotoxic** *CD8 positive T-killer cells* bind to an antigen and release enzymes or chemicals that help to destroy target cells. These substances include monokines and lymphokines, which have a variety of functions that heighten the immune response and inflammation. Destroyed cells are removed by phagocytic cells. *Helper CD4 positive T cells* facilitate the immune response, with *memory T cells* (a subgroup) remaining for

Antigens

Antigens (immunogens) are either human cell surface antigens or foreign substances. When they are not foreign substances, they are unique to every individual except for identical twins. Usually made of polysaccharides or complex proteins, or combinations such as **glycoproteins**, they activate the immune system to produce *matching antibodies.*

Self antigens are present on cell membranes, coded by genes inherited from a person's parents. It is not likely that two individuals could have identical antigens because so many gene combinations are possibly inherited from each person's parents. Major histocompatibility complex (MHC) is an antigen that has an essential role in the activation and regulation of the immune response and intercellular communications. MHC detects changes in cell membranes changed by viruses or cancers. It is also known as human leukocyte antigen because of its initial detection on leukocyte cell membranes. These antigens are used for matching tissues between donors and tissue recipients. The immune system is activated by the presence of cells that have different MHC molecules. The immune system tolerates self antigens, not recognizing them as foreign.

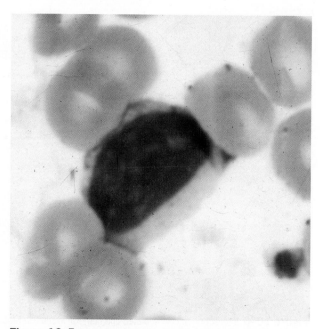

Figure 10–5 Structure of mature lymphocyte in the peripheral blood (original magnification X 1,000).

years in the lymph nodes to reactive the response if the same invader returns.

In AIDS, T-helper cells and T-killer cells play vital roles. By secreting "messenger" cytokines the cells regulate all cells of the immune system. However, HIV destroys the CD4 cells to weaken the entire immune system. CD4 cells normally occur twice as often as CD8 cells. This ratio is closely monitored in AIDS patients to diagnose the infection's progress.

B lymphocytes (B cells) control *humoral immunity* by producing *antibodies* (*immunoglobulins*), also shown in **Figure 10–6**. They are believed to mature in the bone marrow and then move to the spleen and lymphoid tissue. After antigen exposure they become antibody-producing plasma cells, acting mostly against bacteria and viruses that are outside body cells. B-memory cells form, which provide for repeated antibody production. *Natural killer cells* are distinct from the B and T lymphocytes. Without prior exposure and sensitization, they destroy tumor cells and those infected with viruses.

RED FLAG

Cytokine is a general term for any protein that functions as an intercellular messenger after being secreted by cells. Cytokines influence cells of the immune system. They are secreted by macrophages and monocytes (*monokines*), lymphocytes (*lymphokines*), and other cells.

Antibodies or Immunoglobulins

Antibodies (immunoglobulins) are proteins produced by plasma cells that have unique structures. All various types of antibodies have the same basic structure: two light chains and two heavy chains. The light chains are pairs of "half chains,"

whereas heavy chains are longer (**Figure 10–7**). The *variable portions* of antibodies bind to antigens and are attached to common bases. Each common base is a *constant region* that attaches to macrophages. As antibodies bind to matching antigens, they destroy them. This is significant in the development of immunity to specific diseases. Antibodies exist in the general circulation. They form the globulin portion of both plasma proteins and lymphoid structures.

Complement System

During immune reactions, with IgG or IgM, the **complement** system is often activated. *Complement* involves inactive proteins that circulate in the blood; these proteins are numbered from *C1* to *C9*. The way in which these proteins act is similar to the blood-clotting cascade. When an antigen–antibody complex binds to an initial complement component (C1), the sequence of activation begins. It ultimately results in destruction of the antigen by lysis when the cell membrane is damaged. Sometimes, a complement fragment may

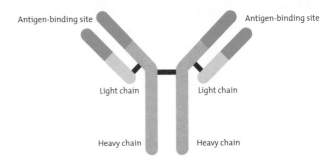

Figure 10–7 Structure of an immunoglobulin molecule.

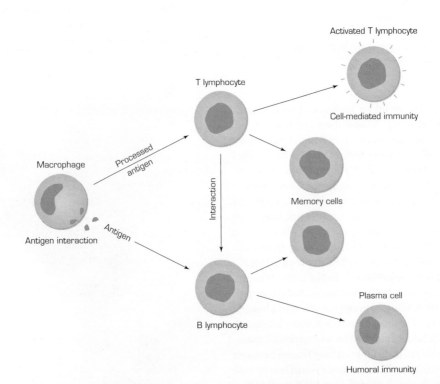

Figure 10–6 Interaction of cell-mediated and humoral immunity. Macrophage processes and presents processed antigen fragments to T lymphocyte; B lymphocyte processes intact antigen and displays fragments of the same antigen on its cell membrane. T lymphocyte, which has responded to the same antigen, stimulates the B lymphocyte to proliferate, mature into plasma cells, and make antibodies.

attach to a microorganism that marks it for phagocytosis. An inflammatory response is also initiated by the complement activation.

Chemical Mediators

In an immune reaction a variety of chemical mediators may be involved, including interleukins or histamine. The type of chemical mediators involved depends on the specific circumstances occurring. These mediators may have various functions, including causing cellular damage or signaling cellular responses.

Diagnostic Tests

Diagnostic tests used for immune function may qualitatively or quantitatively measure serum immunoglobulins. They may also assess the measure (*titer*) of certain antibodies. Antibody identification may help to detect Rh blood incompatibility, screen for HIV infection, detect the presence of German measles in pregnant women, monitor the level of hepatitis B infections, and assist in many other situations. Lymphocytes may be counted and characterized to determine disease states. Other tests provide the framework in determining compatibility for tissue transplantation.

Acquiring Immunity

Humans are not susceptible to diseases that affect many other animals, and vice versa. *Natural immunity* is specific to each species. *Innate immunity* is specific to certain genes, controlled by race. Usually, a person will have only one episode of a bacterial or viral disease because the specific antibody is "remembered" by the body. As the body ages from early childhood into later childhood, the amount of infections usually decreases as a result. However, certain bacteria and viruses have more than 100 causative organisms and slightly different antigens, to which a person cannot easily adapt. This explains the reoccurrences of colds and "the flu." Various strains can **mutate** (change slightly over time). Therefore, a new influenza vaccine is made each year, and its composition is based on the current antigenic forms of the virus that will likely cause a "flu" epidemic.

Recommendations for all types of vaccines are established by the Centers for Disease Control and Prevention. Via vaccinations, many diseases, including measles and polio, have been greatly reduced in occurrence. Smallpox is another example of a nearly eradicated disease. Today, continued research is moving toward more effective treatment against malaria, AIDS, and other conditions. Types of vaccinations include *toxoids*, which use altered or weakened bacterial toxins that act as antigens, or *boosters*, which are additional immunizations that "remind" the immune system of an antigen to promote a more effective secondary response.

Transplant Rejection

Today, transplantation of many different body parts occurs on a regular basis. These include transplantation of corneas, kidneys, lungs, hearts, bone marrow, and skin. **Table 10–4** lists the various types of tissue or organ transplants.

The most common type of transplantation is the allograft (homograft), from one human to another. The immune system of the recipient reacts to the transplanted tissue as

TABLE 10–4	Transplantation of Tissues and Organs	
Type	**Explanation**	**Example**
Allograft (homograft)	Transferred between members of the same species, with possible genetic differences	Between one human and another human
Isograft	Transferred between two bodies that are genetically identical	Between identical twins
Autograft	Transferred from one part of the body to another part of the same individual patient	From skin to bone
Xenograft (heterograft)	Transferred from a member of one species to a member of a different species	From pig to human

"foreign" and attempts to reject and destroy the tissue. This primarily involves a type IV cell-mediated hypersensitivity reaction. It also involves a humoral response. The results are inflammation and tissue necrosis. In most cases transplanted organs must be replaced after just a few years.

When the match is excellent, however, survival time of the transplanted tissue is increased. This is also improved when the donor is living, meaning the donated tissue is less likely to be damaged. Immunosuppressive drugs, taken on a regular basis, also improve the process. Transplanted cartilage and corneas usually work well because they lack a blood supply and therefore rejection is not a problem. As surgeries and drug therapies improve, transplants last for longer periods of time. Neonates and young infants are more likely to be able to receive heart transplants even when there is not a good tissue match, with rejection not occurring because their immune systems are immature and unable to respond to foreign tissue.

Rejections of tissue may occur as follows:

- *Hyperacute rejection*: Occurs immediately after transplantation, usually when preexisting antibodies are present; blood vessels are affected, resulting in lack of blood flow to the transplanted tissue
- *Acute rejection*: Develops after several weeks, usually because unmatched antigens cause a reaction
- *Chronic* or *late rejection*: Occurs after months or years, as blood vessels gradually degenerate

Immunosuppression techniques reduce immune response to prevent rejection. This involves drugs such as azathioprine, cyclosporine, and the glucocorticoid known as prednisone. Dosages must be carefully monitored, with the major concern being the potential heightened risk of infection. Because normal body defenses become limited, **opportunistic** infections may occur as normally harmless microbes become able to harm the body. Patients with diabetes are usually at higher risk of these infections.

> **RED FLAG**
> When working with immunosuppressed patients, the physical therapist assistant (PTA) needs to wear personal protective equipment such as gowns and masks so he or she does not transmit any pathogens to them.

Other potential results of immunosuppression are certain cancers (such as lymphomas, skin cancer, oral cancer, and Kaposi's sarcoma) and gingival hyperplasia.

Autoimmune Disorders

When a patient develops antibodies to his or her own cells or cellular material, the antibodies can then attack the body tissues. This is known as an autoimmune disorder. The term **autoantibodies** refers to antibodies formed against self antigens. Common autoimmune disorders include hematopoietic disorders, collagen disorders, neurologic disorders, and renal disorders. Less common autoimmune disorders include thyroiditis (Hashimoto's disease), systemic lupus erythematosus (SLE), myasthenia gravis, rheumatic fever, pernicious anemia, scleroderma, and rheumatoid arthritis. **Table 10–5** summarizes the major clinical manifestations of autoimmune disorders. SLE is discussed in more detail below.

Mechanism

Although the exact cause is unknown, patients may lose immune tolerance after tissue destruction occurs and large amounts of self antigens are released into the circulation to form antibodies. The condition may be age related and genetically linked. The immune system usually tolerates self antigens with no reaction, but once self-tolerance is lost the immune system cannot differentiate self from foreign. The immune reaction is then triggered by autoantibodies, causing inflammation and tissue necrosis (**Figure 10–8**).

Role of the PTA in Patients with Autoimmune Disorders

The PTA must understand the needs of patients with the many different types of autoimmune disorders and provide appropriate therapy interventions based on the established plan. **Table 10–6** lists the most important factors for each of the most common autoimmune disorders concerning physical therapy.

TABLE 10–5 Clinical Manifestations of Autoimmune Disorders

Disorder	Major Clinical Manifestations
Addison's disease	Localized disease of the adrenal glands (involving inadequate production of cortisol and aldosterone); causes muscle fatigue, weight loss, skin darkening, low blood pressure, hypoglycemia, vomiting, muscle and joint pain, depression
Ankylosing spondylitis	Inflammation of joints between spinal bones and between the spine and pelvis
Autoimmune blood diseases	Anemia, leukopenia, or thrombocytopenia
Autoimmune hepatitis	Localized, chronic disease that leads to progressive liver damage; more common in younger women, it usually causes fatigue, nausea, abdominal pain, joint aches, itching, and jaundice
Celiac disease	Localized disease characterized by an inappropriate immune response to dietary proteins found in wheat, rye, and barley; causes abdominal pain and distention, anemia, bleeding, bloody stool, bone and joint pain, changes in dental enamel, diarrhea, fatigue, changes in stool, oral ulcers, weakness, and weight loss
Crohn's disease	Localized inflammatory bowel disease that may affect any part of the gastrointestinal system; common symptoms include abdominal cramps, fever, fatigue, loss of appetite, pain with passing stool, persistent and watery diarrhea, and unintentional weight loss
Diabetes mellitus (type 1)	Diabetes mellitus due to insulin deficiency; type 1 diabetes mellitus is a localized disease affecting the beta cells of the pancreas and their production of insulin; common symptoms include flu-like symptoms, weight gain or loss, blurred vision, slow healing, frequent infections, nerve damage, irritated gums, frequent urination, excessive thirst or hunger, fatigue, and irritability
Glomerulonephritis	A condition involving renal glomeruli inflammation, which affects the kidneys' filtration abilities; common symptoms include blood in the urine, foamy urine, and swelling of the face, eyes, ankles, feet, legs, or abdomen
Goodpasture's syndrome	Systemic disease that affects the lungs and kidneys to cause blood to be coughed up, pain upon urination, fatigue, nausea, difficulty breathing, paleness, and proteinuria
Graves' disease (diffuse toxic goiter)	Localized disease that is the most common cause of hyperthyroidism; caused by an autoantibody, it causes weight loss, increased appetite, hand tremors, heat sensitivity, sweating, nervousness, increased heart rate, enlarged thyroid, and protruding eyes
Guillain-Barré syndrome	Acute systemic condition involving progressive muscle weakness or paralysis, with inflammation that damages the myelin sheath coverings of nerves; common symptoms include loss of reflexes, poor blood pressure control, numbness, sensation changes, tenderness or muscle pain, and uncoordinated movement
Hashimoto's thyroiditis	Localized disease that is the most common form of thyroiditis that is the most frequent cause of hypothyroidism; results from an autoimmune attack on the thyroid gland and may also cause bouts of hyperthyroidism; common symptoms include weight gain, depression, mania, temperature sensitivity, paresthesia, fatigue, panic attacks, heart rate changes, high cholesterol, reactive hypoglycemia, constipation, migraines, muscle weakness, cramps, memory loss, infertility, and hair loss
Juvenile arthritis	Chronic condition appearing in children that causes joint inflammation, pain, swelling, redness, and stiffness
Multiple sclerosis	Still not fully believed to be an autoimmune disease; a localized, chronic disorder affecting the central nervous system; causes inflammation and destruction of myelin, resulting in abnormal nerve transmission, lack of muscular control, and a variety of motor, sensory, and psychological symptoms

TABLE 10–5 Clinical Manifestations of Autoimmune Disorders (*Continued*)

Disorder	Major Clinical Manifestations
Myasthenia gravis	Muscle weakness from inadequate transmission of impulses from nerves to muscles; common symptoms include difficulty breathing, difficulty chewing or swallowing, difficult body movements or talking, drooping head, facial paralysis, fatigue, vocal changes, and eye muscle weakness
Pernicious anemia	Macrocytic anemia and nervous system damage from inadequate absorption of vitamin B_{12}; common symptoms include diarrhea or constipation, fatigue, loss of appetite, pale skin, concentration problems, shortness of breath, gum abnormalities, and nerve damage
Polymyalgia rheumatica	System disease that causes pain and weakness in the neck, shoulder muscles, and pelvis, as well as morning stiffness; it usually affects women over age 50
Primary biliary cirrhosis	Localized disease that commonly causes abdominal pain, enlarged liver, fatigue, fatty deposits under the skin, fatty stools, itching, jaundice, and soft yellow spots on the eyelids
Rheumatic fever	Heart and joint inflammation that manifests with symptoms including abdominal pain, fever, heart problems, joint pain and swelling, nosebleeds, skin nodules or rash, and Sydenham's chorea (which includes uncoordinated muscle movements and emotional instability)
Rheumatoid arthritis	Systemic disease with degeneration and inflammation of joints; other common symptoms include fatigue, loss of appetite, low fever, swollen glands, weakness, and, eventually, serious deformity of the joints
Scleroderma	A group of systemic connective tissue disorders associated with thickened, hardened skin, fibrosis, inflammation, blood vessel degeneration, and tissue damage
Sclerosing cholangitis	Localized disease that causes common symptoms such as fatigue, jaundice, itching, loss of appetite, enlarged liver or spleen, and repeat episodes of cholangitis (abdominal pain, chills, fever, clay-colored stools, dark urine, nausea, and vomiting)
Sjögren's syndrome	The body reacts to the tissue in glands that produce moisture such as tear and salivary glands, often progressing to a systemic disorder; characterized by decreased tears, saliva, and drying of other mucous membranes
SLE and other collagen-related diseases	Systemic disease manifesting in several organs; common symptoms include butterfly-shaped rash on the face, fatigue, fever, weight changes, various lesions, and more
Temporal arteritis	Localized disease that causes chronic inflammation and damage of large arteries in the face and head; resulting symptoms include headache, scalp tenderness, loss of vision, and facial pain; also known as "giant cell arteritis"
Ulcerative colitis	Localized disease that causes rectal pain, inflammation, and bleeding, bloody diarrhea, abdominal cramps, weight loss, fatigue, colon rupture, and toxicity
Various skin conditions and diseases	Loss of skin pigment (vitiligo) or skin blistering that results from loss of intercellular skin connections
Vasculitis	Various types of blood vessel inflammation and damage that interferes with function and blood supply to tissues
Wegener's granulomatosis	Systemic disease that affects the blood vessels, sinuses, lungs, and kidneys to cause frequent sinusitis, fever, night sweats, fatigue, malaise, chronic ear infections, loss of appetite, kidney problems, and eye problems

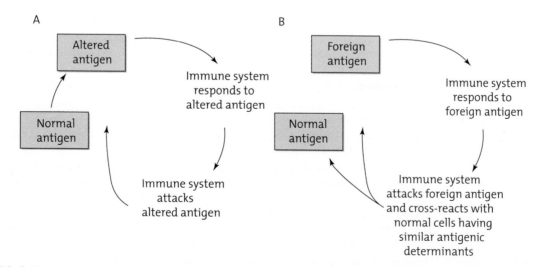

Figure 10–8 Two mechanisms postulated to induce autoimmunity. (A) Normal self antigens altered, generating an immune response. (B) Immune response directed against foreign antigen cross-reacts with similar antigenic determinants in normal self antigens.

TABLE 10-6 Physical Therapy Factors for Autoimmune Disorders

Autoimmune Disorder	Physical Therapy Factors
Addison's disease	Light activities focused on muscle strengthening due to altered contractile properties and decreased endurance; physical stress should be minimized; aquatics should be avoided because of heat and humidity issues; constant monitoring of vital signs; monitoring for impending Addisonian crisis; refer back to physician if any signs of an infection
Ankylosing spondylitis	Low-impact exercise will prevent or slow development of stooped posture and maintain joint movement and flexibility; stretching, strengthening, and deep-breathing exercises are also recommended
Autoimmune blood diseases	Blood counts must be monitored before physical therapy; all efforts to prevent falling are essential; for patients hospitalized long term, the ability for locomotion must be maintained as the goal of physical therapy
Autoimmune hepatitis	Physical therapy is not a significant factor in the treatment of autoimmune hepatitis
Celiac disease	Physical therapy is not a significant factor in the treatment of celiac disease
Crohn's disease	Regular exercise is recommended to combat the fatigue caused by this disease
Diabetes mellitus	Exercise, along with diet, is an essential component of the treatment of diabetes mellitus; it helps to lower blood sugar levels significantly and to encourage weight loss, which is important for successful treatment
Glomerulonephritis	Physical therapy is aimed at lowering hypertension, which is extremely important to treat this disease
Goodpasture's syndrome	Physical therapy is not a significant factor in the treatment of Goodpasture's syndrome
Graves' disease (diffuse toxic goiter)	Avoid heavy exercise due to the strain placed upon heart muscle by the disease; heat tolerance created by exercise is worsened by this condition, as is exophthalmos; heart rate should be monitored to avoid overexertion
Guillain-Barré syndrome	To rebuild weakened muscles, isometric, isotonic, and resistance exercises are recommended; rest is important to avoid persistent fatigue; comfortable shoes and socks are required during exercise
Hashimoto's thyroiditis	Exercise is important with this disease to relieve stress and reduce weight; in combination with diet modification, exercise is significant in the treatment of this disease; whole body approaches to exercise are recommended; avoid too much repetition of exercises to keep trauma to the musculoskeletal system to a minimum
Juvenile arthritis	Exercise restores lost motion to joints; range-of-motion exercises keep joints flexible, while strengthening exercises build muscle, endurance, and strength; exercises are recommended to be done daily, even if difficult; other physical therapies include hot baths or packs as well as hot wax or cold treatments before exercise
Lupus erythematosus and other collagen-related diseases	Exercise is required to keep muscles and joints active and for muscles to remain toned; isometric aerobic exercise is recommended; patients should be instructed to avoid exercise when SLE is flaring
Multiple sclerosis	Exercise is important but should not be overdone; allow time to warm up and cool down before and after exercise; avoid hazards that could cause falling; make sure supports are nearby in case of loss of balance; stop exercise if any strain or pain is felt; recommended activities include water aerobics, swimming, tai chi, and yoga
Myasthenia gravis	Light exercise is recommended, including walking, swimming, cycling, bowling, gymnasium exercise machines, and tennis; maintain hydration at all times; avoid temperature extremes; stop if any signs of fatigue occur
Pernicious anemia	Because of decreased exercise capacity, only light exercise is recommended
Polymyalgia rheumatica	Regular exercise helps to reduce pain, including swimming, walking, and riding stationary bicycles; moderate stretching helps keep muscles and joints flexible; start slowly with exercise and build up to a comfortable level
Primary biliary cirrhosis	Regular exercise is recommended to combat fatigue
Rheumatic fever	Light exercise is recommended only; avoid all extremely strenuous exercise due to potential heart problems resulting from rheumatic fever
Rheumatoid arthritis	Exercises designed for arthritic conditions provide pain relief and build muscle strength and also keep bones strong and increase the ability to live and move normally
Scleroderma	Range-of-motion exercises require a general warm-up period and should involve the arms, hands, legs, and feet; facial exercises should include stretching, augmentation, and manual exercises including the lips, tongue, and palate
Sclerosing cholangitis	Exercise helps to cleanse the body of toxins related to this condition; recommended activities include mini-trampoline use, walking, jogging, tai chi, chi gong, yoga, martial arts, dancing, aerobics, gymnastics, stretching, swimming, and light weight lifting; avoid exhaustion and exercising immediately after eating
Sjögren's syndrome	Exercise of all types helps to relieve inflammation and reduce the psychological stressors that can complicate this disease

TABLE 10-6 Physical Therapy Factors for Autoimmune Disorders (*Continued*)

Autoimmune Disorder	Physical Therapy Factors
Temporal arteritis	Exercise strengthens the heart and lowers blood pressure; it is important to begin slowly and work up to a comfortable level using an individualized physical therapy plan
Ulcerative colitis	Physical therapy is not a significant factor in the treatment of ulcerative colitis
Various skin conditions and diseases	Exercise may help certain skin conditions to heal faster; however, contact transmission must be avoided by wearing personal protective equipment
Vasculitis	Regular aerobic exercise, such as walking, can prevent the condition from worsening; it should be started slowly and increased to a comfortable level
Wegener's granulomatosis	Exercise can improve and sometimes suppress this disease; it also improves the mood symptoms that may be related

Hematopoietic Disorders

Hematopoietic disorders include anemia, neutropenia, neutrophilia, thrombocytopenia, thrombocythemia, eosinophilia, monocytosis, pancytopenia, leukemia, and tumors.

Renal Disorders

Renal disorders such as Goodpasture's syndrome may have lymphatic system effects. Goodpasture's syndrome actually consists of three interrelated features: hemorrhage, glomerulonephritis, and antibody activity.

Goodpasture's Syndrome

The manifestations of this disorder include diffuse pulmonary hemorrhage, glomerulonephritis, and circulating antiglomerular basement membrane antibodies.

Signs and Symptoms

Goodpasture's syndrome may be indicated by the features mentioned above and by hemoptysis, chills, fever, nausea, vomiting, weight loss, chest pain, anemia, arthralgias, tachypnea, inspiratory crackling, cyanosis, hepatosplenomegaly, hypertension, and skin rash.

Etiology

Goodpasture's syndrome is an autoimmune disorder with renal components. The hemorrhage component of this disorder may be caused by the broad antigen serotype called HLA-DR2, organic solvents, hydrocarbons, smoking, infections, cocaine use, and exposure to metal dusts.

Diagnosis

A variety of blood tests (including complete blood count, erythrocyte sedimentation rate, electrolyte, blood urea nitrogen, and creatinine tests) may be given to diagnose this condition. Other tests include urinalysis, serologic antibody tests, chest x-rays, and various pulmonary tests.

Treatment

Treatment for Goodpasture's syndrome mainly involves **plasmapheresis**, immunosuppressive medications, and removal of the agents that may have started the disease process. The role of the PTA is limited because physical therapy is not a significant factor in the treatment of Goodpasture's syndrome.

Prognosis

Prognosis is good with early diagnosis and the avoidance of lung hemorrhaging. The degree of kidney damage, however, can result in the need for dialysis or a kidney transplant. Immunosuppressive medications can also cause opportunistic infections with lethal potential.

Collagen Diseases

Collagen is the main component of connective tissue, which is found in all body structures. Collagen is an insoluble, fibrous protein and makes up about 30% of the body's total protein. Collagen diseases are autoimmune disorders wherein the immune system malfunctions and attacks itself. When connective tissue is damaged, the structures involved may be weakened to the point of failure. These disorders can only be treated by inhibiting the overactive immune system. The collagen diseases discussed in this chapter include SLE, scleroderma, rheumatoid arthritis, and polymyositis.

Systemic Lupus Erythematosus

There are two types of lupus erythematosus: cutaneous (discoid) and systemic (diffuse). SLE is much more severe because it affects many body systems. This disorder affects about 1 of every 2,400 people and occurs 10 times more frequently in women than in men.

SLE, commonly referred to simply as "lupus," affects many body systems. It causes a characteristic, butterfly-shaped facial rash that resembles the facial markings of a wolf, hence the name *lupus*, which means "wolf" in Latin (**Figure 10–9**). As SLE can now be identified earlier in the disease process, prognosis is improving. Side effects of certain medications can also cause lupus-like symptoms.

SLE primarily affects women between the ages of 20 and 40 years, with incidence higher in African Americans, Asians, Hispanics, and Native Americans. Although the actual lupus gene has not been identified, causes of SLE include genetically linked, hormonal, and environmental factors. Research is ongoing to determine the familial relationship to lupus.

> **RED FLAG**
>
> The clinical implications of SLE for the PTA include maintaining strength and joint mobility through regular exercises.

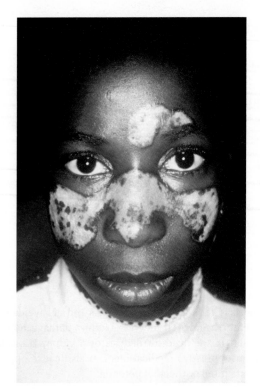

Figure 10–9 Butterfly rash of lupus.

Pathophysiology

SLE involves large amounts of circulating autoantibodies against deoxyribonucleic acid (DNA), erythryocytes, platelets, nucleic acids, and other nuclear materials. Immune complexes become deposited in connective tissues throughout the body, which activate complement and cause inflammation and necrosis. Inflammation of blood vessels (vasculitis) impairs blood supply to tissues and organs. Inadequate oxygen (ischemia) causes increased inflammation and tissue destruction. Common areas include the kidneys, heart, brain, lungs, joints, skin, and digestive tract. Diagnosis is made when there is a minimum of four areas of disease involvement and based on laboratory tests.

Signs and Symptoms

The signs and symptoms of SLE are greatly varied. Often, skin rashes and joint inflammation occur first, which progress to kidney or lung conditions. This disease has a progressive course, often with sporadic relapses and remission. Significant bone loss may occur because of this condition if the bones are not used regularly. **Table 10–7** lists the common manifestations of SLE.

Diagnostic Tests

SLE is indicated by the presence of numerous antinuclear antibodies, especially anti-DNA, in the serum. Another positive indication is the presence of lupus erythematosus cells, which are mature neutrophils that contain nuclear material (**Figure 10–10**). Other indications include low complement levels and a high erythrocyte sedimentation rate. Often, erythrocyte, leukocyte, lymphocyte, and platelet counts are low. Diagnosis may be confirmed by additional immunologic tests for various antibodies, and all organs and body systems needed to be examined for inflammation and damage.

Treatment

Physicians known as *rheumatologists* commonly treat SLE with prednisone. This glucocorticoid reduces the immune response and inflammation. Doses depend on whether the disease is in a state of exacerbation or remission. Other treatments include nonsteroidal anti-inflammatory drugs, the antimalarial drug *hydroxychloroquine*, and other therapies. It is critical to limit damage to the vital organs and minimize exacerbations by avoiding causative factors. Treatment of acute episodes and avoiding sun exposure or excessive fatigue also assists in preventing exacerbations of SLE. Warning signs of an impending exacerbation include increased fatigue, pain, fever, headache, and rash. Today's treatments for SLE usually allow most patients to live an active life and to have a normal life span. This is truer with early diagnosis.

Aerobic exercise is preferred to maintain muscle integrity and tone. Isometric exercises should be used with caution because they cause the release of autoantigen, nucleic acids, and other proteins into the blood. With lupus patients, exposing the immune system to such proteins causes it to react even more strongly to reexposure. It is important to remember that SLE patients should not exercise when their condition is flaring up.

RED FLAG

PTAs can assist patients with SLE in alleviating the effects of stress by teaching patients about healthy lifestyle choices and personal behaviors that allow them to deal more effectively with their condition.

TABLE 10–7 Signs and Symptoms of SLE

Body Area	Conditions	Comments
Blood vessels	Raynaud's phenomenon	Periodic vasospasm and pain in fingers and toes
Bone marrow	Blood related	Anemia, leukopenia, thrombocytopenia
Central nervous system	Brain related	Depression, mood changes, psychoses, seizures
Heart	Carditis	Inflammation of (usually) the pericardium, though any layer may be affected
Joints	Polyarthritis or arthralgia	Swollen, painful joints, without damage
Kidneys	Glomerulonephritis	Antigen–antibody deposits in glomeruli, with inflammation, marked proteinuria, and progressive renal damage
Lungs	Pleurisy	Inflammation of the pleural membranes, resulting in chest pain
Skin	Butterfly rash and other rashes, hair loss	Erythema on cheeks and over nose or other parts of skin, photosensitivity that is exacerbated with sun exposure, ulcerations in oral mucosa

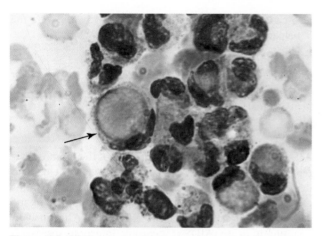

Figure 10–10 Positive test for lupus erythematosus. Spherical mass derived from damaged nucleus (arrow) engulfed by neutrophil (original magnification X 1,000).

Muscle aches and fatigue will occur, indicating the patient should not be exercising at this time.

Scleroderma

Scleroderma is an autoimmune disorder characterized by hardened, thickened, and shrunken connective tissues, including the skin. The disorder has periods of exacerbation and remission. It usually progresses very slowly, but if it does develop rapidly, it can affect body organs, usually causing death because of kidney failure.

Signs and Symptoms
Scleroderma causes the skin and joints to appear thick, shiny, and tight, similar to leather. Raynaud's phenomenon may be the first symptom, with the mouth becoming wrinkled and "pursed," making eating difficult.

Etiology
Scleroderma appears to start with skin and connective tissue, attracting lymph cells, which stimulate collagen production, leading to the disorder. Milder forms affect women, whereas more severe forms affect men and elderly people of both sexes. The severe form also attacks the internal organs, including the heart, lungs, and kidneys, limiting their ability to function.

Diagnosis
Clinical examination and tissue biopsy confirm the diagnosis, but it mimics other diseases such as bursitis and arthritis. Other signs that may aid in diagnosis include capillary changes near the fingernails and calcium deposits under the skin. Blood tests for anticentromere antibodies usually provide a positive diagnosis.

Treatment
No current treatment halts the progression of scleroderma. Anti-inflammatory agents, immunosuppressives, and antibiotics can be helpful. To maintain muscle strength and joint mobility, stretching and strengthening exercises may be used.

The role of the PTA includes physical therapy involving breathing exercises, stretching, strengthening, and relaxation therapy. Many exercises can be done while sitting or lying down. The focus of an exercise program should be on general strengthening of the arms, legs, and face.

Prognosis
Prognosis is not favorable, especially in severe cases, because there is no cure. Earlier diagnosis for mild cases is much better due to the slow progression of symptoms. Milder cases may have a better prognosis because symptoms worsen very slowly.

Rheumatoid Arthritis

Rheumatoid arthritis severely affects the joints, causing deformity and disability. It is a chronic inflammatory disease affecting over 2 million people in the United States, with women three times more likely to develop rheumatoid arthritis than men. The disease may begin at any age but usually appears when patients are in the third or fourth decade of life. Rheumatoid arthritis is discussed in greater detail in Chapter 16.

Prognosis
Prognosis varies depending on when a diagnosis is made (the earlier the better) and implementation of treatment. Without treatment, the disease progresses with poor outcomes.

Polymyositis

Polymyositis is a muscle disease involving muscle inflammation near the trunk or torso. It is a chronic condition resulting in severe weakness. Polymyositis is discussed in greater detail in Chapter 16.

Immunodeficiency Disorders

Immunodeficiency is caused by a loss of function of one or more immune system components. This can lead to increased risk of infection and cancer. Examples include inherited X-linked **hypogammaglobulinemia** (low antibody levels due to a B-cell defect). Secondary or acquired immunodeficiency can be caused by (particularly) viral infections, **splenectomy** (removal of the spleen), malnutrition, liver disease, **hypoproteinemia**, use of immunosuppressive drugs in patients with organ transplants, and radiation or chemotherapy for cancer treatment.

Immunodeficiency and its causes may be acute or chronic, with deficits classified by component or etiology. Changes in function vary greatly and may lead to the development of other diseases and conditions.

Signs and Symptoms
The development of *opportunistic infections* may occur because of immunodeficiency. These infections may be very severe and difficult to treat successfully. Often, resident *fungi* or *Candida* species may cause infections when normal body defenses become impaired. Organisms that are not normally pathogenic, such as *Pneumocystis carinii*, may become so, resulting in severe, life-threatening infections.

Anyone in an immunodeficient state should receive **prophylactic antimicrobial** drugs (also known as *preventative antibiotics*) before undergoing any invasive procedure. This includes any procedure that has direct access to the blood or tissues, such as tooth extraction. Because the body's immune surveillance may be decreased, there is an increased incidence of cancer because the body cannot destroy malignant cells as quickly as it should.

Etiology

Immunodeficiency may result from a partial or total loss of function. This may affect one or more immune system components and lead to increased risk of infections or cancers. **Table 10–8** lists examples of immunodeficiency disorders.

Primary deficiencies involve basic developmental failures, such as in the bone marrow and its production of stem cells. These deficiencies are often first noticed in infants and children and may be associated with other organ or systemic problems. X-linked hypogammaglobulinemia is defined as low antibody levels due to a B-cell defect. It is an example of a primary deficiency, as is hypoplasia of the thymus (called *DiGeorge's syndrome*).

Secondary deficiencies are acquired immunodeficiencies. Immune response is lost from certain specific causes that can occur any time during life. These include viral infections (and other infections), removal of the spleen (splenectomy), malnutrition, liver disease (such as hypoproteinemia), and use of immunosuppressive drugs, radiation, or chemotherapy. All these depress the production of leukocytes by the bone marrow. Glucocorticoids may cause this, as well as lymph node atrophy and immune response suppression.

Severe emotional or physical stress is believed to cause a temporary immunodeficiency state because of high levels of glucocorticoid secretion. AIDS or HIV infection may also cause secondary immunodeficiency by affecting the T-helper cells.

Treatment

Gamma globulin is often used as a replacement therapy for antibodies. Other treatments include the less-proven transplantation of bone marrow or the thymus gland.

AIDS

AIDS involves progressive impairment of the immune system. It is caused by HIV (**Figure 10–11A and B**). This virus destroys helper T lymphocytes to cause loss of immune response and increased chances of secondary infections and cancer. Many organ systems are affected by AIDS, usually resulting in death. AIDS is a chronic infectious disease. It develops over a long, latent period, followed by active infection (**Figure 10–12A, B, and C**).

The term *HIV positive* describes the presence of the virus but little to any clinical signs of the condition. Once the infection has become active, it is described as *AIDS*. It is possible to be HIV positive for many years, and current treatments have extended this period of time. Eventually, active infection develops. Unusual infections may be seen, such as pneumonia or cancers, with no other pathology, signifying the presence of active HIV infection and the need for testing.

TABLE 10–8 Immunodeficiency Disorders		
Immune Deficit	**Primary Disorder**	**Secondary Disorder**
B cell (humoral)	Congenital hypogammaglobulinemia	Kidney disease with globulin loss
T cell (cell mediated)	Thymic aplasia DiGeorge's syndrome	Hodgkin's disease, which is cancer of the lymph nodes Temporary disorders with some viruses, though it may also be related to AIDS (HIV infection)
B and T cell	Inherited combined immunodeficiency syndromes	Cytotoxic drugs (cancer chemotherapy), immunosuppressive drugs, radiation
Complement system	Inherited deficiency of one or more components	Cirrhosis (liver disease), malnutrition (decreased synthesis)
Phagocytes	Inherited chronic granulomatous diseases	Diabetes (decreased chemotaxis), immunosuppression (glucocorticoid drugs, neutropenia)

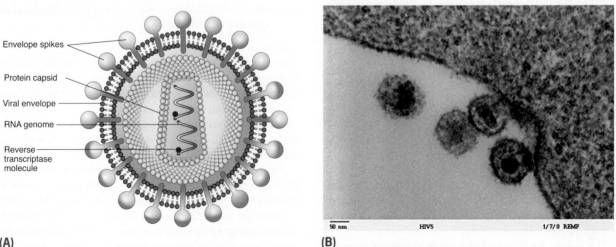

(A)

Envelope spikes

Protein capsid

Viral envelope

RNA genome

Reverse transcriptase molecule

50 nm   HIV5   1/7/0 REMF

(B)

Figure 10–11 The human immunodeficiency virus. (A) The virus consists of two molecules of RNA and molecules of reverse transcriptase. A protein capsid surrounds the genome. (B) A micrograph of the virus.

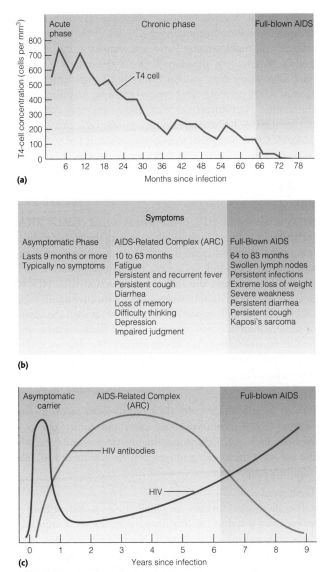

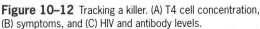

Figure 10–12 Tracking a killer. (A) T4 cell concentration, (B) symptoms, and (C) HIV and antibody levels.

The clinical manifestations of HIV differ between adults and children but basically include the following:

- Asymptomatic stage: No symptoms in general, although some patients develop a condition that appears similar to mononucleosis or a viral-like syndrome. Latency may persist for 10 years or more. Normal life is generally unaffected during this stage, although some patients experience swollen, firm lymph glands.

- Early symptomatic stage: Adenopathy, diarrhea, fatigue, night sweats, fevers, weight loss, neurologic symptoms related to HIV encephalopathy, and opportunistic infections may occur. If present, cytomegalovirus may cause peripheral neuropathy or HIV retinitis. Pneumonia may develop, with many pulmonary symptoms. Toxoplasmosis may affect the central nervous system. Multiple medications used for treatment can cause adverse side effects. More than 50 percent of patients in this stage report fatigue that greatly affects their normal activities.

- HIV advanced disease: May involve the central, peripheral, and autonomic nervous systems. Encephalopathy may lead to dementia, incontinence, and paraplegia. A variety of skin conditions may develop, such as seborrheic dermatitis, Kaposi's sarcoma, and scabies. Nutritional disorders may change the appearance of hair and nails. A variety of infections usually manifests. Painful sensory peripheral neuropathy is also commonly reported. Neuromuscular diseases may include osteomyelitis, bacterial myositis, and infectious arthritis. Lipodystrophy, or lipodystrophic syndrome, may cause central fat accumulation with visceral fat deposition and is related to *highly active antiviral therapy*. AIDS-related lymphomas may include Hodgkin's or non-Hodgkin's lymphomas and Burkitt's lymphoma. Many patients with HIV/AIDS die from resulting cardiopulmonary diseases.

To reduce the chance of transmission of HIV and AIDS, it is important to avoid unprotected sexual behavior involving multiple partners and sharing needles used to inject illegal drugs. Precautions that can be taken include using latex condoms during sex because other types may allow transmission of the HIV/AIDS virus. Blood transfusions are another method of transmission of the virus, although steps are now in place in the health care system to ensure that no contaminated blood is ever used for transfusion.

The role of the PTA when working with patients with AIDS or those who are immunosuppressed includes low impact physical therapy to maintain strength, prevent atrophy, and maintain endurance. The level of fatigue should help to determine the amount of physical activity that can be tolerated. The goals of physical therapy are to reduce pain, improve mobility, and promote independent activities of daily living. Other physical therapy interventions used for patients with HIV/AIDS include ultrasound, transcutaneous nerve stimulation, soft tissue massage, manual therapy, myofacial release, and craniosacral therapy.

The PTA should take special precautions when working with patients with HIV/AIDS. Personal protective equipment should be used, making sure that any part of the body likely to be exposed to blood, semen, or vaginal fluids is covered. After physical therapy all surfaces contacted by the patient should be disinfected with approved medical cleaning solutions.

RED FLAG

For the PTA and other health care professionals, protective personal equipment should be used at all times when dealing with HIV/AIDS patients. Universal precautions must be followed, and all body fluids must be considered "infected" and handled accordingly.

RED FLAG

AIDS was first discovered in 1981 and is considered a worldwide pandemic. It affects all individuals, including children. Life span after diagnosis has increased (because of advanced treatments) from 6 months to many years. AIDS has affected millions of people across the world and is still multiplying in sub-Saharan Africa and Asia.

Pathophysiology

HIV is a **retrovirus** (containing ribonucleic acid [RNA]) with two types, type 1 or 2. It develops slowly, with HIV-1 primarily seen in America and Europe and HIV-2 primarily seen in central Africa. It primarily affects the CD4 T-helper lymphocytes, also attacking macrophages and central nervous system cells. In early stages it affects lymphoid tissue and continues to use this tissue as a reservoir as the infection proceeds.

The core of HIV contains two RNA strands and the *reverse transcriptase* enzyme, with a spiked envelope of glycoproteins. The spikes help the virus to attach to human cells. Once inside the host cells, the viral RNA is converted into viral DNA, which integrates with human DNA. The virus can then control the human cells, using their resources to produce more viral cells.

The host cells eventually die, and new viruses "bud" out of them. Antibodies to the virus are delayed in appearing in the blood (usually taking between 3 and 7 weeks). Antibodies form more quickly during transmission into the blood and develop very slowly from sexual transmission.

Tests to indicate HIV use antibodies, and their slowness in developing creates difficulty in timely test results. Repeated testing is usually required. Antibodies fail to destroy all virus cells, probably because of the following:

- The HIV virus hides inside host cells in lymphoid tissue during the latent phase.
- There are frequent, slight mutations to the viral envelope, causing the antibodies to be less effective.
- Progressive T-helper cell and macrophage destruction eventually harms the entire immune system.

HIV must find entry into the patient's circulating blood and may be also transmitted in various body fluids, including semen and vaginal secretions. Blood contains the highest concentrations, with semen being next in concentration. Donated blood is tested for the virus. Organ donors who are HIV positive may also transmit the infection to recipients. Transmission to health care workers from infected patients may occur by accidental injury or the presence of open skin lesions. There is a higher risk of transmitting other infections such as hepatitis B from body fluid contact.

Highest risk patients for HIV include intravenous drug users and those with multiple sexual partners. The greatest increase in HIV cases is now seen in women, who may transmit the disease to their fetus (especially if AIDS is fully developed). Azidothymidine has been used in HIV- or AIDS-positive pregnant women to decrease risk of transmission of the disease to the infant. During nursing, breast milk can also transmit the virus to the infant. HIV is not transmitted by casual contact (such as touching or kissing an infected patient), sneezing, coughing, insect bites, toilet seats, or eating utensils.

The virus may survive up to 15 days at room temperature but is killed in temperatures over 60 degrees Celsius. Agents that kill the virus include autoclaving, disinfectants such as alcohol and bleach, and 2% glutaraldehyde.

RED FLAG
Exposure to HIV while working must be immediately followed by evaluation of the exposure source and by postexposure prophylaxis.

Signs and Symptoms
Patients with HIV are usually asymptomatic for years, although within 1 to 2 weeks of exposure they may experience a sore throat, fever, and body aches. As HIV progresses, symptoms include lymphadenopathy, weight loss, diarrhea, fatigue, and night sweats. Various malignant tumors in the body's systems may develop. Kaposi's sarcoma is a malignant skin lesion that was once rare but is now commonly seen in AIDS patients. This type of sarcoma may also affect the mouth, gastrointestinal tract, and respiratory system. It is characterized histologically by *spindle cells* mixed with vascular tissue. Frequent infections persist as the condition worsens, and malignancies often occur. In the later stages encephalopathy and various malignancies lead to dementia and death.

Etiology
AIDS is caused by HIV, or retroviruses that contain RNA. HIV attacks helper T lymphocytes, leaving the body defenseless against infection, malignancy, and nervous system damage. More than 33 million people are currently infected with the AIDS virus, and the time from infection with HIV to death is approximately 10 years. There is no cure or effective vaccine. It is usually spread by direct contact with the blood or semen of an infected person. Infected females can transfer the disease to their fetuses or infants. The disease is also commonly transferred through the use of needles shared by intravenous drug users.

Diagnosis
HIV is usually diagnosed via a blood test known as the *enzyme-linked immunosorbent assay* and confirmed by a *Western blot test*. Additional diagnostic methods include the constant monitoring of lymphocyte counts to evaluate immunocompetence.

Treatment
Although there is no cure for AIDS, the goal of treatment is to maintain a stable, healthy immune status via immunizations and anti-infective therapy. Nucleoside inhibitors and protease inhibitors are combined (known as highly active antiretroviral therapy, or HAART) for this purpose. However, these medications have serious adverse effects and toxicities. When malignancy exists, surgery is recommended to prolong life and provide as much comfort as possible. Health care practitioners must use protective clothing and equipment when working with HIV/AIDS patients due to the serious possibility of transmission.

Prognosis
Prognosis is only fair because AIDS is ultimately fatal but is improving due to the better medications that have been developed. Patients are living longer and experiencing less severe symptoms until they reach the final stages of disease.

X-Linked Agammaglobulinemia

Also known as Bruton agammaglobulinemia, this disease is a condition of severe B-cell deficiency.

Signs and Symptoms
This type of agammaglobulinemia primarily affects male infants. It causes severe, recurrent infections such as bacterial otitis media, bronchitis, and meningitis, usually after 4 to 6 months of age. Other symptoms include conjunctivitis, dental caries, and symptoms that mimic rheumatoid arthritis.

Etiology

X-linked agammaglobulinemia is caused by a defect in the Bruton tyrosine kinase found in B cells and myeloid and erythroid cells. Immunoglobulins are absent, and circulating B cells and T cells are abnormally missing or low. Because the disease is genetic, parents of a child with this condition should be counseled about having more children.

Diagnosis

This condition is diagnosed based on clinical findings, age of patient at onset, and family history (of anyone who died from a severe infection). Tests include *immunoelectrophoresis*, which shows decreased immunoglobulin levels, but this form of testing is not usable until 6 to 8 months of age. Other tests include finding normal T-cell levels when B cells are entirely missing or low.

Treatment

Treatment for X-linked agammaglobulinemia strives to improve immune defenses, control infections, and relieve the arthritic symptoms. Intravenous immune globulins are given every 2 to 4 weeks, as are (sometimes) fresh frozen plasma infusions. Antibiotics are also sometimes used. *NOTE: Children with this condition must never be immunized with live virus vaccines, and immunosuppressive drugs or corticosteroids must never be administered.*

Prognosis

Although incurable, regular immune globulin infusions may allow a nearly normal lifestyle.

Thymic Hypoplasia

Also known as *DiGeorge's syndrome*, this condition involves a congenital immunodeficiency caused from a small or absent thymus.

Signs and Symptoms

Thymic hypoplasia causes specific structural anomalies in the body: eyes that are wide set and downward slanted, ears that are low set with notched pinnas, a smaller than normal mouth, and cardiovascular defects. Also, the parathyroid glands are absent or underdeveloped. Other conditions that may be present include tetany, hypocalcemia, and/or hypoparathyroidism. There is often some cognitive impairment and higher susceptibility to severe infections.

Etiology

Thymic hypoplasia is caused by abnormal development of the pharyngeal pouches, causing thymus developmental defects. There are both complete and partial forms of this disease. This means the thymus is either absent or very small, influencing T-cell and B-cell counts and normal antibody production. Most patients show abnormal development of chromosome 22.

Diagnosis

Diagnosis is established through reduced T-cell levels and two of these three features: cardiovascular defects, hypocalcemia lasting more than 3 weeks, and a microdeletion of chromosome 22. Radiographic studies show thymus gland defects. Low serum calcium levels, high serum phosphorus levels, and lack of parathyroid hormone show hypoparathyroidism.

Treatment

Treatment involves intravenous infusion to replace calcium depletion and restore electrolyte balance. Also, parathyroid hormone and vitamin D may be replaced. Intravenous immune globulin may be helpful, and repair of cardiac defects may be attempted. Thymus transplant may be indicated. Parents are instructed to keep the infant from any exposure to people with symptoms of infection.

Prognosis

The complete form of this condition is usually fatal in early childhood. Those with the partial form may actually see their immune function improve with age.

Hypersensitivity Reactions

Hypersensitivity or allergic reactions from normally harmless substances may occur (rarely), although they have the potential to be quite damaging. They stimulate an inflammatory response in the body and include four basic types (**Table 10–9**).

Type I: Allergic Reactions

Allergies, particularly in young children, appear to be on the increase and may result in hay fever, skin rashes, anaphylaxis, and vomiting. Allergies are often inherited, with familiar allergies referred to as *atopic hypersensitivity reactions*. Antigens are usually referred to as *allergens*, which may be chemicals, foods, drugs, or pollens. Allergies can be singular or multiple and can change over time. Common foods that are often allergenic include nuts, shellfish, and strawberries. Drugs that often cause hypersensitivities include aspirin, penicillin, local anesthetics, and sulfa drugs. Cross-allergies may cause an individual allergic to a certain drug to become allergic to other drugs from the same drug class or family.

Mechanism

When a patient is exposed to a certain allergen and develops IgE antibodies from B lymphocytes, a type I hypersensitivity begins. The antibodies attach to **mast cells** in various

TABLE 10–9	Types of Hypersensitivities	
Type	**Example**	**Mode and Effects**
I	Anaphylaxis, hay fever	IgE is bound to mast cells, histamine and chemical mediators are released, causing immediate inflammation and pruritus
II	ABO blood incompatibility	IgG or IgM reacts with cell antigen, activating complement, causing cell lysis and phagocytosis
III	Autoimmune disorders such as glomerulonephritis and SLE	Antigen–antibody complex deposits in tissues, activating complement to cause inflammation and vasculitis
IV	Contact dermatitis, transplant rejection	Antigen binds to T lymphocytes, sensitizing them to release lymphokines and cause delayed inflammation

locations to create *sensitized* mast cells (**Figure 10–13**). Mast cells are connective tissue cells found in large numbers in the respiratory and digestive mucosa. When reexposure to an antigen occurs, the allergen attaches to the IgE antibody on the mast cell. This stimulates release of chemical mediators such as histamine, causing an inflammatory reaction, vasodilation, and increased capillary permeability at the site, with swelling and redness of local tissues.

Initial histamine release may irritate nerve endings to cause mild pain or itching. Prostaglandins and leukotrienes, released in a second phase of reaction, can cause similar effects. If the respiratory mucosa of the lungs becomes sensitized, **bronchoconstriction** may occur, releasing mucus that obstructs the airways. This condition is commonly referred to as *asthma*.

Signs and Symptoms

An allergic reaction's signs and symptoms occur on the second or any subsequent reexposure to a specific allergen. The first exposure just causes formation of antibodies and sensitized mast cells. The target area becomes swollen and red, with possible **vesicles** or blisters, and an itchy (**pruritic**) sensation. The types of allergic reactions include hay fever (allergic rhinitis), food allergies, eczema (atopic dermatitis), and asthma. The following list summarizes these types of allergic reactions:

- *Hay fever (allergic rhinitis)*: Frequent sneezing, increased watery nasal secretions, itching of the nose and its passages, reddening of the eyes, watering of the eyes, and itching of the eyes. Hay fever may be seasonal due to plant pollens or can occur any time throughout the year.
- *Food allergies*: Nausea, vomiting, diarrhea, rash (hives), and, in severe cases, the hives may appear on the pharyngeal mucosa to obstruct airflow. It is vital to watch for respiratory difficulties associated with skin rash.
- *Eczema (atopic dermatitis)*: Chronic, often genetically linked skin condition common in infants and young children. Skin rash may occur on face, trunk, or extremities and is associated with foods, fabrics, and a dry atmosphere. Eczema may recur during childhood or even adulthood.

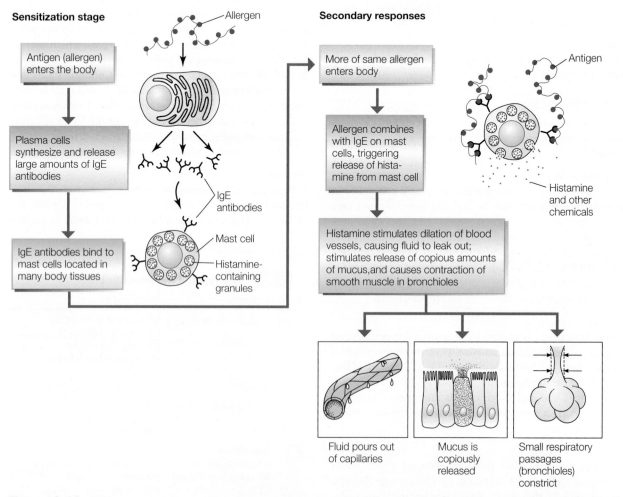

Figure 10–13 Allergic reaction. Antigen stimulates the production of massive amounts of IgE, a type of antibody produced by plasma cells. IgE attaches to mast cells. This is the sensitization stage. When the antigen enters again, it binds to the IgE antibodies on the mast cells, triggering a massive release of histamine and other chemicals. Histamine, in turn, causes blood vessels to dilate and become leaky. This triggers the production of mucus in the respiratory tract. In some people, the chemicals released by the mast cells also cause the small air-carrying ducts in the lungs to constrict, making breathing difficult.

- *Asthma*: Lung disorder resulting from allergic response in the bronchial mucosa, interfering with airflow. Often seen in families, three atopic conditions may occur: asthma, eczema, and hay fever.

Anaphylaxis or Anaphylactic Shock

Anaphylaxis is a severe systemic condition that may be life threatening. It causes airway obstruction, decreased blood pressure, and severe hypoxia. Anaphylaxis may result from eating nuts and shellfish, from insect stings, from administration of penicillin, or from injection of local anesthetics. These types of reactions usually occur within minutes of exposure.

In anaphylaxis, large amounts of chemical mediators (histamines) are released from mast cells into the systemic circulation. This quick release results in systemic vasodilation and a sudden, severe decrease in blood pressure. Edema of the lung mucosa and constriction of the bronchi and bronchioles occur, to obstruct airflow. Loss of consciousness occurs within minutes due to a marked lack of oxygen.

Initial symptoms of anaphylaxis include generalized itching or tingling, coughing, and difficulty in breathing. Additional symptoms that may quickly develop include weakness, dizziness, fainting, fear, and panic (**Table 10–10**). The eyes, lips, tongue, hands, and feet may show signs of edema (**Figure 10–14**). Hives (urticaria) may appear on the skin, with general collapse within minutes.

> **RED FLAG**
> Anaphylactic shock is a severe, generalized IgE-mediated hypersensitivity reaction characterized by marked respiratory distress and hypotension.

Treatment
Anaphylaxis is treated immediately with an epinephrine injection, which acts as the normal hormone called *adrenaline*. In the early stages of an allergic reaction, antihistamines or chlorpheniramine are useful. For severe or prolonged reactions, glucocorticoids or cortisone derivatives may be used.

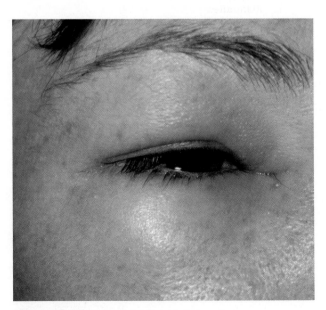

Figure 10–14 The effects of anaphylaxis.

Body Area	Signs and Symptoms	Comments
TABLE 10–10 Anaphylaxis Signs and Symptoms		
Skin	Hives, pruritus, tingling, warmth	Chemical mediators and histamine irritate sensory nerves
Respiration	Cough, difficulty breathing, tight feeling, wheezing	Chemical mediators cause smooth muscle contraction in the bronchioles, edema, and increased secretions; this leads to lack of oxygen and narrow airways
Cardiovascular	Decreased blood pressure with rapid or weak pulse that may be irregular	Chemical mediators cause generalized vasodilation, which leads to low blood pressure; the heart rate is increased by the sympathetic nervous system
Central nervous system	Early anxiety and fear, then dizziness, weakness, and loss of consciousness	Sympathetic response occurs early; followed later by lack of oxygen to the brain because of low blood pressure and respiratory obstruction

Glucocorticoids may be administered orally, by injection, or topically.

To determine the specific cause of an allergy, skin tests can be performed. A very small amount of antigen is injected intradermally. The patient's skin is observed for any **erythema** (redness), indicating a positive skin reaction. Once the causative antigen has been identified, the patient should avoid all contact with it. Another method of treatment involves desensitization, wherein repeated injections of very small amounts of an antigen are given. These injections create a "blocking antibody" that can reduce the allergic response.

Type II: Cytotoxic Hypersensitivity

This type of hypersensitivity occurs because of an antigen present on a cell membrane, which may be a normal or foreign component. As circulating IgG antibodies react, the cell is destroyed by phagocytosis or the release of cytolytic enzymes that are related to complement activation.

An incompatible blood transfusion is an example of a type II (cytotoxic) hypersensitivity reaction. Type A blood means a patient has type A antigens on the red blood cells, with anti-B antibodies in the blood. If type B blood is transfused into a type A patient, the antigen–antibody reaction destroys red blood cells in type A blood. A related type of blood incompatibility is the Rh factor.

Type III: Immune Complex Hypersensitivity

A type III reaction is defined as an antigen combining with an antibody to form a complex that is deposited in tissue. This usually occurs in blood vessel walls and activates complement. Inflammation and tissue destruction result.

Diseases believed to be caused by immune complexes include glomerulonephritis, rheumatoid arthritis, and serum sickness. Serum sickness occurs less today because of the reduced use of animal serum for passive immunization. Another example of a type III reaction is an *Arthus* reaction, wherein localized inflammation and tissue necrosis occur when an immune complex lodges in a vessel wall, causing vasculitis. An example is "farmer's lung," caused by inhalation of particles from a mold that grows on hay.

Type IV: Cell-Mediated or Delayed Hypersensitivity

Type IV hypersensitivity is described as a delayed response by sensitized T lymphocytes to antigens. Chemical mediators such as lymphokines are released, causing an inflammatory response and destruction of the antigen. This type of reaction is used when testing for tuberculosis. Another example is organ transplant rejection.

A type IV reaction causes contact dermatitis via chemicals such as cosmetics, dyes, metals, soaps, or plant toxins. Other examples include reactions to rubber or latex products, which are signified by rashes within 48 to 96 hours. However, it should be noted that *serious* reactions to rubber or latex are considered type I, which are more serious (and may result in anaphylaxis).

SUMMARY

The immune system is an important defense system for the body. When it is weakened or compromised, the body cannot adequately defend itself against invading microorganisms. Primary immune disorders are classified as hypersensitivity disorders or immune deficiency disorders. Hypersensitivity disorders include allergies and autoimmune disorders. The immune deficiency disease known as AIDS is one of the most common and debilitating fatal conditions of the immune system. It is caused by HIV. Those at highest risk for contracting HIV/AIDS include intravenous drug users and those having unprotected sex with multiple sexual partners. Diagnostic testing for immune disorders includes skin testing, complete blood cell counts, and some specific antibody studies. Treatment for immune disorders varies with the specific disorder. Some immune disorders are severe, requiring long-term therapy, whereas others are very mild.

REVIEW QUESTIONS

Select the best response to each question.

1. Serum sickness is defined as which type of hypersensitivity?
   a. I
   b. II
   c. III
   d. IV
2. Antigens are usually made of which of the following?
   a. complex proteins
   b. glycoproteins
   c. polysaccharides
   d. all of the above
3. Macrophages develop from what type of cells?
   a. mast cells
   b. monocytes

c. helper T cells
   d. basophils
4. Which of the following cells play vital roles in the development of AIDS?
   a. T-helper cells
   b. monocytes
   c. T-killer cells
   d. both A and C
5. The most common antibody found in the blood is
   a. IgG
   b. IgA
   c. IgM
   d. IgE
6. Transplantation of tissues or organs between members of the same species is called
   a. a xenograft
   b. an autograft
   c. an allograft
   d. an isograft
7. ABO blood incompatibility is an example of which hypersensitivity type?
   a. I
   b. II
   c. III
   d. V
8. A butterfly-shaped facial rash is a characteristic of what disease process?
   a. rheumatoid arthritis
   b. pernicious anemia
   c. myasthenia gravis
   d. lupus erythematosus
9. A primary disorder involving B-cell immune deficit is known as what?
   a. congenital hypogammaglobulinemia
   b. DiGeorge's syndrome
   c. an inherited deficiency of one or more components
   d. an inherited chronic granulomatous disease
10. HIV can survive for how long at room temperature?
   a. 30 minutes
   b. 90 minutes
   c. 3 days
   d. 15 days

CASE STUDIES

Karen Coupe, PT, DPT, MSEd

Case 1

A 31-year-old woman was diagnosed with SLE 10 years ago. She was referred to outpatient physical therapy. Complications include Raynaud's phenomenon. The PT evaluation reveals the beginning stages of ulnar deviation deformity of the bilateral wrists with swan neck deformity on the second and third digits of the right hand, bilateral knee flexion contractures, and decreased gait cadence and step and stride length. Plan of care includes modalities, splinting, range of motion, strengthening, gait training, and education in energy conservation.

1. What is the etiology and pathogenesis of SLE?
2. What are the common clinical manifestations?
3. This patient has Raynaud's phenomenon. How does this present? What modalities need to be avoided?
4. Why would you suspect the patient has decreased cadence and step and stride length during gait?
5. Explain the rationale behind the PT plan of care for energy conservation techniques. List some examples.

Case 2

A 58-year-old man was referred to outpatient PT for general strengthening, gait, and balance activities. Patient was HIV positive for 10 years and was diagnosed with AIDS 8 years ago. Patient is on a combination of antiretroviral medications and presents with the following complications: left extremity peripheral neuropathy, left extremity weakness, gait ataxia, and mild short-term memory loss. Current level of function: Ambulates with a front-wheeled rolling walker with dyspnea after 15 feet. Requires minimal to moderate assistance for cooking, cleaning, dressing, bathing, and grooming activities.

1. Explain the general etiology and pathogenesis of HIV. What determines when HIV progresses to AIDS?
2. What are the transmission methods of HIV/AIDS? What are the myths surrounding the methods of transmission?

3. Based on the method of transmission, what standard precautions should be used by the PTA?
4. This patient has dyspnea with ambulation. What would you suspect is the reasoning behind this problem? How would you adjust your treatment for this issue?
5. How would the patient's short-term memory loss affect therapy sessions? What would you do to assist the patient in this matter?

WEBSITES

http://aids.gov/

http://pathmicro.med.sc.edu/ghaffar/hyper00.htm

http://www.biology-online.org/1/11_cell_defense_2.htm

http://www.healthline.com/search?q1=immune+disorders

http://www.hmc.psu.edu/healthinfo/i/immunodeficiency.htm

http://uhaweb.hartford.edu/BUGL/immune.htm

http://www.lupusny.org/

http://www.merck.com/mmpe/sec13/ch163/ch163b.html

http://www.nlm.nih.gov/medlineplus/ency/article/000821.htm

http://www.sciencedaily.com/articles/t/transplant_rejection.htm

Pathology of the Body Systems

Cardiovascular Disorders

LEARNING OBJECTIVES

After completion of the chapter the reader should be able to

1. Compare atherosclerosis and arteriosclerosis.
2. Describe myocardial infarction and common diagnostic tests.
3. Discuss congestive heart failure.
4. List risk factors causing coronary artery disease.
5. Explain rheumatic fever and its effects on the heart.
6. Distinguish endocarditis, myocarditis, and pericarditis.
7. Describe phlebitis, thrombophlebitis, and varicose veins.
8. Distinguish Raynaud's disease and Buerger's disease.

KEY TERMS

Afterload: Force against which cardiac muscle shortens.

Angioplasty: Repair of a narrowed blood vessel via surgery or other angiographic procedures

Anoxia: A total lack of oxygen in tissue.

Arteriosclerosis: Hardening of the arteries.

Asystole: Absence of contractions of the heart, also known as "cardiac standstill."

Atheroma: Athermatous plaque; a plaque-like deposit of material in the coronary arteries.

Atherosclerosis: A type of arteriosclerosis wherein fatty deposits collect along the walls of arteries that may harden and eventually block them.

Auscultation: A diagnostic technique of listening for sounds within the body.

Bolus: A single, relatively large dose of a drug.

Bruit: An abnormal sound heard during auscultation; it results from blood flowing through a narrow or partially occluded artery.

Cardiomegaly: Enlargement of the heart.

Cardiomyopathy: Chronic disease of the heart muscle, wherein it is abnormally enlarged, thickened, or stiffened.

Coronary artery disease: A condition characterized by blockage of the blood vessels (coronary arteries) that supply the heart muscle.

Defibrillation: Process of using an electronic device to shock the heart to stop rapid, irregular heartbeat and restore normal rhythm.

Depolarization: Reduction of a membrane potential to a less negative value.

Diaphoresis: Sweating.

Ejection fraction: Fraction of the total ventricular filling volume that is ejected during each ventricular contraction.

Hemoptysis: Spitting up blood.

Holter monitor: A portable device used for recording cardiac activity over 24 hours or longer; the patient wears it throughout the day and keeps a journal of stressful events, which is compared with the monitor's record.

Hypovolemia: A decrease in the volume of blood

KEY TERMS CONTINUED

plasma, which decreases overall blood volume.

Ischemia: Insufficient supply of blood to an organ, usually because of a blocked artery.

Ligate: To tie or bind with a ligature.

Microcirculation: Flow of blood or lymph through the smallest vessels of the body (usually the venules, capillaries, and arterioles).

Murmurs: Blowing sounds heard when listening to the heart or blood vessels with a stethoscope.

Myocardium: The middle, thickest layer of the heart composed of cardiac muscle.

Perfusion: Delivery of oxygen and other nutrients to the tissues by the blood.

Plaque: A deposit of hardened material lining a blood vessel.

Repolarization: Restoration of a resting potential across a membrane.

Resect: To cut out part or all of an organ or other body

structure.

Sclerosing: Hardening, as of a body part.

Stroke: Sudden death of brain cells in a localized area due to inadequate blood flow.

Thromboembolism: Obstruction of a blood vessel with thrombotic material carried by the blood from another site in the body.

Thrombosis: Formation or presence of a thrombus.

Thrombus: A stationary blood clot along the wall of a blood vessel.

Toxic: A state of being poisoned or poisonous.

Ultrasonography: Imaging of deep body structures by recording the echoes of pulses of ultrasonic waves directed into the tissues.

Vasospastic: Related to, or an agent that produces spasms of the blood vessels.

Overview

As part of the cardiovascular system, the circulatory system transports oxygen and nutrients needed for metabolic processes to the tissues. It also carries waste products from the cellular metabolism to the kidneys and other excretory organs for elimination. Another function is the circulation of electrolytes and hormones needed to regulate body function. Cardiovascular disorders are the number one cause of morbidity and mortality in the United States. There are many disorders of the heart and blood vessels, but this chapter focuses on the most common of these disorders.

Anatomy and Physiology

The cardiovascular system consists of the heart and blood vessels. The heart pumps blood through the pulmonary and systemic circulations (**Figure 11–1**). The heart lies within the *mediastinum* between the lungs and is composed of a double-walled *pericardial sac*. It is anchored to the diaphragm by an outer, fibrous *pericardium*. The pericardial cavity contains a lubricating fluid between the layers. The cardiac muscle (**myocardium**) is the middle layer. The heart's inner layer (*endocardium*) also forms the four valves of the heart, which separate the four chambers and only allow a *one-way flow* of blood.

The four chambers in the heart are the left atrium, left ventricle, right atrium, and right ventricle (**Figure 11–2**). The atria are separated from the ventricles by the atrioventricular (AV) valves. On the right side the AV valves comprise the tricuspid valve (with three cusps) and on the left side, the

mitral (bicuspid) valve (with two cusps). The aortic and pulmonary valves found at the exits to the large arteries from the ventricles are called "semilunar valves," and each has three cusps (**Figure 11–3A and B**). The interventricular *septum* separates the heart's left and right sides.

Blood enters the heart from the inferior and superior vena cava into the right atrium and then enters into the right ventricle. When the right ventricle is filled, unoxygenated blood passes the pulmonary valve into the pulmonary artery and travels to the lungs, where carbon dioxide and oxygen are exchanged. The oxygenated blood returns to the heart through the pulmonary vein and empties into the left atrium through the mitral valve into the left ventricle. After filling the left ventricle, the blood flows into the aorta and out to the body tissues (Figure 11–2).

The cardiac conduction system consists of specialized cardiac muscle cells. Its components include the sinoatrial (SA) node, the AV node, the AV bundle (bundle of His), the bundle branches, and the Purkinje fibers (**Figure 11–4**). A complete phase of atrial contraction and ventricular contraction, followed by relaxation, makes up the cardiac cycle. On an electrocardiogram this appears as the "PQRST" segment. The P wave represents the contraction and **depolarization** of the atria. The QRS complex correlates with the contraction of the ventricles. The T wave represents the recovery (**repolarization**) of the ventricles (**Figure 11–5**). One cardiac cycle comprises one heartbeat. In normal adults this occurs about 60 to 100 times per minute.

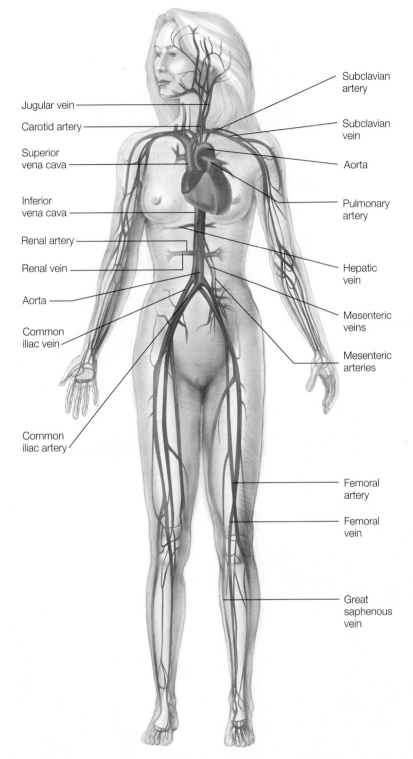

Jugular vein

Carotid artery

Superior
vena cava

Inferior
vena cava

Renal artery

Renal vein

Aorta

Common
iliac vein

Common
iliac artery

Subclavian
artery

Subclavian
vein

Aorta

Pulmonary
artery

Hepatic
vein

Mesenteric
veins

Mesenteric
arteries

Femoral
artery

Femoral
vein

Great
saphenous
vein

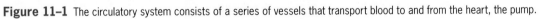

Figure 11–1 The circulatory system consists of a series of vessels that transport blood to and from the heart, the pump.

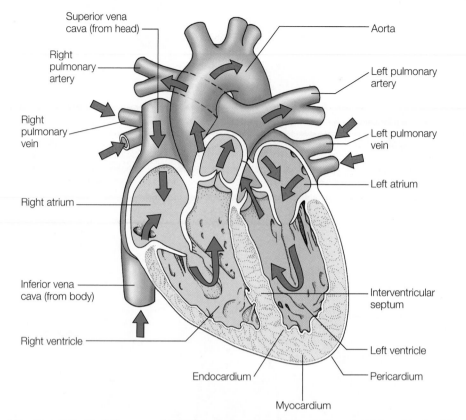

Superior vena
cava (from head)

Aorta

Right
pulmonary
artery

Left pulmonary
artery

Right
pulmonary
vein

Left pulmonary
vein

Left atrium

Right atrium

Inferior vena
cava (from body)

Interventricular
septum

Right ventricle

Left ventricle

Endocardium

Pericardium

Myocardium

Figure 11–2 Blood flow through the heart. Deoxygenated (carbon dioxide–enriched) blood (blue arrows) flows into the right atrium from the systemic circulation and is pumped into the right ventricle. The blood is then pumped from the right ventricle into the pulmonary artery, which delivers it to the lungs. In the lungs, the blood releases its carbon dioxide and absorbs oxygen. Reoxygenated blood (red arrows) is returned to the left atrium, then flows into the left ventricle, which pumps it to the rest of the body through the systemic circuit.

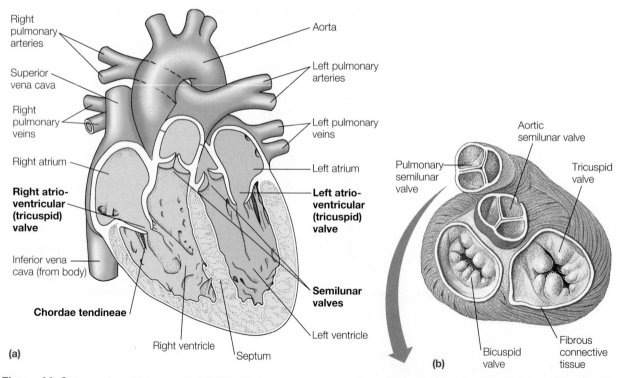

Right
pulmonary
arteries

Aorta

Superior
vena cava

Left pulmonary
arteries

Right
pulmonary
veins

Left pulmonary
veins

Right atrium

Left atrium

**Right atrio-
ventricular
(tricuspid)
valve**

**Left atrio-
ventricular
(tricuspid)
valve**

Inferior vena
cava (from body)

**Semilunar
valves**

Chordae tendineae

Left ventricle

(a)

Right ventricle

Septum

Aortic
semilunar valve

Pulmonary
semilunar
valve

Tricuspid
valve

(b)

Bicuspid
valve

Fibrous
connective
tissue

Figure 11–3 Heart valves. (A) A cross section of the heart showing the four chambers and the location of the major vessels and valves. (B) A view of the heart from above, with the major vessels removed to show the valves.

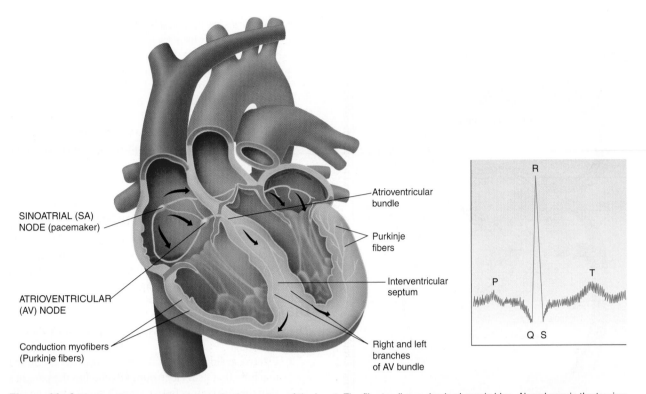

Figure 11–4 The impulse generation and conduction system of the heart. The fibrotendinous ring is shown in blue. Also shown is the tracing of an EKG. The P wave corresponds to atrial depolarization, the QRS complex to ventricular depolarization, and the T wave to ventricular repolarization.

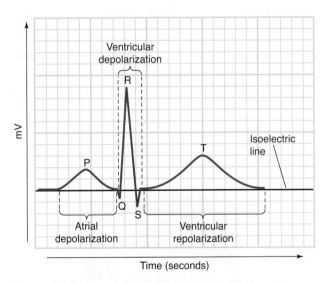

Figure 11–5 Characteristic features of a normal electrocardiogram.

Cardiac function can be measured as follows:

- *Cardiac output* is the volume of blood ejected by a ventricle in 1 minute: it depends on heart rate and *stroke volume*. Stroke volume is defined as the volume pumped from one ventricle in one contraction. At rest, the heart pumps an amount equal to the total blood volume in the body every minute and can increase output up to five times the minimum volume when required.
- Stroke volume varies with sympathetic stimulation and venous return. During exercise, stress, or infection cardiac output increases greatly.
- *Cardiac reserve* refers to the heart's ability to increase blood output in response to increased demand.
- *Preload* refers to venous return and is defined as the pressure of blood entering the heart from the general circulation.
- *Afterload* is defined as the pressure the heart must push against when it ejects blood into the circulation system. It is controlled by the *peripheral resistance* to the opening of the semilunar valves, which are involved with the ejection of blood from the ventricles.

Blood distribution throughout the body involves a closed system made up of arteries, capillaries, and veins:

- Pulmonary circulation allows the exchange of oxygen and carbon dioxide in the lungs.
- Systemic circulation provides for the exchange of nutrients and wastes between the blood and body cells.
- Arteries transport blood away from the heart to the lungs or body tissues.
- Arterioles branch off of arteries to control the amount of blood flowing into the capillaries via the degree of contraction (vasoconstriction) or relaxation (vasodilation) of vessel walls.

Figure 11–6 depicts the two sections of the circulatory system.

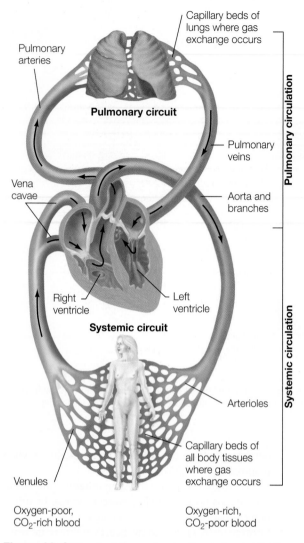

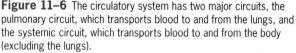

Figure 11–6 The circulatory system has two major circuits, the pulmonary circuit, which transports blood to and from the lungs, and the systemic circuit, which transports blood to and from the body (excluding the lungs).

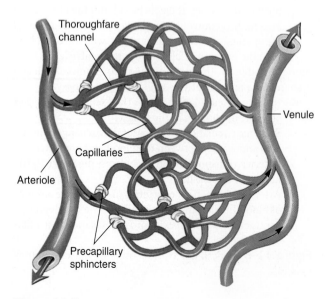

Figure 11–7 A network of capillaries.

- Capillaries are tiny vessels that form the **microcirculation** via numerous networks, with very slowly moving blood flow (**Figure 11–7**).
- Small venules conduct blood from the capillaries to veins, flowing toward the heart.
- Veins collect blood from the venules, storing up to 70% of the body's blood at any given time: the veins therefore act as "capacitance vessels," with venal blood flow depending on skeletal muscle action, respiration, and gravity.
- Valves in the larger veins (in the arms and legs) help keep blood flowing to the heart.

Common Signs and Symptoms

Signs and symptoms of cardiovascular disorders include arrhythmias, dysrhythmias, chest pain, edema, shock, fever, kidney disorders, circulation problems, breathing problems, bluish skin discoloration, fainting, and fatigue.

Diagnostic Tests

The following are basic diagnostic tests used for cardiovascular disorders:

- Electrocardiogram (ECG): An electrocardiograph is a machine that uses electrodes attached to the patient's skin that are connected to wires through which amplified electrical impulses from the heart are transmitted (**Figure 11–8**). The results of these impulses are printed onto a paper record known as an electrocardiogram. It is used to diagnose arrhythmias, myocardial infarction (MI), infection, and pericarditis. The patient may also wear a **Holter monitor** to record ECGs during daily activities. A Holter monitor is a portable system for recording a patient's cardiac activity over a 24-hour period or longer. It can be programmed to record cardiac information continuously or periodically (**Figure 11–9**). A *transthoracic echocardiogram* (an ultrasonic procedure) is commonly used to measure valve functions such as **ejection fraction** of the left and right ventricles.

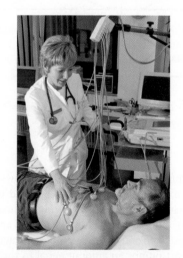

Figure 11–8 An electrocardiograph is a machine that uses electrodes attached to the patient's skin that are connected to wires through which amplified electrical impulses from the heart are transmitted.

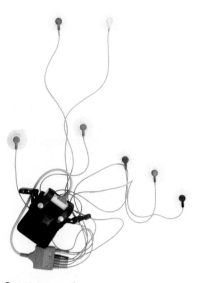

Figure 11–9 A Holter monitor.

- **Auscultation**: A stethoscope is used to detect valvular abnormalities or abnormal shunts of blood that cause *murmurs* and recorded by a phonocardiograph. It is very useful for evaluating lung, heart, and abdominal sounds.
- *Stress tests*: Used to assess general cardiovascular function and to check for exercise-induced problems. These tests are often used to evaluate an individual's health risks for insurance purposes. Stress tests are designed to diagnose heart disease that a standard, resting ECG cannot detect, to determine the patient's energy performance capacity, and to prescribe a specially designed exercise plan. During stress tests a cardiologist must be present. The patient either walks on a treadmill or rides a stationary bicycle while attached to an electrocardiograph. A *thallium stress test* is usually done along with a basic stress test. It is useful in determining how well blood flows to the heart muscle via the injection of a radioactive contrast medium known as thallium.
- *Chest x-rays*: Used to show the heart's shape, size, and possible evidence of pulmonary congestion. *Nuclear imaging* involves the use of radioactive substances (such as thallium) to better see within the heart. *Tomographic studies* illustrate various levels of a tissue mass within the heart.
- *Positron emission tomography scans*: These are nuclear medicine imaging techniques that produce three-dimensional body images. Gamma rays are used via computerized scanners that reproduce body images in great detail. The patient is injected with a radioactive isotope and lies on a movable table. The scan is accomplished as the table moves through a circular scanning device.
- *Cardiac catheterization*: Involves passing a catheter through a specific blood vessel (usually in the leg) into a ventricle to determine heart function, including pressure, valve action, central venous pressure, and pulmonary capillary wedge pressure. Contrast dye is injected, and fluoroscopy is used to monitor blood movements and to visualize any abnormalities.

- *Coronary angiography*: An x-ray visualization of the blood vessels; during this procedure the patient is given a sedative and a local anesthetic into the inguinal region of the abdomen. Then, a catheter is threaded into a peripheral artery toward the head. A contrast medium is injected, and video fluoroscopic studies are recorded as the patient lies completely still for up to 1 hour. It is used to visualize blood flow in the coronary arteries (**Figure 11–10**) and assess any obstructions to determine which other procedures can be used.
- *Doppler* ultrasonography: Process of examining structures within the body by the use of high-frequency sound waves. It is used to assess blood flow in peripheral vessels via a handheld transducer that records blood flow sounds when placed over a blood vessel. This technique is used to monitor moving substances or body structures such as the blood or the heart. Doppler ultrasonography is commonly used to image heart functions, locate vessel obstructions, localize the placenta, and observe fetal sounds. It is also called *Doppler scanning*.
- *Blood tests*: Used to assess serum triglyceride and cholesterol levels as well as other blood components. For example, the most important tests related to MI include those that measure serum enzymes and isoenzymes, including lactic dehydrogenase type 1, creatine phosphokinase with M and B subunits, and aspartate aminotransferase. Other indicators are abnormal levels of serum electrolytes such as potassium and sodium. For cardiovascular disorders, other common tests include those to determine C-reactive protein levels and the erythrocyte sedimentation rate test.

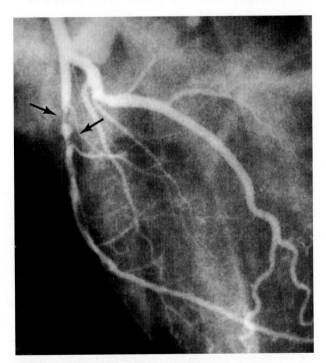

Figure 11–10 A coronary angiogram illustrating segmental narrowing (arrows).

■ *Arterial blood gas determination*: Used in shock or MI to check current oxygen levels, carbon dioxide levels, and acid-base balances (pH). The test determines how well the lungs are moving oxygen into the blood and removing carbon dioxide from the blood.

Cardiovascular Rehabilitation

A patient with a cardiovascular condition is treated with three general phases of physical therapy. These phases are listed in **Table 11–1**.

Common Diseases of the Cardiovascular System

Common diseases of the cardiovascular system include those that affect either the heart or the blood vessels. Diseases of the heart include coronary artery disease, angina pectoris, MI, arrhythmia, hypertension, congestive heart failure, cardiomyopathy, rheumatic heart disease, carditis, and valvular heart disease. Diseases of the blood vessels include phlebitis, varicose veins, hemorrhage, and shock.

Diseases of the Heart

Cardiovascular diseases include many varied disorders of both the heart itself and the circulatory system. Some disorders cause the rhythm of the heartbeats to become irregular, whereas others result in chest pain, heart failure, shock, fever, breathing difficulties, discoloration, edema (swelling), fatigue, and fainting. Nearly one-third of all deaths in Western countries are attributed to heart disease, usually either coronary artery disease or hypertension. Many heart diseases can lead to premature death.

Coronary Artery Disease

Coronary artery disease (CAD) involves the arteries supplying the myocardium. The arteries are marked by atherosclerotic deposits with a thrombus blocking them, causing temporary cardiac **ischemia** and eventually a MI (**Figure 11–11**).

Signs and Symptoms

The first symptom of CAD is usually angina pectoris. As the disease progresses, the more severe pain of MI is described as burning, squeezing, or crushing, with subsequent

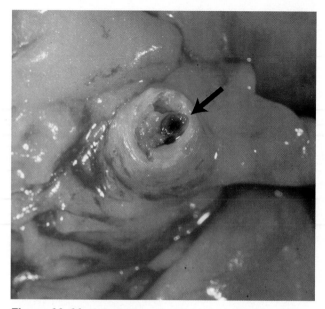

Figure 11–11 Marked atherosclerosis of coronary artery with thrombus blocking artery (arrow).

radiation to the arm, neck, or jaw. It may then cause nausea, vomiting, and weakness. An ECG can show visible changes when this occurs.

Etiology

Arteries narrow and develop **atherosclerosis** because of deposits of fat-containing substances called **plaque** in the interiors of arteries (**Figure 11–12**). The myocardium must have adequate blood supply to function. Atherosclerosis causes constriction of the coronary arteries, resulting in many consequences. The plaque-like deposit of material is called an *atheromatous plaque* or **atheroma**. The plaques, which become surrounded by fibrous tissue, are called *stable plaques*. Therefore, the small artery becomes permanently narrowed (**Figure 11–13**).

> **RED FLAG**
> CAD may produce no symptoms in older adults due to a decrease in sympathetic response. Dyspnea and fatigue are two key signals of ischemia in active, older adults. CAD may manifest slightly differently in men compared with women, with women usually experiencing more fatigue than men.

TABLE 11–1 Phases of Cardiovascular Rehabilitation

Phase	Location	Type of Rehabilitation
I	Inpatient setting	Ankle pump exercises to prevent deep vein thromboses Encouraging positive family support Gait training Patient education about life changes that may occur because of a cardiovascular condition Teaching how to transfer with assistance Teaching the importance of following cardiac precautions concerning the condition Teaching the patient bed mobility skills
II	Outpatient settings	Patient education to self-monitor vital signs Patient education about activities of daily living Low intensity/impact endurance training (stationary bicycle riding, treadmills, etc.) Low intensity strengthening exercises (upper body, legs)
III	After discharge from outpatient settings	Continuing fitness programs and activities (often offered by inpatient facilities), whether in the community or at home

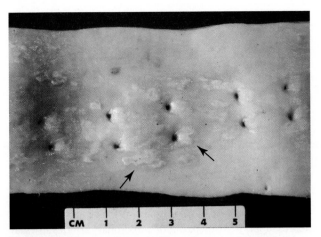

Figure 11–12 Interior of aorta, illustrating early atheromatous plaque formation. Two plaques are indicated by arrows. Circular openings are orifices of intercostal arteries.

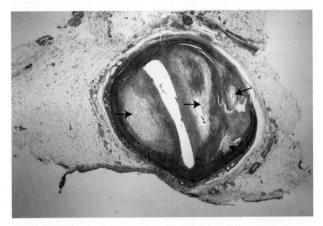

Figure 11–13 Low-magnification photomicrograph of coronary artery in cross-section illustrating several stable atheromatous plaques (arrows) surrounded by dense fibrous issue. Atheromatous deposits reduce lumen of artery to a narrow slit (original magnification X 40).

Arteriosclerosis is commonly called "hardening of the arteries." It is most common in the elderly and in diabetics, involving loss of elasticity and cardiac ischemia. Eventually, cells of the myocardium weaken and die, interfering with the heart's pumping ability and leading to heart failure. Risks for CAD are higher because of the following circumstances or factors:

- Genetic predisposition
- Age over 40 years
- Male gender
- Postmenopausal women
- White race
- History of smoking
- Urban residence
- Hypertension, diabetes, or obesity
- History of elevated serum cholesterol or reduced serum high-density lipoprotein levels
- Lack of exercise
- Stress

Diagnosis

Once coronary arteries are about three-fourths occluded, chest pain begins to develop. Often, collateral circulation develops to supply the tissue with needed oxygen and nutrients. If an ECG is undertaken, it shows ischemia and sometimes arrhythmias. Other methods of diagnosing CAD include treadmill testing, thallium scan, cardiac catheterization, and angiotensins to detect insufficient oxygen supply and confirm the diagnosis. Another reliable test is a coronary angiogram to illustrate segmental narrowing of a coronary artery.

Treatment

CAD treatment involves attempts to restore adequate blood flow to the myocardium, often by using vasodilators. To open constricted arteries, **angioplasty** is often attempted (**Figure 11–14**). Coronary angioplasty is a technique in which a guiding catheter is introduced through the skin into a large artery in the arm or leg. It is then threaded, by using fluoroscopic control, into the narrowed coronary artery and positioned at the site of narrowing. Then, the balloon catheter is threaded through the guide catheter until the balloon lies within the narrowed area. After it is properly positioned, the balloon is

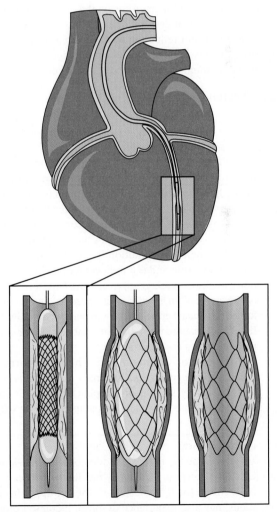

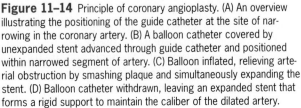

Figure 11–14 Principle of coronary angioplasty. (A) An overview illustrating the positioning of the guide catheter at the site of narrowing in the coronary artery. (B) A balloon catheter covered by unexpanded stent advanced through guide catheter and positioned within narrowed segment of artery. (C) Balloon inflated, relieving arterial obstruction by smashing plaque and simultaneously expanding the stent. (D) Balloon catheter withdrawn, leaving an expanded stent that forms a rigid support to maintain the caliber of the dilated artery.

inflated briefly under very high pressure, which forces the plaque toward the arterial wall.

Drugs used to reduce plaque buildup include hypolipidemic drugs. Beta-blockers and anticoagulants are used to prevent blood clots from breaking off and becoming lodged in cerebral arteries. If these therapies fail, coronary artery bypass surgery may be required to restore circulation.

Physical therapy for CAD may include developing a treatment protocol of exercises, verifying that the patient is taking his or her medications correctly, and increasing awareness of common signs and symptoms of CAD. Exercises should progress gradually, based on oxygen needs and the stage of cardiac rehabilitation. Risk factors should be reduced and vital signs monitored before, during, and after exercise. The patient's diet should be assessed, and, if necessary, a dietitian should be contacted.

Prognosis

The prognosis of CAD depends on how the patient responds to treatment. Patients who smoke have a much less favorable prognosis than nonsmokers. Altering the diet to one that is low in salt, fat, and cholesterol helps to improve outcomes. Regular exercise and reduction of stress are also indicated. The patient needs to be reminded that immediate medical care should be sought when symptoms of MI occur.

Angina Pectoris

Angina chest pain is defined as "chest pain after exertion" and results from reduced oxygen supply to the myocardium. There are three types of angina:

- Stable (exertional) angina: The most common form, it occurs when a coronary artery is narrowed due to severe buildup of plaque. When demand for oxygen is low, enough blood reaches the heart, but when physical activity is more strenuous, pain occurs due to lack of sufficient oxygen. Rest improves the symptoms.
- Unstable angina: A condition that can occur without physical exertion and is unrelieved by rest or medications; it requires emergency treatment. Unstable angina occurs more often in older adults, possibly signifying an impending heart attack (in 10–20 percent of patients). It is usually caused by blood clots that partially or completely block a coronary artery.
- Prinzmetal's or variant angina: The rarest form, it is caused by a spasm in a coronary artery. This narrows the artery, slowing or stopping blood flow to the heart. This type may occur in patients with or without CAD.

Signs and Symptoms

Angina pectoris usually causes a sudden onset of left-sided chest pain after exertion, which may radiate to another part of the body (often the left arm, jaw, or the left upper back). The patient may also experience dyspnea, increased blood pressure, and arrhythmias.

It is important to differentiate if a complaint of chest pain is a life-threatening occurrence or simply heartburn. The physical therapist assistant (PTA) should educate patients about this. The differences are basically as follows: whereas heartburn causes slight pain and burning that may radiate

outward, signs of cardiac problems include more severe symptoms, such as:

- Sudden pressure, tightening, squeezing, or crushing pain in the center of the chest for more than a few minutes
- Pain spreading to the back, neck, jaw, shoulders, or arms (especially the left arm)
- Shortness of breath, sweating, dizziness, or nausea
- Symptoms occurring as a result of physical activity or emotional stress

Etiology

Physical exertion requires increased blood flow to supply more oxygen, but because of atherosclerosis the vessels may not be able to supply it. Also, spasms of the coronary arteries also may be a causative factor. The pain of angina pectoris may also be caused by the cardiac ischemia that results from severe prolonged tachycardia, anemias, and respiratory diseases.

Diagnosis

To diagnose angina pectoris, the patient's prior history of chest pain should be reviewed. During an anginal episode an ECG may be performed to confirm ischemia. Similar diagnostic measures to those used for CAD may also be performed.

Treatment

Treatment of angina pectoris includes ceasing strenuous activity, sitting or lying down, and placing nitroglycerin tablets under the tongue. Nitroglycerin is a vasodilator used for many different heart conditions. Immediate medical attention is required when angina persists after three tablets have been taken (5 minutes apart). Transdermal nitroglycerin may be used to prevent angina on a longer-term basis.

The PTA should be aware of the many treatment implications when working with a patient who has angina. For stable and unstable angina, which are related to CAD, patients need to progress gradually with their physical exercises. Exercises should be appropriate for phase I, II, or III of cardiac rehabilitation. The patient should be educated about reduction of risk factors and monitoring of vital signs before, during, and after exercise routines. The PTA must be aware of all medications the patient is taking, including their adverse effects and how they relate to exercise. The PTA should also be aware of the patient's oxygen requirements and dietary restrictions. Frequent rest periods between exercises and activities are usually required.

Prognosis

Prognosis of angina pectoris depends on the amount of arterial blockage. Patient compliance in modifying diet, exercise, and lifestyle may improve the prognosis. These modifications are similar to those suggested for CAD.

Myocardial Infarction

MI is a "sudden death of a segment of the heart muscle caused by an abrupt interruption of blood flow to part of the heart." MI is caused by an occlusion of a coronary artery, resulting in ischemia and infarct (death) of the myocardium (**Figure 11–15**).

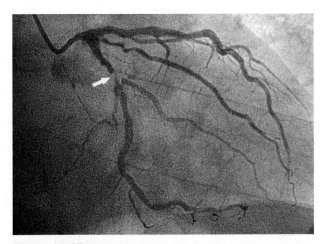

Figure 11–15 Infarcted heart muscle.

Signs and Symptoms

The pain of MI is crushing and causes a sudden feeling of massive substernal or left-sided chest constriction and pain that may radiate to the left arm, back, or jaw and may or may not be relieved by rest or use of nitroglycerin. Other signs and symptoms include dyspnea, irregular heartbeat, and **diaphoresis**. Many patients deny what is happening and experience severe anxiety.

> **RED FLAG**
>
> Many older adults do not have chest pain with MI but experience certain atypical symptoms such as dyspnea, falls, confusion, and syncope.

> **RED FLAG**
>
> It is important to note that the signs and symptoms for MI are not identical between men and women. Whereas most men experience the symptoms listed above (plus nausea, vomiting, and anxiety), women often describe their symptoms as being shortness of breath, weakness, indigestion, and fatigue.

Etiology

MI results from insufficient oxygen supply, often due to occlusion by atherosclerotic plaque, **thrombus**, or myocardial muscle spasm. If ischemia is not reversed within 6 hours, the cardiac muscle dies. Coronary **thrombosis** is the most common cause of MI. MIs can range from relatively small events (causing few long-term effects) to massive events (causing immediate death).

Diagnosis

Diagnosis of MI includes a thorough history, ECG, chest radiographic studies, and laboratory testing for cardiac enzyme levels. Enzyme changes may indicate death of cardiac tissue, resulting in a study of cardiac isoenzymes. Creatine kinase is an enzyme that is important in muscle contraction. Creatine kinase isoenzymes are found in elevated amounts in cardiac muscle after an MI.

Treatment

For MI, treatment begins with the administration of oxygen and then morphine to control pain. Aspirin is given to reduce the risk of additional damage from ischemia. Vasodilation is attempted with a nitroglycerin drip. Lidocaine is given by intravenous drip, after a leading **bolus**, to help control arrhythmias. As soon as possible after diagnosis, thrombolytic drugs may be administered unless contraindicated. Within 6 hours an attempt may be made to use angioplasty to open the occlusion and restore blood flow, or coronary artery bypass surgery may be indicated.

After a patient has had an MI, and cardiac rehabilitation is required, the role of the PTA may include monitoring vital signs throughout treatment; starting the patient out with only light exercise and working up to more aggressive exercise as tolerated; patient education about lifestyle and diet, smoking cessation, alcohol use, lowering high blood pressure, and cardiac precautions; and providing emotional as well as social support.

Prognosis

Nearly 65% of deaths from MI occur in the first hour after the infarction begins. Prognosis is determined by immediate defibrillation for ventricular fibrillation. Eventual death from MI depends on how much damage or complications have occurred, but sudden death is typically due to a fatal arrhythmia.

Arrhythmia

Arrhythmias are defined as any deviation from normal heartbeat (normal sinus rhythm) and are commonly referred to as "irregular heartbeats."

Signs and Symptoms

Arrhythmias result from interference with the heart's conduction system. Symptoms include palpitations, tachycardia or bradycardia, skipped heartbeats, syncope, and fatigue.

Etiology

Arrhythmias can be caused by conduction disturbances, including those affecting the SA or AV node, the bundle branches, or the Purkinje fibers. They also may be caused by various medications or ischemia as well as failure of the SA node.

Diagnosis

Diagnosis of arrhythmias is made by using a 12-lead ECG. Echocardiography may be used to help confirm certain arrhythmias. For example, **Figure 11–16** shows both atrial and ventricular fibrillation. Also, the patient may be required to wear a Holter monitor (also known as an "ambulatory ECG") to capture any arrhythmic event.

Treatment

Treatment of arrhythmias depends on the cause. Those that are related to medications or other drugs usually stop on their own once the substance is stopped. Anticoagulants may be given to prevent possible **thromboembolism**, which is occasionally a related condition. Ischemia should respond to oxygen administration. Less serious arrhythmias may be treated with a mild electric shock to the heart to restore normal rhythm. The goal of this treatment is to enable the heart to return to a normal state, enough to allow discontinuation of antiarrhythmic medications. However, if the heart rhythm does not stabilize, the arrhythmia can be fatal.

The role of the PTA with arrhythmia includes being aware of current rhythm status and any precautions for exercises.

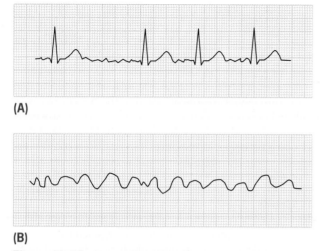

(A)

(B)

Figure 11–16 (A) Atrial fibrillation illustrating absence of distinct P waves together with irregular ventricular rate, usually 140 to 160 beats per minute. (B) Ventricular fibrillation illustrating extremely abnormal chaotic cardiac rhythm without any evidence of synchronized electrical impulses.

If exercise is too aggressive, the patient risks an episode of syncope. It is important for the PTA to know the physician's protocol and ensure the patient follows the guidelines of his or her physician and physical therapist.

Prognosis
Prognosis of arrhythmias varies depending on the type and cause.

Cardiac Arrest

The sudden, unexpected cessation of cardiac activity is described as "cardiac arrest" and is a true life-threatening emergency. If a person is discovered with the signs and symptoms of cardiac arrest, 911 should be called immediately and cardiopulmonary resuscitation (CPR) initiated (and defibrillation if available).

> **RED FLAG**
> If you aware that a patient has previously chosen not to be resuscitated in this type of situation and legal paperwork has been correctly filed (sometimes called a "living will"), you cannot proceed with CPR or calling 911.

Signs and Symptoms
In cardiac arrest the patient is unresponsive, with no palpable pulse and no respiratory effort.

Etiology
Cardiac arrest can be caused by arrhythmia, respiratory arrest, MI, drowning, electrocution, massive hemorrhage, severe trauma, or drug overdose. It results from **anoxia** or interruption of the electrical stimuli to the heart.

Diagnosis
Diagnosis of cardiac arrest is based on the absence of respiratory effort and lack of palpable pulse. The ECG shows ventricular fibrillation or **asystole**.

Treatment
Within 4 to 6 minutes after cardiac arrest CPR must be initiated. Cardiac defibrillation should be attempted by people trained in advanced life support techniques. Medications used to treat cardiac arrest include epinephrine, isoproterenol, dobutamine, and antiarrhythmic drugs such as lidocaine and bretylium.

Cardiac rehabilitation is a specialized intervention for patients with serious cardiovascular conditions such as cardiac arrest. It crosses many disciplines and may involve the PTA, PT, physician, nurse, occupational therapist, nutritionist, social worker, and exercise physiologist. Cardiac rehabilitation begins in the hospital as phase I, continues on an outpatient basis as phase II, and follows the patient until he or she is back at home (phase III) and beginning to resume normal activities (Table 11–1).

Prognosis
Prognosis after cardiac arrest depends on the amount of time that has elapsed before the patient is resuscitated. People have a greater chance of survival if CPR and **defibrillation** are administered earlier in the event rather than later. Respiratory efforts cease within 1 to 2 minutes after cessation of cardiac activity. Brain cells begin to die at 4 to 6 minutes after cessation of cardiac activity. After 10 minutes the brain dies with no chance of reversal of the condition.

Hypertension

Essential (primary) hypertension is a condition of abnormally high blood pressure in the arterial system. It may develop silently with no symptoms until permanent damage has occurred.

Signs and Symptoms
Hypertensive patients may experience *epistaxis* (nosebleed), headaches, lightheadedness, or syncope. Hypertension is usually found when the blood pressure is taken during a physical examination and is more common as a factor of increased age. If accompanied by hyperlipidemia, it may lead to atherosclerosis.

Etiology
The etiology of hypertension is unknown, but stress (the major factor), age, family history, race, and "type A" personality may all contribute to its occurrence. Lifestyle factors include excessive calorie intake and obesity, high sodium intake, excessive alcohol consumption, physical inactivity, and low potassium intake. In women predisposed to hypertension, oral contraceptives may also increase the risk. Other risk factors for hypertension include smoking and a diet high in saturated fats and cholesterol.

> **RED FLAG**
> African Americans are at an increased risk for primary hypertension based on predisposition to low plasma renin levels, which diminishes the ability to excrete excess sodium.

Diagnosis
Hypertension is usually first diagnosed based on elevated blood pressure; a systolic reading of greater than or equal to 140 mm Hg and a diastolic reading of greater than or equal to 90 mm Hg indicate hypertension. Borderline hypertension is considered to exist when systolic readings are between 121 and 139. Diagnosis is based on a

> **RED FLAG**
> Hypertension develops at an earlier age and is more severe in African Americans than in Whites.

series of blood pressure readings with consistently elevated pressures, followed by a thorough medical history, physical examination, and laboratory tests. Classifications of adult blood pressure are summarized in **Table 11–2**.

Treatment

Hypertension is often treated with *diuretics*, beta-adrenergic blockers, vasodilators, calcium channel blockers, and *angiotensin-converting enzyme (ACE) inhibitors*. These drugs may also be prescribed in combination with each other for varied effects. Each patient is different and requires a specific drug regimen. Additional suggested measures include limiting ~~~~~ment, reduction of weight, reg-~~~~~ss, and smoking cessation.

> **RED FLAG**
>
> Throughout all phases of rehabilitation for hypertension, it is important to allow heart rate to gradually return to normal by cooling down slowly after exercise. Regular monitoring of blood pressure is important.

working with patients who have hypertension involves patient education about sodium intake, healthy diet, smoking cessation, and adequate forms of exercise. Also, the PTA may be involved with monitoring and education about the many types of medications used to treat hypertension. Massage may be indicated to help patients cope with stress, although the PTA would not do this because it is not billable for cardiac conditions. Education about stress management is important. Aerobic conditioning is often indicated. **Table 11–3** shows the four phases of rehabilitation for hypertensive patients who need physical therapy for any reason.

Prognosis

The prognosis is varied, depending on the patient's response to drugs and lifestyle changes.

Malignant Hypertension

Malignant hypertension is a severe form of hypertension that is a life-threatening condition. Those who were previously diagnosed with essential hypertension may complain of sudden severe symptoms that signify the onset of malignant hypertension and require prompt medical intervention.

Signs and Symptoms

Signs and symptoms of malignant hypertension may be sudden, including severe headache, blurred vision, and dyspnea.

Etiology

The etiology of malignant hypertension is unknown, although extreme stress is considered to be a major contributing factor. It may possibly be linked to genetic disposition or family history.

Diagnosis

Marked blood pressure elevation (as high as 200/120 in severe cases) indicates malignant hypertension.

Treatment

Aggressive intervention techniques must be used, including intravenous vasodilators (diazoxide and sodium nitroprusside), followed by constant blood pressure monitoring and drug therapy throughout life. The PTA often does not see these patients until they are stable, but the roles of the PTA are more controlled in malignant hypertension. They must ensure the patient follows the basic guidelines of physical therapy for lesser forms of hypertension, monitors blood pressure, and maintains a strict regimen as dictated by physician protocol and the physical therapy plan.

TABLE 11–2 Classifications of Blood Pressure for Adults

Classification	Systolic Blood Pressure (mm Hg)	Diastolic Blood Pressure (mm Hg)
Normal	<120	<80
Prehypertension	121–139	81–89
Stage 1 hypertension	140–159	90–99
Stage 2 hypertension	≥160	≥100

TABLE 11–3 Phases of Physical Therapy for Hypertensive Patients

Phase	Location	Comments
1	Inpatient setting	Low levels of intensity with monitoring of vital signs Focus is on preventing dangers associated with bed rest, reducing episodes of orthostatic hypotension, and maintaining overall body mobility Exercise intensity is increased until discharge Activities include stationary bicycles and stair climbing
2	Outpatient setting	Similar exercises to those in phase 1 but with increased intensity Therapy is focused on improving function and increasing endurance Heart activity is monitored by a continuous electrocardiograph during all exercise PTs and PTAs will keep a log of blood pressure, heart rate, and cardiac rhythm
3	Outpatient setting, from 3 to 12 months after start of rehabilitation (usually lasts from 3 to 6 months)	Daily log continues to be kept, and electrocardiograph may also be continued This phase may last for several months up to a full year, and the patient may not be able to return to a full work schedule Higher level exercises may include swimming, hiking, light jogging, and cycling
4	Home or outpatient setting	Long-term maintenance of performance levels that have been previously reached Aerobic exercises emphasized These include brisk walking, jogging, running, swimming, stair climbing, and cycling

Prognosis

Prognosis is varied, based on response to drug therapy. Malignant hypertension may cause strokes (cerebrovascular accidents) and irreversible renal damage. If drug therapy is not successful, death may occur due to a **stroke**.

Congestive Heart Failure

Congestive heart failure (CHF) is the acute or chronic inability of the heart to pump enough blood to meet the body's demands for homeostasis.

Signs and Symptoms

CHF usually develops silently, with gradually increasing dyspnea. Anxiety begins as cardiac and respiratory rates increase. Eventually, veins in the neck distend and edema occurs in the ankles. With right-sided heart failure the liver and spleen enlarge, with peripheral edema becoming more prominent. When right-sided heart failure is caused by pulmonary disease, it is referred to as *cor pulmonale*. Left-sided CHF causes increased pulmonary congestion and more pronounced respiratory problems. The two types have differing etiologies. Left-sided CHF may be caused by aortic valve stenosis, hypertension, hyperthyroidism, or infarction of the left ventricle. Right-sided CHF may be caused by infarction of the right ventricle, cor pulmonale, or pulmonary valve stenosis. **Table 11–4** shows the four classifications of heart failure.

> **RED FLAG**
> An individual with CHF experiences reduced tolerance to exercise, reduced quality of life, and a shortened life span.

> **RED FLAG**
> CAD is the most common cause of heart failure. It occurs in adults, infants, and children with congenital and acquired defects.

Etiology

CHF may be caused by underlying conditions, resulting in heart failure and inadequate **perfusion**. These underlying conditions can include MI, hypertension, CAD, chronic obstructive pulmonary disease, cardiac valve damage, arrhythmias, and **cardiomyopathy**.

Diagnosis

Diagnosis of CHF occurs after a thorough history and physical examination. In CHF the presence of fluid in the lungs is indicated by radiographic film evidence, and the patient will have diminished breath sounds. An ECG can help to discover underlying causes (such as hypertrophy, ischemic changes, or infarction). An echocardiogram will help evaluate the extent of myocardial disease and may reveal left ventricular hypertrophy, dilation, and abnormal contractility. Catheterization can be used to monitor circulation pressures. Laboratory tests may reveal abnormal liver function and elevated blood urea nitrogen or creatinine levels. Prothrombin time may be prolonged as congestion impairs the liver's ability to synthesize procoagulants.

Treatment

Treatment for CHF is directed at reducing the heart's workload and increasing its efficiency. Heartbeat can be strengthened and slowed by administering digitalis preparations. To increase blood flow in general circulation, beta-blockers and ACE inhibitors are used. The volume of fluid in the body can be reduced by diuretics, and vascular pressure can be

TABLE 11–4	Classifications of Congestive Heart Failure
Class	**Description**
Class I: minimal	No limitations Ordinary physical activity does not result in excess fatigue, dyspnea, palpitations, or angina
Class II: mild	Slightly limited physical activity Patient is comfortable when resting Ordinary physical activity results in fatigue, dyspnea, palpitations, or angina
Class III: moderate	Very limited physical activity Patient is comfortable when resting Activity that is below normal levels produces symptoms
Class IV: severe	Patient cannot perform physical activity without discomfort Angina or cardiac inefficiency symptoms may develop when resting

reduced by vasodilators. Fluid and sodium intake should be restricted.

The role of the PTA is to carefully monitor patients with CHF while they are being treated. Based on heart rate history, aerobic exercise should include large muscle activities three times per week. If approved, strength training should include circuit training with high repetitions and low resistance three times per week. Exercises 2 to 3 days per week may be prescribed for both upper and lower extremities.

Prognosis

Acute CHF usually responds to medical interventions, with a good prognosis. Chronic CHF, however, is vulnerable to major organ impairment and complications.

Cardiomyopathy

Cardiomyopathy is a noninflammatory disease of the cardiac muscle. It results in enlargement of the myocardium and ventricular dysfunction. It occurs in three main forms: hypertrophic, dilated, and restrictive cardiomyopathy. It is the second most common direct cause of sudden death.

Signs and Symptoms

Cardiomyopathy causes symptoms of CHF, including dyspnea, fatigue, palpitations, tachycardia, and (occasionally) chest pain. Other symptoms may include hepatic congestion, peripheral edema, cardiac murmurs, or peripheral edema. The type (and cause) of cardiomyopathy influences the signs and symptoms that occur.

Etiology

Although usually of unknown cause, cardiomyopathies are divided into either dilated, hypertrophic, or restrictive types. Dilated cardiomyopathy can be caused by chronic alcoholism, autoimmune conditions, or viral infections. This type results in degeneration of myocardial fibers, followed by a decrease in contractile effort. Hypertrophic cardiomyopathies are considered genetic. They cause hypertrophy of the left ventricular wall and septum, resulting

> **RED FLAG**
> Dilated cardiomyopathy results from extensively damaged myocardial muscle fibers.

in shrinking of the left ventricle and possible aortic valve obstruction. Restrictive cardiomyopathies occur when any infiltration of the heart leads to fibrosis and myocardial thickening.

Diagnosis

Diagnosis of cardiomyopathy includes a thorough patient history and physical examination. At various stages **cardiomegaly** will be present as well as various cardiac murmurs. This is confirmed by x-rays and ECG. The type of cardiomyopathy is identified by echocardiogram and cardiac catheterization. In some cases, a *biopsy* may be required for diagnosis.

> **RED FLAG**
>
> It is recommended that all adolescents be screened before beginning any sporting activities to determine the possibility of cardiomyopathy.

Treatment

Treatment of cardiomyopathy depends on the type. Dilated and hypertrophic cardiomyopathies are treated similarly to CHF. Treatment of restrictive cardiomyopathy also includes reducing the heart's workload, but changes in the cardiac muscle due to this form are irreversible, with a poor prognosis. ACE inhibitors are used as first-line therapy to reduce **afterload** through vasodilation. Administering diuretics along with ACE inhibitors can reduce fluid retention. With these therapies digoxin will not improve myocardial contractility.

The role of the PTA in cardiomyopathy is to implement as much exercise as possible, based on the PT's evaluation and monitoring of objective findings. This is because of the many other conditions often present concurrently with cardiomyopathy. Response to exercise must be monitored closely, because certain patients may react negatively to physical therapy. Stationary bicycles, walking, treadmill usage, and general strengthening exercises are the most common methods of exercise for these patients.

Prognosis

The prognosis of patients with cardiomyopathies is better with use of approved medications. However, certain types can be fatal, with the only chance for survival involving heart transplantation.

Rheumatic Heart Disease and Rheumatic Fever

Rheumatic heart disease is damage to the heart from rheumatic fever, a systemic inflammatory and autoimmune disease that involves the joints and cardiac tissue. It is a systemic inflammatory disease of childhood.

Signs and Symptoms

Symptoms begin with a sore throat caused by streptococcus bacteria, followed by rheumatic fever (usually occurring in childhood). Patients with rheumatic fever experience joint pain, edema, redness, and reduced motion. Rheumatic heart disease involves acute endocarditis, valve damage, CHF, dyspnea, tachycardia, edema, nonproductive cough, and cardiac **murmurs**.

Etiology

Rheumatic fever is caused by group A beta-hemolytic streptococcal pharyngitis.

Diagnosis

Diagnosis of rheumatic heart disease is based on history of rheumatic fever and cardiac murmurs. Laboratory testing may reveal an elevated white blood cell count and elevated erythrocyte sedimentation rate during the acute phase. C-reactive protein levels may be abnormal, especially during the acute phase. *Antistreptolysin-O titer* may be elevated in patients within 2 months of onset. This is a blood test used to measure antibodies against *streptolysin-O*, which is produced by *group A streptococcus* bacteria. Echocardiograms show vegetations or resulting valvular damage. Chest x-rays may show normal heart size or cardiomegaly, pericardial effusion, or heart failure.

Treatment

Prompt treatment of all group A beta-hemolytic streptococcal pharyngitis should be undertaken with the use of oral penicillin V or intramuscular penicillin G benzathine. Salicylates may be used to relieve fever and pain and to minimize joint swelling. Treatment of rheumatic heart disease is aimed at reducing stenosis of heart valves and

> **RED FLAG**
>
> Secondary prevention of rheumatic fever, which begins after the acute phase subsides, involves monthly intramuscular injection of penicillin G benzathine for at least 5 years, or until the age of 21.

preventing resultant damage, and surgery may be required in some cases. Good dental hygiene is important to prevent gingival infections, which can cause further bloodborne infection and valve damage. Prophylactic antibiotics are given to patients before any dental procedures.

The role of the PTA in rheumatic heart disease is to implement physical therapy after symptoms of carditis have subsided. Both physical and occupational therapy may be indicated. ECG and daily logs of vital signs are used to gauge the patient's response to exercise. ECG may be discontinued as stamina improves. Pain ranking is used to determine the amount and intensity of suitable exercise. Treadmill usage, stationary bicycling, and other forms of aerobic exercise are often recommended.

Prognosis

Prognosis varies according to the extent of heart valve damage. Recurrences of rheumatic heart disease are common, and valve replacement may be required to improve the patient's prognosis.

Carditis

Carditis is an inflammation of heart tissue. It may be due to infection or an immune system problem. Carditis is divided into several forms: pericarditis, myocarditis, and endocarditis. Pericarditis is an acute or chronic inflammation of the pericardium (serosa), the sac that encloses and protects the heart. Myocarditis is inflammation of the muscular walls of the heart. Endocarditis is inflammation of the lining and valves of the heart.

Signs and Symptoms

Pericarditis results from blood or inflammatory exudate being released into the pericardial sac or pericardial space, resulting in friction and irritation. Other symptoms include fever, malaise, chest pain, dyspnea, and chills. Myocarditis involves damage by pathogenic invasion or **toxic** insult, which may be acute or chronic, and occurs at any age. Symptoms include palpitations, fatigue, dyspnea, fever, arrhythmia, and chest tenderness. Endocarditis is usually secondary to infection elsewhere in the body, preexisting heart disease, or because of abnormal immune reactions. Symptoms include fever, chills, night sweats, weakness, anorexia, and fatigue.

Etiology

Pericarditis is idiopathic (of unknown origin) or a result of other infections, including those caused by viruses, bacteria, trauma, rheumatic fever, and malignant neoplastic disease. Myocarditis is often a viral, bacterial, fungal, or protozoal infection or a complication of diseases such as influenza, diphtheria, mumps, or rheumatic fever. Endocarditis is often caused by bacteremia, intravenous drug use, or rheumatic disease.

Diagnosis

History reveals recent febrile upper respiratory infection. For pericarditis, blood studies may lead to the identification of the causative organism, and an echocardiogram will confirm the presence of pericardial fluid or a thickened pericardium. For myocarditis, diagnostic findings can include elevated white blood cells, increased erythrocyte sedimentation rate, elevated cardiac enzyme levels, ventricular enlargement, and an abnormal ECG. For endocarditis, a complete blood count may indicate leukocytosis, with an elevated erythrocyte sedimentation rate present. Chest x-rays may show an enlarged heart and pulmonary vascular congestion. Echocardiography may demonstrate left ventricular dysfunction to certain degrees. Radionuclide scanning may identify inflammatory and necrotic changes that are characteristic of myocarditis.

Treatment

Treatment of pericarditis is directed at managing the underlying systemic disease and at reducing inflammation and pain. When infection is the underlying cause, appropriate anti-infection agents are used to treat myocarditis. In endocarditis, identification of the causative organism dictates the anti-infective therapy (usually intravenous antibiotics), usually continuing for several weeks. Limited exercise is indicated with carditis, which should be closely monitored.

Prognosis

Acute pericarditis usually resolves with complete recovery, although the pericardium may have to be **resected**. With myocarditis, prognosis for complete recovery is favorable unless the condition is chronic and damages the cardiac muscle. For endocarditis, early diagnosis and treatment with antibiotics usually result in complete recovery. However, untreated cases can have a poor prognosis.

Valvular Heart Disease

Valvular heart disease is an acquired or congenital disorder, potentially harming any of the heart's four valves. It can exist in the form of insufficiency (failure of the valves to close completely) or stenosis (hardening of the cusps of the valves, preventing complete opening or impeding blood flow). It most often affects the mitral valve (**Figure 11–17**) but may also affect the aortic valve.

Mitral insufficiency is an abnormality of the mitral *leaflets* (the parts of the valve that actually open and close). Blood from the left ventricle flows back into the left atrium during systole. This causes the atrium to enlarge to accommodate the backflow. As a result the left ventricle also dilates to

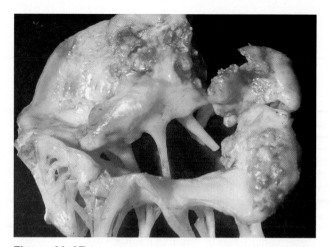

Figure 11–17 A poorly functioning scarred and calcified mitral valve resulting from valve damage caused by prior rheumatic fever. The valve was excised and replaced by an artificial heart valve.

accommodate the increased blood volume from the atrium and to compensate for diminishing cardiac output. Ventricular hypertrophy and increased end-diastolic pressure result in increased pulmonary artery pressure. This eventually leads to left-sided and right-sided heart failure.

Mitral stenosis is a narrowing of the valve due to valvular abnormalities, fibrosis, or calcification that obstructs blood flow from the left atrium to the left ventricle. Aortic insufficiency is defined as when blood flows back into the left ventricle during diastole. This causes fluid overload in the ventricle, which dilates and hypertrophies.

Aortic stenosis is defined as when increased left ventricular pressure attempts to overcome the resistance of the narrowed valvular opening. The added workload increases the demand for oxygen. Diminished cardiac output causes poor coronary artery perfusion, ischemia of the left ventricle, and left-sided heart failure.

Signs and Symptoms

Mitral stenosis causes exertional dyspnea and fatigue as well as cough, palpitations, **hemoptysis**, and, sometimes, cyanosis. Mitral insufficiency causes dyspnea, fatigue, and heart murmurs. Aortic stenosis causes chest pain, fainting on exertion (syncope), and labored breathing on exertion due to heart failure. Aortic insufficiency causes a thrusting apical pulsation, bounding apical pulse, and diastolic murmur.

Etiology

Most mitral stenosis cases are caused by rheumatic heart disease. Most mitral insufficiency cases are caused by either rheumatic heart disease or mitral valve prolapse. Aortic stenosis is usually caused by congenital malformation of the aortic valve. Aortic insufficiency may result from aortic valve abnormalities or from dilation and distortion of the aortic root.

Diagnosis

Symptoms of mitral stenosis may be insidious (occurring silently over time) or acute, with cardiac murmurs occurring. Mitral insufficiency is based on a thorough patient history of, especially, sore throat or rheumatic fever and heart murmur. Aortic stenosis is diagnosed by cardiac catheterization and

Doppler echocardiography. Aortic insufficiency is diagnosed by cardiac catheterization, aortic angiography, and Doppler echocardiography. Chest x-rays and electrocardiography can also be used.

Treatment

In mitral stenosis limitation of sodium intake, along with administration of digoxin or diuretics, helps reduce the heart's workload. Treatment for mitral insufficiency includes bed rest, oxygen therapy, and antibiotics. Treatment for aortic stenosis includes bed rest, fluid restriction, diuretics, supplemental oxygenation, digoxin, vasodilators, and surgical repair or replacement. Treatment for aortic insufficiency includes treating underlying endocarditis or syphilis, limiting strenuous physical activity, fluid restriction, diuretics, supplemental oxygenation, digoxin, and early elective valve surgery (repair or replacement).

> **RED FLAG**
> Prophylactic antibodies before and after surgery or dental care to prevent endocarditis must be given to patients who have valvular heart disease.

The role of the PTA in valvular heart disease is to assist with a program of aerobic exercise, including walking, jogging, swimming, and cycling. Heart rate should be monitored, and exercise should cease if symptoms of lightheadedness or tachycardia occur.

Prognosis

The prognosis of mitral stenosis improves with surgical intervention. The prognosis of mitral insufficiency is generally good, but the disease can lead to right ventricular hypertrophy. The prognosis for asymptomatic aortic stenosis is excellent, but once symptomatic, survival rate is less than 50 percent, improved greatly based on the timing and effectiveness of surgery. The prognosis for aortic insufficiency is excellent unless it progresses to become symptomatic.

Diseases of the Blood Vessels

Diseases of the arteries and veins are more common in the elderly. They are more serious in patients with other chronic disorders such as diabetes mellitus.

Aneurysms

The weakening and resulting local dilation of the wall of an artery is called an *aneurysm*. An aneurysm may be signified by a pulsating mass in the abdomen. Several types of aortic aneurysms can occur:

- *Saccular aneurysm*: When increased arterial pressure pushes out a pouch or bulge on one side of the artery (**Figure 11–18**)
- *Fusiform aneurysm*: When the arterial wall weakens around its circumference, creating a spindle-shaped aneurysm

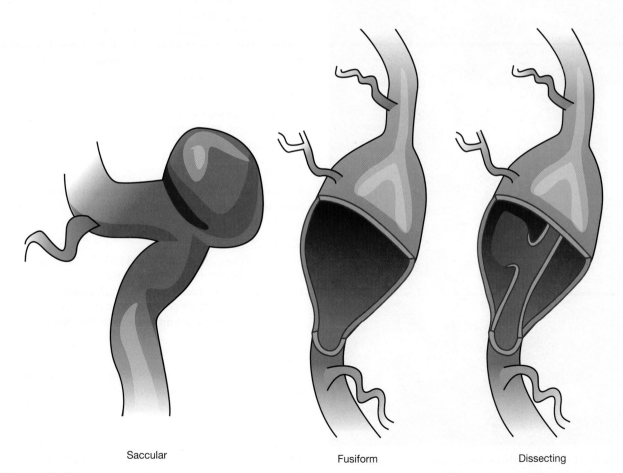

Saccular   Fusiform   Dissecting

Figure 11–18 Types of aneurysms.

■ *Dissecting aneurysm*: When blood is forced by layers of the arterial wall, causing them to separate and create a false lumen.

Signs and Symptoms

An aneurysm can have either an insidious or sudden onset. Symptoms vary based on location and size, with an abdominal aortic aneurysm being the most common form. As it enlarges the patient may experience abdominal or back pain, and a pulsating mass is observed in the abdomen. If a rupture occurs, the patient exhibits signs of hemorrhagic shock.

Etiology

Aneurysms are commonly caused by the buildup of atherosclerotic plaque that weakens the vessel wall (**Figure 11–19**). Other causative factors include trauma, infection, inflammation, and congenital tendencies.

Diagnosis

For abdominal aneurysm pulsation may be observed, and the aortic mass is noted mid-abdomen. A **bruit** may be heard on auscultation of the area. Cerebral aneurysms are usually found after they rupture, with severe consequences. Diagnosis is confirmed via radiographic studies (**Figure 11–20**), **ultrasonography**, computed tomography, and magnetic resonance imaging.

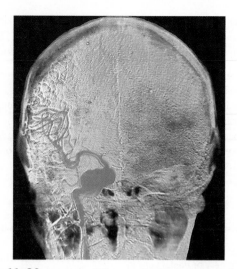

Figure 11–20 Aneurysm. This x-ray shows a ballooning of one of the arteries in the brain. If untreated, an aneurysm can break, causing a stroke.

Treatment

Treatment for aneurysms depends on the size, location, and chance of rupture. Usually, surgery is required to repair aneurysms before they leak or rupture. Immediate surgical intervention is required if the aortic wall has been damaged. Usually, a synthetic graft is installed. If small, constant monitoring of the aneurysm is indicated.

If exercise is recommended, the role of the PTA with a patient who has had an aneurysm is to implement exercises lightly, progressing slowly to more rigorous physical activity as dictated by the monitoring of the condition.

Prognosis

Prognosis is varied based on location and size. Surgical intervention greatly improves the prognosis, as does the speed of emergency intervention.

Phlebitis

Phlebitis is inflammation of a vein. It mostly occurs in the lower legs, though any vein (including those in the cranium) may be affected.

Signs and Symptoms

Signs and symptoms of superficial phlebitis are in pain and tenderness, becoming more severe over time. Swelling, redness, warmth, and eventually the development of a tender cord-like mass under the skin can occur. Deep venous inflammation affects the tunica intima with the formation of clots (thrombophlebitis).

Etiology

The cause of phlebitis is uncertain, but the condition can appear for apparently no reason. Possible causes are believed to include venous stasis, obesity, blood disorders, injury, and surgery.

Diagnosis

The clinical picture and history of a preceding phlebitis condition help establish the diagnosis.

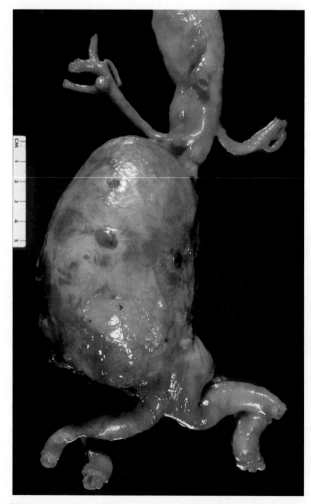

Figure 11–19 Large arteriosclerotic aneurysm extending from renal arteries (above) to iliac arteries (below).

Treatment

Analgesics are given for the pain of superficial phlebitis. The affected area should not be massaged, because this type of action can stimulate clot formation or release formed clots as emboli. The role of the PTA in phlebitis is to inform patients that daily exercise is important in preventing the development of the condition. This may include walking, dancing, swimming, cycling, yoga, and other forms of exercise. It is vital for the patient to move as much as possible during work activities and at home; changing positions often and avoiding sitting or standing still for long periods are also very helpful.

Prognosis

The prognosis for phlebitis is usually positive with treatment.

Thrombophlebitis

Thrombophlebitis occurs because of inflammation of a vein and the formation of a thrombus on the vessel wall.

Signs and Symptoms

Thrombophlebitis interferes with blood flow and results in edema. Similar to phlebitis, patients experience pain, heaviness, swelling, and warmth in affected areas, as well as chills and fever. The affected area may be tender to the touch.

Etiology

The occurrence of thrombophlebitis may be related to venous stasis, blood disorders causing a hypercoagulable state, and injury to the venous wall. The formation of clots may be linked directly to the deep venous inflammation of phlebitis, which affects the tunica intima.

Diagnosis

Thrombophlebitis is suggested by extreme edema in one leg compared with the other, with the affected area tender to palpation. Diagnosis is confirmed by imaging of the vessel with radiographic venography and ultrasonography.

Treatment

Thrombophlebitis requires immediate intervention, involving immobilization of the affected part to prevent the thrombus from spreading and dislodging to become an embolus. Heparin or low–molecular weight heparin is used to prevent the clot from enlarging. Antibiotics are used to prevent infection. If surgery is required, early mobilization after surgery reduces the likelihood of complications.

The role of the PTA in thrombophlebitis is to assist with aerobic exercise. This may include walking, swimming, and cycling, as well as other forms of exercise selected by the PT and physician.

Prognosis

Prognosis is good if prompt intervention occurs, with the condition usually resolving and requiring no further treatment. If it does not, surgical intervention may be required to **ligate** the affected vessel. Collateral circulation then develops. During immobilization and reduced physical activity, preventing the formation of deep vein thrombosis is essential.

Varicose Veins

Varicose veins are swollen, twisted, and knotted veins that usually occur in the lower legs (**Figure 11–21**).

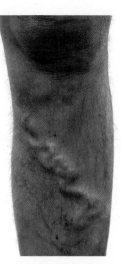

Figure 11–21 Varicose veins. Any restriction of venous blood flow to the heart causes veins to balloon out, creating bulges commonly known as varicose veins.

Signs and Symptoms

Symptoms develop gradually, with a feeling of fatigue in the legs and then a continuous dull ache. Varicose veins may cause nighttime leg cramps and swelling of the ankles. Eventually, the veins thicken and feel hard to the touch. The pain can worsen until it has a stabbing quality.

Etiology

Varicose veins are of no clearly identifiable cause. It is suspected that valves in the veins are either defective or absent, and prolonged standing or sitting can cause pressure on them, especially in the lower legs. Normal leg movement causes muscles to contract and relax to move the blood upward. When standing or sitting for extended periods, gravity pushes blood downward, increasing pressure on the valves. Lack of exercise stresses the valves until they are no longer able to function normally, followed by blood stasis and vein swelling. Pregnancy also frequently results in varicose veins due to increased pressure on the leg and pelvic veins, compromising free flow of venous blood.

Diagnosis

Varicose veins are easy to diagnose based on their appearance and on patient history regarding pregnancy or prolonged standing or sitting. Advanced varicosities cause a brown discoloration of the skin around the affected veins.

Treatment

Rest periods, with the patient elevating the feet higher than the heart, give relief in mild cases. Exercise or submerging the legs in warm water increases blood flow. Support stockings may help to encourage return flow of blood. When varicose veins progress, they may require surgical intervention (vein ligation and stripping) or injection of **sclerosing** solutions to harden and eventually atrophy the affected veins. Collateral circulation develops, augmenting blood return to the heart.

The role of the PTA involves assisting the patient who has varicose veins with moderate exercise, to promote circulation and improve muscle tone. Moderate exercises include walking, weight training, low-impact aerobics, and swimming.

Basically, any form of exercise that strengthens the legs will help relieve varicose veins.

Prognosis

Venous ligation or injection of sclerosing solutions usually relieves symptoms.

Deep Vein Thrombosis

Deep vein thrombosis mostly affects the lower legs, thighs, and pelvis, with the danger of clots that occur in the femoral and pelvic veins becoming emboli (which is very common).

Signs and Symptoms

Deep vein thrombosis is mostly asymptomatic until embolization occurs, often resulting in a pulmonary embolism that may be fatal.

Etiology

Risk factors for deep vein thrombosis include immobility, dehydration, varicose veins, leg surgery, pelvic surgery, obesity, and pregnancy.

Diagnosis

An initial indication of the condition is provided via Well's criteria as an evidence-based practice of assessing deep vein thrombosis:

- Active cancer
- Bedridden recently for more than 3 days or major surgery within 4 weeks
- Calf swelling of more than 3 centimeters compared with the other leg
- Collateral (nonvaricose) superficial veins present
- Entire swelling of leg
- Localized tenderness along the deep venous system
- Pitting edema that is greater in the symptomatic leg
- Paralysis, paresis, or recent plaster cast on the leg
- Previously documented deep vein thrombosis
- Alternative diagnosis to deep vein thrombosis as likely or more likely

If the squeezing of the posterior calf also causes pain, deep vein thrombosis is indicated. The most widely used test to evaluate the disease is ultrasonography.

Treatment

Treatment is aimed at reducing formation of more clots and preventing embolization. Bed rest with elevation of the affected area has been shown to improve blood flow in some patients. Anticoagulants are used to decrease potential thrombus formation. Precautions concerning deep vein thrombosis are as follows:

- Minimizing airplane or jet flights, and using leg exercises if flying is unavoidable
- Minimizing long trips by automobile, and using regular stops during trips to exercise the legs if they are unavoidable
- Exercising as much as possible after surgical operations that require long-term bed rest
- Exercising as much as possible if a condition such as a clotting disorder, systemic lupus erythematosus, pregnancy, obesity, heart failure, or a circulatory problem exists
- Exercising after certain types of chemotherapy are administered

- Closely monitoring health if you are taking oral combination contraceptives
- Closely monitoring health if you are elderly, a smoker, or are a female taking hormone replacement therapy

The role of the PTA in deep vein thrombosis commences after the physician determines that exercise is safe to begin. Regular cardiovascular exercise is indicated, as are lower calf exercises. If the patient is cleared for air travel, it is important that he or she be taught exercises that can be done while flying: ankle pumps, elbow bends, shoulder rolls and stretches, forward bends, knee-to-chest lifts, neck rolls, upper body stretches, and thigh tightening (which is an isometric exercise that helps to increase blood flow).

> **RED FLAG**
> If you suspect a patient has developed a deep vein thrombosis, you must seek **immediate emergency medical attention**. If you delay, it is possible for a clot to dislodge and travel to the lungs, causing a fatal pulmonary embolism. **Do not squeeze or stretch the affected area!!!**

Prognosis

Prognosis depends on the causes and complications of the blood clot. Precautions that are taken can reduce likelihood of reoccurrence by 50 percent, which include wearing compression garments, such as knee or thigh high stockings.

Raynaud's Disease

Raynaud's disease is a **vasospastic** condition occurring bilaterally that usually affects the hands or, less commonly, the feet. It is characterized by episodic vasospasm in the small peripheral arteries and arterioles. This condition is precipitated by exposure to cold or stress.

Signs and Symptoms

Raynaud's disease is precipitated by cold, causing a white discoloration, then a blue discoloration as venous blood returns, and resulting in a red or purple discoloration when circulation is restored (**Figure 11–22**). It is often triggered by stress and is much more common in women. It is called "Raynaud's phenomenon" when secondary to another disease. Severe cases cause ulceration of the fingers or toes.

> **RED FLAG**
> *Raynaud's phenomenon* is usually associated with scleroderma, systemic lupus erythematosus, or polymyositis.

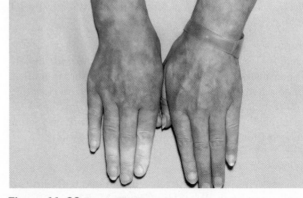

Figure 11–22 Raynaud's phenomenon.

Etiology

Although family history is a risk factor, the cause of this disorder is unknown. It is also made worse by smoking cigarettes or other tobacco products.

Diagnosis

Diagnosis is based on severity of symptoms and a history of numbness or paleness in the affected areas. Normal arterial pulses should be present. Antinuclear antibody titer is used to identify autoimmune disease as an underlying cause of Raynaud's phenomenon. Arteriography rules out arterial occlusive disease. Reduced blood flow may be shown by Doppler ultrasonography if symptoms result from arterial occlusive disease. The condition mostly affects women between puberty and age 40. Smokers show a higher incidence.

> **RED FLAG**
> Cutaneous gangrene may occur as a result of prolonged ischemia, requiring amputation of one or more digits.

Treatment

Treatment involves applying warmth to the affected areas, smoking cessation, avoiding exposure to cold, and avoiding any stressors that precipitate the attacks. Drugs used to dilate vessels and increase blood flow include vasodilators, alpha-adrenergic blockers, and calcium channel blockers, but their effects must be closely monitored. The role of the PTA in Raynaud's disease is, in the primary form of the disease, to encourage the patient to participate in regular exercise and to provide patient education. It is crucial for the patient to warm all portions of the body before exercise.

Prognosis

Prognosis is good in most cases, unless signs and symptoms are severe and treatment does not provide adequate relief.

Buerger's Disease

Buerger's disease, also known as *thromboangiitis obliterans*, is an inflammation of the peripheral arteries and veins of the extremities, with the formation of clots. Incidence is highest among men of Jewish ancestry, aged 20 to 40, who smoke heavily.

Signs and Symptoms

This condition causes intense pain in the affected area (usually the legs or instep of the foot). Initial symptoms include coldness, cyanosis, and numbness of the feet during exposure to low temperatures. This results from diminished blood flow. Later symptoms include redness, heat, and tingling. It is often aggravated by exercise and relieved by rest. If circulation is not restored, it can result in atrophy, ulcers, and gangrene (**Figure 11–23**).

Etiology

Although the cause of Buerger's disease is unknown, it is primarily caused by the effects of long-term smoking. Inflammation and clot formation advance to obliterate the vessels and completely compromise circulation. It causes tissue death and gangrene, affecting mostly males of Jewish descent.

Diagnosis

Buerger's disease is diagnosed after reports of intense pain in the commonly affected areas, followed by Doppler

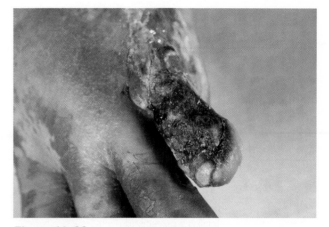

Figure 11–23 Thromboangiitis obliterans.

ultrasonography to show diminished circulation in the peripheral vessels. Arteriography may be used to locate lesions and rule out atherosclerosis.

Treatment

Smoking cessation is the first step in treatment of Buerger's disease. This usually reduces inflammation and restores partial circulation. Progressive ambulation has been found to be beneficial up to the preclaudication threshold. Surgical intervention can be used to establish "detours" or to cut a pathway through the clot itself. If gangrenous, amputation must be performed. The role of the PTA in Buerger's disease is to encourage the patient to get adequate exercise and to provide education about the condition, skin monitoring, and any changes that may occur.

Prognosis

There is no known cure for Buerger's disease. Prognosis is fair if the patient stops smoking and receives any required surgical intervention.

Shock

Shock is basically defined as extremely low blood pressure that leads to decreased tissue perfusion. It is not a disease but rather a clinical syndrome leading to reduced tissue and organ perfusion. Eventually, shock leads to organ dysfunction and failure. Types of shock include anaphylactic, cardiogenic, hypovolemic, neurogenic, and septic shock.

Signs and Symptoms

Patients who are in shock exhibit pale, cold, and clammy skin; cyanosis, tachycardia; altered mental status; tachypnea; syncope; unconsciousness; anuria; and oliguria.

Etiology

Vasodilation causes a state of **hypovolemia**. It depends on the type of shock. **Table 11–5** shows the various causes of shock.

Diagnosis

Diagnosis of shock is usually established by a thorough medical history, physical examination, and blood pressure of less than 90/50.

Treatment

Treatment of shock depends on the type. Common treatment measures include laying the individual on his or her back,

TABLE 11-5   Types and Causes of Shock

Type of Shock	Causes
Anaphylactic	ABO-incompatible blood Contrast media Foods Medications, vaccines Venom
Cardiogenic	Arrhythmias Cardiomyopathy Heart failure MI (most common cause) Obstruction Pericardial tamponade Pulmonary embolism Tension pneumothorax
Hypovolemic	Ascites Blood loss (most common cause) Burns Fluid shifts Gastrointestinal fluid loss Hemothorax Peritonitis Renal loss (adrenal insufficiency, diabetes insipidus, diabetic ketoacidosis)
Neurogenic	Hypoglycemia Medications Severe pain Spinal anesthesia Vasomotor center depression
Septic	Gram-negative bacteria (most common cause) Gram-positive bacteria Microorganisms (fungi, viruses, parasites, *Rickettsiae*, protozoa, yeast, or mycobacteria)

keeping the patient warm and quiet, and elevating the feet and legs above heart level to improve vascular return.

Prognosis

Untreated shock can be fatal. Prompt assessment and treatment for shock as well as its underlying causes greatly improves prognosis. Drug therapy may include epinephrine or dopamine. If of a cardiogenic nature, atropine may be used.

SUMMARY

The cardiovascular system controls the pumping of blood throughout the body and its cells and tissues. Over 64 million Americans are affected by cardiovascular disease. It is a significant cause of death in older adults, with risks that can be reduced by changing lifestyle and behaviors. Common symptoms include pain, fatigue, difficulty breathing, tachycardia, cyanosis, and edema. The most common cardiovascular disorders include CAD, heart attack, hypertension, arteriosclerosis, and varicosities such as varicose veins. The number one cause of death in older adults is heart disease.

Carditis is an inflammation of heart tissue that may be caused by infection or immune system problems. Mitral insufficiency is an abnormality of the mitral leaflets that causes abnormal blood flow resulting in the enlargement of

the atrium. Aortic insufficiency is when blood flows back into the left ventricle during diastole, causing fluid overload in the ventricle, which dilates and hypertrophies. Shock is a clinical syndrome leading to reduced tissue and organ perfusion, organ dysfunction, and organ failure.

REVIEW QUESTIONS

Select the best response to each question.

1. Pulmonary arteries do which of the following?
   a. transfer blood to the brain
   b. transfer low-oxygen blood away from the heart
   c. transfer oxygenated blood away from the heart
   d. send blood toward the heart
2. Which of the following terms is defined as "inflammation of the inner membrane or lining of the heart"?
   a. vasculitis
   b. pericarditis
   c. endocarditis
   d. myocarditis
3. Thrombophlebitis occurs most commonly in which of the following areas?
   a. lower legs
   b. lower arms
   c. lower abdomen
   d. lungs
4. An area of dead cells caused by lack of oxygen is called
   a. gangrene
   b. atresia
   c. ischemia
   d. infarction
5. Angioplasty is defined as which of the following?
   a. surgical excision of a vein
   b. surgical repair of a blood vessel
   c. surgical incision of the heart
   d. surgical excision of an artery
6. Which of the following chambers of the heart receives oxygenated blood from the pulmonary veins?
   a. right atrium
   b. left atrium
   c. right ventricle
   d. left ventricle
7. Which of the following is defined as a collapse of the cardiovascular system that results in a dangerous reduction of blood flow throughout the body?
   a. cardiac tamponade
   b. rheumatic fever
   c. acute endocarditis
   d. shock
8. A noninflammatory disease of the cardiac muscle that results in enlargement of the myocardium and ventricular dysfunction is called
   a. cardiomyopathy
   b. myocarditis
   c. myocardial infarction
   d. carditis
9. The most common cause of mitral stenosis is which of the following?
   a. congestive heart failure
   b. coronary heart disease

c. rheumatic heart disease

d. hemorrhage

10. The first symptom of coronary artery disease is usually which of the following?

a. diaphoresis

b. headache

c. peripheral edema

d. chest pain

CASE STUDIES

Karen Coupe, PT, DPT, MSEd

Case 1

A 56-year-old woman was hospitalized secondary to a severe episode of shortness of breath 2 days previously. Echocardiogram results indicate left CHF. Patient medical history includes hypertension, diabetes, bilateral knee osteoarthritis, and mild obesity. Prior level of function: Ambulation with a cane, independent in all activities of daily living. PT evaluation reveals the need for patient assistance with bed mobility, transfers, and ambulation. The PT plan of care is for bed mobility, transfers, and progressive ambulation beginning with a walker and progressing to a cane.

1. When comparing signs and symptoms of left versus right CHF, what type of symptoms does the PTA need to watch for during treatment?

2. The PTA is working on bed mobility and notes the patient has orthopnea if the head of the bed is below the semi-Fowler's position. Explain why this occurs.

3. The patient is on a pulse oximeter. What is considered the minimal percentage of O_2 saturation rate permissible to continue treatment?

4. What other types of monitoring are vital for this patient?

5. How does the patient's medical history contribute to her diagnosis?

Case 2

A 68-year-old woman is currently being seen in physical therapy secondary to a venous stasis ulcer on the posterior aspect of the right medial malleolus. Patient medical history: Chronic venous insufficiency and history of deep vein thrombosis with the most recent 4 months ago. Plan of care is for wound care and patient education.

1. Describe what you would observe in the lower extremities of a patient who has chronic venous insufficiency. Why do the legs appear this way? What is the pathogenesis?

2. This patient has a history of deep vein thrombosis. Why would you suspect this is true?

3. A PTA must be aware of any potential complications. What would alert you to the fact that a patient may have a deep vein thrombosis?

4. As part of patient education would you tell the patient to elevate her lower extremities or keep them in a dependent position? How would this differ if a patient had arterial disease?

5. Compression stockings and/or gradient wraps are a common treatment of chronic venous insufficiency. Explain the rationale behind this treatment.

WEBSITES

http://www.americanheart.org/presenter.jhtml?identifier=4481

http://www.emedicinehealth.com/phlebitis/article_em.htm

http://www.hypertensionsymptom.net/hc3.asp

http://www.mayoclinic.com/health/heart-failure/DS00061

http://www.medicinenet.com/heart_attack/article.htm

http://www.merck.com/mmpe/sec07.html

http://www.nhlbi.nih.gov/health/dci/Diseases/Cad/CAD_WhatIs.html

http://www.nlm.nih.gov/medlineplus/aneurysms.html

http://www.webmd.com/heart-disease/tc/deep-vein-thrombosis-topic-overview

Blood Disorders

LEARNING OBJECTIVES

After completion of this chapter the reader should be able to

1. Describe the composition of blood.
2. List various types of anemia.
3. Identify the significance of blood-clotting disorders.
4. List the common diagnostics used to determine blood disorders.
5. Describe the important signs and symptoms of various anemias.
6. Compare polycythemia vera with leukemia.
7. Discuss the causes of disseminated intravascular coagulation.
8. Describe and compare hemophilia with sickle cell anemia.

KEY TERMS

Achlorhydria: Lack of hydrochloric acid in the stomach.
Aplastic anemia: Type of anemia in which bone marrow does not produce sufficient new cells to replenish blood cells.
Cooley's anemia: Beta-thalassemia major; it occurs when similar gene defects affect production of the beta globin protein, with both parents having the defective gene.
Cyanotic: A bluish discoloration of the skin and mucous membranes resulting from inadequate oxygenation of the blood.
Diapedesis: Outward passage of blood cells through intact vessel walls.
Dyspnea: Increased efforts to breathe.
Erythrocytosis: Secondary polycythemia, which involves increased erythrocytes in response to prolonged hypoxia and increased erythropoietin secretion.
Erythropoietin: A hormone secreted by the kidneys that stimulates the production of erythrocytes in the red bone marrow as a response to insufficient oxygen.
Glossitis: Inflammation or infection of the tongue.
Hemarthrosis: Bleeding into joint spaces.
HbA$_2$: Hemoglobin alpha 2; a gene that is coded for the alpha globin chain of hemoglobin.
HbF: Fetal hemoglobin; the main fetal oxygen transport protein.
Hematocrit: The proportion of cells (mostly red blood cells) in blood.
Hematopoiesis: Development of blood cells.
Hepatomegaly: Enlargement of the liver.
Hypochromic: Paler than normal (cells).
Leukocytes: White blood cells.
Leukocytosis: An increase in circulating white blood cells.
Leukopenia: A decrease in leukocytes, often caused by certain viral infections, radiation, and chemotherapy.

KEY TERMS CONTINUED

Lymphadenopathy: Disease of the lymph nodes.

Malabsorption: A state caused by abnormal absorption of food nutrients across the gastrointestinal tract.

Microcytic: Unusually small (cells).

Morphology: Size and shape of cells.

Myelotoxins: Toxins that destroy bone marrow cells.

Occult: Hidden, such as when bleeding occurs internally.

Pallor: Paleness of the face.

Pancytopenia: A reduction in the number of red blood cells, white blood cells, and platelets.

Panhypoplasia: Inability of the bone marrow to produce red blood cells, white blood cells, and platelets.

Petechiae: Pinpointed skin hemorrhages.

Phlebotomy: Act or practice of opening a vein by incision or puncture to remove blood.

Plasma: Clear yellowish fluid that remains after the cells are removed.

Plethoric: Characterized by an overabundance of blood.

Reticulocyte: Immature red blood cell.

Rh factor: The human blood grouping system that is clinically the most important after the ABO system. The term specifically refers to the "D" antigen.

Serum: Fluid and solutes that remain after the cells and fibrinogen are removed.

Splenomegaly: Enlargement of the spleen.

Stomatitis: Oral mucosa ulcers.

Syncope: Fainting.

Tachycardia: Higher than normal heart rate.

Thrombocytopenia: Presence of relatively few platelets in the blood.

Overview

Blood is the fluid component of the cardiovascular system. Circulating blood provides nutrients, oxygen, glucose, electrolytes, hormones, and a way of removing wastes in the body. The blood also transports specialized cells that defend peripheral tissues from infection and disease. The primary action of red blood cells (RBCs) is to carry oxygen, white blood cells (WBCs) mostly fight pathogens, and platelets are used for clotting. The blood assists in controlling body temperature by distributing heat through the peripheral tissues. *Hemostasis* depends on clotting factors in the circulating blood. Stable pH (between 7.35 and 7.45) is maintained by buffer systems in the blood. Disorders of the blood are common yet varied.

Nature of Blood

Blood is a connective tissue that contains cellular and liquid components. The blood volume of the adult male is 5–6 liters and in an adult human female, is 4–5 liters, which accounts for 8 percent of body weight. It is made up of water and dissolved solutes (collectively termed *plasma*, discussed below). The remainder (45 percent) is composed of blood cells or formed elements. The proportion of cells (mostly the erythrocytes, which are also called RBCs) in blood is called hematocrit. This component indicates the viscosity of the blood, with males having a higher hematocrit (averaging 48 percent) than females (averaging 42 percent). Elevated hematocrit levels may indicate dehydration or an excess of RBCs. Low hematocrit levels can occur due to blood loss or anemia. The fluid and solutes that remain after the cells and fibrinogen are removed are collectively termed **serum**.

Plasma proteins in the blood include albumin (which maintains the blood's osmotic pressure), globulins (antibodies), and fibrinogen (needed for blood clot formation). **Figure 12–1** summarizes blood components and functions.

Red Blood Cells

Red bone marrow in the body is the site of origination of all blood cells. During hemopoiesis or **hematopoiesis**, various blood cells develop from a stem cell. The cells proliferate and mature to provide specialized functional cells required by the body. In adults, the only site of blood cell production is the red bone marrow.

RBCs are also called *erythrocytes*. Mature erythrocytes do not have nuclei and contain hemoglobin. Each hemoglobin molecule has 2 alpha chains and 2 beta chains of polypeptides. The RBCs are biconcave, highly flexible disks (**Figure 12–2A and B**) and can easily pass through small capillaries.

The kidneys secrete a hormone called **erythropoietin**, which stimulates the production of erythrocytes in the red bone marrow as a response to insufficient oxygen (hypoxia). For example, when a person who lives in a city that is at sea level takes a vacation in the Rocky Mountains, their red blood cells will increase in number. The level of erythropoietin in the blood may also rise during anemia, hemorrhage, and when blood flow to the kidneys is disrupted. RBCs normally live 120 days. As aging occurs they become rigid and fragile. They are phagocytized in the spleen or liver. These RBCs are broken down into globin and heme, with globin further broken down into amino acids. The iron in these cells is returned to the bone marrow and liver.

> **RED FLAG**
>
> Hemoglobin is a protein chain (globin) within RBCs, composed of an iron–porphyrin complex (heme), which is able to exchange carbon dioxide and oxygen.

White Blood Cells

WBCs, or **leukocytes,** are a part of the body's defense against infection. Leukocytes do not have hemoglobin, and they

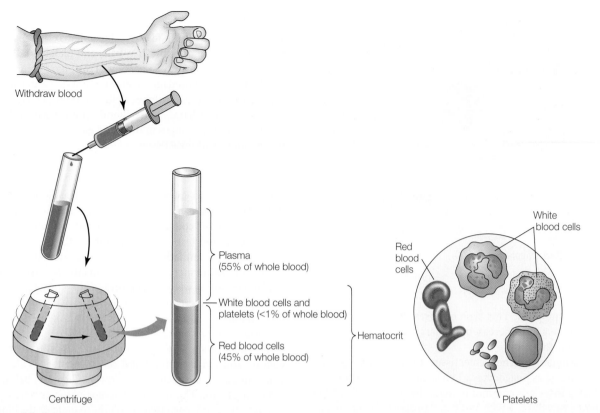

Figure 12–1 Blood composition. lood removed from a person can be centrifuged to separate plasma from the cellular component. Red blood cells constitute about 45% of the blood volume, except at higher altitudes where they make up about 50% of the volume to compensate for the lower oxygen levels.

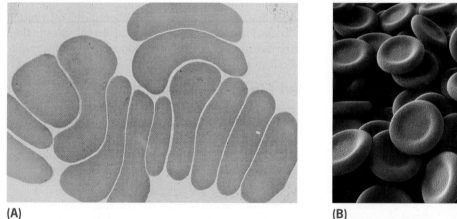

(A)

(B)

Figure 12–2 Red blood cells. (A) Transmission electron micrograph of human RBCs showing their flexibility. (B) Scanning electron micrograph of human RBCs.

move through capillary walls by **diapedesis**. They are classified into two groups: granulocytes and agranulocytes. Granulocytes have large granules in their cytoplasm. Examples are neutrophils, basophils, and eosinophils. Agranulocytes do not have these granules; examples are lymphocytes and monocytes.

Leukocytes vary in structure and function. Some of them are visible as large nucleated cells (via a purple stain) in the blood smear (**Figure 12–3**). There are five types of leukocytes:

- Neutrophils: The most common leukocytes, making up 50 percent to 60 percent of WBCs, but surviving only 4 days; immature neutrophils are called *bands* or *stabs*; they increase in number in response to bacterial infections.
- Lymphocytes: These make up 30 percent to 40 percent of WBCs.
- Basophils: They migrate from the blood to enter tissue and become mast cells capable of releasing histamine and heparin.

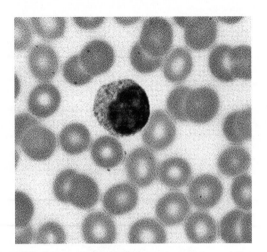

Figure 12–3 Lymphocyte (X 600).

- Eosinophils: This type opposes the effects of histamine and is increased by allergic reactions and parasitic infections.
- Monocytes: These enter tissue to become *macrophages*, acting as phagocytes when tissue damage occurs.

Diagnoses are commonly made by using a *differential count* procedure, which indicates proportions of specific types of WBCs in the blood. Bacterial infections or inflammatory conditions cause neutrophils to increase, whereas allergic reactions or parasitic infections cause eosinophils to increase.

Platelets

Platelets are also called *thrombocytes* and are vital for blood clotting and hemostasis (**Figure 12–4**). They are not cells but rather cell fragments from large megakaryocytes. Platelets adhere to damaged tissue and each other, forming a platelet plug to seal small blood vessel breaks. They can also adhere to foreign material and rough surfaces. Their ability to adhere is reduced by drugs such as aspirin. Thrombocytes can also begin the coagulation process.

Megakaryocyte   Platelets

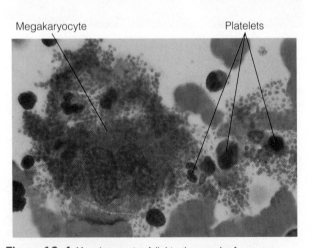

Figure 12–4 Megakaryocyte. A light micrograph of a mega-karyocyte, a large, multinucleated cell found in bone marrow; the megakaryocyte fragments, giving rise to platelets.

Plasma

The blood **plasma** is a fluid extracellular matrix that suspends the formed elements (RBCs, WBCs, and platelets). Plasma makes up approximately 55 percent of the blood volume and is a clear, straw-colored liquid. Plasma contains water, amino acids, carbohydrates, proteins, lipids, vitamins, electrolytes, hormones, and cell fragments. Blood volume varies with the size of the body, changes in fluid and electrolyte levels, and the amount of adipose tissue.

Diagnostic Tests

A complete blood count is taken to test the blood for total RBCs, WBCs, platelets, **morphology** (size and shape of cells), differential WBC count, hemoglobin, and hematocrit. This and other blood tests are important for diagnosing many conditions. Inflammation or infection is often signified by **leukocytosis** (an increase in WBCs in circulation). Certain viral infections, as well as radiation and chemotherapy, cause **leukopenia**, a decrease in leukocytes. Size, shape, uniformity, maturity, and amounts of cells and hemoglobin are very important when a blood smear is analyzed.

Hematocrit shows the percentage of RBCs in the blood volume and indicates fluid and cell content. It is checked when anemia is suspected, with low RBC counts being the indicating factor. The amount of hemoglobin per cell is illustrated by the mean corpuscular volume to indicate the blood's oxygen-carrying capacity. The **reticulocyte** count helps to assess bone marrow function, and other tests can determine the blood's levels of iron, vitamin B_{12}, folic acid, cholesterol, urea, and bilirubin.

Bleeding time tests can determine specific blood-clotting disorders. Prothrombin time or partial thromboplastin time can be measured to determine the function of various coagulation factors.

Red Blood Cell Disorders

Common blood diseases (dyscrasias) include the various anemias (including iron deficiency anemia, pernicious anemia, aplastic anemia, hemolytic anemia, sickle cell anemia, and thalassemia) and polycythemia.

Anemias

The term *anemia* has been used incorrectly as a diagnosis. It actually denotes a complex group of signs and symptoms. The "type" of anemia defines its pathophysiologic mechanism and its essential nature, allowing for appropriate therapy. Blood loss may be acute or chronic. Acute blood loss carries a risk for hypovolemia and shock. Chronic blood loss does not affect blood volume but instead leads to iron deficiency anemia when iron stores are depleted. Anemias affect the body by reducing oxygen transport in the blood because of decreased hemoglobin. This leads to the following sequence of events:

- Cell metabolism and reproduction are diminished, and the cells have less energy.

> **RED FLAG**
> Anemia is a decrease in hemoglobin or RBCs, or both. The physical therapist assistant (PTA) needs to understand that anemia affects the patient's ability to tolerate physical therapy and exercise.

- Tachycardia and peripheral vasoconstriction occur to compensate.
- Signs and symptoms include fatigue, **pallor** (paleness of the face), **dyspnea** (increased efforts to breathe), and **tachycardia**.
- Inflammation of the digestive tract occurs, leading to **stomatitis** (oral mucosa ulcers), drying and inflammation of the lips, dysphagia (difficulty swallowing), and less lustrous hair and skin.
- Severe anemia can lead to angina during stress and, eventually, to congestive heart failure.

The causes of anemia include nutrient deficiencies, impaired bone marrow function, excessive blood loss, and excessive destruction of RBCs. **Table 12–1** summarizes various types of anemia.

Iron Deficiency Anemia

Iron deficiency anemia is a common worldwide cause of anemia, affecting people of all ages. It results from increased demands on the stored iron in the body that exceed the amount the body can supply. Lack of iron impedes hemoglobin synthesis, reducing oxygen transport in the blood. **Microcytic, hypochromic** erythrocytes are the result (**Figure 12–5A and B**). About one of every five women is affected, with higher amounts of pregnant women experiencing the disorder. Iron deficiency anemia often occurs because of another underlying condition.

Signs and Symptoms

Iron deficiency anemia manifests with the general signs and symptoms of other anemias, as described above, but with additional symptoms such as cold intolerance, irritability, concave or ridged nails, **glossitis**, menstrual irregularities, delayed wound healing, palpitations, and **syncope** (fainting).

Etiology

Iron deficiency anemia may be caused by less than adequate iron in the diet, chronic blood loss, hemorrhoids, cancer, or excessive menstrual flow. Disorders that can impair iron absorption include **malabsorption** syndromes such as regional ileitis, **achlorhydria** (lack of hydrochloric acid in the stomach), gastrectomy procedures, severe liver disease, and protein deficits. In men the most frequent cause of iron deficiency anemia is chronic **occult** bleeding, usually from the gastrointestinal tract.

TABLE 12–1	Types of Anemia		
Type	**RBC States**	**Etiology**	**Effects**
Iron deficiency anemia	Hypochromic, microcytic, decreased hemoglobin production	Decreased dietary intake, malabsorption, blood loss	Only effects of anemia
Pernicious anemia	Megaloblasts, short life span	Deficit of intrinsic factor due to immune reaction	Achlorhydria and neurologic damage
Aplastic anemia	Normal cells (often), pancytopenia	Bone marrow damage or failure	Excessive bleeding, multiple infections
Sickle cell anemia	Elongated and hardened RBCs into "sickle" shape when oxygen levels are low, short life span	Recessive inheritance	Painful crises with multiple infarctions, hyperbilirubinemia

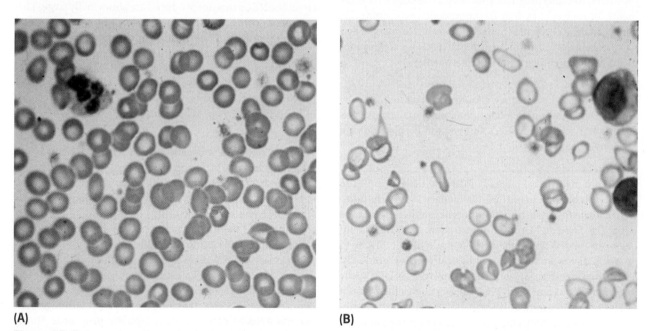

(A)   **(B)**

Figure 12–5 Comparison of normal red cells (A) with those of hypochromic microcytic anemia (B) caused by chronic iron deficiency (original magnification X 400).

Diagnosis

Iron deficiency anemia is indicated in laboratory tests by low values for hemoglobin, hematocrit, mean corpuscular volume, mean corpuscular hemoglobin, serum ferritin, serum iron, and transferring saturation. Under a microscope the RBCs appear hypochromic and microcytic. *Poikilocytosis* (irregular shape) and *anisocytosis* (irregular size) are also present.

Treatment

Treatment depends on the actual cause of this type of anemia. Iron-rich foods or supplements may be given. Iron supplements should be taken with food to reduce gastric irritation and nausea, and their use may lead to constipation. If given as an oral solution, a straw should be used to avoid staining teeth or dentures. The role of the PTA in iron deficiency anemia is to assist with suggested exercises after the patient has started taking iron supplements.

Prognosis

Prognosis is good as long as the underlying cause of iron deficiency anemia is identified.

Folate Deficiency Anemia

Also known as "folic acid deficiency anemia," this type of megaloblastic anemia results when insufficient amounts of folic acid are available for DNA synthesis.

Signs and Symptoms

Folate deficiency anemia causes tiredness, lightheadedness, forgetfulness, difficulty in concentration, loss of appetite, weight loss, and agitation.

Etiology

The most common causes of folic acid deficiency are malnutrition or dietary lack of folic acid. This is especially common in the elderly or because of alcoholism. Malabsorption of folic acid may be due to syndromes such as *sprue* or other intestinal disorders. Because pregnancy increases the body's requirements for folic acid by 5 to 10 times, deficiency commonly occurs. During pregnancy poor dietary habits, anorexia, and nausea also may cause folic acid deficiency. This type of anemia is clinically similar to pernicious anemia.

Diagnosis

A complete medical history should be taken, followed by blood tests to show deficiency of folic acid, to diagnose this condition. Lack of both RBCs and vitamin B_{12} also indicate the condition.

Treatment

Treatment involves taking daily folic acid tablets or pills to bring levels back up to normal. On January 1, 1998 the addition of folate to cereal grain products became a requirement of the U.S. Food and Drug Administration. After the patient has been treated with folic acid, the role of the PTA is to ensure patients increase their physical exercise gradually. There are no restrictions on physical exercise as long as the patient does not feel tired. Physical exertion to the point of fatigue must be avoided. If the patient experiences numbness, balance problems, or visual disturbances the physician should be contacted.

Prognosis

Prognosis is good as long as folic acid supplementation is administered. Lack of sufficient folic acid in pregnant women can cause neural tube defects, such as spina bifida, in the developing spines of fetuses.

Pernicious Anemia

Pernicious anemia is a progressive, megaloblastic, macrocytic anemia that results from a lack of intrinsic factor essential for cyanocobalamin (vitamin B_{12}) absorption in the ileum. As a result the maturation of RBCs in bone marrow becomes disordered. Pernicious anemia is a chronic condition of reduced hemoglobin levels. It is also known as *Addison's anemia*. Deficiency of vitamin B_{12} inhibits the growth of RBCs. This leads to the production of insufficient and deformed RBCs with poor oxygen-carrying capacity.

Signs and Symptoms

Patients with pernicious anemia complain of extreme weakness, numbness and tingling in the extremities (paresthesia), fever, pallor, anorexia, and weight loss. Other symptoms include an enlarged, red, sore, and shiny tongue; gastric discomfort including nausea and diarrhea; loss of coordination; and ataxia.

Etiology

Pernicious anemia occurs because of two causes, inadequate intake or poor absorption of vitamin B_{12}. Inadequate intake may result from dietary deficiencies. Failure to absorb this vitamin occurs from a deficiency in intrinsic factor. Pernicious anemia is significantly more common in patients with autoimmune-related disorders (such as thyroiditis, myxedema, and Graves disease). Gastric resection can also result in the absence of intrinsic factor.

Diagnosis

Megaloblastic anemia is the form of anemia that is most linked to vitamin B_{12} deficiency. When vitamin B_{12} is deficient, the RBCs that are produced are abnormally large. This is because of excess RNA production of hemoglobin and structural protein. The cells have immature nuclei and show evidence of cellular destruction. Bone marrow is hyperactive, with increased megaloblasts. Granulocytes are decreased in number and hypersegmented. Serum vitamin B_{12} is lower than normal. Gastric atrophy is confirmed by the presence of hypochlorhydria or achlorhydria.

Treatment

Pernicious anemia is usually treated with cyanocobalamin injections and folic acid and iron therapy. Oral supplements are recommended prophylactically for pregnant women and vegetarians. Cardiac stress and neurologic damage can occur without proper early treatment.

The role of the PTA in pernicious anemia follows medical treatment with vitamin B_{12} replacement. Physical therapy is necessary for full recovery of body functions. This may consist of active assistive exercises, range-of-motion exercises, endurance training, and reconditioning. If orthostatic hypotension is present, tilt tables may be used, although their use has decreased. The patient typically progresses slowly in recovering normal body functions, over several months.

Additionally, walking is indicated for pernicious anemia patients along with supervised physical therapy.

Prognosis
Prognosis is good as long as prompt diagnosis and treatment occur.

Aplastic Anemia

The term **aplastic anemia** commonly implies a **panhypoplasia** of the bone marrow. This leads to loss of stem cells and **pancytopenia**. Many serious complications can result. The bone marrow can also become hypocellular with increased fatty tissue.

Signs and Symptoms
Onset of aplastic anemia is usually insidious, often occurring over weeks or months after exposure to a toxin, but occasionally may be acute. Signs vary because of the severity of the pancytopenia. Manifestations of the disease include waxy pallor of the skin and mucous membranes, weakness, dyspnea, leukopenia (with recurrent, multiple infections), **thrombocytopenia** (with **petechiae** [pinpointed skin hemorrhages]), and a tendency for excessive bleeding, especially in the mouth. Uncontrollable infections and hemorrhages become more likely as WBCs and platelets diminish.

Etiology
About half of the cases of aplastic anemia occur in middle-aged patients and are of unknown or idiopathic origin. It may be caused by **myelotoxins**, including excessive radiation, industrial toxins such as benzene, and certain drugs such as chloramphenicol, gold salts, phenylbutazone, phenytoin, and antineoplastic drugs. All these agents can damage the bone marrow. When severe aplastic anemia because of cancer treatment is a risk, stem cells may be harvested before treatment for later transfusion if they are needed. Other causes of aplastic anemia include viruses such as hepatitis C, autoimmune disease such as lupus, and genetic abnormalities such as myelodysplastic syndrome.

Diagnosis
Pancytopenia may be indicated by blood counts, and a bone marrow biopsy may be needed to confirm its cause. Erythryocytes may remain normal in appearance.

Treatment
Prompt treatment of the underlying cause and removal of any bone marrow–suppressing agents are essential. Blood transfusion may be required if stem cell levels are very low. In younger patients bone marrow transplantation may be helpful. Common complications of the use of donated stem cells include damage to the digestive tract, rejection, and infection that can result from immune suppression.

The role of the PTA in aplastic anemia is based on the progression of the condition. If advanced, physical exertion must be reduced. Even mild exertion often results in fatigue (due to the overworking the heart) and shortness of breath. The PTA should instruct the patient to avoid contact sports in order to avoid wounds that may lead to bleeding because of low platelet counts. Low impact, regular exercise is usually acceptable for patients with aplastic anemia.

> **RED FLAG**
> New techniques allow harvesting of stem cells from the peripheral blood instead of the bone marrow.

Prognosis
Prognosis is not as good as other types of anemia and is entirely based on prompt treatment and whether the bone marrow can be returned to normal.

Sickle Cell Anemia

Sickle cell anemia is a genetic disorder that results in abnormalities of the hemoglobin molecule of RBCs. It is more common in African Americans than in other groups in the United States. Sickle hemoglobin (HbS) is transmitted by recessive inheritance and can manifest as the sickle cell trait. Sickle cell disease occurs when the patient is a *homozygote* (having two HbS genes). Approximately 10 percent of Black Americans carry the trait for this disease, but only 0.1 percent to 0.2 percent of patients develop the actual disease. The RBCs that contain more HbS than HbA are prone to sickling when exposed to decreased oxygen tension in the blood. They become more elongated, with a "sickle" shape (**Figure 12–6A and B**). Once "sickled," RBCs are more rigid, fragile, and rapidly destroyed. Sickle cell anemia is the most common type of megaloblastic anemia.

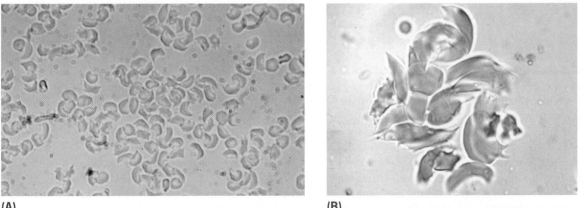

(A)   **(B)**

Figure 12–6 Distortion of red cells containing sickle hemoglobin when incubated under reduced oxygen tension. (A) Overview of cells under low magnification (X 100). (B) Higher magnification view (X 400) of red cell distortion caused by sickle hemoglobin.

Sickled cells cannot flow easily through tiny capillary beds and may become clumped and cause obstructions. The obstructions can lead to ischemia and necrosis, which produce the major clinical manifestations of pain. Serious crises may occur in individuals who have lung infections or dehydration when basic oxygen levels are reduced. Multiple infarctions can then occur throughout the body to affect the brain, bones, or organs. Many organ systems can experience loss of function over time. The high rate of hemolysis leads to hyperbilirubinemia, jaundice, and gallstones.

Signs and Symptoms

Once a child with sickle cell anemia is about 1 year old, fetal hemoglobin (HbF) is replaced by HbS, leading to pallor, weakness, tachycardia, dyspnea, hyperbilirubinemia with jaundice, gallstones, **splenomegaly**, adult fibrotic spleen, vascular occlusions and infarctions, leg or foot ulcers, bone or kidney necrosis, seizures or hemiplegia resulting from strokes, intense pain, acute chest syndrome with pain and fever, hand–foot syndrome with pain and swelling, delayed growth and development, late puberty, late tooth eruption, hypoplasia, impaired intellectual development, congestive heart failure, frequent infections, poor wound healing, pneumonia, and death.

> **RED FLAG**
> Symptoms of sickle cell anemia do not develop until age 6 months because fetal hemoglobin protects the infant for the first few months after birth.

Etiology

The recessive HbS gene is common in African and Middle Eastern patients. Clinical signs may only occur with severe hypoxia such as in pneumonia or at high altitudes. This is called the *sickle cell trait*. About 1 in 12 African Americans have the trait, and 1 in 600 have sickle cell anemia.

Diagnosis

A simple blood test known as hemoglobin electrophoresis can detect carriers of the defective gene. Prenatal diagnosis can be checked by DNA analysis of fetal blood. Children older than 1 year can be diagnosed via the presence of sickled cells in peripheral blood and the presence of HbS. Many states mandate neonatal screening of all newborns, regardless of their ethnic origin. Their bone marrow displays hyperplasia, with more immature RBCs being released into the blood circulation.

Treatment

There is no known cure for sickle cell anemia. Treatment to reduce symptoms includes pain medications, hydration, and management of complications. The drug known as hydroxyurea reduces the frequency of sickling crises and prolongs life span. Patients should avoid severe physical activity or high altitudes. Supportive measures include prevention of dehydration, acidosis, infection, and exposure to cold. Children should be immunized against pneumonia, influenza, and meningitis. Prophylactic penicillin may be required for young children and adults with severe cases. Prophylactic penicillin should begin in children as early as 2 months of age and continued until at least 5 years of age. Maintaining full immunizations is recommended.

The role of the PTA in sickle cell anemia includes educating patients about consuming large amounts of fluids with exercise. When exercising the patient should avoid aggressive activities, because this condition has been known to cause under-hydrated patients to die during very strenuous physical activity. The goal of exercise for sickle cell anemia patients is to improve their endurance. Exercises that use large muscle groups are preferred, but only at a moderate level. Exercise should be stopped immediately if the patient complains of pain developing in various areas of the body because this may progress to full body pain relatively quickly.

Prognosis

Prognosis for sickle cell anemia is relatively poor. Most children with sickle cell anemia are at risk for fulminant septicemia and death during the first 3 years of life. Many patients do not live past age 20.

Thalassemia

Thalassemia is also a type of hemolytic anemia. It usually results from a genetic defect and may vary from moderate to severe. The amount of hemoglobin synthesized and the number of RBCs that develop is reduced. Thalassemia *alpha* refers to a reduction in, or lack of, alpha chains (there are normally two alpha and two beta chains in hemoglobin). Thalassemia *beta* refers to a decrease, or lack or, beta chains. Thalassemia major is a severe form, and thalassemia minor is a mild form. This condition causes the bone marrow to be hyperactive as it attempts to compensate for the anemic state.

Signs and Symptoms

Thalassemia exhibits, aside from the normal signs and symptoms of anemia, the following:

- Beta-thalassemia minor is clinically asymptomatic.
- Beta-thalassemia major (**Cooley's anemia**) presents with symptoms of severe anemia. Patients are jaundiced, and leg ulcers and cholelithiasis occur. Splenomegaly is common, and the spleen may be several times its normal size.

> **RED FLAG**
> Bone marrow hyperactivity causes thickening of the cranial bones, and long bone involvement makes pathologic fractures common.

Etiology

Thalassemia results from unbalanced hemoglobin synthesis caused by decreased production of at least one globin polypeptide chain (alpha or beta). Thalassemia beta, the most common form, occurs frequently in patients from Mediterranean countries (such as Greece or Italy). The alpha form is most often found in Indians, Chinese, or southeastern Asians.

Diagnosis

Quantitative hemoglobin studies are used for routing clinical diagnosis. When a test shows elevated **HbA$_2$**, beta-thalassemia minor is indicated. In β-thalassemia major, **HbF** is usually increased, up to 90 percent. HbA$_2$ is usually elevated by 3 percent. The percentages of HbF and HbA$_2$ are generally normal in alpha-thalassemia.

In beta-thalassemia major, x-ray findings are characteristic of chronic bone marrow hyperactivity. The skull and long bones are thinned, and the marrow space is widened. Tests show microcytic RBCs of varied size, with low hemoglobin. There are increased erythropoietin levels and, often, an overload of iron.

Treatment

The outlook is varied for the different types of thalassemia. Life expectancy is normal for persons with beta-thalassemia minor. Some patients with beta-thalassemia major only live to puberty, whereas others live beyond it. The only effective treatment is blood transfusion. Multiple blood transfusions, however, may cause iron overload in patients. Iron chelation therapy can remove excess iron from numerous transfusions. Splenectomy may be required. Very severe forms may cause death during childhood.

The role of the PTA in thalassemia is to implement a specifically designed exercise plan for each patient. Generally, thalassemia patients should engage in 20- to 30-minute exercise sessions four times per week. Weight-bearing activities are indicated, including brisk walking, jogging, running, aerobics, step classes, dancing, and circuit training.

Prognosis

Prognosis is good with prompt and effective treatment, although severe forms have the ability to cause death if treatment is not adequate.

Polycythemia

Polycythemia is a chronic disease characterized by overproduction of total RBC mass with a hematocrit greater than 50 percent. Primary polycythemia (polycythemia vera) is a proliferative disease of the bone marrow stem cells. It also is accompanied by elevated WBC and platelet counts. Polycythemia vera is accompanied by splenomegaly and is neoplastic, with low serum erythropoietin levels. Secondary polycythemia (**erythrocytosis**) involves increased erythrocytes in response to prolonged hypoxia and increased erythropoietin secretion. In the primary form, there is increased blood volume and viscosity, with blood vessel distention and sluggish blood flow. Frequent thromboses and infarctions may result, with elevated blood pressure and hypertrophy of the heart. Hemorrhage is frequent with spleen and liver congestion and enlargement. Bone marrow may become fibrotic, resulting in anemia. Leukemia can develop in later stages if treatment has involved chemotherapy.

Signs and Symptoms

Patients appear **plethoric** and **cyanotic** with dark skin tones and mucosal darkening. The face may be red, and the retinal veins engorged. **Hepatomegaly** and splenomegaly are present, and pruritus is common. Blood pressure increases, with resulting effects, possibly leading to congestive heart failure.

Etiology

Primary polycythemia is of unknown cause. It most commonly develops in men between ages 40 and 60 years. Secondary polycythemia can result from a physiologic increase in erythropoietin levels, often as a compensatory response to hypoxia. Conditions that may cause hypoxia include high altitudes, chronic heart or lung disease, and smoking. When erythropoietin is released from the kidneys, it causes increased RBC formation in the bone marrow. Secondary polycythemia may also be caused by neoplasms that secrete erythropoietin.

Diagnosis

Tests may show increased cell counts, hemoglobin values, and hematocrit. In the primary type erythrocytes become abnormal or malignant. Red bone marrow may replace some fatty marrow, and hyperuricemia is present due to the high cell destruction rate.

Treatment

Bone marrow activity may be suppressed by drugs or radiation, which can lead to fibrosis or leukemia. Periodic removal of the blood, via **phlebotomy**, can minimize thromboses or hemorrhages. Treatment of secondary polycythemia is focused on relieving the causative hypoxia.

The role of the PTA in polycythemia involves education of the patient about acceptable activities, such as walking (which improves blood circulation and reduces the chances for blood clots). Moderate exercise is indicated to safely increase the heart rate of the patient. Leg and ankle stretching exercises are also indicated. It is important to ensure the patient does not develop any sores on the feet. Sores on the feet must be reported to the patient's physician. Therefore, it is important to teach the patient about correct self-inspection of the skin.

Prognosis

Prognosis depends on the time taken to diagnose the condition and begin proper treatment. Without treatment, 50 percent of symptomatic patients die within 18 months of diagnosis. With treatment, the median survival period is 7 to 15 years. Thrombosis is the most common cause of death, followed by complications of hemorrhage and the development of leukemia.

Transfusion Therapy and Incompatibility Reaction

Different types of anemias are treated with transfusions of whole blood or RBCs only when oxygen delivery to the tissues is compromised. This is based on measures of oxygen transport and use, hemoglobin, and hematocrit. It is currently recommended that a transfusion be undertaken when hemoglobin levels are less than 7 to 8 g/dL, but this depends on age, illness, risk factors, and surgical procedures.

When there is acute massive blood loss, a whole blood transfusion is usually indicated. However, most anemias are treated with transfusions of red cell concentrates. This supplies the patient with RBCs (the only blood component that is deficient). ABO blood group compatibility is essential for effective transfusion therapy. This requires knowledge of ABO antigens and antibodies. The four major ABO blood groups are differentiated by the presence or absence of the two red cell antigens (A and B).

Patients who have neither A nor B antigens are classified as having "type O" blood. Those with "A" antigens are classified as having "type A" blood. Those with "B" antigens have "type B" blood, and those with both types of antigens have "type AB" blood (**Table 12–2**). **Figure 12–7** further explains the ABO blood group and the compatibilities between each type of blood.

Transfusion incompatibility reaction can result when blood or blood products that have been transfused contain antibodies to the recipient's RBCs or if the recipient has antibodies to the donor's RBCs. If transfusion incompatibility reaction occurs, the recipient will react immediately. This is usually fatal (**Figure 12–8**).

	RECEIVERS							
DONORS		AB+	AB–	A+	A–	B+	B–	O+	O–
O–	✔	✔	✔	✔	✔	✔	✔	✔
O+	✔		✔		✔		✔	
B–	✔	✔			✔	✔		
B+	✔				✔			
A–	✔	✔	✔	✔				
A+	✔		✔					
AB–	✔	✔						
AB+	✔							

Figure 12–7 Antigens and antibodies of the ABO blood group.

TABLE 12–2 Blood Typing

Blood Type	Red Cell Antigens	Serum Antibodies	Transfuse To	Transfuse From
O	None	A and B	All	O
A	A	B	A, AB	A, O
B	B	B	B, AB	B, O
AB	A and B	None	AB	All

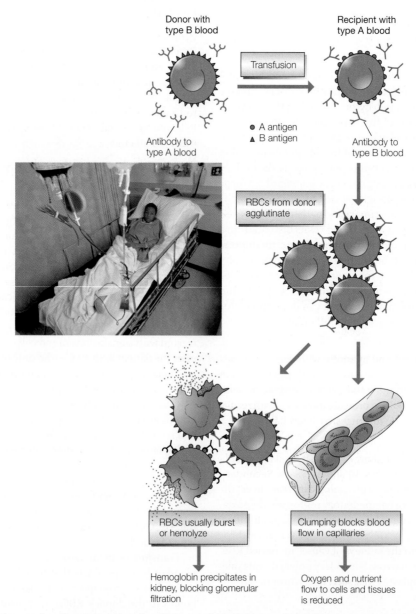

Figure 12–8 Transfusion reaction. Type B blood transfused into an individual with type A blood results in a transfusion reaction, characterized by agglutination and hemolysis, the breakdown of RBCs.

The **Rh factor** must also be considered in blood transfusions. This antigen is so named because it was first identified in rhesus monkeys. People who have the Rh antigen are said to be "Rh-positive," and those without it are "Rh-negative." In this blood typing system antibodies are produced when Rh-positive blood is transfused into the bloodstream of an Rh-negative person. Although the first such transfusion does not result in a transfusion reaction, the second transfusion does.

During pregnancy, problems can arise if an Rh-negative mother has an Rh-positive baby. Because small amounts of fetal blood enter the maternal bloodstream, the mother forms antibodies against the baby's Rh factor. Within 72 hours after an Rh-negative mother gives birth to an Rh-positive baby, she is injected with antibodies to fetal Rh-positive RBCs that bind to Rh-positive RBCs from the fetus before the mother's immune system can respond to them. The woman is therefore not sensitized, and a future pregnancy will not be in danger. Rh-positive babies born to Rh-negative mothers are likely to have brain damage, and may even die, if no measures are taken to counteract the effects of the Rh factor. **Figure 12–9** explains how the Rh factor interacts with pregnancy.

Signs and Symptoms
This reaction can range from mild to fatal, with severe reactions characterized by hemolysis or agglutination. Signs and symptoms include chills, fever, tachycardia, severe back pain, vomiting, diarrhea, hives or rash, dyspnea, a tightness below the sternum, hypotension, circulatory collapse, bleeding, blood in the urine, and, eventually, renal failure.

Etiology
ABO- and Rh-incompatible blood causes an antibody-antigen reaction that produces hemolysis or agglutination (clumping of RBCs). Histamine and serotonin release triggers disseminated intravascular coagulation (DIC).

Diagnosis
Any of the above-listed signs and symptoms should alert healthcare professionals to this type of reaction. Blood and urine specimens, along with the used blood, should be examined to confirm the incompatibility as well as any present hemolysis or activated coagulation.

Treatment
The patient's vital signs must first be taken several times over a 15-minute period. This monitoring of vital signs should continue at intervals throughout the procedure, wherein the blood transfusion is immediately stopped, and blood and urine samples are obtained for laboratory testing. Mild reactions are treated with antihistamines. Anaphylaxis is aggressively treated according to standard institutional procedures. The patient should not begin any exercise program after treatment for this disease until approved by his or her physician.

Prognosis
Prognosis varies based on how much blood has been transfused, the causative factors, and the speed of intervention.

White Blood Cell and Lymphoid Tissue Disorders
WBCs (and lymphoid tissues where they originate) mature and function to protect the body against invasion by foreign agents. WBC disorders include a deficiency of leukocytes (leukopenia) and proliferative disorders. These disorders may be reactive (such as when they occur due to infection) or neoplastic (such as with leukemias and lymphomas).

Neutropenia (Agranulocytosis)
Neutropenia (agranulocytosis) is a blood dyscrasia. It is signified by extremely low levels of leukocytes. It damages the immune system to reduce the body's response to bacterial infections. It affects females more than males.

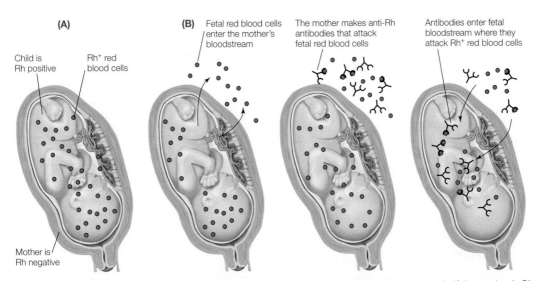

Figure 12–9 The Rh Factor and pregnancy. (A) Rh-positive cells from the fetus enter the mother's blood at birth. If the mother is Rh-negative, her immune system responds, producing antibodies to the Rh-positive RBCs and destroying them. (B) Problems arise if the mother becomes pregnant again and has another Rh-positive baby. If the mother was not treated the first time, antibodies to Rh-positive RBCs cross the placenta and destroy fetal RBCs.

Signs and Symptoms

Neutropenia may be of rapid onset, causing severe fatigue and weakness followed by a sore throat, dysphagia, oral mucosa ulcerations, fever, chills, and weak, rapid pulse.

Etiology

This condition is usually caused by hypersensitivity or drug toxicity. Causes include chemotherapy agents, benzene, chlorpromazine, propylthiouracil, chloramphenicol, phenytoin, and phenylbutazone. Neutropenia may also accompany aplastic or megaloblastic anemia, tuberculosis, malaria, or uremia. Pathogens usually invade the body through the oral or pharyngeal mucosa.

Diagnosis

Neutropenia is diagnosed via blood tests, bone marrow studies, patient history, and cultures (of blood, urine, and/or oral mucosa). Cultures are usually taken several times to monitor growth of microorganisms.

Treatment

Aggressive antimicrobial therapy is initiated to eliminate causative microorganisms. If caused by a drug or chemical, exposure to the substance must be eliminated. The role of the PTA in neutropenia is to assist with a slowly increasing physical therapy regimen designed to improve overall fitness and enhance resistance to disease. Fatigue and activities that cause a rapid heartbeat should be avoided. Exercise should be stopped if chest pain or shortness of breath occurs. Excessive exercise is contraindicated.

Prognosis

Prognosis is good only if treated within 1 week; otherwise, it may be fatal.

Leukemias

Leukemias are malignant diseases of the blood-forming organs, involving WBCs in the bone marrow and lymphatic tissues. Leukemias affect 30,000 new patients in the United States each year, including 2,500 children. Overall survival rates are only about 45 percent. In leukemia, WBCs multiply without control in the bone marrow to be released into the general circulation. These cells infiltrate the lymph nodes, spleen, liver, brain, and other organs. Onset of acute leukemia is usually abrupt. Chronic leukemias have more mature cells, insidious onset, mild signs, and a better prognosis. There are four major types of leukemia:

- Acute lymphocytic leukemia
- Chronic lymphocytic leukemia
- Acute myelogenous leukemia
- Chronic myelogenous leukemia

Acute myelogenous leukemia is the most common *acute form* of adult leukemia. Also, two of three children who develop acute leukemia have acute lymphocytic leukemia. An additional two types of leukemia are acute monocytic leukemia and hairy cell leukemia. The proliferation of leukemia cells in bone marrow suppresses production of other normal cells. As malignant cells develop, they cause

RED FLAG
In leukemia patients, death often occurs from a complication such as a massive infection or hemorrhage.

congestion and enlargement of lymphoid tissue, **lymphadenopathy**, splenomegaly, and hepatomegaly.

Chronic lymphocytic leukemia is the most common overall form of leukemia in adults in the United States and involves the B lymphocytes (B cells). **Table 12–3** describes the various types of leukemias in greater detail.

Signs and Symptoms

Onset of leukemia, when acute, is often marked by an infection that is unresponsive to treatment or by excessive bleeding. Signs and symptoms include multiple infections; severe hemorrhage; signs of anemia; bone pain; weight loss; fatigue; fever; enlarged lymph nodes, spleen, and/or liver; headache; visual disturbances; drowsiness; and vomiting. Chronic leukemia has more insidious onset with milder signs but includes fatigue, weakness, and frequent infections.

Etiology

The exact cause of acute leukemia is unknown, but there are several risk factors. Overexposure to radiation, even years before the development of the disease (particularly if the exposure was prolonged), is a major risk factor. Chronic leukemias are more common in older adults. Other risk factors include chemicals, chemotherapy, and certain viruses. Chromosomal abnormalities in children, such as Down syndrome and albinism, may also play a part.

Diagnosis

Peripheral blood smears show immature leukocytes and greatly increased numbers of WBCs, many of which are abnormal in appearance. RBCs and platelets appear in less than normal quantities. Bone marrow biopsy confirms the diagnosis.

Treatment

Leukemia is treated with chemotherapy, biologic therapy such as interferon, good nutrition and hydration, antacids to prevent kidney stones, and bone marrow transplantation. The role of the PTA in leukemia is to encourage and monitor as much exercise as the patient can tolerate. Exercise is proven to combat symptoms of fatigue, which are a major component of all forms of leukemia. Exercise equipment must be specially treated so that no infections may be transmitted to

TABLE 12–3 Types of Leukemias

Type	Primary Affected Patients	Malignant Cell
Acute lymphocytic leukemia (ALL)	Young children ages 2–4 years	B lymphocytes
Acute myelogenous (or myelocytic) leukemia (AML)	Adults	Granulocytic stem cells
Chronic lymphocytic leukemia (CLL)	Adults older than 50 years	B lymphocytes
Chromic myelogenous leukemia (CML)	Adults ages 30–50 years	Granulocytic stem cells
Acute monocytic leukemia	Adults	Monocytes
Hairy cell leukemia	Men older than 50 years	B lymphocytes

the patient due to his or her weakened immunity. Approved physical therapy for leukemia patients includes aerobic exercise, resistance exercise, core strengthening exercises, and light stretching.

Prognosis

Prognosis is excellent in young children with acute lymphocytic leukemia, which responds well to drug therapy. The best prognosis is found in children between the ages of 1 and 9 years. The more rapid the response to drug therapy, the more positive the outlook. Chemotherapy is less successful in adults with acute myelogenous leukemia. Individuals with chronic leukemia may live up to 10 years with treatment. Prognosis is often related to WBC counts and the proportion of blast cells present at the time of diagnosis.

Blood-Clotting Disorders

These disorders may be signified by spontaneous or excessive bleeding after minor tissue trauma. Warning signs can occur from many other conditions but include viral infections, autoimmune reactions, hepatomegaly, splenomegaly, certain drugs, chemotherapy, radiation, cancers, uremia, vitamin K deficiency, liver disease, malabsorption, inherited clotting factor conditions, hemorrhagic fever, and interactions with anticoagulants. Blood-clotting disorders include hemophilia A and DIC.

Clotting is stimulated by the release of *thromboplastin* from injured cells that line damaged blood vessels (**Figure 12–10A**). Thromboplastin is a lipoprotein that acts on the inactive plasma protein called *prothrombin* and converts it into its active form, *thrombin*. This acts on the blood protein called *fibrinogen*, which is converted into *fibrin*. When a blood vessel is damaged, a web-like network of fibrin traps RBCs and platelets to form a platelet plug, stopping blood flow to the tissue (**Figure 12–1B**). Additional thromboplastin is released, causing more fibrin to reinforce the network of fibers.

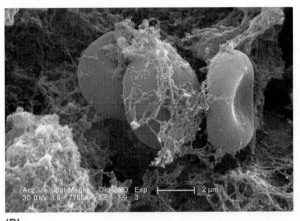

(B)

Figure 12–10 A scanning electron micrograph of a fibrin clot that has already trapped platelets and RBCs, plugging a leak in a vessel. The RBCs are red, and the fibrin network is turquoise.

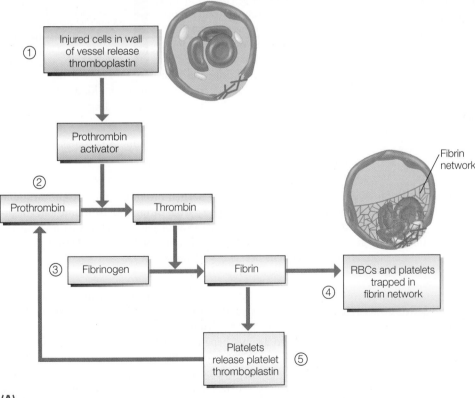

(A)

Figure 12–10 Blood clotting simplified. (A) Injured cells in the walls of blood vessels release the chemical thromboplastin (1). Thromboplastin stimulates the conversion of prothrombin, found in the plasma, into thrombin (2). Thrombin, in turn, stimulates the conversion of the plasma protein fibrinogen into fibrin (3). The fibrin network captures RBCs and platelets (4). Platelets in the blood clot release platelet thromboplastin (5), which converts additional plasma prothrombin into thrombin. Thrombin, in turn, stimulates the production of additional fibrin.

Thrombocytopenia

Thrombocytopenia (or *thrombocytopenia purpura*) consists of a decrease in platelets, which can lead to an inability of normal blood clotting.

Signs and Symptoms

Thrombocytopenia is characterized by abnormal skin bleeding, as well as bleeding in the mucous membranes and internal organs. Small hemorrhagic spots (petechiae) or larger ones (ecchymoses) may appear. The term *purpura* describes purple-colored areas of the skin. Other symptoms include gastrointestinal hemorrhage, nosebleeds, and hematuria.

Etiology

Thrombocytopenia can be caused by abnormal platelet production or destruction, with platelet life reduced to only hours instead of days. Causes are basically unknown. This condition is also sometimes called *idiopathic thrombocytopenia purpura*.

Diagnosis

Diagnosis is based on patient history as well as platelet count and bleeding time tests. Low platelet counts or extended bleeding times can indicate the disease.

Treatment

Treatment of thrombocytopenia includes avoiding additional tissue trauma, administration of vitamin K, and transfusion of platelets. Persistent disease requires a splenectomy, which is very effective but usually the last treatment of choice. The role of the PTA in thrombocytopenia is to assist and educate patients about low-impact methods of exercise they may undertake, while monitoring for any hazards that could injure the patient and cause bleeding.

Prognosis

Prognosis is fair with proper treatment, although this condition may indicate underlying cancers and other blood cell conditions. It requires constant, thorough medical monitoring that must be ongoing.

Disseminated Intravascular Coagulation

DIC is a potentially life-threatening condition of excessive bleeding and clotting. It causes multiple thromboses and infarctions but also consumes available clotting factors and platelets while stimulating the fibrinolytic process. This eventually leads to hemorrhage, hypotension, and/or shock.

Signs and Symptoms

Clinical effects of DIC depend on the underlying cause. Hemorrhage is usually the critical problem.

Etiology

DIC may be caused by obstetric complications, amniotic fluid embolus, abruptio placentae, infections, carcinomas, major trauma, and deposits of antigen-antibody complexes.

Diagnosis

The disorder is indicated by low plasma fibrinogen levels, thrombocytopenia, and prolonged bleeding time, prothrombin time, and thrombin time.

Treatment

In life-threatening cases of DIC treatment is difficult, depending on whether hemorrhage or thromboses dominate. Underlying causes must be successfully treated as well. If bleeding is severe, replacement therapy is indicated. Platelet concentrates and fresh frozen plasma should be used for thrombocytopenia. The role of the PTA in DIC is to assist with as much exercise as the patient can tolerate after treatment is successful. It is important that patients with DIC avoid exercise until the condition is stabilized.

Prognosis

Prognosis depends on the severity of the primary underlying cause.

Hemophilia

Classic hemophilia (hemophilia A) is a deficit or abnormality of clotting factor VIII, which manifests in men but is carried by women. Ninety percent of hemophiliacs have this type. About 400 infants are born each year with hemophilia in the United States. About 70 percent of affected individuals have the severe type wherein bleeding can occur without significant trauma. Hemophilia B (factor IX deficiency) has identical clinical manifestations and shows similar abnormalities in screening tests.

Signs and Symptoms

A patient with a factor VIII or IX level less than 1 percent of normal has severe bleeding episodes throughout life. Minor trauma results in prolonged or severe hemorrhage. This may occur into joints (**hemarthrosis**) and can cause painful, crippling deformities due to recurring inflammation. Blood may appear in the urine or feces due to internal bleeding.

> **RED FLAG**
> Bleeding into the base of the tongue, causing airway compression, may be life threatening and requires prompt, vigorous replacement therapy.

Etiology

The causative defect for hemophilia is transmitted as an X-linked recessive trait.

Diagnosis

Blood tests reveal normal bleeding time and prothrombin time but prolonged partial thromboplastin time and coagulation times. Low serum levels of factor VIII or IX exist. Generation time of thromboplastin differentiates between deficits of factor VIII and factor IX.

Treatment

Hemophiliacs should avoid using aspirin. Regular dental care is essential to avoid tooth extractions and other dental surgery. Newly diagnosed hemophiliacs should be vaccinated against hepatitis B. Replacement therapy for factors VIII and IX are available by using fresh frozen plasma. Some individuals have, however, developed immune reactions to repeated replacement therapy. A new recombinant DNA product called Advate shows great signs of positive treatment outcomes because it does not contain any ingredients than can provoke immune responses.

The role of the PTA in hemophilia is to assist the patient with exercise intended to help strengthen and condition his or her joints and muscles. Range-of-motion, strength, and *proprioception* (position changing) exercises are focused on the knees, ankles, and elbows. Muscle exercises are focused on strengthening or lengthening muscles that have become tight due to bleeding or in response to joint bleeding. Most muscle exercises for hemophiliacs focus on the hips, calves, hamstring muscles, forearms, and quadriceps.

Prognosis

Prognosis varies based on age of the patient and responses to treatment.

SUMMARY

Blood and blood vessels transport oxygen and nutrients to cells, help prevent infection, and remove wastes. The other major structures of this system include the lymph nodes, bone marrow, liver, and spleen. Blood-related conditions often cause fatigue, shortness of breath, bleeding, lesions, increased susceptibility to infections, and pain. Anemia is the most common RBC-related disorder, and all types of anemia share common symptoms. Leukemia is a common disorder of the WBCs. Platelet disorders include bleeding diseases such as hemophilia. Older adults may develop hematologic disorders that are actually related to disorders of other body systems.

REVIEW QUESTIONS

Select the best response to each question.

1. Stimulation of erythropoietin is caused by what condition?
   a. tissue hypoxia
   b. hypervolemia
   c. inflammation
   d. infection

2. Overproduction of erythrocytes, leukocytes, and platelets, accompanied by splenomegaly, signifies which of the following conditions?
   a. chronic lymphocytic leukemia
   b. acute monocytic leukemia
   c. acute myelogenous leukemia
   d. polycythemia vera

3. What is the primary risk to thalassemia major patients who receive frequent and multiple blood transfusions?
   a. iron overload
   b. polycythemia
   c. hyperviscosity
   d. all of the above

4. Neutropenia can be observed in which of the following?
   a. bone marrow injury
   b. nutritional deficiency
   c. increased destruction and utilization
   d. all of the above

5. The most common type of anemia in the United States is which of the following?
   a. sickle cell anemia
   b. pernicious anemia
   c. folate deficiency anemia
   d. iron deficiency anemia

6. Hemophilia B may occur because of a lack of which clotting factor?
   a. Factor V
   b. Factor VII
   c. Factor VIII
   d. Factor IX

7. The most common form of chronic leukemia is which of the following?
   a. myelogenous
   b. lymphocytic
   c. monocytic
   d. eosinophilic

8. The failure of bone marrow to produce erythrocytes, leukocytes, and platelets is called
   a. hemolytic anemia
   b. aplastic anemia
   c. sickle cell anemia
   d. leukemia

9. The chronic hereditary form of anemia found predominantly in Blacks is known as
   a. sickle cell
   b. hemolytic
   c. pernicious
   d. aplastic

10. Malabsorption of vitamin B_{12} due to lack of intrinsic factor may cause which condition?
    a. iron deficiency anemia
    b. polycythemia
    c. pernicious anemia
    d. aplastic anemia

CASE STUDIES

Karen Coupe, PT, DPT, MSEd

Case 1

A 67-year-old woman is hospitalized with complaints of chronic fatigue and unexplained bleeding and bruising. Blood testing and a bone marrow biopsy confirm a diagnosis of chronic lymphocytic leukemia. Complications include hemolytic anemia and thrombocytopenia. The patient began chemotherapy but has become very weak and developed pneumonia. Prior level of function: Independent in ambulation up to 20 feet before fatigue, independent bed mobility and transfers, required assistance with household chores of cooking and cleaning. PT plan of care is for ambulation with front-wheeled rolling walker, bed mobility, and transfers.

1. Explain the etiology and clinical manifestations of chronic lymphocytic leukemia.
2. When reviewing lab results for this patient and the diagnosis, what blood test values would be high or low? Is it important for the PTA to check these values before treatment? Why or why not?
3. What is hemolytic anemia? How might it affect the patient during therapy?
4. What is thrombocytopenia? What precautions should be taken with a patient during therapy?

5. Would this patient be considered immunocompromised? What precautions should be taken if this is true?

Case 2

A 32-year-old woman was admitted to the hospital after a car accident. The patient suffered a fractured right humeral neck and underwent an *open reduction internal fixation*, in addition to a ruptured spleen with severe internal bleeding and subsequent splenectomy with blood transfusion. Patient medical history: PT plan of care is for bed mobility, transfers, therapeutic exercise, and ambulation with axillary crutches.

1. Explain the role of the spleen. Will this have any effects on physical therapy treatment?
2. The patient underwent a blood transfusion. What are some signs and symptoms that could present if the patient has a reaction to the transfusion?
3. Before seeing the patient in the afternoon after the morning PT evaluation, the PTA is reviewing the chart and notes a hemoglobin level of 12 g/dL. Would the PTA continue with the treatment? What levels would put treatment on hold? Why?

4. Before seeing the patient on the second day the PTA is reviewing the chart and notes the blood lab values indicate leukocytosis. What could this mean? Should the PTA continue with treatment?
5. On the third day the patient developed DIC and therapy was put on hold. What does this mean?

WEBSITES

http://generalmedicine.suite101.com/article.cfm/ blood_clotting_disorders

http://www.funsci.com/fun3_en/blood/blood.htm

http://www.healthline.com/channel/abo-incompatibility-reaction.html

http://www.leukemia.org/hm_lls

http://www.merck.com/mmhe/sec14.html

http://www.nia.nih.gov/HealthInformation/Publications/ AgingHeartsandArteries/chapter04.htm

http://www.nlm.nih.gov/medlineplus/ency/article/000560 .htm

http://www.oncologychannel.com/leukemias/index.shtml

Lymphatic Disorders

OUTLINE

LEARNING OBJECTIVES

After completion of this chapter the reader should be able to

1. Discuss the major functions of the lymphatic system.
2. Describe the common signs and symptoms of lymphatic system disorders.
3. Distinguish between lymphangitis and lymphedema.
4. Explain Reed-Sternberg cells in lymphoma.
5. List the other name for multiple myeloma and discuss how it affects older adults.
6. List the causative virus for mononucleosis and how the disease is transmitted.
7. Distinguish Hodgkin's disease and non-Hodgkin's lymphoma.
8. Describe the Bence-Jones protein.

KEY TERMS

Antigens: Specific invading substances or structures the body senses as "foreign."

Bence-Jones protein: A monoclonal globulin protein found in the blood or urine that is often suggestive of multiple myeloma.

B lymphocytes: Those lymphocytes that play a central role in the humoral immune response, creating antibodies against specific antigens.

Filarial parasites: Long, round, thread-like worms that may invade lymphatic structures and vessels, soft tissues, and skin; they are most common in tropic and subtropic regions.

Heterophil: A neutrophil that can recognize antigens other than the one it is expected to attack.

Larvae: Juvenile forms of various types of animals, including insects.

Lymph nodes: Masses of lymphoid tissues that create lymphocytes, remove noxious agents, and are believed to help produce antibodies.

Lymphocytopenia: A deficiency of lymphocytes.

Lymphocytosis: An unusually large concentration of lymphocytes in the blood; it is often seen during allergic reactions or infections.

Lymphomas: Neoplastic growths of lymphoid tissue.

Remissions: Disappearances of diseases as a result of treatment.

Thymus: A lymphatic gland that shrinks as the body ages; it serves primarily to begin the body's immunity during childhood.

Overview

The lymphatic system contains lymphatic vessels and organs. Common lymphatic disorders include **lymphomas**, multiple myeloma, and infectious mononucleosis. Lymphomas are malignant neoplasms. Non-Hodgkin's lymphomas are on the increase, partly because they are associated with HIV infection. The immune system responds to substances and structures that are perceived as foreign to the body. **Antigens** or immunogens provoke immune responses via antibodies. The lymphocyte is the primary cell in the immune response. Immunity is acquired in four ways: actively, passively, naturally, or artificially.

Anatomy and Physiology

The lymphatic system is made up of the lymphatic vessels, **lymph nodes**, and lymphoid tissue (including the palatine and pharyngeal tonsils, the spleen, and the **thymus** gland). **Figure 13–1** depicts the lymphatic system. Lymph fluid flows through the structures of this system and is similar to plasma but contains more lymphocytes. This system returns excess interstitial fluid and protein to the blood, filters and destroys unwanted materials, and initiates the immune response.

When infection occurs, regional lymph nodes often become swollen and tender. Enlarged nodes in the neck, for example, signify an upper respiratory infection. Body fluids are constantly monitored by lymph nodes situated along every lymphatic and blood vessel. Lymph nodes are also essential to the immune response and for the sensitization of the *B* and *T lymphocytes*.

Lymphatic circulation works in the following ways:

- Excess interstitial fluid flows in capillaries as tissue pressure increases.
- Lymphatic capillaries form larger vessels that have valves, creating a one-way flow of fluid.
- *Lymph nodes* are located at various points in the lymphatic vessels to filter the lymph and release more lymphocytes into it (**Figure 13–2**).
- The body's upper right quadrant empties lymph into the right lymphatic duct, which returns it to the general circulation via the right subclavian vein.
- The rest of the body's lymphatic vessels drain into the thoracic duct in the upper abdomen and thoracic cavity and then into the left subclavian vein.
- In the intestinal villi, lymphatic capillaries absorb and transport most lipids as chylomicrons.

Common Signs and Symptoms

When the body has an infection, a common sign is enlargement of the lymph nodes or glands. Other symptoms include fatigue, fever, and weight loss. Blood conditions that may occur include **lymphocytosis** and **lymphocytopenia**.

Diagnostic Tests

To determine lymphatic and immune deficiency disorders, a complete blood count with white blood cell differential is often used. Another test is the lymphangiography, which involves the injection of a contrast dye and taking x-rays. Other tests include computed tomography (CT) and magnetic resonance imaging (MRI). Additionally, biopsy of lymph nodes and glands can help in determination of a lymphoma.

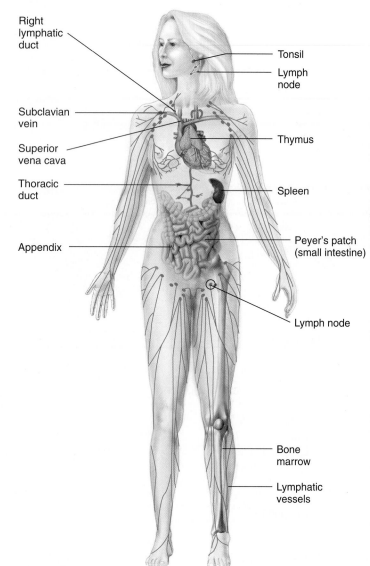

Figure 13–1 Human lymphatic system.

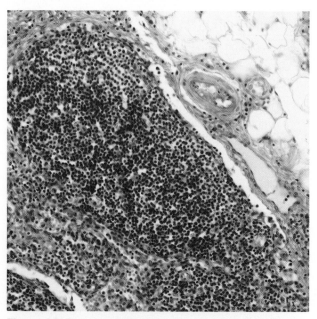

Figure 13–2 Lymph node, cortical region (original magnification X 200).

Lymphatic Disorders

Common lymphatic disorders include lymphadenopathy, lymphangiopathy, lymphomas (including Hodgkin's disease/Hodgkin's lymphoma and non-Hodgkin's lymphoma), multiple myeloma or plasma cell myeloma, and infectious mononucleosis.

Lymphedema

Lymphedema is an abnormal collection of lymph fluid in soft tissues. This usually occurs in the extremities but may occur in the trunk. The two broad categories are primary (idiopathic) and secondary (acquired) lymphedema. Stages of lymphedema are as follows:

- Stage 0 (latent): Reduced lymph transport capacity with no clinical edema
- Stage I: Protein-rich pitting edema, reversible with elevation, increases with activity, heat, or humidity
- Stage II: Protein-rich pitting edema with connective scar tissue, irreversible, with clinical fibrosis; when stage II is severe, skin changes are present
- Stage III (lymphostatic elephantiasis): Severe protein-rich nonpitting edema with significant increase in connective and scar tissue, with fibrosis; atrophic changes include hardening of dermal tissue, skin folds, skin papillomas, and hyperkeratosis

Signs and Symptoms

Swelling and heaviness in the arms, hands, fingers, legs, feet, and toes are the common signs of lymphedema. Lymphedema of the lower extremities begins with mild swelling of the foot that extends to the entire limb (**Figure 13-3A and B**). The infection may spread to the bloodstream.

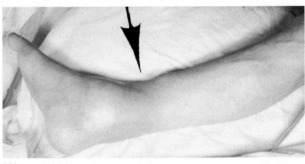

(A)

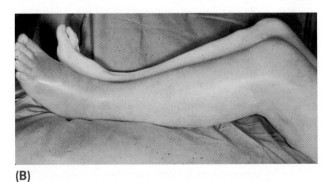

(B)

Figure 13-3 (A) Marked pitting edema of leg (arrow) as a result of chronic heart failure. (B) Localized edema of left leg caused by venous obstruction. Right leg appears normal.

Etiology

Lymphedema is most often caused by inflammation, obstruction, or removal of lymph channels. Other causes include surgical removal of lymph channels, mastectomy, obstruction of lymph drainage due to malignant tumors, or infestation of lymph vessels with adult **filarial parasites**. These parasites are long, round worms with a thread-like appearance. They are most often found in tropic and subtropic regions. They usually enter the body as microscopic **larvae** after the bite of an insect, most commonly a mosquito. *Filariasis* results, characterized by occlusion of the lymphatic vessels, causing the affected limb to swell and become painful.

It is possible for this condition to cause a leg to swell so it weighs much more than other parts of the body. This condition is called *elephantiasis*. Elephantiasis is the end-stage lesion of long-term filariasis and is characterized by extensive swelling, most commonly of the legs and external genitalia (**Figure 13-4**). The overlying skin darkens, thickens, and becomes coarse. Congenital lymphedema is a hereditary disorder caused by chronic lymphatic obstruction. Secondary lymphedema may follow this condition.

> **RED FLAG**
> Lymphedema is aggravated by pregnancy, prolonged standing, obesity, warm weather, and the menstrual period.

Diagnosis

Patient history as well as physical examination of affected areas (often with physical therapist or occupational therapist evaluation), followed by CT or MRI scans, confirm the diagnosis of lymphedema. If a patient is diagnosed with cancer involving the lymph nodes and surgery is indicated, the patient can take steps to prevent or reduce secondary lymphedema from occurring (see Treatment, below).

> **RED FLAG**
> Physical or massage therapists may use lymph drainage therapy to help clear lymphatic obstructions and provide relief from pain and swelling. This technique is a large part of preventing recurrence of lymphedema.

Treatment

Treatment depends on the cause of lymphedema. This may include antibiotics, raising the affected area above heart level,

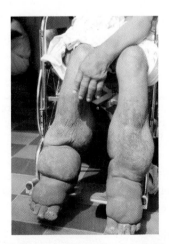

Figure 13-4 Elephantiasis. A parasitic worm that invades the body stimulates the production of scar tissue, which blocks the flow of lymph through the nodes, causing tissue fluid to build up. This condition is known as elephantiasis.

exercise, wearing looser clothing, compression therapy, and surgery.

For secondary lymphedema the patient can reduce risks of developing the condition with the following steps:

- Protecting the arms or legs from cuts, scrapes, and burns
- Resting the arms or legs during recovery
- Avoid applying heat to the arms or legs
- Elevating the arms or legs
- Avoid tight clothing
- Keep the arms and legs clean, including the nails, to avoid infection

It is also important that the limb with lymphedema should not be used for any clinical tests or for measuring vital signs, such as blood pressure, or needle sticks. Secondary lymphedema is managed long term with the use of compression garments.

Prognosis

Prognosis depends on the causative factors and whether treatment is correctly given.

Lymphadenitis

Lymphadenitis occurs when a lymph node becomes overwhelmed by an infection and becomes infected. It can be classified as acute or chronic. When acute, lymphadenitis is usually located in the cervical region and is related to tooth or tonsil infections. It may also be located in the axillary or inguinal regions due to infections in the extremities. Lymphadenitis, when chronic, may result in scarring of the lymph nodes and replacement of them with fibrous connective tissue.

Signs and Symptoms

Lymphadenitis is characterized by swelling of the lymph glands, nodes, or both. Pain and tenderness are also common.

Etiology

Lymphadenitis is usually caused by a primary infection elsewhere in the body, with swelling developing because of drainage of bacteria or toxic substances.

Diagnosis

Physical examination that reveals swollen lymph nodes is indicative of lymphadenitis. Blood cultures may determine spread of infection to the bloodstream, confirmed by biopsy.

Treatment

Antibiotic treatment is generally helpful to cure primary bacterial infections. Maintaining overall good health is helpful in preventing infections.

Prognosis

Prompt antibiotic treatment usually results in complete recovery. Swelling may take weeks or months to disappear. Recovery is based on the underlying cause.

Lymphangitis

Lymphangitis is a condition involving swelling of the lymph vessels because of inflammation.

Signs and Symptoms

It is often characterized by a red streak where bacteria have entered the lymph vessel, extending to the nearby lymph nodes. Other symptoms include chills, fever, headache, malaise, cellulitis, and leukocytosis. Cellulitis is a common skin infection caused by bacteria that often accompanies lymphatic conditions.

Etiology

The inflammation of one or more lymphatic vessels is usually caused by an acute streptococcal infection of one of the extremities, which follows some form of localized trauma.

Diagnosis

It may be diagnosed quickly based on the red streaks below the skin surface, combined with high fever. Complete blood count and blood culture indicate if bacteria are present in the bloodstream, and a biopsy determines the type of causative bacteria.

Treatment

Lymphangitis is usually treated with antibiotics (penicillins), hot and moist packs, and elevation of the affected area. If concurrent cellulitis develops, it requires immediate action to avoid dangerous outcomes. Antibiotics are indicated to treat cellulitis as well as other underlying infections. Physical therapy must be evaluated carefully because some patients experience increased pain caused by exercise.

Prognosis

Prognosis is good as long as treatment guidelines are followed and good hygiene and general health are maintained.

Lipedema

Lipedema is defined as a symmetric swelling of both legs that extends from the hips to the ankles. It is caused by deposits of subcutaneous adipose tissue. Lipedema is described in several stages, with stage I causing nodular skin changes that may be palpated. In stage II the skin becomes more nodular and tough, with large fatty lobules forming.

Signs and Symptoms

In lipedema fat in the lower extremities extends to "flap over" the feet, which are not affected themselves. Usually, fatty bulges exist in the medial proximal thigh and medial distal thigh, just above the knee. Patients often complain of pitting edema during

> **RED FLAG**
> Onset of lipedemic swelling is often around puberty.

the daytime hours, which is relieved by prolonged leg elevation overnight. Hypersensitivity may occur over the anterior tibial area. Skin color changes may occur in the lower legs. Lipedema is also occasionally found in the arms. Regardless of location, lipedema can decrease the elasticity of the epidermis and dermis, thicken the basement membrane of vessels, and disturb vasomotion. Increased venous or blood capillary pressure causes increased ultrafiltration. Lymph flow may or may not be affected.

Etiology

The underlying etiology of lipedema remains unknown. The condition is often confused with bilateral lower extremity lymphedema. Lipedema occurs almost entirely in women, is usually accompanied by hormonal disorders, and may have an associated family history. It occurs rarely in men, always accompanied by a serious hormonal disorder.

Diagnosis

Lipedema is diagnosed in part by its symmetric swelling, with the subcutaneous tissues feeling "rubbery." Diagnosis is otherwise difficult compared with lymphedema because common characteristics resemble each disease.

Treatment

No effective medical treatment for lipedema is available. The condition can be improved by treatment of the hormonal disturbance and altering diet to prevent additional weight gain. Without treatment, the individual becomes more embarrassed by the condition, and hypersensitivity often affects the ability to walk or exercise without pain. This unfortunately leads to further weight gain.

> **RED FLAG**
> It is important that lipedema patients be given support for needed exercise as well as counseling for their mental outlook.

Group sessions are often very helpful as patients can share their insights and problems in alleviating this condition. It is important for the physical therapist assistant (PTA) to understand that adipose fat that accumulates in the areas targeted by lipedema will never be lost by diet and exercise. Any physical therapy is targeted at overall improvement of health and mental outlook.

Prognosis

Prognosis for lipedema is guarded based on treatment of the underlying hormonal disturbance. Lower grade compression garments may be helpful, but heavier types should be avoided. Later stage lipedema is often accompanied by lymphedema, making prognosis less hopeful.

Mononucleosis

Mononucleosis affects lymphocytes and is caused by the Epstein-Barr virus. It is common in adolescents and young adults and is usually mild but may involve complications. It is transmitted by direct contact with infected saliva and has been commonly named "the kissing disease." It is also transmitted by airborne droplets and blood. Epstein-Barr virus invades the epithelial cells of the nasopharynx and oropharynx, penetrating lymphoid tissue and targeting B lymphocytes. It normally takes between 4 and 6 weeks to incubate.

Signs and Symptoms

Signs and symptoms include sore throat, headache, fever, fatigue, malaise, enlarged lymph nodes, enlarged spleen, a rash on the trunk, increased lymphocytes and *monocytes* in the blood, and the presence of atypical T lymphocytes. Possible complications include hepatitis, ruptured spleen, and meningitis.

Etiology

Epstein-Barr virus is responsible for nearly 90 percent of all cases of infectious mononucleosis. Cytomegalovirus may also be associated. Etiology of Epstein-Barr virus is mostly unknown.

Diagnosis

Infectious mononucleosis is diagnosed by a positive **heterophil** antibody test (Monospot test). Tests are first given to rule out strep throat, and microscopic examination of blood cells reveals an atypical appearance of certain lymphocytes (**Figure 13–5**). Blood chemistry tests may also reveal the presence of abnormal liver function.

Treatment

Supportive treatments are indicated, including bed rest. The disease is usually self-limiting. Antiviral medications are not useful in treating symptoms of "mono" (its common name). Acetaminophen can be given to make the patient more comfortable, but sleep and resting as much as possible during waking hours lend the best results.

The role of the PTA in infectious mononucleosis is to educate the patient about the need to avoid sports, physical activity, or exercise of any kind until cleared to do so by the physician. Sports should be avoided because of the contagious nature of this disease. Also, if the patient's spleen is enlarged, excessive movement may cause the organ to rupture. Generally, the patient must avoid exercise and physical therapy until 3 to 4 weeks after diagnosis with mononucleosis. After recovering from the condition, physical activities usually begin with low impact exercise, increasing slowly as the patient's body returns to normal.

Prognosis

Recovery may be prolonged, with persistent fatigue and malaise. Those who have experienced a ruptured spleen as a result of this disease should avoid strenuous exercise or sports activities until the spleen has returned to its normal size.

Lymphomas

Lymphomas are malignant neoplasms involved in the proliferation of lymphocytes in the lymph nodes. The two common types are Hodgkin's lymphoma and non-Hodgkin's lymphoma, which constitute a group of lymphomas differentiated by lymph node biopsy. A third form, *Burkitt's lymphoma*, is rare in North America but relatively common in Central Africa. Clinicians attempt to classify them based on whether the tumor is aggressive or slow-growing (indolent). There is no specific etiology known for lymphomas.

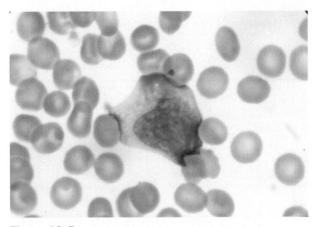

Figure 13–5 Large lymphocyte from subject with infectious mononucleosis, illustrating characteristic morphologic abnormalities (original magnification X 1,000).

Hodgkin's Disease/Hodgkin's Lymphoma

The incidence of this condition has been on the decline, but it still occurs primarily in adults between 20 and 40 years of age, with no preference for gender. Another peak occurrence appears in men over 50 years of age. In the early stages of disease, when the *malignancy* is localized, prognosis is excellent.

Hodgkin's lymphoma usually involves a single lymph node in the neck and then spreads to adjacent nodes in a very ordered fashion, moving on to organs via the lymphatic system. In this condition the lymphocyte count is decreased and T lymphocytes appear to be defective. The *Reed-Sternberg cell*, which is very large, is sought in the lymph node as a marker for diagnosis of the condition (**Figure 13–6A and B**).

There are four subtypes of Hodgkin's disease, which are based on cells found during biopsy. They are called: *nodular sclerosing, mixed-cellularity, lymphocyte-rich,* and *lymphocyte depleted* Hodgkin's disease (or lymphoma). The stages of lymphoma development are as follows:

- Stage I: Affecting a single lymph node or region
- Stage II: Affecting two or more lymph node regions on the same side of the diaphragm or in a relatively localized area
- Stage III: Involves nodes on both sides of the diaphragm and the spleen
- Stage IV: Represents diffuse extralymphatic involvement, usually in the bones, lungs, or liver

The typical spread of Hodgkin's lymphoma is shown in **Figure 13–7**.

Signs and Symptoms

Usually, the first indicator is a lymph node in the neck that is large, painless, and nontender. Then, splenomegaly and enlarged lymph nodes in other areas may cause pressure, such as enlarged mediastinal nodes that can compress the esophagus. The next occurrences are general cancer symptoms such as anorexia, anemia, low-grade fever, night sweats, and fatigue. Generalized pruritus may occur. Because abnormal lymphocytes interfere with the immune response, recurrent infections are common.

Etiology

The cause of Hodgkin's disease/lymphoma is unknown. It is believed to occur because of genetic, environmental, infectious, and immune deficiency conditions.

Diagnosis

Initial diagnosis often results from abnormalities in a chest x-ray that may have been performed because of nonspecific symptoms. A medical history is then obtained to check for the presence of symptoms, and a complete physical examination helps to confirm the diagnosis. A lymph node biopsy may also be used. The result is positive if the biopsy reveals a *Reed-Sternberg cell.*

> **RED FLAG**
>
> The atypical cell used as a marker for diagnosis of Hodgkin's lymphoma is the Reed-Sternberg cell, a giant cell present in the lymph nodes.

Treatment

Treatment for Hodgkin's disease/lymphoma consists of radiation, chemotherapy, and surgery. One of the most effective

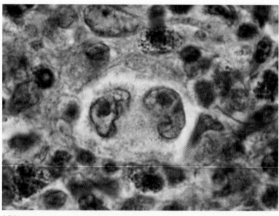

(A)

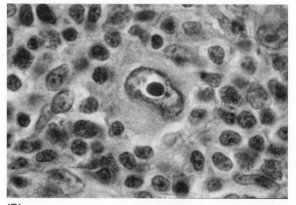

(B)

Figure 13–6 Characteristic appearance of Reed-Sternberg cells. (A) Binucleate cell. Note the mirror image nuclei with prominent nucleoli. (B) Cell with single nucleus illustrating prominent nucleolus and perinuclear halo (original magnification X 400).

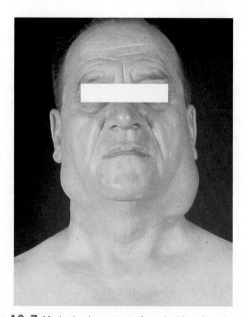

Figure 13–7 Marked enlargement of cervical lymph nodes as a result of malignant lymphoma.

combination drugs is "ABVD," which consists of Adriamycin (generic name, doxorubicin), Blenoxane (bleomycin), Velban or Velsar (vinblastine), and DTIC-Dome (dacarbazine). Patients in stage II need to receive three courses of chemotherapy at 4-week intervals, followed by reevaluation. In advanced stages **remissions** are common, with some occurrence of secondary cancers.

The role of the PTA in various types of lymphomas is to assist the patient with as much regular exercise as is tolerable. Light activities are indicated, including range-of-motion and resistance training. The Borg Rating of Perceived Exertion is used to determine the intensity of exercise the patient can tolerate. Stretching is also indicated for lymphoma patients.

Prognosis

Prognosis is based on the type of lymphoma, the stage of development, and other factors such as the patient's age, health, and response to treatment. The overall 5-year survival rate for Hodgkin's lymphoma is approximately 84.9 percent.

Non-Hodgkin's Lymphomas

Non-Hodgkin's lymphomas are on the increase, partially because of those associated with HIV infection. Nearly 80 percent of cases involve **B lymphocytes**.

Signs and Symptoms

The initial manifestation involves enlarged but painless lymph nodes. Clinical signs and stages are similar to Hodgkin's lymphoma. Non-Hodgkin's lymphomas are distinguished by multiple node involvement throughout the body and a nonorganized pattern of *metastasis*.

Etiology

Although the cause of this disease is unknown, substantial evidence suggests a viral cause. Risk factors include immunodeficiency, *Helicobacter pylori* infection, exposure to certain chemicals, and previous treatment for Hodgkin's lymphoma. Non-Hodgkin's lymphomas are the second most common type of cancer in HIV/AIDS patients.

Diagnosis

The presence of widespread metastasis is often the basis for diagnosis. Intestinal nodes and organs are frequently involved in the early stage. Common diagnostic techniques include chest x-ray, CT scans, blood tests, HIV tests, MRI of the spine, and lymph node or *bone marrow* biopsy.

Treatment

Treatment for non-Hodgkin's lymphomas is similar to that of Hodgkin's lymphoma. However, it is more difficult to treat when tumors are not localized. Treatment includes chemotherapy, radiation, or a combination of both; the use of monoclonal antibodies; and stem cell transplantation. The role of the PTA is consistent with physical therapy for Hodgkin's lymphoma.

Prognosis

Prognosis is improving as the condition is studied in more depth, and newer medications are developed. Prognosis is worse for those with T-cell lymphomas rather than B-cell lymphomas. Survival has improved with the use of rituximab. The major risk factors considered when determining outcomes include age (over 60), poor performance status to therapies,

elevated lactate dehydrogenase, more than one extranodal site, and stage III or IV disease. Patients with four or five of the above risk factors have a 50 percent 5-year survival rate, but others have a much higher rate.

Multiple Myeloma

Multiple myeloma occurs mostly in older adults and involves plasma cells (mature B lymphocytes) that replace bone marrow and erode the bone (**Figure 13–8**). Multiple myeloma is also called *plasma cell myeloma*. Blood cell production, and the production of antibodies, becomes impaired. Multiple tumors develop in the vertebrae, ribs, pelvis, and skull, with bone fractures often resulting. Hypercalcemia develops as bones are broken down. Tumor cells can spread into lymph nodes and infiltrate many organs.

Signs and Symptoms

Onset is usually insidious, with malignancy becoming very advanced before it can be diagnosed. Initial signs may include frequent infections, followed by bone pain, which is not alleviated by rest. Pathologic fractures may occur as bones weaken (**Figure 13–9**), and anemia and bleeding are common due to affected blood cell production. Kidney function is interrupted, leading to proteinuria and kidney failure.

Etiology

Etiology is unknown. Nuclear industry workers have been shown to experience higher than normal rates of developing this disease. Farmers and other workers exposed to dichlorodiphenyltrichloroethane, or DDT, and other pesticide-type chemicals have also shown increased risk. Also, herpesvirus type 8 may be related to this condition.

Diagnosis

Extensive testing is needed to diagnose multiple myeloma. Conditions that may prompt the diagnosis of multiple myeloma include pancytopenia, abnormal coagulation, hypercalcemia, azotemia, elevated alkaline phosphatase, elevated erythrocyte sedimentation rate, and hypoalbuminemia. Electrophoretic analysis will reveal increased levels of immunoglobulin in the blood, the **Bence-Jones protein**, or both (**Figure 13–10**). All patients suspected of having

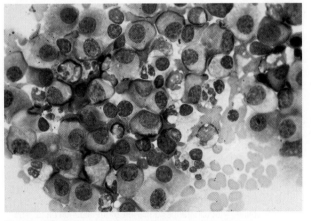

Figure 13–8 Photomicrograph illustrating aspirated bone marrow from a patient with multiple myeloma. Almost all cells are immature plasma cells containing large eccentric nuclei and abundant cytoplasm (original magnification X 400).

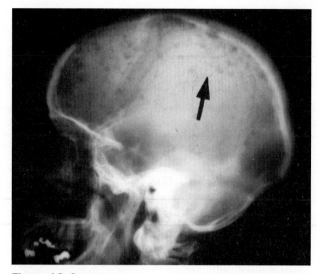

Figure 13–9 A skull x-ray from a patient with multiple myeloma. Multiple punched-out areas in skull bones (arrow) result from bone destruction caused by nodular masses of neoplastic plasma cells growing in bone marrow.

this condition must undergo a 24-hour urinalysis by protein electrophoresis. MRI is very accurate at depicting multiple myeloma tumors.

Treatment

Multiple myeloma treatment includes chemotherapy, analgesics for bone pain, treatment for kidney impairment, and, in the later stages, blood transfusions. The role of the PTA in multiple myeloma is assisting with regular weight-bearing exercise, designed to improve bone strength. Certain high-impact exercises such as tennis or jogging may be dangerous due to the potential for bone fracture. Walking and low-impact aerobics are indicated.

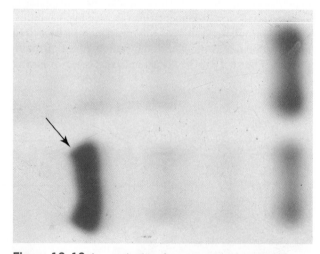

Figure 13–10 An examination of serum proteins by a special technique (electrophoresis) that separates serum proteins into various fractions. The upper pattern is from normal serum, with the dense albumin band at the far right in the photograph and the less intensely stained globulin bands to the left of the albumin band. The lower pattern is from a patient with multiple myeloma. The arrow indicates densely stained homogeneous globulin band representing large amounts of a single type of globulin protein produced by the abnormal plasma cells.

Prognosis

Prognosis for multiple myeloma is based on staging. Stage I prognosis is just over 5 years, stage II prognosis is just under 4 years, and stage III prognosis is 2½ years.

SUMMARY

The lymphatic system helps the body to fight infection and maintain immunity. It is made up of lymph, lymph nodes, and lymph vessels. Aside from lymph, this system also transports fluid that has leaked into interstitial areas located between blood vessels. Lymphatic diseases are usually caused by infections or neoplasms, ranging from mild to severe.

Lymphedema is an abnormal collection of lymph fluid in soft tissues, usually occurring in the extremities. Lymphadenitis occurs when a lymph node becomes overwhelmed by an infection and becomes infected. Lymphangitis is a condition involving swelling of the lymph vessels because of inflammation. Although treatments for lymphatic conditions vary, common symptoms include fatigue, fever, enlarged lymph nodes, and weight loss.

REVIEW QUESTIONS

Select the best response to each question.

1. Multiple myeloma involves which of the following cells?
   a. B lymphocytes
   b. T lymphocytes
   c. mast cells
   d. monocytes
2. Bence-Jones protein is found in the blood or urine of patients with which of the following disorders?
   a. multiple myeloma
   b. lymphedema
   c. lymphoma
   d. Hodgkin's disease
3. How many stages of lymphedema exist?
   a. one
   b. two
   c. three
   d. four
4. The Reed-Sternberg cell is a marker for the diagnosis of which of the following conditions?
   a. multiple sclerosis
   b. Hodgkin's lymphoma
   c. rheumatoid arthritis
   d. myasthenia gravis
5. An abnormal collection of lymph in the extremities is called which of the following conditions?
   a. multiple myeloma
   b. lymphoma
   c. lymphangitis
   d. lymphedema
6. Lipedema differs from lymphedema because of which of the following?
   a. one or both legs may be affected
   b. fat tends to "flap over" the feet
   c. it commonly affects the neck
   d. it is exclusively found in men

7. Lymphadenitis can be confirmed by which of the following diagnostic tests?
   a. biopsy
   b. blood tests only
   c. urine tests
   d. x-rays
8. Which of the following activities is appropriate for the PTA when working with patients who have lymphomas?
   a. educating them about side effects of medications
   b. assisting them with hydrotherapy
   c. assisting them in as much regular exercise as possible
   d. educating them about dietary needs
9. Which of the following disorders is caused by the Epstein-Barr virus?
   a. Hodgkin's disease
   b. systemic sclerosis
   c. Goodpasture's syndrome
   d. infectious mononucleosis
10. Which of the following terms may also be called "immunogens"?
   a. complements
   b. antibodies
   c. antigens
   d. immunoglobulins

CASE STUDIES

Karen Coupe, PT, DPT, MSEd

Case 1

A 54-year-old woman was referred to outpatient physical therapy for decongestive physical therapy. Patient was diagnosed with a melanoma on the right popliteal region. A surgical procedure removed the melanoma and several inguinal lymph nodes. Patient is currently cancer free but has recently developed lymphedema in the right lower extremity. Patient medical history: type 1 diabetes.
1. Why would this patient develop lymphedema?
2. Decongestive physical therapy is a specialized therapy specifically for patients with lymphedema. Look up decongestive physical therapy and report on your findings.
3. When working with this patient the PTA notes the patient has on sweat pants with an elastic band at the ankle and is wearing a tight anklet. What type of patient education should the PTA provide regarding tight clothing and wearing jewelry on the affected side?
4. During treatment the patient informed the PTA that she injects her insulin into the right thigh and has for years. Should this be addressed? What could develop?

5. The patient reports she likes to use a heating pad if she gets muscle soreness and asks the PTA if she can continue to use the heating pad. What is your response?

Case 2

A 45-year-old woman was referred to physical therapy with a diagnosis of rheumatoid arthritis. Patient was diagnosed at age 21. Patient medical history: right TKR 2 years ago, right THR 4 years ago, MP joint arthroplasty of digits 2, 3, 4 on the right and 2, 3 on the left. Patient underwent a left TKR 3 weeks ago. Prior level of function: Independent ambulation with a cane, independent in all activities of daily living. Current level of function: Independent ambulation with a rolling walker. Requires assistance in all other activities of daily living. Plan of care is for range-of-motion, strengthening, gait activities, and education in joint protection.
1. Compare and contrast the etiology and pathogenesis of rheumatoid arthritis with osteoarthritis.
2. What are the clinical manifestations of rheumatoid arthritis on the musculoskeletal system?
3. List and explain how rheumatoid arthritis affects other systems in the body. How could this affect the plan of care?
4. Would the patient's previous surgical procedures have any effect on the current plan of care?
5. Based on the disease process, why would a patient with rheumatoid arthritis need instruction in joint protection? What are some educational statements for protection?

WEBSITES

http://pathmicro.med.sc.edu/ghaffar/hyper00.htm
http://www.aahf.info/sec_exercise/section/lymphatic.htm
https://www.caremark.com/wps/portal/HEALTH_RESOURCES?topic=prchematopoiesis
http://www.koshland-science-museum.org/exhib_infectious/vaccines_10.jsp
http://www.lymphnet.org
http://www.medicinenet.com/connective_tissue_disease/article.htm
http://www.merck.com/mmhe/sec03/ch037/ch037a.html
http://www.nlm.nih.gov/medlineplus/ency/article/000816.htm
http://www.umm.edu/ency/article/000815.htm
http://www.webmd.com/a-to-z-guides/infectious-mononucleosis-topic-overview

Nervous System Disorders

OUTLINE

LEARNING OBJECTIVES

After completion of this chapter the reader should be able to

1. List the structures of the brainstem and diencephalon.
2. Name the cranial nerves and their functions.
3. Differentiate between cerebrovascular accident and transient ischemic attack.
4. Describe the etiology of meningitis and the most common cause.
5. State the possible causes for the development of Parkinson's disease and characterize its manifestations.
6. Describe the manifestations of epilepsy.
7. List the common causes of insomnia.
8. Differentiate between concussions and contusions, and describe the best treatment of each.

KEY TERMS

Akinesia: Impaired body movement.

Amnesia: Lack of memory about specific events.

Arachnoid: The middle layer of the meninges, covering the brain and spinal cord.

Astrocytomas: Types of common primary childhood brain tumors.

Brain: Main component of the nervous system along with the spinal cord, it is protected by and contained within the skull.

Brainstem: The portion of the brain divided into the midbrain, pons, and medulla that contains nerves and helps control respiration, swallowing, wakefulness, and other activities.

Cauterize: To burn with electricity; used to stop bleeding from tissues.

Central nervous system: The brain and spinal cord; it communicates with organs and body systems via the peripheral nervous system.

Cephalgia: Headache.

Cerebellum: Portion of the brain that helps to control fine motor movements and coordination.

Cerebrum: Primary portion of the brain, divided into two lobes, each of which have specialized lobes.

Chorea: Continuing and rapid complex body movements.

Convulsions: Abnormal muscle contractions.

KEY TERMS CONTINUED

Diencephalon: Portion of the brain that houses the thalamus and hypothalamus.

Dura mater: Outermost layer of the meninges, covering the brain and spinal cord.

Dysphagia: Difficulty swallowing.

Dysphasia: Impaired ability to use and understand language.

Epidural: Between the skull and dura mater.

Epilepsy: A chronic brain disease caused by intermittent electrical activity, involving seizures or convulsions.

Gliomas: Common types of primary brain tumor in adults that originate in glial (supportive) cells in the brain or spinal cord.

Hemiparesis: Weakness on one side of the body.

Insomnia: A chronic inability to sleep or to remain asleep throughout the night.

Meninges: Membranes that cover the brain and spinal cord that are divided into three layers: the dura mater, arachnoid, and pia mater.

Meningiomas: Common types of primary brain tumor in adults that usually originate in the dura mater of the meninges.

Nervous system: Brain, spinal cord, and nerves; it is subdivided into the central and peripheral nervous systems.

Paraplegia: Paralysis of the lower part of the body.

Quadriplegia: Paralysis of the arms and legs. Also called "tetraplegia."

Seizure: A sudden attack that is commonly indicative of a convulsive seizure.

Shingles: An acute infection caused by the varicella-zoster virus that causes a painful rash and sharp stabbing pains along the path of sensory nerves.

Sleep apnea: A condition that involves more than five periods of interrupted breathing, each lasting for at least 10 seconds, during every hour of sleep; it affects nearly one-third of adults in the United States.

Spinal cord: Portion of the nervous system that runs from the brain through the vertebral column, stopping near the tailbone; it transmits motor and sensory impulses.

Subdural: Between the dura mater and the arachnoid layer.

Tetanus: An acute, potentially fatal infection of the central nervous system.

Transient ischemic attack (TIA): An episode of cerebrovascular insufficiency, usually due to partial occlusion of a cerebral artery.

Overview

The nervous system is very complex, allowing communication between the brain and the body. Both intellectual and physical responses to stimuli require nervous system activity. Because this system is interconnected with every other body system, nervous disorders can affect potentially all normal functions of an individual. Brain and spinal cord damage is often irreversible. Nervous system disorders are often severe, with potentially permanent effects.

Anatomy and Physiology

The brain, spinal cord, and nerves comprise the **nervous system**, which is divided into the central nervous system and peripheral nervous system. **Figure 14–1** shows the components of the nervous system.

Central Nervous System

The **central nervous system** comprises the brain and spinal cord. It communicates with the organs and body systems via the peripheral nervous system. The **brain** is protected and contained within the skull. The divisions of the brain include the cerebrum, cerebellum, and brainstem. There are two hemispheres of the **cerebrum**, each of which is divided into lobes with specialized functions (**Figure 14–2**).

The gray matter (basal ganglia) makes up the deeper portions of the hemispheres of the cerebrum. Another portion is called the **diencephalon**, which is where the thalamus and hypothalamus are located. These structures help to control the sleeping and wakefulness patterns of the body and assist the functions of the pituitary gland. In the lower back portion of the brain, the **cerebellum** helps to control fine motor movements and coordination. The final portion of the brain is the **brainstem**, which is divided into the midbrain, pons, and medulla. It contains nerves and helps in the control of respiration, swallowing, wakefulness, and other activities. **Figure 14–3** shows a cross-section of the human brain.

The **spinal cord** runs from the brain through the vertebral column, stopping near the tailbone (**Figure 14–4**). It is composed of both gray and white matter. Separate ascending and descending pathways transmit information. The impulses that travel from the brain to the spinal cord are known as *motor impulses* (used for the movement of muscles). The impulses that travel from the spinal cord to the brain are known as *sensory impulses* (used to sense stimuli such as pain, temperature, and touch). The brain and spinal cord are covered in **meninges**, which are membranes divided into three layers: the outer portion (dura mater), middle layer (arachnoid), and inner layer (pia mater). The meninges protect and support the structures of the central nervous system.

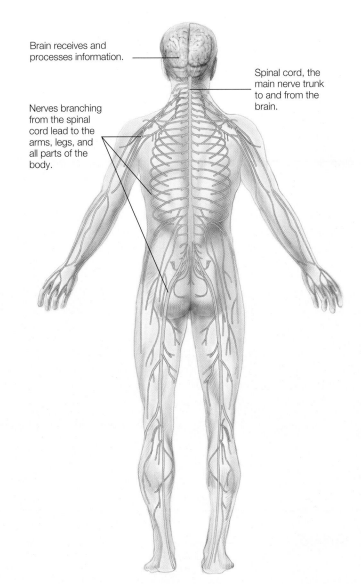

Figure 14–1 The nervous system. The human nervous system is a network of nerves connected to the brain and spinal cord. Nerves comprise the peripheral nervous system. The spinal cord and brain make up the central nervous system.

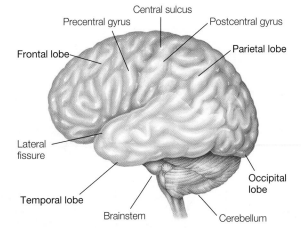

Figure 14–2 The various lobes of the brain. The cerebral cortex consists of the lobes shown here. The lobes, in turn, can be divided into sensory, association, and motor areas (not shown).

Peripheral Nervous System

The peripheral nervous system is composed of the autonomic nervous system, cranial nerves, and spinal nerves. The autonomic nervous system innervates cardiac and smooth muscle and controls how the body's organs function. It is divided into the sympathetic and parasympathetic nervous systems. The sympathetic system controls changes in the body that are required to respond to stress by increasing the blood pressure or heart rate (known as the "fight-or-flight" response). The parasympathetic system controls changes in the body that are required to respond to stress in an opposite manner (known as the "rest-and-digest" response). **Table 14–1** lists the 12 pairs of cranial nerves and their functions, and **Figure 14–5** shows the cranial nerves.

There are 31 pairs of spinal nerves, with each nerve innervating specific areas (*dermatomes*) of the skin. The 31 pairs are divided into 8 cervical pairs, 12 thoracic pairs, 5 lumbar pairs, 5 sacral pairs, and 1 coccygeal pair. Each spinal nerve sends sensory impulses from the body organs and skin surfaces to the brain. Motor impulses return impulses from the brain via the spinal cord.

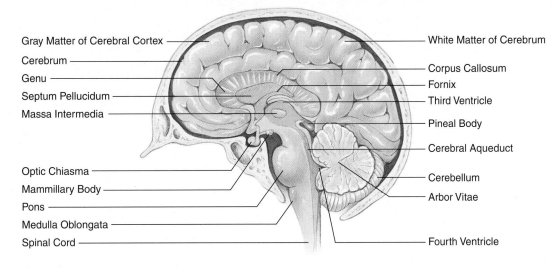

Figure 14–3 A cross-section of the human brain.

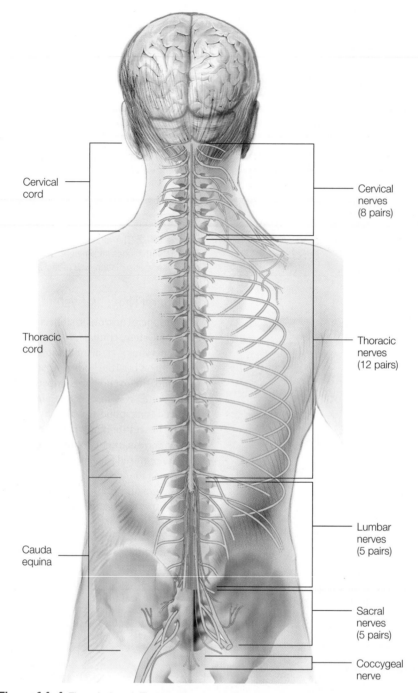

Figure 14–4 The spinal cord. The spinal cord extends from the brain to the upper lumbar region.

TABLE 14-1 Cranial Nerves and Their Functions

Cranial Nerve	Name	Function
I	Olfactory	Smell
II	Optic	Sight
III	Oculomotor	Eyeball, pupil, and eyelid movement
IV	Trochlear	Eyeball movement
V	Trigeminal	Face and mouth pain, temperature, and touch; chewing
VI	Abducens	Eyeball movement
VII	Facial	Taste; facial movement; saliva secretion
VIII	Auditory	Hearing; balance
IX	Glossopharyngeal	Swallowing; saliva secretion; taste; sensation in mouth and pharynx
X	Vagus	Pharyngeal, laryngeal, chest, and gastrointestinal system movement and sensation
XI	Accessory	Head and shoulder movement
XII	Hypoglossal	Tongue movement

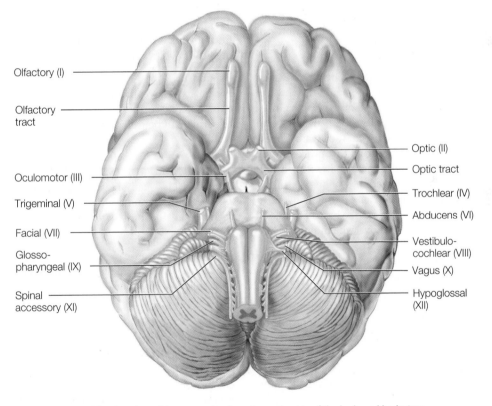

Figure 14–5 Cranial nerves. The 12 pairs of cranial nerves arise from the underside of the brain and brainstem.

Common Signs and Symptoms

Nervous system disorders often cause the following signs and symptoms: headache, nausea and/or vomiting, mood swings, fever, and weakness. Disturbances in motor function include inability to move body parts, paralysis, seizures or convulsions, and stiffness in various body areas. Disturbances in sensory function include inability to speak, paralysis, and visual problems. When cognitive function or mental alertness is altered, it may become apparent because of amnesia or forgetfulness, drowsiness, stupor, unconsciousness, or coma.

Diagnostic Tests

Because the signs and symptoms of nervous system conditions may involve motor functions, sensory functions, and mental functions, neurologic examination commonly involves related tests. Motor tests check gait, posture, and reflexes. Sensory tests check the ability to feel (using pin pricks, hot or cold temperatures, or vibrations), smell, and/or see. Cognitive or mental tests include asking simple questions involving the patient's name, location, job, and other questions about current events, or even simple mathematics. Analyzing the cerebrospinal fluid (CSF) is the most important laboratory test because microscope examination can reveal bacteria, leukocytes, neoplastic cells, red blood cells, and other components.

CSF is obtained by lumbar puncture. The patient must lie on his or her side and bring the knees up to the chest to widen the spaces between the vertebral discs. A spinal needle is inserted into the meningeal space that surrounds the spinal cord. The CSF is then withdrawn. Intracranial pressure (ICP) can also be measured during this procedure by connecting a manometer to the spinal needle. Raised ICP may indicate brain hematoma, infection, swelling, or tumor. Increased pressure in the brain may cause it to actually move down through the foramen magnum at the base of the skull, leading to coma and death due to overwhelming pressure on the brainstem.

Diagnostic tests used to detect various nervous system conditions also include x-rays, myelogram (spinal cord picturization), angiogram, electroencephalogram (EEG), computed tomography (CT), and magnetic resonance imaging (MRI). The skull and vertebral column are commonly tested via x-rays and various radiologic examinations. Myelogram may reveal herniated discs, nerve root compression, and spinal tumors. Angiogram may help diagnose hematomas and vessel occlusion. EEG measures electrical activity in the brain and brain death.

Nervous System Disorders

Nervous system disorders or diseases can range widely and may be only mild or very severe. Some of them are influenced by the age of the patient. However, many nervous system disorders can affect all ages of patients.

Infectious Diseases

Nervous system infections are more common in younger patients, but they may occur at any age. Infections involving the nervous system are more successfully treated when correct diagnosis is achieved early in their development. When this does not occur, permanent neurologic deficits or death may result.

Encephalitis

Encephalitis is defined as "inflammation of the brain tissue." Because it may be commonly carried by mosquitoes, people should take precautions to reduce the likelihood of mosquito bites.

Signs and Symptoms

Encephalitis may cause fever, headache, and stiffness in the back and neck. It can also intensify to cause lethargy, mental confusion, and coma.

Etiology

Encephalitis may be caused by bacteria and viruses (carried by insects, animals, or other humans). Additionally, it may be the result of chickenpox, measles, or mumps.

Diagnosis

Encephalitis is usually diagnosed by examining the CSF via lumbar puncture. Other tests include EEG, CT, MRI, CSF culture, and radionuclide scans.

Treatment

Encephalitis is commonly treated with supportive antiviral medication with varying degrees of effectiveness.

Prognosis

Prognosis of encephalitis is guarded due to varying severity of its different forms. Some forms kill most patients or lead to permanent neurologic impairment.

Meningitis

Meningitis is an inflammation of the brain and the spinal cord *meninges*. It is usually a result of a bacterial infection (**Figure 14–6**). Such inflammation may involve all three meningeal membranes (the dura mater, arachnoid, and pia mater).

Signs and Symptoms

Meningitis may cause high fever, chills, photophobia, severe headache, vomiting, and neck stiffness. Further progression of the disease may cause drowsiness, stupor, seizures, and coma.

Etiology

Meningitis is most frequently caused by bacterial or viral agents. Meningitis is almost always a complication of bacteremia, especially from otitis media, sinusitis, pneumonia, osteomyelitis, or endocarditis. Bacterial meningitis is usually caused by *Neisseria meningitidis*, *Haemophilus influenzae*, *Streptococcus pneumoniae*, and *Escherichia coli*. Neonates with meningitis are usually affected by a group B or D *streptococci* or *E. coli*. Infants and children (between ages 1 month and 10 years old) develop meningitis usually because of *H. influenzae*, pneumococci, or meningococci. In adults the most common causes of bacterial meningitis are pneumococci or meningococci.

The condition of meningitis may also follow trauma or invasive procedures, including penetrating head wounds, skull fracture, lumbar puncture, and ventricular shunting. Aseptic meningitis may result from a virus or another organism. Sometimes no causative organism can be detected.

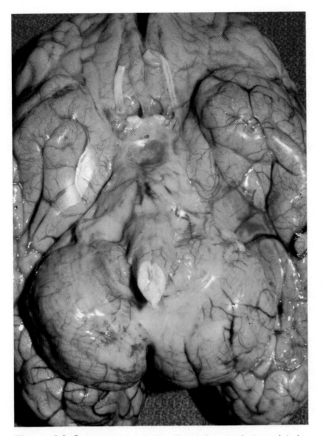

Figure 14–6 Bacterial meningitis, illustrating purulent exudate in the meninges. Exudate is most noticeable over the pons (middle of photograph) and cerebellum.

Diagnosis

Meningitis is diagnosed by a lumbar puncture, which shows cloudy or milky-white CSF, elevated CSF pressure, decreased glucose level, and high protein level. Cultures of the blood, nasal secretions, and urine may reveal the causative organism.

Treatment

Bacterial meningitis usually responds well to appropriate intravenous antibiotic treatment. Additional forms of treatment include anticonvulsives and antipyretics and keeping the patient in a quiet and dark environment. Proper hand-washing procedure can help prevent meningitis from spreading. Precautions for dealing with meningitis patients include wearing masks, semi-isolation, prophylactic antibiotics, and vaccinations.

The physical therapist assistant (PTA) is concerned with long-term physical therapy that certain meningitis patients may require. This can help them to recover abilities that were lost because of the disease. Occupational and emotional therapies are also indicated.

RED FLAG

The most critical treatment for bacterial meningitis is the rapid initiation of antibiotic therapy. For those who have been exposed to the condition, prophylactic antibiotics should be administered.

Prognosis

If the disease is recognized early and the infecting organism responds to treatment, the prognosis is good and complications are rare. The prognosis is poorer for infants and elderly patients. If untreated, the mortality rate from meningitis is 70 percent to 100 percent.

Poliomyelitis

Poliomyelitis is less common today than in previous years. It is caused by polio virus entering the body via the gastrointestinal tract and manifesting in the spinal cord and brainstem. As the anterior horn cells of the motor neurons are destroyed by the disease, muscles become paralyzed due to lack of nerve impulses and muscle atrophy. The virus is attracted to the gray matter of the spinal cord, hence its name (*polios* = gray). Immunization against polio on a widespread basis has virtually eliminated poliomyelitis in most developed countries. Efforts are now being made to immunize people in Third World countries, which may bring about a worldwide cure.

Patients who have survived the initial poliomyelitis event may experience progressive neurologic problems and muscle decline later in life. Known as the "postpolio syndrome," it affects muscles secondary to those primary muscles that were initially affected. No medical treatment restores function to muscles that have already become weakened and atrophied. The role of the PTA is to assist with mild exercise, patient education, and energy conservation. Activities include swimming, range-of-motion and stretching exercises, and various types of light cardiovascular exercise. Treatments to improve pulmonary function may be needed if the respiratory muscles have been affected.

Rabies

Rabies is a form of encephalomyelitis that may be fatal. It is an acute viral disease of the central nervous system that affects humans and other animals. It is transmitted from animals to people through infected saliva. Rabies is also referred to as "hydrophobia" or a "fear of water."

Signs and Symptoms

The incubation period for rabies ranges between 10 days and 1 year. It is followed by a prodromal period, characterized by headache, malaise, myalgia, and paresthesia. Several days after this period delirium, severe encephalitis, muscular spasms, seizures, and paralysis ensue, leading to coma and death.

Etiology

Rabies is caused by a virus that usually only affects animals. However, it may be spread to humans by the bite of an infected animal. The virus moves slowly from the bite wound to the brain and spinal cord, and the location of the wound is significant in the disease's progression.

Diagnosis

Diagnosis of rabies is based on patient history and physical examination that checks for muscle spasms, pain, and stiffness.

Treatment

Treatment involves immediate washing of the bite wound with soap, water, and a disinfectant. If the wound is deep, it may be cauterized, and immune globulin is injected directly into the base of the wound. The animal that bit the patient should be found and examined. If the animal is a domestic animal and appears normal over 10 days, there is little danger of rabies developing from the bite. Immunizations are therefore not recommended.

If the bite is from a wild animal, once captured it will be killed, with the brain sent for microscopic examination. A positive result means rabies immunizations must start immediately. Active immunization requires a series of five intramuscular injections of the rabies vaccine. The first vaccine is given immediately, followed by vaccines on days 3, 7, 21, and 28. These injections are required in a series to stop the virus from reaching the brain. There is no cure for the disease once it has progressed to the brain. Muscle relaxants may reduce convulsions, although death usually occurs because of respiratory arrest.

> **RED FLAG**
> The most critical treatment is the rapid initiation of antibiotic therapy for bacterial meningitis.

Prognosis

Prognosis is good as long as the full series of rabies injections are given in time. If not, untreated cases end with severe convulsions and death within 2 to 5 days after the symptoms of rabies begin.

Shingles

Shingles is an acute infection caused by the varicella-zoster virus and mainly affects older adults. Nearly half of shingles patients have experienced an episode of "chickenpox" (which is also caused by the herpes zoster virus).

Signs and Symptoms

Shingles causes an itching, painful, red-colored rash. It may also cause small blisters or vesicles that follow along the path of one of the sensory nerves (**Figure 14–7**). The disease causes sharp, stabbing pain due to inflammation of the sensory nerve affected. Symptoms may last between 10 days and several weeks. Most often, shingles affects the trunk of the body but can also appear on the face and other parts of the body.

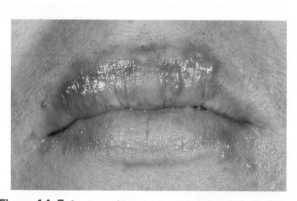

Figure 14–7 One type of herpes virus infection (called shingles or herpes zoster) characterized by clusters of vesicles that occur in a segment of skin (dermatome) supplied by a sensory nerve. The subject was photographed beside a mirror in order to illustrate the band-like distribution of the rash in the segment of skin supplied by a spinal nerve.

Etiology

Herpes zoster is the causative virus, attacking children to cause chickenpox and attacking immune-compromised adults to cause shingles. It is believed that a dormant herpes zoster virus may return later in life to cause shingles. Aging, trauma, stress, and other disease processes may exacerbate shingles.

Diagnosis

The appearance of lesions aids in the diagnosis of shingles, confirmed by a viral culture or blood test for the herpes zoster virus.

Treatment

Treatment of shingles is based on severity of symptoms, usually involving antivirals, antipruritics, and analgesics. In 2006 the U.S. Food and Drug Administration approved the first vaccination for adults over age 60 to prevent shingles. Precautions to be taken when dealing with shingles patients are influenced by whether or not the health care provider has ever had chickenpox. Once the lesions break open, the likelihood of transmitting the virus is increased. Proper hand washing is required at all times. All health care providers working with these patients should wear masks, gloves, and gowns. The role of the PTA may include assisting with pain management for patients who have secondary musculoskeletal pain.

Prognosis

Prognosis is generally good with proper treatment for shingles.

Tetanus

Tetanus is an acute, potentially fatal infection of the central nervous system. It is a disease for which lasting immunity cannot be conferred. Booster doses of tetanus vaccine must be given regularly through life (recommended every 10 years).

Signs and Symptoms

Tetanus is characterized by irritability, headache, fever, and painful spasms of the muscles resulting in "lockjaw" and laryngeal spasm. Eventually, every muscle of the body experiences tonic spasm.

Etiology

Tetanus is caused by *Clostridium tetani*, a bacterium that releases an exotoxin that attacks the central nervous system to cause voluntary (skeletal muscle) contraction. This toxin is a *neurotoxin* and one of the most lethal poisons known.

Diagnosis

Diagnosis of tetanus is based on a "spatula test," which involves the use of a soft-tipped instrument to touch the back of the patient's throat. A positive diagnosis is indicated by an involuntary contraction of the muscles, causing the patient to bite down on the instrument.

Treatment

Because tetanus is transmitted via wounds (especially puncture-type wounds), any time the skin is cut, punctured, or otherwise broken it should be cleaned promptly with appropriate substances. If an individual has not been immunized against tetanus in the past 5 years, an antitoxin should be injected. Tetanus toxoid is commonly administered to children as part of the DPT (diphtheria, pertussis, tetanus) immunization. Tetanus boosters should be given throughout life, every 7 to 10 years. Treatment of tetanus symptoms includes antibiotics and muscle relaxants. The disease process normally lasts from 6 to 8 weeks.

Prognosis
Unfortunately, once tetanus has developed it is usually fatal due to respiratory failure. When treatment is adequate, tetanus does not leave any permanent disability.

Vascular Disorders

Vascular disorders affecting the nervous system may be prevented or reduced by making substantial lifestyle changes. When they occur, however, they can result in long-term disability.

Cerebrovascular Accident

Also known as a *stroke* or *brain attack*, cerebrovascular accident (CVA) is more common in people over age 50. CVA is a major cause of death in this age group. A CVA is a sudden impairment of cerebral circulation in one or more blood vessels. This event interrupts or lessens oxygen supply, usually causing serious damage or necrosis in brain tissue (**Figure 14–8A and B**). The effects of a CVA depend on its location and the extent of ischemia.

> **RED FLAG**
> Although strokes may occur in younger persons, most patients experiencing strokes are over age 50. The risk of stroke doubles with each passing decade after age 55.

Signs and Symptoms
CVA may cause sudden unconsciousness, permanent neurologic disability, or death. Those who survive may have either no functional disability or ongoing problems ranging widely in severity.

CVA may cause numerous symptoms, based on the part of the brain affected and how severe the occurrence actually is. Common symptoms include **dysphasia**, **dysphagia**, confusion, poor coordination, and **hemiparesis**.

Etiology
Stroke typically results from one of three common causes: cerebral embolism, thrombus, or hemorrhage. An embolism usually occurs because of a small piece of a thrombus or arterial plaque that has broken loose and traveled in an artery until it becomes wedged, blocking blood flow suddenly. A thrombus usually travels from another part of the body and lodges in a brain artery and is the most common cause of vessel occlusion, occurring gradually over time. A common thrombus is from deep vein thrombosis in a leg that travels to the lung or brain.

Hemorrhage is the rupture of an artery that fills surrounding tissue with blood, usually due to arteriosclerosis and hypertension but sometimes caused by aneurysm (**Figure 14–9**). Symptoms are very sudden. Risk factors that have been identified as predisposing a patient to stroke include hypertension and family history of stroke or transient ischemic attacks (discussed below). Other factors include acute myocardial infarction, diabetes, cigarette smoking, familial hyperlipidemia, increased alcohol intake, obesity, and a sedentary lifestyle.

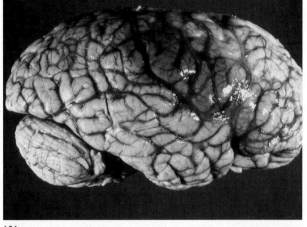

(A)

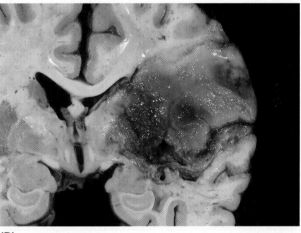

(B)

Figure 14–8 Large recent infarct of right cerebral hemisphere caused by thrombosis of middle cerebral artery. (A) External surface of brain illustrating the swollen, dark, infarcted area in the right hemisphere. (B) Coronal section through hemispheres at level of basal ganglia. Cerebral tissue is necrotic and discolored and involves a large part of the hemisphere.

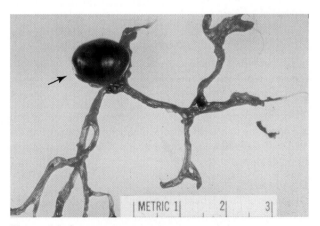

Figure 14–9 Dissection of vessels from the brain of a person with large congenital cerebral aneurysm.

Diagnosis

The diagnosis of a stroke may be confirmed by a physical examination combined with an EEG as well as a CT or MRI scan. If hemiparesis is present, it may indicate the location of damaged brain tissue. Left-side body systems are indicative of right-side brain damage, and right-side body systems are indicative of left-side brain damage.

Treatment

Treatment of stroke varies with severity of symptoms but commonly includes anticoagulant and hypertensive medications. Patients who have physical disabilities due to stroke may require long-term physical and speech therapy. The role of the PTA in stroke is to assist patients in reestablishing body control and movements that were lost due to the CVA. Different physical therapy or rehabilitation interventions may need to be developed to retrain patients to move as normally as possible. Repetitive practice is highly effective, especially in teaching patients how to live normally when use of one hand is affected or when speech is compromised.

Ideally, physical therapy may begin within 24 to 48 hours, while the patient is still in acute care, and is based on individual case specifics. Passive or active limb movements are encouraged to help patients prevent contractures and to improve control and range of motion. Physical therapy is focused on increasing difficulties of movements and actions based on the needs of daily living. Physical therapy commonly lasts from months to years or may continue throughout the patient's entire lifetime.

Prognosis

Prognosis for those surviving a stroke varies widely with its severity and the areas of the brain affected.

Transient Ischemic Attack

A **transient ischemic attack (TIA)** is an episode of cerebrovascular insufficiency, usually associated with partial occlusion of a cerebral artery by an atherosclerotic plaque or an embolus.

Signs and Symptoms

The symptoms are varied, depending on which part of the brain that is affected. Common symptoms, however, include dizziness, weakness of limbs, numbness, slurring of speech, and brief or mild loss of consciousness; usually, there is not a total loss of consciousness. Symptoms usually subside in less than an hour, with full return of normal functions.

> **RED FLAG**
> The effects of a TIA are not long-lasting, unlike those caused by most strokes.

Etiology

TIAs are warning signs that a stroke may be impending and are often due to arteriosclerotic plaque that is causing arteries to narrow. They are caused by insufficient blood supply to the brain.

Diagnosis

Diagnosis of TIAs is based on patient history, physical exam, and neurologic exams. Blood pressure is checked to determine if hypertension exists. Blood flow irregularities may be assessed by using a stethoscope to listen to the neck veins.

Vessel blockage or occlusion can be located via arteriograms, and CT scans of the head may be required. However, because all symptoms usually resolve with a TIA, arteriograms and CT scans are not often needed.

Treatment

If an arteriogram indicates a blocked blood vessel, surgery may be used to open the vessel or bypass the blockage. A common surgery to correct blood flow for TIA is a carotid endarterectomy. The role of the PTA is similar to physical therapy indicated for stroke.

Prognosis

Prognosis is improved if the patient avoids or quits smoking and improves lifestyle habits concerning general health, exercise, and diet.

Functional Disorders

Functional disorders of the nervous system are among the most common. Causes of these disorders are often unknown, and treatment is aimed at relieving symptoms and maintaining as normal a life as possible.

Bell's Palsy

Bell's palsy affects the seventh cranial nerve (the facial nerve) to cause one-sided (unilateral) paralysis of the face. It usually affects people between 20 and 60 years of age of both genders. People at highest risk are pregnant women, diabetics, those with influenza or herpes simplex virus, and patients with upper respiratory infections. However, Bell's palsy can affect any individual.

Signs and Symptoms

The signs and symptoms exhibited by Bell's palsy patients usually result from interference in motor function associated with the seventh cranial nerve. Bell's palsy usually produces aching pain around the angle of the jaw or behind the ear and drooping of the eye and mouth on one side of the face. Patients cannot close the affected eye and may drool saliva from the corner of the affected side of the mouth. The face appears distorted, and common functions of the face are impaired.

Etiology

Bell's palsy is of idiopathic origin but may be caused by viral diseases (herpes simplex virus or herpes zoster virus), Lyme disease, hypertension, diabetes mellitus, hemorrhage, meningitis, tumor, local trauma, sarcoidosis, and autoimmune disorders.

Diagnosis

Diagnosis is based on patient history and clinical presentation: distorted facial appearance and inability to raise the eyebrow, close the eyelid, show the teeth, smile, or puff out the cheek on the affected side. To understand the effects of the disorder fully, electromyography and MRI may be used, especially when there is another existing condition.

Treatment

Analgesics and anti-inflammatory medications (such as corticosteroids) may be used to treat Bell's palsy. The affected eye should be protected with an eye patch and artificial tear medication. Facial muscle atrophy can be prevented by applying warm, moist heat, as well as massage and/or electrotherapy. The role of the PTA focuses on retraining of the use of facial muscles based on the individual characteristics of the disease development.

Prognosis

Prognosis for Bell's palsy is good. Most cases resolve within 8 weeks. However, chronic conditions may require plastic surgery to correct facial deformities.

Epilepsy

Epilepsy is a chronic brain disease caused by intermittent electrical activity. About 2.5 million people in the United States have epilepsy, with a higher incidence during childhood and among elderly people.

Signs and Symptoms

Epilepsy involves recurring seizures that can be classified as partial, generalized, status epilepticus, or unclassified. Some patients may be affected by more than one type. Abnormal muscle contractions are termed **convulsions**. A **seizure** actually means "a sudden attack" that is commonly indicative of a convulsive seizure; however, not all seizures are characterized by convulsions. Also, not all convulsions are caused by epilepsy (such as those caused by excessive temperature, hypocalcemia, hypoglycemia, and drug or alcohol toxicity).

> **RED FLAG**
>
> Status epilepticus results when more than six seizures occur in 24 hours or when the patient progresses from one seizure to the next without resolution of the postictal period.

Etiology

About half of all seizure disorder cases are idiopathic. Possible causes of other conditions include birth trauma, anoxia, perinatal infection, encephalitis, meningitis, brain tumors, or scar tissue that is due to stroke or trauma.

Diagnosis

Clinically, the diagnosis of epilepsy is based on the occurrence of one or more seizures. Epilepsy may be diagnosed via EEG, CT, and skull x-rays. Altered brain activity or structure, tumors, and altered blood flow may all indicate this condition. Hypoglycemia or toxicities may be revealed by blood tests.

Treatment

Epilepsy is usually treated with anticonvulsive medications, individualized per patient. Family and friends of epileptics should be educated about what they can do when an epileptic attack occurs. Few people with epilepsy require physical therapy. For those who do, treatment usually involves movement and coordination exercise such as stretching, low-impact aerobics, and various levels of needed skill development.

Prognosis

Prognosis is based on the effectiveness of medications and the severity of the condition. Generally, the prognosis is good if the patient adheres strictly to the prescribed treatment. The main goal for epileptics is to achieve as normal a lifestyle as possible.

Headache

Headache (**cephalgia**) is usually a symptom of another disease state, including meningitis, sinusitis, encephalitis, hypertension, anemia, constipation, premenstrual tension, and tumors. In general, a headache is caused by tense facial, scalp, and neck muscles and by dilation or constriction of the vessels inside the head. Types of headache include cluster, migraine, tension, and post–lumbar puncture headache. A cluster headache occurs at night after falling asleep and is caused by emotional trauma, stress, or from unknown reasons. A migraine headache is severe, incapacitating, and often accompanied by visual disturbances, nausea, and vomiting. A tension headache is caused by stress, strain, and tension on the muscles of the head and neck. A post–lumbar puncture headache occurs in 40 percent of individuals after a lumbar puncture procedure.

> **RED FLAG**
>
> Migraine headache is a primary headache syndrome that is an episodic vascular disorder with or without a common aura.

Signs and Symptoms

Headaches can differ in which parts of the head they affect and may be acute or chronic. The level of pain varies widely. Because there are no sensory fibers in the brain, the sense of pain from a headache actually comes from pain receptors in the scalp, meninges, and facial tissue.

Etiology

Headaches may be caused by allergies, noise, stress, lack of sleep, toxic fumes, and consumption of alcohol.

Diagnosis

There is no test available to diagnose migraine headaches. Patient history and physical examination assist in proper diagnosis of headaches. The following tests may be necessary for differential diagnosis: skull x-rays, EEG, CT, MRI, cranial nerve testing, arteriogram, lumbar puncture, and CSF testing.

Treatment

Treatment of headaches is related to cause, frequency, and severity. Many over-the-counter medications exist for headache, including acetaminophen and ibuprofen. Improving diet, exercise, and sleep often reduce incidence and severity of headaches. In some cases antinausea or prescription pain medications are used. Most patients can have their migraine headache managed by pharmacology. Dietary modification may decrease symptoms, such as reducing the intake of caffeinated beverages, monosodium glutamate, sausage, citrus fruit, red wine, and cheese.

Prognosis

Prognosis is good except in cases of extreme headache, which may indicate a severe underlying cause. Physical therapy plays a big role, because exercise is useful for pain management.

Parkinson's Disease

Parkinson's disease is one of the most common disabling diseases in the United States. It more commonly affects men in their late 50s or 60s compared with women and involves slow and progressive brain degeneration. Parkinson's disease characteristically produces progressive muscle rigidity, **akinesia**, and involuntary tremor. **Figure 14–10** shows the classic posture of Parkinson's disease.

Signs and Symptoms

Parkinson's is commonly signified by rigid and immobile hands, slow speech, fine tremor of the hands with a "pill rolling" motion of the fingers, infrequent eye blinking, an expressionless facial appearance, flexed arms, a "bent-forward" posture, and a walking gait that consists of short, quick steps. The characteristic walk is due to the abnormal posture, which often causes the patient to stumble forward and fall.

Common issues with Parkinson's disease include the following:

- Bradykinesia: Slowed ability to start and continue movements as well as impaired ability to adjust the body's position
- Cognitive changes: May affect thinking, memory, language, reasoning, attention, and mood (various levels including possible depression)
- Festinating gait: Short, jerky steps as well as difficulty in starting to walk or stopping; these symptoms are related to muscle hypertonicity
- Flat affect: The face appears "flattened," with infrequent blinking and widened palpebral fissures (the separations between the upper and lower eyelids)
- Freezing of gait: Often a "late" feature of Parkinson's disease; the patient is suddenly unable to start walking or fails to continue to move forward (akinesia)
- Shuffled gait: Short, uncertain steps, with minimal flexion and dragging of the toes
- Stiffness of trunk: May result in stooped posture but may be helped by core strength training
- Tremors: Most commonly affect the hands, fingers, feet, or jaw; it often occurs at rest and either may be on only one side of the body or affect it completely; later progression may include tremors in the head, lips, and tongue
- Visual perception changes: Decreased blink rate, irritation of eye surfaces, alteration in tear film, visual hallucinations, decreased eye convergence, blepharospasm, difficulty in moving the eyes, and limitations in gazing upward

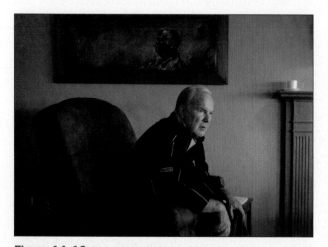

Figure 14–10 The classic posture of Parkinson's disease.

Etiology

The actual cause of Parkinson's disease is unknown, but studies have shown that dopamine deficiency prevents affected brain cells from performing their normal inhibitory function in the central nervous system. Some cases are caused by exposure to toxins such as manganese dust or carbon monoxide, and chemicals and by head injuries.

> **RED FLAG**
> Recent advances in genetics have demonstrated that Parkinson's disease has strong genetic influences.

Diagnosis

Diagnostic tests are usually of little value in identifying Parkinson's disease. Diagnosis is based on the patient's age, history, and characteristic signs and symptoms. Urinalysis may support diagnosis by revealing decreased levels of dopamine. Neurologic patient evaluations are designed to assess the levels of sensory neuron and motor responses, especially reflexes, and include the following:

- Balance: Understanding the patient's ability to maintain balance and equilibrium is vital in helping to prevent falls.
- Presence of hypertonicity or hypotonicity: Hypertonicity is increased muscle tension, causing rigid movements. Hypotonicity is decreased muscle tension, causing inhibited movements because the muscles may not be able to support the body adequately.
- Proprioception: The sense of the relative position of various body parts. Without normal proprioception, the patient cannot judge how various body parts are being coordinated, and this may influence his or her ability to walk, stand, sit, or otherwise move normally.
- Quality of movement: The ability of the body to conduct adequate movements to handle the normal activities of daily life.

Treatment

Treatment is symptomatic, usually involving dopamine replacement, which helps reduce symptoms but cannot cure the disease. Physical therapy may alleviate muscle pain and provide many other benefits to the patient with Parkinson's disease. The role of the PTA is to assist the patient in learning new movement techniques, strategies, and the use of medical equipment. Fall prevention and balance exercises are important. Specific exercises can promote flexibility and strengthen muscles. The goal of physical therapy is to promote function and maintain the ability to live as normally as possible. It can assist with balance problems, lack of coordination, fatigue, gait, immobility, and weakness. Local heat therapy is sometimes indicated for pain management.

Prognosis

Prognosis is poor because the disease is progressive but can be managed and slowed with medications.

Dementia

Dementia is defined as a loss of mental ability because of loss of brain cells or neurons. With aging, senile (old) dementia commonly occurs as the cells degenerate naturally. Although senile dementia is not the same as Alzheimer's, the terms are often interchanged. Vascular dementia is considered a form of senile dementia because it usually occurs in older adults.

Alzheimer's Disease

Alzheimer's disease is a degenerative disorder of the cerebral cortex, especially the frontal lobe, which accounts for more than half of all cases of dementia. It is characterized by death of neurons and their replacement by microscopic plaques. This is the most common cause of dementia in older adults, usually affecting people aged 70 or older. More than 50 percent of people over age 85 are affected by this condition. Some studies indicate that avoiding high-fat diets is of some help in preventing the development of this disease. Vitamin and mineral supplements also appear to be of help.

Signs and Symptoms

The disease begins with slight mental impairment and short-term memory loss. There may be an inability to concentrate and minor personality changes. Communication skills and word usage progressively become impaired. The patient may become irritable because they are often aware of their progressive decline in mental acuity. Late-stage Alzheimer's takes up to 10 years to develop, with severe mental and physical effects. The patient may become unable to control his or her thoughts, speech, and writing. There is increasing difficulty in abstract thinking and judgment, and personality changes often occur. Communication skills are poorer, and the ability to make eye contact is reduced.

Etiology

The exact cause of Alzheimer's disease is unknown. Factors linked to its development include heredity, autoimmunity, aluminum or manganese toxicity, and viral infections. Head trauma is also linked to Alzheimer's.

Diagnosis

Only an autopsy can positively confirm the diagnosis, but CT and MRI scans have the potential to reveal microscopic plaques and the brain atrophy characteristic of Alzheimer's. While alive, a patient may be diagnosed based on the ruling out of other brain diseases.

RED FLAG

Patients with Down syndrome eventually develop dementia that is similar to Alzheimer's if they live long enough.

Treatment

No cure or definitive treatment exists for Alzheimer's disease. Treatment is only supportive because the disease is progressive. Caregivers must assume continually increasing methods of support, including issues related to nutrition, hydration, hygiene, and safety. Emotional support of family and friends is important in making the life of the Alzheimer's patient as comfortable as possible.

The role of the PTA is to assist Alzheimer's patients in exercises designed to increase fitness, endurance, and strength. Regular exercise has been shown to maintain motor skills, decrease falls, and actually reduce the rate of decrease of mental skills. Improved memory and behavior, as well as better communication skills, have been shown to occur because of regular exercise in Alzheimer's patients.

Prognosis

Prognosis is poor because there is no cure for Alzheimer's. Once the late stages of the disease are reached, the patient usually dies from a secondary cause, commonly an infection.

Head Trauma Dementia

Head trauma can cause a large variety of other conditions to develop, including dementia. Most head injuries occur to males between 14 and 24 years of age, but young children usually have the worst outcomes due to the relative softness of their skulls. Protective measures that may prevent head trauma include using seat belts, helmets, and safety equipment and removing hazards in the home and workplace.

Signs and Symptoms

Head trauma dementia may result in an extended or even permanent decrease in cognitive function and mental intellect. Often, the individual cannot remember, reason, or demonstrate appropriate behaviors and emotions. Their personality may change, and they may also experience depression, mania, anxiety, and posttraumatic stress disorder.

Etiology

Head trauma causes brain cell death, either directly from the trauma or because of increased intracranial pressure (ICP) or edema. Cells in the brain die when blood flow is impaired or stopped.

Diagnosis

Patient history, x-rays, MRI, and CT may be used to diagnose head trauma dementia.

Treatment

Treatment is aimed at preserving existing brain tissue and preventing further damage. Damage is permanent because brain cells that have died cannot be replaced. Rehabilitative therapy may be required to regain as much function as is realistically possible, but many head trauma patients must be institutionalized on a long-term basis.

Prognosis

Prognosis is entirely based on the extent of damage to the brain cells.

Substance-Induced Dementia

Substance abuse may cause a temporary form of dementia that is often curable. It also may cause severe depression that only appears to be dementia.

Signs and Symptoms

Decreased mental or cognitive ability related to substance abuse can be temporary or permanent, worsening as time passes.

Etiology

Drugs and toxins may cause brain cell death and, therefore, this type of dementia. Common substances that cause this condition include alcohol, cocaine, heroin, lead, mercury, and fumes from toxic products such as paint thinner. Dementia may persist long after exposure to the causative substance has ceased.

Diagnosis

It is often hard to diagnose whether dementia comes from a certain substance. Patient history, physical examination, and family or caregiver history are often helpful. Mental exams are often given as well.

Treatment

Substance-induced dementia is often successfully treated by removing the toxin.

Prognosis

Prognosis is good if there has not been excessive brain cell damage. If prolonged exposure to toxins has occurred, the prognosis is worse.

Vascular Dementia

Decreased blood flow is the cause of vascular dementia, due to atrophy and death of brain cells. The best methods for preventing the development of this condition are to avoid smoking, eat well, exercise regularly, and control hypertension.

Signs and Symptoms

The slow development of atherosclerotic plaques causes similar slow development of vascular dementia. This type of dementia may cause changes in judgment, memory, and personality as well as depression, irritability, and sleeplessness. Family members may notice the condition because of a lack of personal hygiene, disorientation, and unfamiliarity with what were once comfortable surroundings.

Etiology

Vascular dementia is age related because atherosclerotic plaque commonly increases as we age, decreasing blood flow to the brain.

Diagnosis

Diagnosis of vascular dementia is made based on patient history, physical exam, and testing of blood flow to the brain. Arteriograms may be taken of the cerebral and carotid arteries that reveal narrowed vessels, arteriosclerotic plaques, and stenosis.

Treatment

Medications may help improve cranial blood flow, including cholinesterase inhibitors and memantine. A carotid endarterectomy is a procedure that cleans out carotid artery plaques. The role of the PTA is to assist with regular physical exercise. This has been proven to help slow mental decline, improve physical function, reduce risk of falls, improve mood, ease stress, calm the patient, improve cardiovascular health, add to daily activities, and improve sleep.

Prognosis

Prognosis depends on the amount of brain cell death and how the patient responds to treatment. If ineffective or insufficient due to the severity of brain cell loss, the patient experiences increasing dementia and may need to be institutionalized.

Sleep Disorders

Sleep disorders are classified by their signs and symptoms rather than by their cause. There are four major classifications of sleep disorders:

- Disorders of initiating sleep
- Sleep-disordered breathing
- Disorders of the sleep–wake schedule
- Dysfunctions of sleep, sleep stages, or partial arousals

Insomnia

Insomnia is defined as a chronic inability to sleep or to remain asleep throughout the night. Insomnia actually describes a variety of conditions, including poor sleep, inability to stay asleep or fall asleep, or waking up too early in the morning.

Chronic insomnia is more common in women, especially in postmenopausal years.

Signs and Symptoms

Symptoms of insomnia include sleeplessness, fatigue, irritability, and anxiety.

Etiology

Insomnia may be caused by pain, stress, depression, fear, cardiovascular problems, thyroid disorders, alcohol, caffeine, bronchodilators, and nicotine.

Diagnosis

Insomnia is diagnosed when sleeplessness has occurred for 1 month, interfering with an individual's normal working and social habits. The patient's sleep history should be taken. If a breathing disorder is discovered, referral to a sleep lab may be of help to the patient.

Treatment

Treatment for insomnia requires that the cause be correctly identified and then removed. Sleep scheduling may be used, with consistent bedtimes and waking times, and stress or anxiety counseling may be indicated. The patient should be instructed that getting the required amount of hours of sleep per day is more important than being able to sleep consistently through the night.

Prognosis

Prognosis is good in general, especially when the patient assumes a healthy lifestyle, with adequate rest times, exercise, reduction of stress, and a good diet.

Sleep Apnea

Sleep apnea is characterized by periods of breathlessness (apnea) during sleep. This disorder is the most common sleep disorder in the United States, affecting nearly one-third of adults to some degree.

Signs and Symptoms

Sleep apnea is defined as more than five periods of apnea that each last for at least 10 seconds during every hour of sleep. The patient may suddenly gasp for air, which can also cause him or her to awaken. Signs of sleep apnea may include severe drowsiness during the day, narcolepsy, extremely loud snoring at night, depression, impotence, and personality changes.

Etiology

Sleep apnea is more common in males and can be related to hypertension, obesity, nasal or throat obstruction (*obstructive apnea*), alcohol intake, smoking, a disorder of the respiratory center of the brain (*central apnea*), or a combination of several of these factors (*mixed apnea*).

Diagnosis

The patient may be diagnosed with sleep apnea by monitoring during sleep for apnea symptoms and low blood oxygen levels.

Treatment

Treatment varies based on the type of sleep apnea that exists. Obstructive and mixed apneas are treated with weight-reduction therapies and surgery for nasal obstruction. Obstructive apnea is also treated with oxygen administration, oral appliances that help to open the airway, airway pressure devices, and continuous positive airway pressure devices. Central apnea is harder to treat and may require medications that stimulate breathing.

Prognosis

Prognosis is improved with weight reduction and avoiding alcohol and tobacco use.

Brain Tumors

Primary brain tumors develop from various tissue types within the intracranial cavity. They are named for the tissue from which they originate. Tumors are commonly described as benign or malignant. All brain tumors may be considered malignant because, without treatment, the patient will die. Besides primary tumors that arise from intracranial tissue, metastatic tumors may also migrate to the area via blood circulation. Brain tumors are found in about 2 percent of routine autopsies. They are most common in young or middle-aged adults but may occur at any age. They appear to be occurring more frequently in elderly patients.

Signs and Symptoms

General manifestations result from increased ICP. Headache and vomiting result, and mental status changes. Drowsiness, seizures, loss of memory, and visual disturbances are the initial symptoms. Headache associated with a brain tumor is most common upon awakening in the morning. In young children increased ICP may enlarge the head.

Etiology

Common primary childhood brain tumors are usually **astrocytomas**. The most common metastatic brain tumors in children are caused by *neuroblastoma* or *leukemia*. In adults primary tumors include **meningiomas**, lymphomas, and **gliomas**. Metastatic tumors in adults arise most commonly from bronchogenic carcinoma, adenocarcinoma of the breast, carcinoma of the colon, and malignant melanoma.

> **RED FLAG**
> Brain tumors are also common in the immunosuppressed population.

Diagnosis

Diagnosis of brain tumors is provided by patient history, symptoms, x-rays, CT, MRI, and biopsy. The type of tumor is best determined by biopsy, with treatment and prognosis improved. Additional studies help determine primary locations of metastatic brain tumors.

Treatment

Brain tumor treatments include chemotherapy, radiation, and surgery, depending on the type and location of the tumor. The role of the PTA is focused on helping patients to recover lost function, improve overall cardiovascular health, and restore feeling and sensation in certain cases. Examples of physical therapies used for brain tumor patients include stretching, massage, heat packs, ultrasound, and electrical nerve stimulation.

Prognosis

Prognosis is heavily based on the stage of the tumor when discovered, its type, and its location within the brain.

Trauma

Trauma to the brain, neck, and spinal cord can cause many types of disabilities and even death. Head trauma can lead to edema, increased ICP, hemorrhage, and infection. All these conditions can lead to brain damage. Paralysis can result from injury to the neck and spinal cord. *Traumatic brain injury* is a complex injury with many symptoms and disabilities. It is classified as either mild or severe. Severe brain injury is associated with loss of consciousness for more than 30 minutes and memory loss after the injury for longer than 24 hours.

Concussions and Contusions

A *concussion* is defined as a head trauma that does not physically bruise the brain tissue. A *contusion* is more serious, defined as a physical bruising of the brain tissue. Contusions often occur when the skull is fractured. Prevention of these types of injuries involves similar precautions to those used to stop head trauma dementia from developing.

Signs and Symptoms

The main symptom of both a concussion and a contusion is unconsciousness. **Amnesia** may also follow the event. Additional symptoms include blurred vision, headache, irritability, and sudden vomiting. A contusion can also lead to a hematoma of the brain, increased ICP, and permanent brain damage. The area of bruised brain tissue is referred to as a coup lesion. If the injury occurs on the opposite side of the brain, often due to a "whiplashing" of the head in an automobile accident, it is referred to as a contracoup lesion. Contracoup injuries are often seen along with a coup injury as well.

Etiology

Concussions or contusions may occur due to a blow to the head from an object, a fall, an automobile accident, or other trauma.

Diagnosis

Diagnosis is made on history of the injury, cranial x-rays, neurologic exam, and CT or MRI scans. The Glasgow Coma Scale and Rancho Los Amigo Scale may be used to assess head injuries, including determining the prognosis of each. The Glasgow Coma Scale is designed to assess many different levels of consciousness. The Rancho Los Amigo Scale is used to assess the level of recovery of brain injury patients and those recovering from coma.

With head injuries it is important for the PTA to understand how cognition and behavioral issues may be affected. The patient's safety must be of primary concern at all times. Patients may seem very different from how they were before the injury. Behavior control must precede cognitive and physical rehabilitation. These patients require a tightly controlled schedule to improve. Better outcomes are achieved when physical therapy occurs in familiar settings.

Treatment

Patients who have had a concussion should rest quietly in bed under direct supervision, awakening them every 2 to 4 hours to check for consciousness changes, size of the pupils, mood, and behavior. Patients with skull contusions should be hospitalized and continually monitored. Individuals with head injures should not receive analgesics, sedatives, or stimulants so symptoms can be clearly seen. The role of the PTA is focused on physical therapy designed to help improve mobility and promote activities of daily living. Occupational therapists may deal with loss of balance, attention deficit, and speech problems due to the concussion.

Prognosis
Prognosis is based on the degree of seriousness of the injury.

Skull Fractures

When the cranial (skull) bone has become broken, a skull fracture has occurred. Skull fractures may damage brain tissue in several ways. Fragments of bone can cut the brain and its vessels, resulting in a hematoma. Fractures have the potential to cause temporary or permanent brain damage.

Signs and Symptoms
The area of the skull that is fractured causes specific symptoms that differ from skull fractures of other areas. Fractures near the bottom (base) of the skull can cause injury to the respiratory center of the brain, resulting in cessation of breathing. Other symptoms of different skull fractures include hemiparesis, seizures, and infection of the brain through the actual fracture site.

Etiology
Skull fractures are commonly caused by automobile accidents, falls, severe blows to the head, and injuries from playing sports.

Diagnosis
Skull fractures are diagnosed based on patient history, physical exam, x-rays, and CT scan.

Treatment
The type and position of the skull fracture determines the method of treatment. If increased ICP exists due to brain swelling, a craniotomy may be performed. If a fractured skull bone is pressing on brain tissue, the skull may be surgically repaired. The patient may need to wear protective helmets or other headgear until the fracture is completely healed.

Prognosis
Prognosis is individual, based on the severity of the fracture and the resultant damage to the brain.

Epidural and Subdural Hematomas

An **epidural** hematoma is defined as a collection of blood between the skull and **dura mater**. A **subdural** hematoma is defined as a collection of blood between the dura mater layer and the **arachnoid** layer. Subdural hematomas are more than twice as common as epidural hematomas. **Figure 14–11A and B** shows both types of hematomas in the skull.

Signs and Symptoms
Epidural hematomas cause dilated pupils, headache, nausea, vomiting, dizziness, and, potentially, increased ICP and loss of consciousness. Subdural hematomas cause symptoms that are related to increased ICP. These include hemiparesis, nausea, vomiting, convulsions, dizziness, and loss of consciousness.

Etiology
Epidural hematomas are most often caused by a blow to the head. Figure 14–11 shows both types of hematomas in the skull. In the epidural hematoma blood vessels rupture and

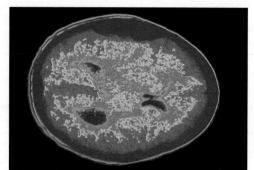

(A)

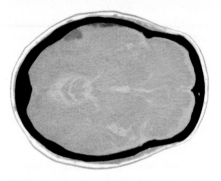

(B)

Figure 14–11 Subdural (A) and epidural (B) hematomas in the brain.

hemorrhage or slowly leak blood between the bony skull and the dura mater. It usually collects quickly over only a few hours and pushes the dura mater away from the inside of the skull.

A subdural hematoma is often caused by the head striking an immobile object, such as when a person falls and hits his or her head on a piece of furniture. This type of hematoma is characterized by slower development, usually over days instead of hours.

Diagnosis
Cerebral hematomas of both types are diagnosed based on patient history, x-ray, CT, and MRI. In general, they are accompanied by some form of skull fracture.

Treatment
The goal of treatment for cranial hematomas is to reduce ICP. A special type of craniotomy (called "burr holes") can be used to drain blood from the brain and **cauterize** (burn with electricity) the tissue to stop any further bleeding.

Prognosis
Promptly treated, ICP has a good prognosis. However, if untreated, ICP can be fatal.

Spinal Cord Injury

When the vertebral column is damaged, there is also the possibility of spinal cord damage. The cervical region of the spinal cord is the most vulnerable section. Paralysis may occur based on the degree of injury to the neck or, in the case of *paraplegia*, to the thoracic or lumbar region. When the lower part of the body is affected, it is called **paraplegia**. When both the arms and legs are affected, it is called **quadriplegia** or, more recently, *tetraplegia* (because it involves the trunk).

Signs and Symptoms

Spinal cord injury often causes loss of feeling and movement below the area of injury. Severe spinal cord damage is usually not reversible. Sometimes, extremities that have lost feeling gain back reflex functions and move in a spasmodic, involuntary manner.

When the C1–3 area of the spinal cord is injured, it is often fatal, due to the breathing centers in the medulla being affected. Quadriplegia (tetraplegia) often occurs from injuries between C1 and C7. Besides paralysis, other symptoms of quadriplegia include loss of bowel, bladder, and sexual function; hypotension; hypothermia; bradycardia; and respiratory difficulties. Although C1–7 injuries results in quadriplegia, injury to just the C5–7 area of the spine leads to differing paralysis of the arms and shoulders. Paraplegia results from injury (involving compression) to the thoracic (below T-1 level) or lumbar section of the spinal cord. Other symptoms of this type of injury include loss of bladder, bowel, and sexual function. **Figure 14–12** depicts various parts of the vertebral column.

Injury Results

- C1–C3 Usually fatal
- C1–C7 Injuries cause quadriplegia
- C5–C7 Injuries lead to differing paralysis of the arms and shoulders
- T1-L5 Paraplegia

Prevention

- Wear helmets during risky activities.
- Do not dive into unfamiliar or shallow water.
- Wear a seat belt at all times in a vehicle.
- Wear protective gear during sports or physical activities.
- Make sure ladders are stable and secure. Do not use the top step or platform to stand on.
- Seek help with climbing activities.

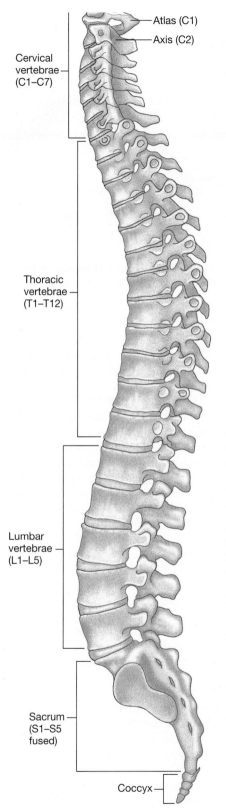

Atlas (C1)
Axis (C2)
Cervical vertebrae (C1–C7)
Thoracic vertebrae (T1–T12)
Lumbar vertebrae (L1–L5)
Sacrum (S1–S5 fused)
Coccyx

Vertebral column (lateral view)

Figure 14–12 Various parts of the vertebral column.

Etiology

The primary causes of spinal cord injury are automobile accidents, followed by gunshot wounds, knife wounds, falls, and recreational or sports injuries. In an automobile accident, neck injuries are commonly caused by the action known as "whiplash," wherein the head and neck are jerked forward and backward as the impact of the accident occurs.

Diagnosis

Diagnosis of spinal cord injuries is made based on history, physical exam, x-rays, CT, MRI, and myelography.

Treatment

If spinal cord injury is suspected, the patient should not be moved until emergency medical personnel have arrived. The head and neck should be kept as immobile as possible. The spine's position should be maintained by using backboards and special collars. Once in the hospital, common treatment methods include medications, emergency surgery, and immobilization with traction-like devices. Further surgery may be required to realign the spinal column and release pressure on the spinal cord. Many other problems can develop due to the patient's immobilization, including contractures, wasting of muscles, bedsores, blood clots, and urinary tract infections. Long-term care involves rehabilitation and physical therapy as well as the possible need for ventilators, wheelchairs, and other equipment.

The role of the PTA is to assist with a variety of helpful therapies for spinal cord injury, such as stretching, computerized traction, range-of-motion exercises, strengthening exercises, and mobility training (either with a wheelchair or a gait trainer, which is a wheeled device that helps the patient relearn to walk correctly).

Prognosis

Prognosis is generally better the earlier proper treatment is started, although the level and severity of injury are factors.

Rare Diseases

The following are rare diseases of the nervous system and are only briefly explained.

Amyotrophic Lateral Sclerosis

Amyotrophic lateral sclerosis, better known as ALS or "Lou Gehrig's disease," is a degenerative disease that affects the upper and lower motor neurons. It is the most common of the motor neuron diseases causing muscular atrophy. Onset is usually between ages 40 and 70. ALS is a chronic, progressively debilitating disease that may be fatal in less than 1 year or may continue for 10 years or more, depending on the affected muscles. The disease affects three times as many men as women.

> **RED FLAG**
> There is no simple reliable laboratory test available that confirms the diagnosis of ALS.

The role of the PTA is to assist with gentle, low-impact exercise, such as walking, swimming, and stationary cycling. Range-of-motion and stretching exercises are also indicated. Helpful equipment may include braces, ramps, walkers, and wheelchairs.

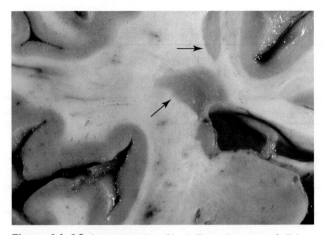

Figure 14–13 Coronal section of brain illustrating areas of glial scarring (arrows) adjacent to ventricle in multiple sclerosis. The demyelinated areas appear much darker than the adjacent normal white matter because of loss of myelin.

Guillain-Barré Syndrome

Guillain-Barré syndrome is an acute, progressive spinal nerve disease of unknown origin. It is suspected to be an autoimmune disorder because it often appears within 21 days after an illness that has caused a fever. Initial symptoms include fever, malaise, and nausea. Within 72 hours muscle weakness, paresthesia, and paralysis usually begin in the legs and move upward, although these symptoms may begin in the face and arms as well. When respiratory muscles are affected, this syndrome can be life threatening. Symptoms can progress to several weeks, and recovery can take up to 1 year. Treatment is supportive, and recovery is most often complete.

The role of the PTA is to assist with range-of-motion exercises to increase muscle flexibility and strength. Muscles must be retrained to develop normal function. The most important thing to remember is that Guillain-Barré patients must have frequent rests between exercises and should go slowly for as long as they can tolerate a physical therapy session. Adequate hydration during exercise is vital.

> **RED FLAG**
> Thirty percent of patients with Guillain-Barré syndrome have respiratory paralysis requiring mechanical ventilation. Complete or substantial recovery is the goal.

Huntington's Chorea

This genetic disease affects half of children in families in which one parent has the dominant gene. Huntington's chorea does not appear until middle age. Symptoms include progressive brain deterioration, loss of muscle control, and **chorea**. There may also be mood and personality changes, loss of memory, and eventually dementia. There is no cure, and treatment is supportive, usually resulting in institutionalization. Genetic counseling should be given to families with this inherited disease.

Multiple Sclerosis

Multiple sclerosis (MS) is a chronic inflammatory disease involving demyelinization of the white matter of the brain and spinal cord. **Figure 14–13** illustrates the effects of MS. MS scars (scleroses) the white matter, causing debilitation. The

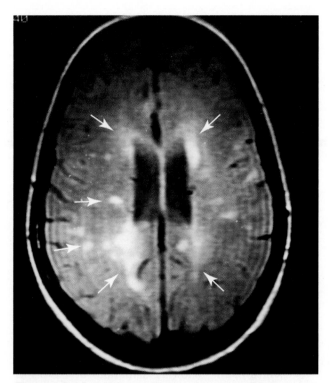

Figure 14–14 Multiple sclerosis demonstrated by MRI. The ventricular system is well demonstrated in the center of the photograph. Dense white areas adjacent to posterior horns of the ventricles and scattered throughout the brain lateral to the ventricles (arrows) are multiple sclerosis plaques.

disease usually affects adults between ages 20 and 40 (women more than men), with periods of remission and exacerbation over several years.

Signs and Symptoms

MS symptoms include lack of coordination, muscle weakness or numbness, unsteady gait, paresthesia, vertigo, difficulty speaking, dysphagia, loss of bladder function, facial numbness or pain, hearing loss, male impotence, fatigue, increased urinary tract infections, emotional disturbances, and visual disturbances such as double vision. The demyelinating lesions vary in location in the body, and this influences the types of symptoms. MS prevents transmission of stimuli to the brain and spinal cord, causing sensory and motor abnormalities.

Etiology

The cause of MS is unknown, but it may be genetically linked because it occurs 15 times as often in first-degree relatives. Immune function and viral infections may also be causative factors. MS may be linked to heredity but is more widely believed to be triggered by an unknown virus that causes the immune system to attack the body's myelin. More cases of MS occur in northern climates than in southern ones, and more Whites are affected than any other race. It usually develops more often in women and in people between ages 20 and 40, but sometimes occurs in people older than 60 years.

Diagnosis

Diagnosis of MS is therefore very difficult because the symptoms are variable and inconsistent. Once a patient has had several episodes of central nervous system dysfunction, the diagnosis is more likely. MRI is extremely useful for evaluating patients with neurologic disease in whom MS is suspected (**Figure 14–14**). MRI is able to find a characteristic cerebral or spinal plaque, and examination of the CSF may indicate elevated immunoglobulin levels.

Treatment

Acute attacks of MS are treated with corticosteroids. Chronic forms are treated with interferons, immune modulators, and antineoplastic agents. Radiation, immune globulins, and cytotoxic drugs may also be used. Muscle relaxants, vitamin supplements, braces, walking devices, and physical therapy are also helpful, along with adequate rest and a well-balanced diet.

The role of the PTA is to assist the MS patient in exercise regimens that are low level and focus on energy conservation. Activities must be monitored to avoid fatigue. The physician and physical therapist should assess each MS patient individually and determine exercises and activities that are appropriate. Warm-up and cool-down periods should be part of the regular exercise regimen, and fall prevention strategies should be implemented. Examples of exercises that work well for MS patients include water aerobics, swimming, tai chi, and yoga.

> **RED FLAG**
> There are no known preventive measures for MS. Individuals must avoid factors that may precipitate an exacerbation, such as stressful life events.

Prognosis

MS has the ability to kill patients soon after onset, though *average* life span is 30 years after onset. It is possible for some patients to live a full lifetime with MS, depending on the variation of the disease that exists. These patients may have one to two episodes and never have another one or may not have another one for many years. Females who develop the relapsing form of MS at a younger age are more likely to live longer, as are patients who have sensory pathway impairment as the initial symptom. Although most individuals live a normal life span, physical therapy and muscle relaxants may be required to reduce spastic movements and maintain muscle tone.

Myasthenia Gravis

Myasthenia gravis is a chronic and progressive neuromuscular disease that appears to develop from the presence of autoantibodies to the acetylcholine receptor.

Signs and Symptoms

Myasthenia gravis causes severe muscular weakness and progressive fatigue but does not cause muscular atrophy. Onset may be gradual or sudden. Symptoms include diplopia, drooping eyelids, and difficulty in speaking, chewing, and swallowing.

> **RED FLAG**
> Myasthenia *crisis* is a condition related to myasthenia gravis that occurs when respiratory muscle weakness produces respiratory insufficiency that may lead to respiratory failure.

Etiology

Myasthenia gravis mainly affects women between ages 20 and 40 and men over age 60. It is believed to arise from faulty transmission of nerve impulses in the neuromuscular junctions of the central nervous system. Most patients have autoantibodies against their acetylcholine receptors and either thymus hyperplasia or thymoma (an epithelial tumor of the thymus).

Diagnosis

Initially, physical examination is used to test for muscle fatigue in various muscle groups. An intravenous administration of a short-acting acetylcholinesterase inhibitor is given to see if its administration improves muscle strength. This is known as a "Tensilon test." Tests are then done to check for antibodies that act against the acetylcholine receptor, and electromyography may also be used to confirm diagnosis.

Treatment

Treatment for myasthenia gravis is symptomatic and supportive, based on the age of the patient and whether pregnancy is a factor. Adequate rest and (sometimes) changing to a soft or liquid diet may be needed. Medications include anticholinesterase drugs and muscle-strengthening agents. If thymoma is present, a thymectomy should be performed. Corticosteroids and immunosuppressive agents may also be used.

The role of the PTA in myasthenia gravis is to assist patients with regular exercise to keep muscles and bones in shape. Many medications used for this condition cause patients to gain weight, making exercise even more useful. Physical therapies may include walking, swimming, cycling, bowling, gymnasium workouts, and tennis. Patients must be advised not to overexert themselves. The body must remain completely hydrated for exercise to be beneficial. Temperature extremes must be avoided. Fatigue or difficulty breathing signifies the patient needs to rest.

Prognosis

Prognosis depends on remissions and reoccurrences of the disease, which is usually a lifelong condition. The effects vary, with some patients remaining functionally independent for a long time, only to become more debilitated because of a later exacerbation of the disease.

SUMMARY

The complex human nervous system controls intellectual and physical actions and reactions. It is responsible for reasoning, interacting, and understanding. The nervous system is divided into the central nervous system and peripheral nervous system. Disorders of the nervous system often affect most other body systems and may cause headache, nausea, vomiting, mood swings, fever, and weakness. Brain, neck, and spinal cord injuries cause many people to become disabled and are often fatal. The brain and spinal cord are covered in meninges, which are membranes divided into three layers. Brain and spinal cord injuries often result in permanent neurologic conditions.

Diagnostic tests used for nervous system conditions include x-rays, myelogram, angiogram, EEG, CT, and MRI. Infectious diseases affecting the nervous system include encephalitis, meningitis, poliomyelitis, rabies, shingles, and tetanus. Vascular disorders related to the nervous system include CVA, TIA, Bell's palsy, epilepsy, headache, and Parkinson's disease. Dementia affects many older adults, with one of the most common forms being Alzheimer's disease.

Other conditions related to the nervous system include sleep apnea, brain tumors, and various forms of trauma (which may result in a wide variety of disorders).

REVIEW QUESTIONS

Select the best response to each question.

1. A 52-year-old contractor presents to a physician's office complaining of a 4-week history of daily headaches. He describes the headache as being pronounced in the morning on awakening, associated with nausea and vomiting. The most likely diagnosis is which of the following conditions?
   a. muscle tension headache
   b. classic migraine headache
   c. brain tumor
   d. meningitis

2. The most common causative organism of meningitis in adults is which of the following?
   a. *Streptococcus pneumoniae*
   b. herpes zoster
   c. *Escherichia coli*
   d. *Neisseria meningitides*

3. Which of the following definitions best explains encephalitis?
   a. inflammation of the brain
   b. inflammation of the meninges
   c. inflammation of the spinal cord
   d. inflammation of the brain and spinal cord

4. Herpes zoster is also called which of the following conditions?
   a. warts
   b. shingles
   c. impetigo
   d. acne

5. What body functions does the hypothalamus control?
   a. body temperature
   b. water balance
   c. sleep
   d. all of the above

6. Which of the following terms describes temporary episodes of impaired neurologic functioning caused by inadequate blood flow to a portion of the brain?
   a. migraine headaches
   b. strokes
   c. transient ischemic attacks
   d. concussions

7. Which of the following is an acute, potentially fatal bacterial infection of the central nervous system caused by a neurotoxin?
   a. Guillain-Barré syndrome
   b. tetanus
   c. rabies
   d. meningitis

8. Which of the following cranial nerves affects chest and gastrointestinal system movement?
   a. vagus
   b. abducens
   c. accessory
   d. hypoglossal

9. Which of the following is the cause of Parkinson's disease?
   a. serotonin deficiency
   b. norepinephrine deficiency
   c. dopamine deficiency
   d. unknown cause
10. Which of the following is *not* one of the four major classifications of sleep disorders?
   a. dysfunction of sleep stages
   b. sleep disorders due to improper digestion
   c. disorders of initiating sleep
   d. sleep-disordered breathing

CASE STUDIES

Karen Coupe, PT, DPT, MSEd

Case 1

A 64-year-old man suffered a left cerebrovascular accident (CVA) of the middle cerebral artery 1 week ago and is currently being transferred to the inpatient rehabilitation unit. Complications include right hemiparesis and Broca's aphasia. Patient medical history: Hypertension (medication controlled), arteriosclerosis obliterans, two transient ischemic attacks (TIAs), both in the past 8 months, mildly obese. Social history: Retired physics teacher, smokes two packs a day, likes to play cards. Prior level of function: Independent in all activities of daily living. Current level of function: Right hemiparesis, bed mobility with min x1, transfers w/mod x1 ambulates with a hemiwalker x 8 ft. w/mod x 2. Plan of care is for bed mobility, transfers, gait training, and strengthening activities.

1. Explain the etiology and pathogenesis of a CVA. Why would damage of the left hemisphere affect the right side?
2. What risk factors, if any, did the patient have?
3. The middle cerebral artery involves portions of the frontal, temporal, and parietal lobes. List the functions of each lobe to determine the potential issues.
4. What is Broca's aphasia? How would this affect treatment? What strategies could the PTA use to assist the patient?
5. While in therapy the patient demonstrates slurred speech and increased weakness and complains of headache. How should the PTA respond?

Case 2

A 75-year-old man is referred to outpatient physical therapy for strengthening and balance activities. The patient was diagnosed with Parkinson's disease 20 years ago. Current issues include bradykinesia, rigidity, and infrequent bouts of akinesia, and the patient admits to falling three to four times a day for the past week. Prior level of function: Independent ambulation with a cane, independent in dressing and grooming, assistance with household cooking and cleaning.

1. What is the etiology and pathogenesis of Parkinson's disease?
2. What is bradykinesia? How does this present? What are the implications of bradykinesia on everyday function?
3. Is it a concern that the patient has admitted to frequent falls? What current issues may be contributing to this postural instability? How does the disease process contribute to postural instability?
4. Secondary complications can include cardiac and pulmonary issues. Look at the types of complications for each system and explain the implications of each during treatment.
5. During treatment the patient admits to the PTA that he has noticed lapses in his memory. The PTA asks for examples and he says he can't find things, forgets he turned on the stove and finds it on later, leaves water running, and so on. How should the PTA respond?

WEBSITES

http://users.rcn.com/jkimball.ma.ultranet/BiologyPages/P/PNS.html

http://www.abta.org/

http://www.beverlyhillsneurology.com/myastheniagravis.html

http://www.braininjury.com/epidural-subdural-hematoma.html

http://www.cordingleyneurology.com/contuseconcuss.html

http://www.medicinenet.com/brain_tumor/article.htm

http://www.merck.com/mmhe/sec06/ch076/ch076e.html

http://www.nlm.nih.gov/medlineplus/dementia.html

http://www.nlm.nih.gov/medlineplus/ency/article/000060.htm

http://www.rush.edu/rumc/page-1098994230654.html

http://www.spinalcord.org/resources/index.php

http://www.webmd.com/sleep-disorders/default.htm

Disorders of the Eye and Ear

LEARNING OBJECTIVES

After completion of this chapter the reader should be able to

1. Describe macular degeneration.
2. Describe the conditions known as cataracts and glaucoma.
3. Explain the differences between "nearsightedness" and "farsightedness."
4. State the causes and treatment of dry eye.
5. List the structures of the external, middle, and inner ear, and explain their actions.
6. List the various conditions that may lead to hearing loss.
7. Explain the characteristics of tinnitus.
8. List three common symptoms of acute otitis media.

KEY TERMS

Achromatic vision: Total color blindness, wherein the patient can see only white, gray, and black.
Amblyopia: "Lazy eye"; characterized by poor or indistinct vision in an eye that is relatively normal. It is not the same as "strabismus."
Astigmatism: A refractive error of the eye in which there is a difference in the degree of refraction in different areas of the eye.
Blepharitis: Chronic inflammation of the eyelid.
Carotenoids: Organic pigments with nutritional value that are found in vegetables and fruits such as carrots, sweet potatoes, spinach, kale, collard greens, and tomatoes.
Cataract: A clouding of the crystalline lens of the eye or its envelope.
Choroid: The middle, vascular layer of the eye, containing connective tissue; also known as the "choroid coat" or "choroidea."
Conjunctivitis: "Pink eye"; an acute inflammation of the conjunctiva (the outermost layer of the eye and innermost layer of the eyelids).

KEY TERMS CONTINUED

Cornea: The transparent front part of the eye that covers the iris, pupil, and anterior chamber.

Cryotherapy: Local or general use of low temperatures to decrease cellular metabolism and other activities; when done as a surgical treatment, it is known as "cryosurgery."

Daltonism: The more common form of color blindness wherein the patient cannot distinguish between the colors red and green.

Diplopia: Double vision; the simultaneous perception of two images of the same object.

Electrocholeography: Recording of the electrical activity produced when the cochlea is stimulated.

Electronystagmography: A test used in evaluating the vestibulo-ocular reflex.

Glaucoma: A disease of the optic nerve involving increased intraocular pressure and potentially progressing to blindness.

Hyperopia: Farsightedness (long-sightedness or hypermetropia); it occurs often when the eyeball is too short or the lens cannot become round enough, causing the individual to be able to see far-off objects more clearly than close-up objects.

Iridotomy: Also known as "laser iridotomy," it is a surgical procedure used to treat angle-closure glaucoma; the procedure involves making a hole in the iris to change its configuration.

Iris: The colored portion of the eye; it controls the diameter and size of the pupil.

Lens: The transparent, bioconvex structure that works with the cornea to refract light that is focused on the retina.

Macula: Also known as the "macula lutea," it is the yellow spot near the center of the retina; it is responsible for central vision.

Macular degeneration: A medical condition that usually affects older adults, resulting in a loss of vision because of damage to the retina.

Myopia: "Nearsightedness"; a refractive error wherein the eyeball is too long or the cornea is too steep, causing far-off objects to appear blurred while close-up objects are clear.

Ophthalmic: Referring to ophthalmology, the branch of medicine that focuses on the eyes; ophthalmologists differ from optometrists in that they are both medically and surgically trained.

Otalgia: Ear pain or an "earache."

Phacoemulsification: A procedure used in modern cataract surgery wherein the eye's internal lens is emulsified with an ultrasonic hand piece; the emulsified cataract is then aspirated from the eye.

Photocoagulation: A type of laser surgery used to treat many eye disorders; a laser is used to cauterize small ocular blood vessels, lowering the risk of severe vision loss.

Photophobia: A symptom of excessive sensitivity to light and the aversion to sunlight or areas of bright lighting.

Premenstrual edema: Fluid retention and tenderness of the breasts occurring shortly before the onset of menstruation.

Presbyopia: "Old eye"; a progressively diminished ability to focus on close-up objects due to aging.

Refraction: The deviation of light waves entering the eye; a "refractive test" may be used to determine the eye's "refractive error" and the best corrective lenses to be prescribed.

Retina: Light-sensitive tissue lining the inner surface of the eye.

Retinal detachment: A disorder in which the retina peels away from the choroid, leading to loss of vision and potential blindness.

Retinopathy: Noninflammatory damage to the retina.

Retrobulbar: Related to the area behind the globe of the eye.

Sclera: The outer, white portion of the eye.

Seborrhea: A chronic, inflammatory skin disorder that affects the sebaceous glands of the head and trunk.

Strabismus: A condition in which the eyes are not properly aligned with each other.

Suppurative: Causing the formation or discharge of pus.

Tinnitus: Perception of sound within the ear when there is no corresponding external sound.

Tonometric: Related to the measurement of tension or pressure; in ophthalmology it is used to determine intraocular pressure.

Tympanic membrane: The "eardrum"; it separates the external ear from the middle ear and transmits sounds from the air to the auditory ossicles.

Vertigo: A type of dizziness wherein there is a feeling of motion when a person is actually stationary.

Xerosis: Pathologic dryness of the skin.

Overview

The sensory receptors detect environmental changes and trigger nerve impulses that travel on sensory pathways into two major categories. Receptors are associated with the *somatic senses* of touch, pressure, temperature, and pain. These receptors are widely distributed throughout the skin and deeper tissues and are structurally simple. Receptors of the second type are parts of complex, specialized sensory organs that provide the *special senses* of smell, taste, hearing, vision, and equilibrium. When sensory function is altered, there may be related dysfunctions of sight, hearing, smell, taste, balance, or coordination.

The eye and ear are the major organs of the special senses. About 70 percent of all sensory receptors are in the eyes. Therefore, this chapter focuses on eye and ear disorders. Almost 17.5 million people in the United States have some degree of visual impairment. Of these, 1.1 million are legally blind. The prevalence of visual impairment increases with age. Alterations in vision can result from disorders of the eyelids and optic globe (conjunctiva, cornea, and uvea), intraocular pressure (glaucoma), lens (cataracts), vitreous humor and retina, visual pathways, extraocular muscles, and eye movements.

The ear is the organ of both hearing and balance (equilibrium). Hearing loss or deafness may be related to ear damage, aging, infections, and central nervous system problems. Hearing loss is one of the most common disabilities experienced by people in the United States, particularly among the elderly.

Anatomy and Physiology of the Eye

The eye "sees" because of three basic concepts: (1) light rays enter the eye to form an image on the retina, (2) the rods and cones of the eye become stimulated, and (3) nerve impulses conduct information to the brain. The optic center of the brain is larger than the centers for each of the other senses.

The outermost layer of the eye is the **sclera**, which is known as the "white of the eye." It is made up of tough, connective tissue and extrinsic muscles that move the eye. The *cornea* is the transparent portion of the front of the eye that helps focus light rays. **Figure 15–1A and B** shows (A) the structures of the eye and (B) the visual pathway.

The middle layer of the eye is the **choroid**, which has cells containing a dark pigment. These cells absorb excess light rays that have the potential to interfere with clear vision. The choroid is continuous with the **iris** and ciliary body. The *ciliary body* contains ciliary muscles that focus the lens of the eye. *Aqueous humor* (a fluid in the anterior part of the eye) is secreted by the ciliary processes. The ciliary body is connected by suspensory ligaments to the **lens**, which changes in shape to allow focusing needed for close vision. The iris is the colored portion of the eye that helps adjust how much light enters the eye. It changes size in reaction to bright or dim light conditions.

The inner portion of the eye is the **retina**. It covers the posterior three-fourths of the eye and has a light-sensitive layer made up of *rods* and *cones*. Rods work best in dim light, whereas cones work best in bright light. Rods allow "night vision," whereas cones detect color and finer details. The optic nerve receives messages from the rods and cones, penetrating the optic disk and continuing to the brain. The *optic disk* is known as the "blind spot" of the eye because it contains no receptors. A yellow spot (the **macula** *lutea*) is lateral to the optic disk, with its center (the *fovea centralis*) producing the sharpest vision.

The *conjunctiva* is a transparent membrane that covers the anterior visible portion of the sclera, beginning at the edge of the **cornea**. It folds to line the inside portion of the *eyelids*. The space between the iris and anterior cornea is the *anterior chamber*. Appropriate eye pressure is maintained by the aqueous humor in this region. The large cavity behind the lens is the *vitreous body*, which contains the jelly-like *vitreous humor* that helps maintain eye shape and refract images.

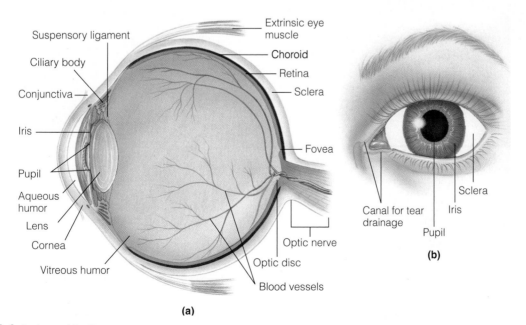

(a)

(b)

Figure 15–1 Anatomy of the human eye.

Contraction and relaxation of the muscles of the ciliary body focuses images. The lens can assume a variety of shapes required for both close and far vision. When the ciliary body relaxes, small tissues called *zonules* are pulled, causing the lens to flatten (which allows for far vision). Light rays enter the eye, pass through the cornea, and continue through the aqueous humor, lens, and vitreous humor. **Refraction** is the process by which light rays bend in the eye. The image that forms on the retina is backward and upside down, conditions that are reversed by the brain. *Accommodation* is the process that changes the shape of the lens to either a flat or bulb-like shape to focus or sharpen an image based on the eye's distance from the object (**Figure 15–2A and B**).

Each eye has six extrinsic muscles located outside the eye that control its movements. These muscles attach to the bony eye socket and to the sclera (**Figure 15–3**). **Table 15–1** lists the extrinsic muscles of the eye and their functions.

Certain eye disorders may be caused by systemic diseases such as diabetes mellitus, autoimmune arthritic diseases, and hypertension. Redness, pain, itching, burning, swelling, drainage, lesions, visual disturbances, and uncontrolled movements are all signs and symptoms of eye diseases.

Disorders of the Eye

There are many disorders of the eye that range from very mild to very severe and also vary in how commonly they occur. The physical therapist assistant (PTA) should take into account any vision problems while assisting patients with physical therapy for other conditions. Poor vision can affect the safety

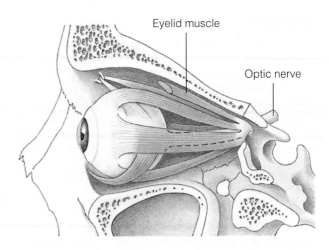

Figure 15–3 Extrinsic eye muscles. These muscles move the eye in all directions. They attach to the bony orbit and the sclera.

of the patient, and the PTA must be aware of potential hazards. The PT must be made aware of any vision problems the PTA discovers not previously addressed.

Blepharitis

Blepharitis is the inflammation of the margins of the eyelids involving glands and hair follicles. It can be ulcerative or nonulcerative. This condition should be evaluated as soon as possible. This condition can be avoided by using proper hygiene to protect the eyes from infection.

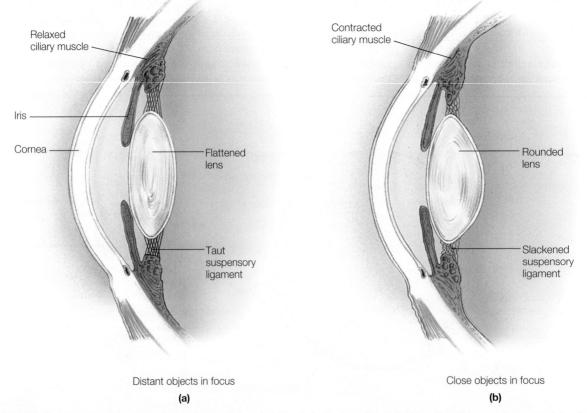

Distant objects in focus
(a)

Close objects in focus
(b)

Figure 15–2 Accommodation. (A) The lens is flattened when the ciliary muscles are relaxed. (B) When the ciliary muscles contract, tension on the suspensory ligaments is reduced and the lens shortens and thickens.

TABLE 15-1 Extrinsic Muscles of the Eye

Eye Muscle	Cranial Innervation	Muscle Function
Inferior oblique	Oculomotor nerve (III)	Rotates eyeball up and out; abducts
Superior oblique	Trochlear nerve (IV)	Rotates eyeball down and out; abducts
Inferior rectus	Oculomotor nerve (III)	Rotates eyeball down and medially; adducts
Lateral rectus	Abducens nerve (VI)	Rotates eye laterally; abducts
Medial rectus	Oculomotor nerve (III)	Rotates eye medially; adducts
Superior rectus	Oculomotor nerve (III)	Allows the eye to look up

Signs and Symptoms

Blepharitis causes chronic redness and crusting of the eyelids. Other symptoms include burning, itching, and the feeling of a foreign object in the eye. Severe blepharitis can cause ulcers to develop on the margins of the eyelids, loss of eyelashes, and flaky scales that can lead to conjunctivitis.

Etiology

Ulcerative blepharitis often results from a staphylococcal infection. Nonulcerative blepharitis can be caused by allergies or exposure to chemicals, dust, or smoke. It can also be secondary to **seborrhea** of the sebaceous glands of the eyelids or recurrent styes or chalazions.

Diagnosis

Blepharitis can be diagnosed via visual examination of the eyelids. If dried secretions are noted, the presence of staphylococci can be determined.

Treatment

Patients should be instructed to clean the eyes twice a day with warm compresses. If improvement is not seen within 2 weeks, antibiotic or sulfonamide **ophthalmic** ointments may be indicated.

Prognosis

Blepharitis can occasionally be resistant to treatment, leading to a chronic condition.

Blepharoptosis

Blepharoptosis is also known as *ptosis*. It is defined as a permanent drooping of the upper eyelid due to a weakness in its muscle (or by inadequate nerve stimulation to the muscle), causing the eyeball to be partially or totally covered. Medical attention should be sought quickly. There is no specific method of prevention.

Signs and Symptoms

Blepharoptosis usually only affects one eye and can be more severe at different times of the day. The condition can occur any time during life, is often genetically linked, and can completely obstruct vision of the affected eye.

Etiology

Blepharoptosis is caused by weakness either of the muscle that raises the eyelid or of the third cranial nerve (oculomotor nerve). It can also occur because of damage to the eyelid muscle or its controlling nerve. Other causes include diabetes mellitus, muscular dystrophy, brain tumor, and myasthenia gravis.

Diagnosis

Ophthalmic examination, blood tests, and imaging (such as computed tomography scan or magnetic resonance imaging) are used to determine the condition and to rule out any underlying diseases.

Treatment

Eyeglasses can be altered with a support that keeps the eyelid raised, or surgery can be used to improve function of the eye muscles.

Prognosis

Prognosis is good if any underlying disease is successfully treated.

Dry Eye

Dryness of the eye may be described as **xerosis**, which occurs because of a lack of tears or conjunctival secretions. Tears prevent the cornea from drying and becoming damaged and are composed of three layers: a superficial lipid layer, an aqueous layer, and a mucinous layer. The cornea requires these three layers to remain sufficiently lubricated and hydrated. The eyes must periodically blink to maintain this "tear surface" over the ocular surface.

The lacrimal glands may diminish in their secretion of tears because of aging or other conditions. This may lead to older adults experiencing irritated eyes after sleeping. Other conditions influencing tear production include congenital defects, infections, irradiation, glandular damage, and medications with antihistamine or anticholinergic actions. Contact lenses may decrease blinking, contributing to the condition. Dry eye may also be caused by *Sjögren's syndrome*, which is seen primarily in women near menopause or with rheumatoid arthritis.

Dry eye causes a gritty sensation, burning, itching, lack of tearing, photosensitivity, pain, redness, and difficulty in blinking. Dry eye may lead to keratinization of the cornea and conjunctival epithelium, corneal ulcerations, and scarring (which can cause blindness).

> **RED FLAG**
> To prevent dry eye artificial tear solutions are often used as well as topical preparations such as ointments.

Chalazion

A *chalazion* is a small, localized, painless swelling on the body or margin of an eyelid, occurring from occlusion of the *meibomian* glands. These glands are sebaceous glands (also known as *tarsal glands*) that supply meibum, an oily substance that prevents evaporation of the eye's tear film. A chalazion can be barely visible or as large as the size of a pea. It may become infected, causing pain, redness, and swelling. A chalazion is diagnosed by a brief visual examination. They usually disappear on their own within 1 to 2 months, although antibiotics may speed healing. Larger chalazions may require surgical removal. Prognosis is good with complete resolution of the condition.

Conjunctivitis

Conjunctivitis is inflammation of the conjunctiva (the mucous membrane that covers the anterior eyeball and also lines the eyelids.) Because it is highly contagious, this condition should be treated by a healthcare provider as soon as possible.

Signs and Symptoms

Conjunctivitis can be unilateral or bilateral. It is a very common condition. Symptoms include redness, itching, and swelling of the conjunctiva and sclera (**Figure 15–4**). Excessive tearing and light sensitivity may persist.

> **RED FLAG**
> Infectious conjunctivitis involves discharge of pus from the eye and is known as "pink eye," which is highly contagious. Therefore, the PTA should follow universal precautions to avoid cross-contamination.

Etiology

Conjunctivitis can be caused by bacterial or viral infection and by allergic or chemical irritation. Transmission of conjunctivitis easily occurs when contaminated fingers, towels, or washcloths come into contact with the eyes.

Diagnosis

Ophthalmic examination shows conjunctival inflammation, and samples of discharge from the eye identify the bacterial or viral origin of the infection.

Treatment

Treatment varies based on cause. Cool compresses should be applied to the eyes three to four per day for 10 to 15 minutes each time. If caused by bacteria, antibiotics are prescribed, either in the form of ophthalmic or systemic preparations. Treatment usually takes 1 to 2 weeks.

Prognosis

Conjunctivitis is usually not serious, and superficial cases have a good prognosis. However, it often recurs. The viral form of the infection is usually self-limiting.

Exophthalmos

Exophthalmos is an abnormal protrusion of the eyeballs (**Figure 15–5A and B**). A complete medical evaluation and ophthalmic examination should be undertaken as soon as possible to assess this condition. There is no known prevention. Patients with exophthalmos have what are termed "bulging" eyes. They may report dryness of the eyes or an abrasive gritty feeling. Additional signs include double vision, blurred vision, and restricted eye movement.

Causes of exophthalmos include enlarged extraocular muscles, edema of the soft tissue lining the eye orbits, **retrobulbar** masses, hyperthyroidism, hypothyroidism, or "euthyroid stare" (in which the thyroid is normal but the exophthalmic condition develops regardless). If exophthalmos occurs suddenly, it is usually because of hemorrhage or inflammation.

> **RED FLAG**
> Exophthalmos is diagnosed by complete ophthalmic examination as well as blood tests, computer tomography scan, echography, and radiographic studies.

Treatment is determined by the underlying condition(s). For example, hyperthyroidism must be treated before the exophthalmic condition can be reduced. For severe cases surgical decompression of the eye orbits may be required. Systemic steroids may be used to control edema. Prognosis depends on the success of treating the cause of this condition.

Ectropion

Ectropion is defined as the lower eyelid everting from the eyeball, leading to drying and irritation of the exposed eyeball and eyelid lining (**Figure 15–6**). Patients should seek prompt medical attention. When ectropion occurs, the conjunctival membrane becomes exposed. Tears run down the cheeks instead of into the tear ducts, and the patient reports eye dryness and tearing. This condition usually affects the elderly due to changes in muscles of the lower eyelid or because of a scar on the eyelid or cheek. It can be easily detected by visual examination. The condition is usually persistent and requires treatment via a minor surgical procedure. Eyedrops or ophthalmic ointment may be helpful. If untreated, it can

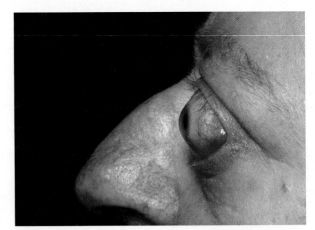

(A)

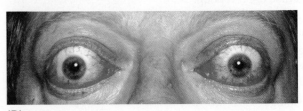

(B)

Figure 15–5 Exophthalmos.

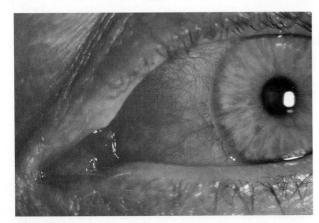

Figure 15–4 Conjunctivitis.

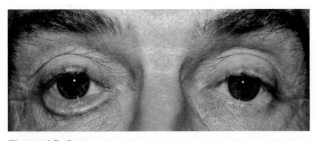

Figure 15–6 Ectropion.

cause development of corneal ulcers and permanent corneal damage.

Entropion

Entropion is defined as the turning inward of the eyelid margins, usually of the lower eyelid (**Figure 15–7**). This causes the eyelashes to rub against the conjunctiva. It can lead to vision problems because of corneal damage. The patient should seek care immediately. This condition causes the sensation of a foreign object in the eye, itching, redness, and tearing. Epithelial defects can lead to conjunctivitis or corneal ulcers. Entropion affects older adults because aging causes the lower eyelid tissues to loosen and the eyelid muscle to contract, turning the eyelids inward. Visual examination reveals inversion of the eyelid, lashes against the conjunctiva, and redness of the eyes due to irritation. Although entropion often resolves on its own, a minor surgical procedure can usually correct the inversion. Treatment usually brings complete relief.

Corneal Trauma

Corneal abrasions may be caused by trauma. Although most heal in a few days because of the epithelial layer's ability to regenerate without scarring, more significant damage slows healing and increases risk of infection. If scar formation occurs, the cornea may become opaque. Impaired light transmission and severely distorted vision occur because the refractive surface is compromised.

Damage to the epithelium or endothelium decreases hydration of the cornea, leading to edema and opacity. Contact lenses are a common cause when they are worn excessively. Corneal edema may also be caused by increased intraocular pressure, causing the cornea to appear dull, hazy, and uneven. It causes visual acuity to decrease and iridescent vision (rainbows seen around light sources) to occur.

Keratitis

Keratitis is any inflammation causing the cornea to be superficially ulcerated (**Figure 15–8**). The patient should see an ophthalmologist promptly. Patients wearing contact lenses should be taught proper lens care and use to reduce risk of infection.

Signs and Symptoms

Keratitis causes decreased visual acuity, irritation, **photophobia**, mild redness of the conjunctiva, and tearing. Another significant sign is pain or numbness of the cornea.

Etiology

Keratitis often follows a herpes simplex virus infection, usually when an upper respiratory tract infection occurs with facial cold sores. It can also be caused by certain bacterial or fungal infections. Additional causes include use of contact lenses, trauma to the cornea, and exposure (of the cornea) to dry air or intense light.

Diagnosis

Cultures may be taken to identify the cause. Examination of the cornea via a "slit lamp" confirms diagnosis of keratitis. Visual acuity decrease may signify the condition, as can a recent upper respiratory tract infection.

Treatment

Eyedrops, ophthalmic ointments, and broad-spectrum antibiotics are used to treat keratitis. If photophobia causes discomfort, an eye patch over the affected eye may be indicated. If fungal infection or contact lenses are the cause, an eye patch should not be used.

Prognosis

Keratitis should be treated promptly to decrease risk of ulceration that can potentially erode the cornea and cause scar tissue to form. Vision can be permanently altered by this condition.

Nystagmus

Nystagmus is an involuntary and constant movement of the eyes that is visible to others but may not be noticed by the affected patient. Nystagmus can affect one or both eyes, and

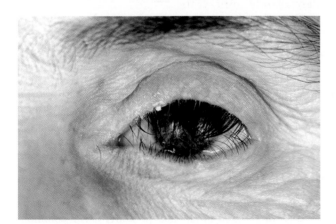

Figure 15–7 Entropion.

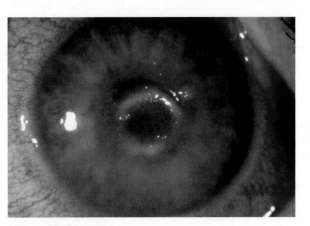

Figure 15–8 Keratitis.

the movements can be in any direction. The only sign is the actual constant movement of the eyes.

Nystagmus may be caused by brain tumors, alcohol abuse, congenital defects, head trauma, or various diseases such as Ménière's disease and multiple sclerosis. Treating the underlying cause is required to relieve the nystagmus condition. Prognosis is only good if the underlying cause is treatable.

> **RED FLAG**
> Congenital nystagmus is often permanent and untreatable.

Uveitis

Uveitis is the inflammation of the uveal tract, which includes the choroid, ciliary body, and iris. It is usually unilateral but may be bilateral. No method of prevention is known.

Signs and Symptoms
Uveitis usually causes pain, blurred vision, papillary constriction, redness, and potentially intense photophobia. Patients should have a complete ophthalmic examination as soon as possible.

Etiology
Uveitis can be related to autoimmune disorders, ankylosing spondylitis, rheumatoid arthritis, syphilis, toxoplasmosis, histoplasmosis, and tuberculosis. It can also be of unknown origin.

Diagnosis
Uveitis can be diagnosed with a simple slit lamp examination and confirmed by skin or blood tests for the causative infection.

Treatment
Each type of uveitis has its own specific treatment, usually consisting of topical agents and sometimes immunosuppressive system agents. The underlying cause should be treated. Inflammation may be reduced by steroids and cycloplegic agents.

Prognosis
Prognosis varies, depending on the type of uveitis and the underlying cause.

Refractive Errors

Refractive errors include astigmatism, hyperopia, myopia, and presbyopia. A perfectly shaped eyeball and cornea result in optimal visual acuity, producing a sharp image in focus at all points on the retinal surface in the posterior part of the eye. However, individual differences in the formation and growth of the eyeball and cornea often result in inappropriate focal image formation.

Astigmatism

Astigmatism is a description of light rays being irregularly focused. Astigmatism causes certain images to appear clear and others blurry. Eye fatigue is common, leading to squinting, headaches, and frequent rubbing of the eyes. Astigmatism is usually caused by the cornea not being spherically shaped. The front of the cornea may be more "egg shaped" instead of spherical. This causes light rays to be unevenly focused across the retina.

Astigmatism is diagnosed by patient eye health history, visual acuity tests, examination via an *ophthalmoscope*, and evaluation of the intensity of the visual deficit. The pupils are usually dilated with eyedrops and then evaluated for refractive error by using a *retinoscope*. The patient is then required to look through corrective lenses of different strengths until the optimal lens is found. All refractive errors may be corrected by use of eyeglasses or contact lenses, and most of them can be corrected by surgery. Laser surgery has replaced *radial keratotomy*, a procedure that reshaped the eye. Laser surgery has fewer complications and offers more precise visual correction. For astigmatism, laser surgery, photorefractive keratotomy, and permanent intraocular contact lenses can be used. Prognosis is good with correctly prescribed eyeglasses, contact lenses, or surgery.

Hyperopia

Hyperopia is also known as "farsightedness." It occurs when light entering the eye is focused behind, rather than on, the retina. This causes the lens to refocus. To counteract hyperopia an external corrective lens must be used to reposition the viewed object on the retina. In hyperopia, far or "distance" vision is usually normal and near vision is impaired. Eye fatigue is common. Hyperopia occurs when the eyeball is abnormally short from front to back (**Figure 15–9A, B, and C**). Prognosis is good with correctly prescribed glasses, contact lenses, or surgery.

Myopia

Myopia is also known as "nearsightedness." It occurs when light rays entering the eye are focused in front of the retina. This causes blurred vision. In myopia near vision is usually normal, whereas far (distance) vision is blurry. Also, the image being viewed cannot be sharpened by the eye's lens. Eye fatigue is also common in myopia. Myopia occurs when the eyeball is abnormally long from front to back (Figure 15–9).

Presbyopia

Presbyopia is also commonly referred to as "old eye." It is the inability of the lens of the eye to focus and refocus quickly enough to accommodate variations in distance. Eye fatigue is also common in presbyopia. Presbyopia manifests slowly, over years,

> **RED FLAG**
> Laser surgery cannot improve presbyopia.

involving farsightedness that progresses with age, difficulty focusing on reading and near objects, and having to hold objects further away to read them. It is sometimes called "age-related hyperopia" or "age-related farsightedness." Presbyopia is caused by a gradual loss of muscle elasticity in the eye, usually due to aging. It usually occurs when a person reaches (approximately) age 45. Diagnosis of presbyopia is similar to that of astigmatism above. For presbyopia, glasses or contact lenses may be used. Prognosis is good with correctly prescribed glasses or contact lenses.

Glaucoma

Glaucoma is defined as damage to the optic nerve, usually because of elevated intraocular pressure. It is a common, severe condition that often causes blindness. It occurs most

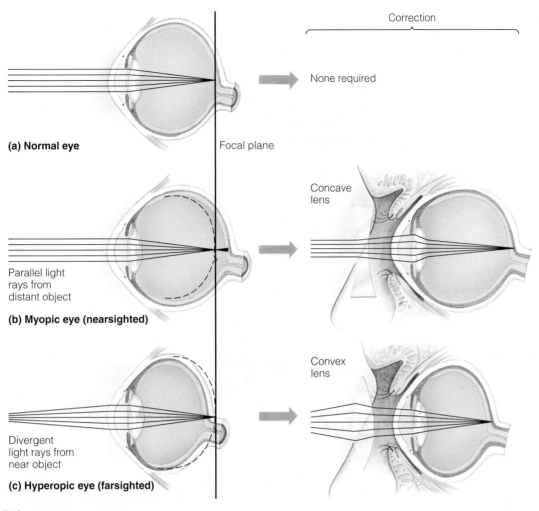

Correction

None required

(a) Normal eye   Focal plane

Concave lens

Parallel light rays from distant object

(b) Myopic eye (nearsighted)

Convex lens

Divergent light rays from near object

(c) Hyperopic eye (farsighted)

Figure 15–9 Common visual problems.

often in patients over age 60. Chronic open-angle and acute angle-closure (narrow- or closed-angle) glaucoma are common forms of the disease (**Figure 15–10**). Patients with the symptoms listed below should seek immediate medical attention. Regular ophthalmic examinations can reveal early signs of glaucoma.

Signs and Symptoms

Signs and symptoms include headache, visual changes, nausea, vomiting, photophobia, and eye pain. Chronic open-angle glaucoma is the most common form and is the most treatable cause of blindness. However, by the time serious symptoms have manifested, considerable damage has occurred. Untreated chronic open-angle glaucoma usually causes loss of peripheral (side) vision first, leading to total blindness. Acute angle-closure glaucoma usually causes blurred vision, headaches, severe pain, eye redness, photophobia, and the perception of "halos" around light sources. More advanced angle-closure glaucoma also causes nausea and vomiting and hazy corneas of the eyes. The intraocular pressure of this type of glaucoma is usually much higher than in open-angle glaucoma.

Etiology

Risk factors for glaucoma include age, family history, near-sightedness, and African-American descent. In chronic open-

angle glaucoma, aqueous humor reabsorption is blocked, leading to increased pressure in the eye. This form may be caused by trauma or overuse of topical steroids. Angle-closure glaucoma is caused by narrowing or complete closing of the drainage system of the eye.

Diagnosis

Patient history, **tonometric** examination of the eyes, optic nerve examination, and visual field analysis lead to diagnosis of glaucoma. Angle-closure glaucoma is diagnosed via a special lens (*goniolens*) that allows viewing of the opening of the draining system of the eye. Also, this type of glaucoma usually causes the eye to be red. The hazy cornea also aids in diagnosis.

Treatment

Early treatment is essential. Vision loss cannot be regained, so the disease must be halted before it can progress extensively. Medications include carbonic anhydrase inhibitors, beta-blockers, alpha-adrenergic agents, and prostaglandin analogues. Laser surgery can assist in opening the eye's drainage system or can bypass the drainage system. Open-angle glaucoma can be controlled with eyedrops. Angle-closure glaucoma is primarily treated with laser **iridotomy**, creating a small opening and allowing drainage in the eye. Additionally, medications that lower intraocular pressure may be prescribed.

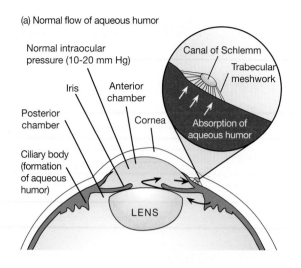

(a) Normal flow of aqueous humor

Normal intraocular pressure (10-20 mm Hg)

Canal of Schlemm

Trabecular meshwork

Iris

Anterior chamber

Posterior chamber

Cornea

Ciliary body (formation of aqueous humor)

Absorption of aqueous humor

LENS

(b) Chronic (open-angle) glaucoma

Degeneration and obstruction of trabecular meshwork and canal of Schlemm decreases absorption of aqueous humor

LENS

(c) Acute (narrow-or closed-angle) glaucoma

Iris in anterior position

Narrow iridoocorneal angle blocks drainage into canal of Schlemm

High intraocular pressure

LENS

Figure 15–10 Types of glaucoma.

Prognosis

Prognosis depends on the type of glaucoma, treating the condition early enough, and continued medical treatment.

Cataracts

A **cataract** is a cloudy or opaque area of the lens of the eye (**Figure 15–11**). They usually develop slowly. Cataracts are the most common cause of age-related visual loss in the world. There are two types: congenital and senile cataracts. A *congenital cataract* is one that is present at birth. A *senile cataract* develops as the patient ages and is the most common cause of age-related vision loss.

Signs and Symptoms

Cataracts cause progressively reduced visual acuity. Blurring and photosensitivity may occur. Advanced cataracts may be easy to see, causing the pupil to have a white, opaque appearance.

Etiology

Cataracts are usually caused by aging, which leads to deterioration of the lens of the eye. Other causes include genetics, trauma, injury from lightning, drug toxicities, diabetes mellitus, or other eye diseases. Cataracts are relatively common.

Diagnosis

Cataracts are often discovered during a routine ophthalmic examination. The eye is dilated and examined with an ophthalmoscope and adequate light.

Treatment

Treatment of cataracts is based on the severity of the condition and the patient's age and health status. There is no effective medical treatment for cataracts. Surgery is the only treatment for correcting cataract-related vision loss. Surgery usually involves lens extraction and intraocular lens implantation. **Phacoemulsification** is used to remove the cataract in most cases, because it requires the least amount of trauma to the eye. This involves the use of an ultrasonic device to emulsify the cataract and then remove it. After surgery the patient will need to have eyeglass prescriptions changed because of the clarity afforded without the cataract. Eye shields may be required during sleep after surgery, and medications may be given to reduce ocular pressure.

Prognosis

Prognosis is usually good, although cataracts can recur. Complications due to surgery are possible.

Diabetic Retinopathy

Diabetic **retinopathy** is a retinal blood vessel disorder (**Figure 15–12**). It usually occurs in both eyes, affecting vision clarity, and is a major cause of blindness. Diabetics should have regular eye examinations to prevent this condition from developing.

Signs and Symptoms

Diabetic retinopathy causes hemorrhages, microaneurysms, retinal vein dilation, and neovascularization (the formation of abnormal new blood vessels in the eyes).

Etiology

This condition usually occurs between 8 and 10 years after diagnosis of diabetes mellitus. It is more likely in diabetic patients who do not control their blood glucose levels. Diabetes commonly causes constriction and death of retinal blood vessels, leakage of blood into the retina, and permanent reduction of vision clarity. If neovascularization develops, vision is markedly reduced due to scar tissue forming on the retina.

Diagnosis

Diabetic retinopathy is diagnosed by a complete ophthalmoscopic examination.

Treatment

Laser **photocoagulation** is usually undertaken to control this condition. Although it may recur, treatment is usually effective. A vitrectomy (removal of some or all of the vitreous humor) may be indicated if there is vitreous hemorrhage or the retinopathy is proliferative.

Prognosis

Prognosis is guarded, although the condition is usually controlled with treatment.

Color Blindness

Color blindness is an abnormal condition characterized by an inability to distinguish colors of the spectrum clearly. In most cases it is not a "blindness" but a weakness in perceiving colors distinctly. There are two forms of color blindness. **Daltonism**, the more common form, is characterized by an inability to distinguish reds from greens. This is an inherited (sex-linked) disorder. Total color blindness (**achromatic vision**) is characterized by an inability to perceive any color at all. In these patients only white, gray, and black are seen. It may be the result of a defect in (or absence of) the cones in the retina. There is no treatment or cure for color blindness or color deficiency.

Macular Degeneration

Macular degeneration is a progressive deterioration of the macula of the retina. It is due to destructive changes of the yellow-pigmented area surrounding the central fovea. Age-related macular degeneration is the most common cause of reduced vision in the United States. It is the leading cause of blindness among people older than 75 years. Regular ophthalmic examinations can detect the condition early.

> **RED FLAG**
> Vitamin therapy and protecting the eyes from ultraviolet rays are helpful in reducing development of macular degeneration.

Signs and Symptoms

The macula lutea is part of the retina located near the optic nerve in the center of the field of vision. Early in the development of macular degeneration, central division may be slightly distorted. This condition develops slowly, usually painlessly, and does not affect peripheral vision. It usually affects both eyes, leading to eventual disappearance of central vision.

Etiology

The cause of age-related macular degeneration is poorly understood. In addition to older age, this condition mostly affects White women, cigarette smokers, and those with a low dietary

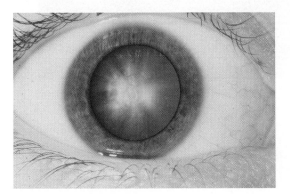

Figure 15–11 Cataracts.

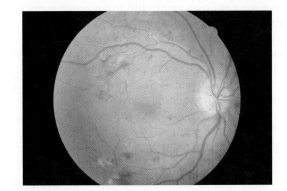

Figure 15–12 Retinopathy in a diabetic patient.

intake of **carotenoids**. There is increasing evidence suggesting that genetic factors may also cause this condition.

Diagnosis

Diagnosis of macular degeneration is made after reviewing patient history and performing an ophthalmoscopy and fluorescein angiography.

Treatment

There is no cure for macular degeneration. There has been recent interest in the effect of supplemental antioxidants (high doses of vitamin C, vitamin E, and beta-carotene) as well as zinc for persons at risk for developing macular degeneration. The FDA approved a drug called ranibizumab (Lucentis®) in 2006 to treat wet age-related macular degeneration. In 2010, the FDA approved implantable micro-sized telescopes to improve vision in patients with end-stage, age-related macular degeneration.

Prognosis

Success of treatment has been limited.

Retinal Detachment

Retinal detachment describes the elevation (separation) of the retina from the choroid in the eye (**Figure 15–13**). There is no specific method of prevention.

Signs and Symptoms

Retinal detachment is a separation of the retina from the retinal pigment epithelium in the back of the eye. Initial signs include the patient seeing light flashes and new "floaters," which are images that sometimes appear as "floating spots." This increases, and a dark shadow will be perceived from the peripheral vision, extending in toward the center vision. Detachment occurs suddenly, without any pain.

Etiology

Severe trauma to the eye, such as a contusion or penetrating wound, may cause retinal detachment. However, in the great majority of cases retinal detachment is the result of internal changes in the vitreous chamber because of aging. It sometimes occurs because of inflammation of the interior of the eye.

Diagnosis

Retinal detachment is easily revealed by an ophthalmoscopic examination.

Treatment

Treatment must occur early and involves either photocoagulation or surgery. Additional portions of the retina may be prevented from detaching if the condition is treated early enough. When the detached area is repositioned, most of its original function returns. Once detachment has reached the macula (the central retina), a certain amount of permanent reduction in central acuity will most likely occur. If the retina is torn but not detached, photocoagulation or **cryotherapy** is effective. Photocoagulation seals retinal tears before detachment occurs—again, requiring very early treatment.

Prognosis

Untreated retinal detachment leads to irreversible blindness.

Strabismus

Strabismus describes the eyes' inability to look in the same direction at the same time. It is usually due to weakness in the nerves that stimulate the muscles that control eye position (**Figure 15–14**). When strabismus develops in adulthood, it usually results in **diplopia**. The adult usually complains of a change in visual perception, usually double vision. If it is of congenital origin, diplopia is usually not present. There is no known prevention for strabismus.

Signs and Symptoms

Strabismus is easily identified by how the eyes appear. There are two forms: esotropia (cross-eye or strabismus), with both eyes turning inward, and exotropia (wall-eye or divergent strabismus), with both eyes turning outward.

Etiology

The esotropic form of strabismus usually develops in infancy or early childhood, possibly related to **amblyopia** that is reversible until about age 8, when the retina becomes fully developed. In adults esotropia usually develops because of another disease or condition, often related to the nerves between the brain and eye muscles. Causative conditions include diabetes mellitus, muscular dystrophy, hypertension, temporal arteritis, aneurysm, intracranial lesion, or trauma.

Diagnosis

A complete ophthalmic examination followed by radiographic studies, and blood and urine tests, usually reveals the underlying cause.

Treatment

Strabismus treatment is more effective earlier in the condition's development. Glasses, treatment of amblyopia, or eye muscle surgery may be indicated.

Prognosis

Children usually respond well to early treatment. Depending on the underlying cause, adults with acquired strabismus have a guarded prognosis.

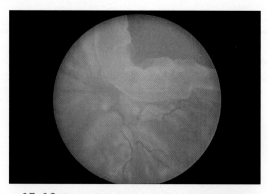

Figure 15–13 Separation of the retina from the choroid layer.

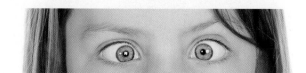

Figure 15–14 Strabismus.

Anatomy and Physiology of the Ear

The ear is responsible for both hearing and equilibrium and is divided into the external (outer), middle, and inner ear. Structures of the external ear include the pinna (auricle) and external auditory canal. The pinna is made up of mostly cartilaginous tissue and smaller amounts of adipose tissue in the earlobes. The 1-inch-long external auditory canal contains glands that produce hair and cerumen. The **tympanic membrane** (eardrum) separates the external and middle ear.

The tympanic cavity (middle ear) contains three tiny bones: the malleus (hammer), incus (anvil), and stapes (stirrup). An *oval window* near the stapes leads to the inner ear, which is the most complex portion of the ear. Equilibrium is controlled in this portion, whereas hearing involves all three portions. Inside its fluid-filled space there is a vestibule, semicircular canals, round window, and cochlea. The semicircular canals assist the body to adjust to position changes, and the contained fluid can cause dizziness when it moves abruptly. The organ of hearing is the *cochlea* (**Figure 15–15A and B**).

Sound waves are picked up by the pinna and sent through the external auditory canal to the tympanic membrane. This membrane vibrates and conducts the vibrations through the middle ear bones, oval window, and cochlear fluid. Receptor

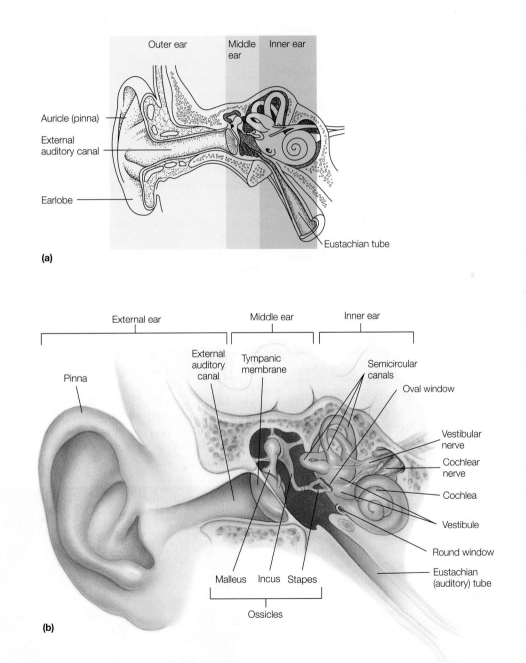

Figure 15–15 The Structures of the ear. (A) Cross section showing the structures of the outer, middle, and inner ears. (B) The receptors for balance and sound are located in the inner ear.

cells convert these vibrations into electrical impulses and transmit them to the brain. In the brain auditory impulses are received in the temporal lobe by the auditory nerve.

Disorders of the Ear

Common disorders of the ear include infections, other diseases, trauma, and conditions that can cause partial or total hearing loss.

Impacted Cerumen

Cerumen is the soft, yellow-brown secretion of the external ear (known as "ear wax"). If it becomes impacted, it is a common cause of hearing loss. Impacted cerumen causes tinnitus, temporary deafness, and itching. An abnormal amount of cerumen may collect in the ear due to excessive hair in the ear, a narrow ear canal, or skin dryness. Another cause is excessive dust buildup in the canal, often due to jobs where dust is prevalent.

Impacted cerumen is confirmed by an otologic examination. Excess cerumen is normally removed during bathing and shampooing the hair. If impacted, cerumen may be removed by using ear irrigations, although the condition often recurs in affected individuals. Prognosis is good as long as the ears are kept clean and/or up to three drops of mineral oil are instilled into the affected ear once a week. The mineral oil should be kept inside for up to 4 minutes and then rinsed out with warm water.

Otitis Externa

Otitis externa is also called "swimmer's ear" or "external otitis" and is the inflammation of the external ear canal. Symptoms include fever, an inflamed and painful ear canal, pruritus (itching), and hearing loss. It may also involve drainage of pus. Commonly affecting people who swim on a regular basis, otitis externa may be caused by ear trauma, by swimming in contaminated water, and by bacterial or fungal infections. Headphone use may encourage microbial growth within the ear as well.

An otologic examination is used to diagnose this condition, and suspected ear infection may require a culture or sensitivity test. Treatment for otitis externa includes analgesics for pain, antibiotics for infection, and keeping the ear canal clean and dry. Prognosis is good as long as the condition is treated promptly.

Mastoiditis

Mastoiditis is the inflammation of the mastoid bone or process. This porous bone is located behind the ear, and the condition often affects children after a middle-ear infection. It is now less common and rarely becomes dangerous. Symptoms include otalgia, tinnitus, fever, and headache. There may also be painful swelling of the mastoid as well as ear drainage. Acute mastoiditis is often the result of a middle-ear infection of *streptococcal* origin.

Diagnosis of mastoiditis is based on examination and otoscopy, mastoid x-ray, bacterial cultures, and computed tomography scan. Mastoiditis is treated with antibiotics. If severe, surgery (a *mastoidectomy*) may be required to remove any infected portions of the mastoid bone. Prognosis is good in general with antibiotic treatment. Most cases do not require mastoidectomy.

Otitis Media

Otitis media is the inflammation in the middle ear. It is common in younger patients and actually may or may not be an infection. The middle ear, normally filled with air, may become filled with serous or suppurative fluid, causing inflammation.

Signs and Symptoms

Symptoms of serous fluid causing otitis media are usually mild, including conductive hearing loss and a feeling of fullness in the ear. Symptoms of suppurative fluid causing otitis media include **otalgia**, nausea, vomiting, fever, chills, **vertigo**, and conductive hearing loss.

> **RED FLAG**
> Children usually outgrow otitis media as their eustachian tubes lengthen and become more vertical due to aging.

Etiology

When serous fluid fills the middle ear, it is clear in appearance and may be caused by allergies, tube obstruction, or a change in middle-ear pressure. In this form there is no infection. **Suppurative** fluid is pus caused by a bacterial infection, usually coming from the eustachian tube because of an upper respiratory tract infection. Forceful blowing of the nose during this condition should be avoided because it can push bacteria up into the middle ear. Another cause is swimming in contaminated water.

Diagnosis

Otitis media is diagnosed via otoscopy that reveals a bulging tympanic membrane. The membrane appears red and swollen, and, if ruptured, the fluid may be cultured for testing. Elevated white blood cells counts signify infection.

Treatment

Both types of otitis media are treated with analgesics to control pain and decongestants, which are designed to help drain the ear(s). Suppurative otitis media requires antibiotics. If chronic, a *myringotomy* may be performed to surgically remove fluid and prevent further infections. Also, a *tympanostomy* can help remove fluid and relieve ear pressure (**Figure 15–16**). This is commonly done in children, wherein pediatric ear tubes are inserted through the tympanic membrane via a procedure called *tympanoplasty*. The tubes usually fall out by themselves or are removed within 6 months to a year.

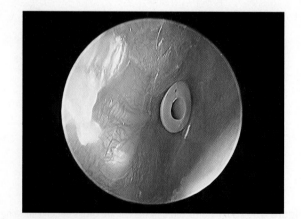

Figure 15–16 Tympanostomy tubes.

Prognosis

Prognosis of both types of otitis media is good with prompt treatment. However, if untreated, chronic otitis media can lead to severe ear damage and irreversible hearing loss.

Otosclerosis

Otosclerosis is defined as the regular ossification that occurs in the ossicles of the middle ear, especially of the stapes, causing hearing loss. This prevents vibrations from being conducted to the inner ear, resulting in conductive hearing loss. It is more common in females (between ages 11 and 30) than males. It may worsen during pregnancy. Otosclerosis is of unknown origin but may be related to genetics.

Diagnosis is made via physical examination, otoscopy, and audiogram (which charts a patient's range of hearing). Otosclerosis may require a procedure called a *stapedectomy*, involving the removal of the stapes bone of the middle ear. The bone is then replaced with an artificial (prosthetic) bone. Hearing is often improved very soon after the procedure. Other treatments include the use of hearing aids. Prognosis is based on success of hearing aids or stapedectomy.

Tinnitus

Tinnitus is the perception of abnormal noises that are not produced by an external stimulus. Although often described as a "ringing in the ears," it may also assume a "buzzing" sound. Tinnitus may be constant or intermittent and unilateral or bilateral. Nearly 37 million people in the United States are estimated to have tinnitus.

> **RED FLAG**
> Tinnitus affects both males and females nearly equally and is most prevalent between ages 40 and 70, although it sometimes affects children.

Tinnitus is usually caused by vascular abnormalities or neuromuscular disorders, with impacted cerumen, medications (such as aspirin), and stimulants (such as nicotine or caffeine) also being causative. Because tinnitus is actually a symptom, the diagnosis of the causative condition relies on the onset, frequency, description, and location of the tinnitus. Treatment is focused on decreasing the symptoms rather than attempting a cure. It includes elimination of causative medications and stimulants as well as cheese, red wine, and the food additive *monosodium glutamate*.

Motion Sickness

Motion sickness describes nausea that is attributed to changes in body position, often related to traveling in cars, airplanes, or boats. It may also be caused by watching large motion picture screens with quick and varied movements shown in a projected film. Motion sickness is signified by nausea, vomiting, diaphoresis, and vertigo. It usually subsides once the motions stop. Motion sickness is caused by abnormal movement of the organs of balance (the semicircular canals) inside the inner ear.

Motion sickness is diagnosed by history and description of symptoms and when they occur. Motion sickness is treated with antihistamines, which calm inner ear stimulation. Nonmedical treatment involves lying down and closing the eyes until symptoms stop. Other techniques include avoiding heavy meals before traveling, avoiding reading while traveling, and avoiding temperature extremes while traveling. Prognosis is good with antihistamine treatment.

Hearing Loss

Hearing loss ranges from mild to severe, culminating in total loss of hearing, otherwise known as *deafness*. The most common form of hearing loss is *sensorineural deafness*, which is due to cochlea or auditory nerve damage. Reducing exposure to loud noises is recommended to keep risk factors for deafness to a minimum. *Presbycusis* is progressive hearing loss due to aging.

Signs and Symptoms

Although congenital hearing loss may produce no obvious signs of hearing impairment at birth, a deficient response to auditory stimuli usually becomes apparent within 2 to 3 days after birth. Gradual loss of hearing is the primary symptom of sensorineural deafness.

> **RED FLAG**
> Presbycusis usually begins after age 50, beginning with higher frequencies being lost first. Conversations become difficult to hear if there is background noise.

Etiology

Deafness may be inherited or acquired (which is more common). Congenital hearing loss may be transmitted as a genetic disorder or as a result of trauma, toxicity, or infection during pregnancy or delivery. Acquired causes include stroke, tumors, infections, certain medications, diseases, and trauma. Exposure to loud noise is the most common type of trauma that causes deafness. Often, this is related to occupational exposure. Playing music loudly is also a common cause. Presbycusis is caused by degenerative changes in the structures of the ear because of aging.

Diagnosis

Diagnosis of sensorineural deafness is based on audiometric testing. Presbycusis is diagnosed after physical examination and medical history are completed to rule out other causes and is confirmed by audiogram.

Treatment

Sensorineural deafness due to auditory nerve or cochlear damage is often permanent. If treatable, the only choices are hearing aids or cochlear implants. Hearing aids consist of devices that fit into the external ear and increase volume to the internal ear. Cochlear implants are implanted behind the ear to directly stimulate the auditory nerve fibers, increasing hearing. For presbycusis hearing aids may help, but they usually become less effective with increased aging.

Prognosis

Prognosis is based completely on the amount of damage.

Vertigo

Vertigo is described as an illusion of motion and is a disorder of vestibular function of the ears. The patient may sense the environment moving around himself or herself (objective vertigo) or that the environment is stationary while he or she is moving (subjective vertigo). It may also manifest as a spinning, falling, or "to-and-fro" sensation. Vertigo is different from faintness, lightheadedness, syncope, or unsteadiness.

Vertigo or dizziness may be caused by either central or peripheral vestibular disorders. Most cases of vertigo are caused by a peripheral vestibular disorder, which are often severe in intensity but may be brief or episodic in duration. The cases caused by central vestibular disorders are usually mild and constant and chronic in duration.

Ménière's Disease

Ménière's disease most often affects people between ages 40 and 60. This condition affects the inner ear, with symptoms that include **tinnitus**, progressive hearing loss, a feeling of "fullness" in the ear, and vertigo. Acute attacks can last from a few hours to a few days. Additional symptoms may include nausea, vomiting, and diaphoresis. Ménière's disease is of unknown origin but may be related to family history, immune disorders, migraine headaches, middle-ear infections, head trauma, and **premenstrual edema**.

Diagnosis is based on detailed patient history, and examination by an otolaryngologist or neurologist may be required. Tests may include magnetic resonance imaging, electroencephalogram, and hearing tests such as **electronystagmography** (which records involuntary eye movements) or transymptomatic **electrocholeography** (which measures excess fluid accumulation in the inner ear). Treatment for acute attacks of Ménière's disease includes diuretics, a low-salt diet, antihistamines, and cessation of smoking. If the disease does not respond to treatment, surgery may be used to correct the inner ear problems; however, surgery is dangerous because of the potential of causing permanent deafness. Prognosis is uncertain and is completely based on the success of treatments.

SUMMARY

The eyes and ears, as well as the other sensory organs, are important for enjoying life. If conditions that affect the sensory organs are diagnosed and treated early enough, they often can be corrected. Disease states such as diabetes can cause a variety of sensory problems. The most common eye disorders are myopia, hyperopia, presbyopia, cataracts, diabetic retinopathy, and glaucoma. The most common ear disorders are otitis media, tinnitus, conductive hearing loss, otosclerosis, and Ménière's disease. The body naturally loses the ability to see and hear as well as it could in earlier life as the aging process continues.

REVIEW QUESTIONS

Select the best response to each question.

1. Rapid movement of the eyeball is known as which of the following?
   a. nystagmus
   b. hordeolum
   c. hyperopia
   d. presbyopia
2. Which part of the ear detects motion and controls balance?
   a. tympanic membrane
   b. semicircular canal
   c. auditory ossicles
   d. cochlea
3. When the eyeball is abnormally short, it is described as which of the following conditions?
   a. strabismus
   b. presbyopia
   c. myopia
   d. hyperopia
4. Which of the following conditions may result in elevated pressure of the eye and eventual blindness?
   a. cataract
   b. uveitis
   c. glaucoma
   d. myxedema
5. Which of the following is not a part of the ear?
   a. incus
   b. iris
   c. stapes
   d. auricle
6. A progressive hearing loss due to aging is known as which of the following conditions?
   a. presbyopia
   b. tinnitus
   c. amblyopia
   d. presbycusis
7. Which of the following is a symptom of mastoiditis?
   a. tinnitus
   b. otosclerosis
   c. headache
   d. ear drainage
8. Which of the following is the cause of Ménière's disease?
   a. cause unknown
   b. smoking
   c. a low-salt diet
   d. low blood cholesterol
9. An irregular ossification that occurs in the bones of the middle ear is known as which of the following conditions?
   a. impacted cerumen
   b. mastoiditis
   c. otosclerosis
   d. tinnitus
10. Motion sickness is caused by which of the following?
    a. an unknown cause
    b. abnormal movement of the organ of balance inside the inner ear
    c. progressive hearing loss and fullness in the inner ear
    d. an abnormal amount of cerumen that may collect in the ear due to excessive hair

CASE STUDIES

Karen Coupe, PT, DPT, MSEd

Case 1

A 75-year-old woman suffers from cerebellar degeneration of unknown cause and was referred to outpatient physical therapy for strengthening, balance, and coordination activities. Patient medical history: Osteoporosis, dry macular degeneration. Prior level of function: Due to macular degeneration patient no longer drives and needs assistance cooking and cleaning. She has recently been losing her balance getting in and out of a chair, walking in her home, is having a great deal of difficulty going up and down the stairs in her house, and finds the task of getting dressed very difficult.

1. What are the functions of the cerebellum? What are some clinical manifestations of a patient with cerebellar degeneration?

2. Relate the cerebellar degeneration to the patient's current issues.

3. Explain macular degeneration. Is there a cure? Will it progress?

4. Stand up, get your balance, and close your eyes for 30 seconds. How did you feel? Still standing, stand on one leg with your eyes open for 30 seconds. Now do the same but close your eyes for 30 seconds. How did you feel? Which was harder? Why?

5. What are the implications for this patient's balance considering she is losing her cerebellar functions and her eyesight? For what does this put her at risk?

Case 2

A 55-year-old woman is attending outpatient physical therapy secondary to a right total knee replacement 2 weeks ago. Patient medical history: Osteoarthritis bilateral knees, type 2 diabetes, bilateral lower extremity peripheral vascular disease, diabetic retinopathy, and Ménière's disease. Previous level of function: Independent in all activities, ambulated with a straight cane. Current level of function: Ambulates with walker w/min x 1 secondary to loss of balance during any turning activities. Plan of care includes right knee range of motion, strengthening, gait training, balance training.

1. Explain diabetic retinopathy. What are the potential effects of this on the plan of care?

2. Many patients have vision issues. What type of educational material could the PTA give to any patient with vision issues to assist in the prevention of falls?

3. During treatment the patient suddenly complains of nausea, dizziness, and the sensation that everything around her is spinning. How should the PTA react to this situation?

4. Looking at the patient's medical history, what could be the potential cause of the above scenario in question 3? Explain the clinical manifestations of your answer.

5. Many patients present with ear problems. Explain the role of the ear in balance. What if the patient's primary issue was difficulty hearing or the loss of hearing? What are some things the PTA could do during treatment to ensure appropriate communication with the patient?

WEBSITES

http://webschoolsolutions.com/patts/systems/ear.htm

http://www.allaboutvision.com/resources/anatomy.htm

http://www.audiologyawareness.com/hearinfo_howhear.asp

http://www.hearingaidscentral.com/howtheearworks.asp

http://www.merck.com/pubs/mmanual_ha/sec1/ch02/ch02c.html

http://www.nia.nih.gov/healthinformation/publications/eyes.htm

http://www.preventblindness.org/vlc/how_we_see.htm

http://www.tedmontgomery.com/the_eye/index.html

Musculoskeletal Disorders

LEARNING OBJECTIVES

After completion of this chapter the reader should be able to

1. List and describe the function of various types of bone cells.
2. Describe osteoporosis and its predisposing factors.
3. Describe common bone tumors.
4. Compare and contrast osteoarthritis and rheumatoid arthritis.
5. Explain factors affecting bone formation and metabolism.
6. Explain the etiology and common signs of gout.
7. Describe risk factors for osteoporosis.
8. Describe muscular atrophy and myasthenia gravis.

KEY TERMS

Achondroplasia: A genetic condition that results in abnormally short stature.

Adhesions: Union of two opposing tissue surfaces, as in the sides of a wound.

Annulus: A ring-like structure or part.

Arthritis: Inflammation of one or more joints.

Articular: Related to joints (articulations).

Avulsion fracture: One in which part of the bone is torn away.

Bone mass density: A measure of the amount of bone tissue in a certain volume of bone.

Bunion: A structural anomaly of the bones and joint between the foot and big toe.

Bursitis: Inflammation of the bursa, which are small fluid-filled pads that act as cushions among bones, joints, muscles, and tendons.

Carpal tunnel syndrome: A painful condition in which the medial nerve becomes pressed or squeezed at the wrist.

Cartilage: Stiff, semi-inflexible connective tissue found throughout the body.

Closed fracture: A broken bone underneath intact skin.

Comminuted fracture: A broken bone that is splintered or crushed into a number of pieces.

Complete fracture: One involving the entire cross-section of a bone.

Compound fractures: Those in which the bone or bones stick through the skin; it is also known as an "open fracture."

Compression: Pressing together.

Compression fracture: A fracture caused by pressing together, often seen in vertebral fractures due to osteoporosis.

Computed tomography: An x-ray procedure that combines many images via computer to generate cross-sectional or three-dimensional views.

Debridement: The act of removing dead, contaminated, or adherent tissue or foreign material.

Diskectomy: Surgery to remove part or all of a spinal disk.

Dislocation: A separation of two bones where they meet at a joint.

Displaced fracture: A fracture in which the two ends of a broken bone are separated from each other.

Dowager's hump: An abnormal curvature of the spine that appears as a rounded hump in the upper back.

KEY TERMS CONTINUED

Dual-energy x-ray absorptiometry: A means of measuring bone mineral density via two x-ray beams with different energy levels.

Electromyography: A technique for evaluating and recording the physiologic properties of muscles while they alternately contract and rest.

Fracture: A separation of a bone into two or more pieces; a fracture may be partial or complete.

Gout: Metabolic arthritis; a disease caused by a buildup of uric acid.

Greenstick fracture: A broken bone that is common in children, wherein the break is incomplete and usually healed easily; it is especially common in children with rickets.

Impacted fracture: A broken bone in which one broken end is wedged into the other broken end.

Incomplete fracture: A fracture that does not extend through the full transverse width of a bone.

Interphalangeal: Between the phalanges (fingers or toes).

Joints: Articulations; connections that allow motion between two bones.

Kyphosis: Hunchback; an abnormal backward curvature of the spine, resulting in a "humped" appearance of the upper back.

Laminectomy: Surgical removal of the posterior arch of a vertebra.

Ligaments: Sheets or bands of tough, fibrous tissue connecting bones or cartilages at a joint or supporting an organ.

Longitudinal fracture: A fracture that follows the long axis of a bone.

Lordosis: An abnormal forward curvature of the spine in the lumbar region; also known as "saddle back" or "hollow back."

Magnetic resonance imaging: A method of viewing the internal body structures by combining magnets with powerful pulses of radio waves; MRI offers fewer health risks than other techniques.

Metacarpophalangeal: Relating to the bones and joints of the hand.

Metatarsophalangeal: Relating to the bones and joints of the foot.

Muscular dystrophy: A group of inherited disorders in which strength and muscle bulk gradually decline.

Nondisplaced: Not displaced; this type of fracture means the bone is cracked but its pieces are still in normal alignment.

Oblique fracture: A break that occurs at an angle across the bone; usually the result of a sharp, angled blow.

Open fractures: Those that involve the bone protruding through the skin (see compound fractures).

Osteoarthritis: Degenerative arthritis; the type caused by the breakdown and eventual loss of the cartilage of one or more joints.

Osteomalacia: Softening of the bones, usually due to demineralization.

Osteomyelitis: An infection of the bones caused primarily by bacteria.

Osteoporosis: A decrease in bone density and strength that commonly results in fractures.

Pathologic: Related to or caused by disease.

Radiologic: Related to radiology, the branch of medicine that uses radiation for the diagnosis and treatment of disease.

Rheumatism: An older term used to describe a variety of painful conditions affecting the muscles, bones, joints, and tendons. Examples of rheumatic conditions include bursitis and tendinitis.

Rheumatoid arthritis: An autoimmune disease that causes chronic inflammation of the joints.

Scoliosis: An abnormal curvature of the spine to the left or right, causing a twisting of the vertebrae.

Simple fracture: An uncomplicated closed fracture (the bones do not pierce the skin).

Spasms: Painful, involuntary muscle contractions.

Spinal orthosis: Orthopedic appliances or apparatuses used to support, align, prevent, or correct spinal deformities or to improve functioning.

Spiral fracture: A torsion fracture, in which the bone has been twisted apart.

Spondylolisthesis: The anterior displacement of a vertebra or the vertebral column in relation to the vertebrae below.

Sprain: Injury to a ligament or ligaments caused by stretching beyond normal capacity or tearing.

Stellate fracture: A bone fracture in which the lines of the break radiate from a point into numerous fissures.

Strain: An injury caused by overuse or overexertion, commonly called a "wrench" of a body structure.

Stress fractures: Those caused by prolonged, repeated, or abnormal stress to bones.

Striations: Stripes or streaks of different colored tissue.

Subluxation: An incomplete or partial dislocation.

Temporomandibular joint syndrome: An incorrect alignment of the lower jaw to the skull that causes pain, nausea, and many other symptoms.

Tendinitis: Inflammation of a tendon or tendons.

Tendons: Fibrous cords of connective tissue that attach muscles to bones or cartilage.

Tennis elbow: Inflammation of the elbow structures caused by repeated, forceful contractions of the wrist muscles of the outer forearm.

Tetany: An abnormal condition of painful muscle cramps, spasms, and numbness.

Tophi: Deposits of sodium urate that develop in fibrous tissue around joints; commonly seen in gout.

Transverse fracture: A fracture that occurs at right angles to the longitudinal axis of a bone.

Overview

The body's structure and movements are provided by the musculoskeletal system. When this system experiences disease conditions, it can affect other body systems. Likewise, diseases of other body systems may affect the musculoskeletal system. The musculoskeletal system is made up of the bones, joints, ligaments, muscles, and **tendons**. Each component interacts with the others to provide mobility and support. Musculoskeletal disorders affect movement and therefore a person's independence and ability to function normally throughout life.

Anatomy and Physiology of the Musculoskeletal System

The *bones* are the body's framework. They serve many other functions: producing blood cells, protecting soft tissues, helping to create body motion, and storing fat and minerals (such as calcium, magnesium, phosphorus, and sodium). Blood circulates through vascular channels in bones. Cells in bones are as follows:

- Osteoblasts: Bone-building cells responsible for the formation of the bone matrix
- Osteoclasts: Bone cells responsible for resorption of bone, removing the mineral content and organic matrix
- Osteocytes: Mature bone cells actively involved in maintaining the bone matrix

Bones are classified by shape (long, short, flat, irregular, etc.) and composition (cortical or cancellous). An example of long bones is the femur of the leg (**Figure 16–1**), of short bones is the finger (metacarpal) bones, of flat bones the skull, and of irregular bones the spinal vertebrae. **Figure 16–2** shows the human skeleton.

Bones are covered by a membrane called the *periosteum*. The *endosteum* is the membrane lining the marrow cavities. It is made up of mostly osteogenic cells. These cells contribute to the growth and remodeling of bone and are required for bone repair.

Several factors are involved in bone formation and mineral metabolism. Calcitonin, parathyroid hormone, calcium, and vitamin D are essential for these processes. Other hormones that influence bone formation (directly or indirectly) include cortisol, growth hormone, sex hormones, and thyroid hormone.

Regarding bone composition, cortical bone is compact, dense, and smooth. Cancellous bone is spongy and contains many open spaces. Bones are connected to other bones and to **joints** (articulations) by fibrous connective tissue **ligaments**.

Bones repair themselves when they are damaged in the following steps:

- Bleeding, clotting, and granulation tissue formation at the site of injury
- Cell proliferation and callus (soft bony deposit) formation over the injury or **fracture**
- Osteoblast bone formation or **cartilage** formation at the site
- Hardening (calcification) of bone at the site via inorganic salt deposits

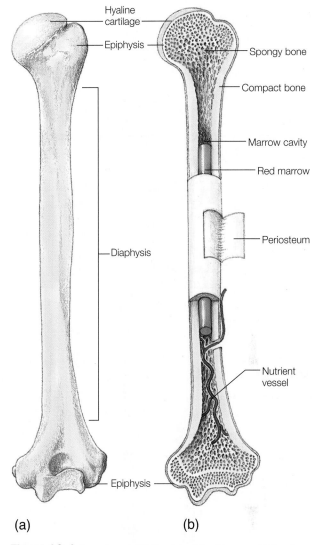

(a)   (b)

Figure 16–1 Long bones. (A) Drawing of the humerus. Notice the long shaft and dilated ends. (B) Longitudinal section of the humerus showing compact bone, spongy bone, and marrow.

- Bone remodeling to assume a required shape to resume function

Joints are areas where two or more bones meet. They are often classified according to the amount of movement they allow (**Table 16–1**). Joints are also classified by structure, as in these examples:

- Cartilaginous: Vertebrae joints, joined by cartilage
- Fibrous: Skull joints, joined by dense irregular connective tissue that is rich in collagen fibers
- Synovial: Knee joints, not directly joined, having a synovial cavity; they are united by dense irregular connective tissue that forms an **articular** capsule normally associated with accessory ligaments

Synovial joints are separated by a fluid-filled cavity. The seven types of synovial joints are as follows:

1. Gliding or plantar, such as the carpals of the wrist
2. Hinge, such as the elbow joint
3. Pivot, such as the atlantoaxial joint, near the atlas bone in the spine

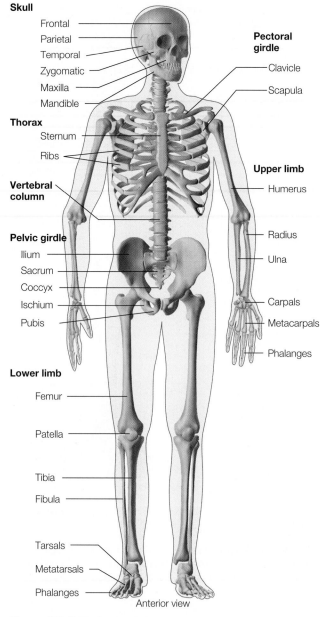

Skull
- Frontal
- Parietal
- Temporal
- Zygomatic
- Maxilla
- Mandible

Thorax
- Sternum
- Ribs

Vertebral column

Pelvic girdle
- Ilium
- Sacrum
- Coccyx
- Ischium
- Pubis

Lower limb
- Femur
- Patella
- Tibia
- Fibula
- Tarsals
- Metatarsals
- Phalanges

Pectoral girdle
- Clavicle
- Scapula

Upper limb
- Humerus
- Radius
- Ulna
- Carpals
- Metacarpals
- Phalanges

Anterior view

Figure 16–2 The human skeleton.

4. Condyloid or ellipsoidal, such as the radiocarpal joint of the wrist
5. Saddle, such as the carpometacarpal joint of the thumb
6. Ball and socket ("universal"), such as the shoulder and hip joints
7. Compound, such as the knee joints

Joint movements most commonly involve the following:

■ Extension: Increasing of a joint angle, such as the extension of the elbow when the hand is brought away from the shoulder

■ Flexion: Decreasing of a joint angle, such as the flexion of the elbow when the hand is brought closer to the shoulder

■ Abduction: Moving away from the body, such as raising the arm so the hand moves away from the side of the body and extends horizontally

■ Adduction: Moving toward the body, such as lowering the arm so the hand moves toward the side of the body from a horizontally raised position

■ Rotation: Turning of a bone on its own axis, such as spinning of a limb either away from the body or toward the midline of the body

■ Circumduction: Moving a limb in a circular fashion; true circumduction can only occur at a ball-and-socket joint, such as the hip or shoulder; this movement pattern combines flexion, extension, abduction, and adduction

■ Elevation: Moving in a superior direction; such as "shrugging the shoulders," which moves them upward; elevation is the anatomic opposite of "depression," which is moving inferiorly or downward

Cartilage supports bones that adjoin each other (known as "articulating bones"). It is made of collagenous tissue and provides cushioning and protection. Cartilage keeps bones from rubbing against each other. It prevents friction by absorbing shock from movement and pressure, reducing stress to the surface of bones. There are three major types of cartilage:

1. Elastic (yellow): Present in the outer ear and epiglottis; its principle protein is *elastin*.
2. Hyaline (blue): Thinly covers the articulating ends of bones, connecting the ribs to the sternum; it supports the nose, trachea, and part of the larynx. It is very elastic and contains no nerves or blood vessels.
3. Fibrocartilage (white): Present in the pubic symphysis, intervertebral disks, meniscus, and temporomandibular joints; it is a mixture of white fibrous tissue and cartilaginous tissue.

The muscles of the body have a variety of functions, such as the provision of movement and structure and producing body heat. **Figure 16–3** shows the major skeletal muscles of the body.

Skeletal muscles appear to have stripes or bands when viewed under a microscope. These marks are called **striations**. Skeletal muscles are also called voluntary muscles. They can be moved by conscious control, whereas other muscles (such as cardiac muscle) cannot. The central nervous system sends signals to skeletal muscles in order for them to move. Muscle fibers are held together by connective tissue.

TABLE 16–1	**Joint Classification by Amount of Movement**	
Joint	**Amount of Movement**	**Classification**
Skull sutures	Little or no movement	Synarthrosis, usually involving fibrous joints
Pelvis or vertebrae	Slight movement	Amphiarthrosis, usually involving cartilaginous joints
Elbow, hip, knee, shoulder, etc.	Varieties of movements	Diarthrosis, always involving synovial joints; subclassifications of diarthrodial joints include nonaxial, uniaxial, biaxial, and triaxial

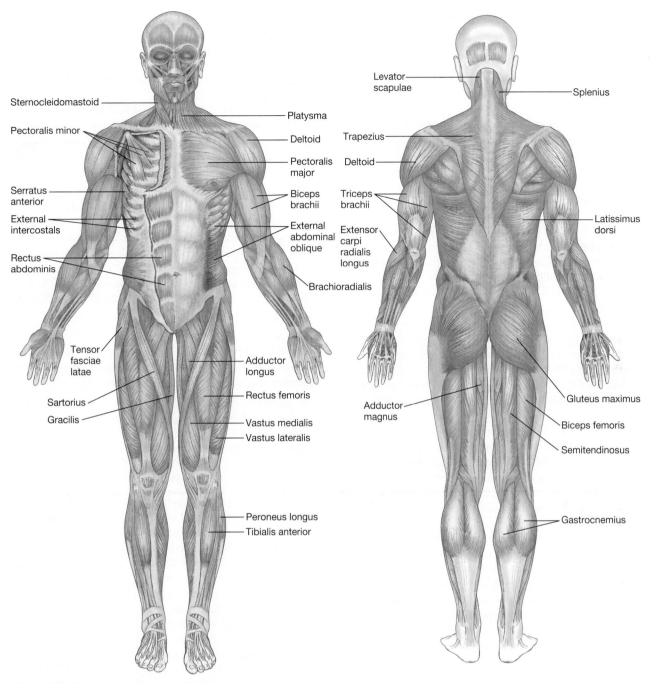

Figure 16–3 Anterior and posterior views of the superficial skeletal muscles.

Muscles are attached to bones by *tendons*. These are fibrous, long, nonelastic connective tissues.

Every muscle fiber of the body is made up of *myofibrils*. These are, in turn, composed of *sarcomeres* that contract and relax. It is this action that provides smooth and elastic muscle movements. Muscles get their energy for movement from metabolizing adenosine triphosphate in their cells. This substance is produced from glucose and *glycogen* (stored glucose) in the cells. Oxygen is also required for this process to occur.

Common Diseases of the Musculoskeletal System

Musculoskeletal diseases commonly cause pain, decreased mobility, swelling, and deformity. Bone fractures are usually easy to recognize because they displace bone and related structures and are usually associated with pain. **Nondisplaced** fractures still cause pain but are not as easy to recognize. Muscle disorders usually cause weakness or atrophy. Common tests used for musculoskeletal disorders are **radiologic** (x-ray) examinations, **computed tomography** (CT) scan, and **magnetic resonance imaging** (MRI). Other tests are **bone mass density** and **dual-energy x-ray absorptiometry** scans. These are forms of a technique called bone *densitometry*. Muscle disorders often require **electromyography**, which records electrical activity within muscles.

Bone Diseases

Bone diseases range from severe to mild and are often more common in older adults. Aging causes a breakdown of many different musculoskeletal structures. Devices that are commonly used by patients with these disorders include crutches, canes, walkers, artificial joints, braces, and pins that may be installed inside the body to offer additional support and strength.

Bone disorders that mostly affect the posture of the spine include **kyphosis**, **lordosis**, and **scoliosis**. Other conditions or disorders can affect any bony structure, such as **osteomalacia**, **osteomyelitis**, and **osteoporosis**.

Kyphosis

Kyphosis is a "humped" curvature of the thoracic spine. It is commonly known as "humpback" or "hunchback." This disorder is common in postmenopausal females with osteoporosis (**Figure 16–4**). Normal curvature in the thoracic spine is a *normal kyphosis*, but kyphosis alone describes an excessive curvature that is abnormal. Different types of kyphosis are as follows:

- Postural: The most common type; it can be corrected by learning proper posture. The "hump" created by postural kyphosis is very round and smooth. When osteoporosis affects the spine, **compression** of the anterior portion of the thoracic vertebrae leads to forward spinal bending, which creates a **Dowager's hump**, located in the upper back.
- Scheuermann's: A type of structural kyphosis that appears during adolescence; it develops when the front of the vertebrae do not grow as quickly as the back of the vertebrae. They become wedge-shaped, and the spine begins to curve excessively as a result.
- Gibbus deformity: A type of structural kyphosis (which is much more angular than seen in postural kyphosis); it appears as a particularly sharp, angular curve.

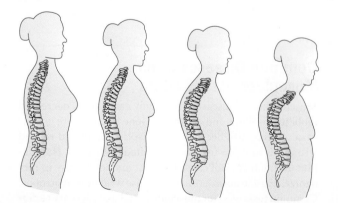

Figure 16–4 Kyphosis and height changes associated with osteoporosis.

- Congenital: A type of structural kyphosis that involves spinal defects that cause it to curve excessively; there may be accompanying heart and kidney problems. This is because the spine, heart, and kidneys develop around the same time, and the abnormalities also develop together.
- Nutritional: A type of kyphosis that may result from childhood nutritional deficiencies, such as a vitamin D deficiency. This softens bones and results in a curving of the spine and limbs under the child's own body weight.

Signs and Symptoms

Signs of kyphosis include an upper spinal area that is curved forward and appears as a "hump." A "bowing" shape of the back is seen, and the demands kyphosis places on the spinal cord and related muscles often result in chronic pain, difficulty standing, difficulty sitting, and general difficulty in most physical activities. The overall posture of the body is described as "slouching." Breathing difficulties may also be present.

Etiology

Kyphosis can be the result of degenerative diseases such as arthritis, developmental problems, osteoporosis with compression fractures of the vertebrae, or trauma.

Diagnosis

Kyphosis is diagnosed by physical examination and sometimes is confirmed by x-rays, which show abnormal vertebral development. X-rays may show potential areas of paralysis of the spine.

Treatment

Treatment of kyphosis depends on the root causes. Physical therapy, medications, and surgery are common treatments. Kyphosis due to osteoporosis must first treat the underlying osteoporosis before the kyphosis can be managed to keep from worsening. The role of the physical therapist assistant (PTA) in kyphosis is to assist with posture correction and exercises that strengthen the spinal muscles. It is often possible to diminish back pain with regular physical therapy. Patients may need to be retrained as to proper sitting, standing, and overall movement. Stretching and strengthening exercises are usually indicated.

Although bracing the back can help with posture, it sometimes results in weakened muscles. Physical therapy for kyphosis is designed to increase spine flexibility and range of motion and to strengthen muscles. For kyphosis caused by spinal compression, strengthening via physical exercise (after healing has occurred) can help prevent additional fractures from occurring. Although physical therapy cannot prevent kyphosis, it can help to strengthen the muscles, thereby potentially preventing its worsening. Exercises for some forms of kyphosis include walking, tennis, and supervised weight lifting.

Prognosis

Congenital kyphosis has a fair prognosis if diagnosed and treated early enough. Spine orthotics (back braces) may improve the outcome if worn during early development. However, kyphosis diagnosed later in life has a poor prognosis and may gradually worsen over time.

Lordosis

Lordosis is often referred to as "swayback," although this term actually describes a condition of *excessive lordosis*. It is defined as an exaggerated inward (anterior) curve of the lumbar spine. Lordosis can affect people of any age. A person can have lordosis and not have swayback, but if he or she has a swayback posture, then lordosis does exist.

Signs and Symptoms

Lordosis causes the abdomen and buttocks to protrude and the lumbar spine to be curved inward. Although frequently without symptoms, sometimes symptoms may exist, which include back pain that makes movement difficult and tingling or numbness.

Etiology

Lordosis usually occurs with pregnancy as a compensatory factor for the weight of the baby, although obesity is also a common cause. Other causes include **achondroplasia**, discitis (inflammations of the spinal disks), kyphosis, **spondylolisthesis**, abdominal weakness, and poor body mechanics. Infrequently, osteoporosis may be related but is more commonly related to kyphosis.

Diagnosis

Lordosis is diagnosed through patient history and examination, including bending the patient forward as well as performing spine range-of-motion tests. Neurologic tests may be indicated.

Treatment

Treatment of lordosis includes exercises (including back strengthening), proper posture, and bracing. For severe cases potential surgeries include spinal instrumentation and artificial disk replacement.

The role of the PTA in lordosis is to assist the patient in a program designed for strengthening, flexibility, and increasing range of motion. The PTA can also educate the patient about exercises done at home. Postural exercises for lordosis may focus on many different areas of the body, including the hips, pelvis, legs, and feet.

Scoliosis

Scoliosis is a lateral curvature of the spine (**Figure 16–5**). It affects females more than males and can occur at any age. However, it mostly affects teenagers when the growth of the body is more rapid. Scoliosis can be structural or functional. Structural scoliosis is often of unknown origin and tends to affect girls more than boys during adolescence. Functional scoliosis describes a structurally normal spine that appears to have a lateral curve.

Signs and Symptoms

Scoliosis usually causes back pain, a rib or shoulder blade "hump," and unaligned hips and shoulders. It often causes clothing to hang lower on one side of the body than the other. The shoulders may not appear to be horizontally level with each other.

Etiology

In most cases scoliosis is of unknown origin, although it appears to be related to genetics. Abnormalities of connective tissue, platelets, skeletal muscle, the spinal column, and the

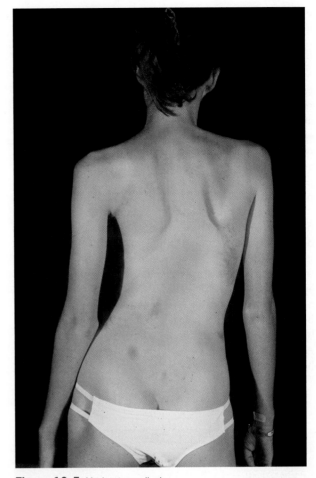

Figure 16–5 Moderate scoliosis.

rib cage may be related, although secondary, to the disease itself.

Diagnosis

Some states have mandated scoliosis screening of children in the school system. During screening the spine is observed as the child bends forward. A positive test is one in which the spine moves to one side with one shoulder blade more prominent.

Treatment

Treatment of scoliosis often includes **spinal orthoses**. Because the condition cannot be prevented, treatment is directed toward keeping the condition from worsening. Idiopathic scoliosis cannot be helped with orthotics or physical therapy. However, functional scoliosis can be helped with physical therapy. Orthoses are usually not indicated until the spinal curvature is between 20 and 30 degrees. In more severe cases surgery may be indicated, but not until the spinal curvature is between 30 and 40 degrees. The role of the PTA in scoliosis is to assist patients in a variety of exercises designed to strengthen and improve flexibility of the spine.

Prognosis

Prognosis is based on early treatment but is poor if the angle of curvature is more than 20 degrees or is left untreated. If so, this condition will have lifelong effects on the body's ability to function (as it affects many other systems) and result in chronic pain.

Rickets and Osteomalacia

Softening of bone due to loss of calcium is referred to as *osteomalacia*, which is sometimes called the adult form of *rickets*, a childhood condition. Osteomalacia may be associated with severe renal disease. It is referred to as "renal rickets" in patients with chronic renal failure. The incidence of osteomalacia is high among the elderly, because their diets are often deficient in calcium and vitamin D. This is compounded by intestinal malabsorption problems that accompany aging.

In vitamin D deficiency bone cannot calcify or harden normally, which results in rickets in infants and young children. Because of vitamin D supplements rickets is now rare in the United States but appears occasionally in breast-fed infants who have not received a vitamin D supplement. It also appears in infants who are fed with a formula that contains a nonfortified milk base. Rickets causes deformities such as bowed legs and "knock-knees" and may also be influenced by a lack of sunshine in locations with less sunlight, such as Alaska. **Figure 16–6** shows the effects of rickets on the leg bones.

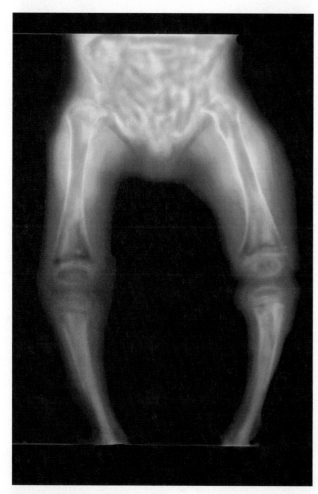

Figure 16–6 Rickets.

Signs and Symptoms

Osteomalacia may be asymptomatic until a fracture occurs. The symptoms of rickets usually are noticed between 6 months and 3 years of age. The child usually has stunted growth, with a height sometimes far below the normal range. Early symptoms are lethargy and muscle weakness, which may be accompanied by convulsions or **tetany** related to hypocalcemia. The skull is enlarged and soft, and closure of the fontanels is delayed.

The clinical manifestations of osteomalacia include bone pain, tenderness, and fractures as the disease progresses. In severe cases muscle weakness is often an early sign and of unknown cause. Osteomalacia is usually accompanied by a compensatory or secondary hyperparathyroidism stimulated by low serum calcium levels.

> **RED FLAG**
> Osteomalacia commonly affects the pelvis, legs, and spine.

Etiology

Osteomalacia and rickets are caused by vitamin D, calcium, and phosphate deficiencies, causing bones to soften and weaken. Bones require all three for normal health. Deficiency of vitamin D develops from inadequate nutritional intake, inadequate exposure to sunlight (which synthesizes vitamin D), or a problem absorbing the vitamin. Prolonged intake of phenobarbital (commonly used to treat seizures) may also cause osteomalacia or rickets.

Diagnosis

Diagnosis is directed toward identifying osteomalacia and establishing its cause. Methods used for diagnosis include x-rays, laboratory tests, bone scans, and bone biopsies. Rickets is primarily diagnosed with x-rays and blood tests, which show a deficiency of vitamin D.

Treatment

Rickets is treated with a balanced diet that is sufficient in calcium, phosphorus, and vitamin D. Exposure to sunlight is also important, especially for premature infants and those fed with artificial milk. Treatment of osteomalacia is directed at the underlying cause. If the problem is related to nutrition, it may be sufficient to restore adequate amounts of calcium and vitamin D to the diet. Elderly patients with intestinal malabsorption may also benefit from vitamin D.

The role of the PTA in rickets and osteomalacia includes assisting the patient with regular exercise. This may include weight-bearing exercises such as walking, which helps to strengthen the bones.

Prognosis

Prognosis is entirely based on correcting the vitamin deficiency and whether severe damage has already been done to the bones.

Osteomyelitis

Osteomyelitis is the inflammation of the bone and adjacent marrow cavity due to infection, which can develop through a wound, a nearby infection, or even from a skin or throat infection. Osteomyelitis represents an acute or chronic pyogenic infection of the bone. It usually affects the long bones of the legs or arms. In children or adolescents it occurs mainly because of a throat infection. Limbs may develop shorter than normal due to osteomyelitis affecting the bones' growth plates.

Signs and Symptoms

Osteomyelitis may cause chills, high fever, malaise, tenderness, and bacteremia. There is often pain upon movement of the affected extremity, loss of movement, and swelling. In adults it often occurs because of trauma to the bones or after implants have been put into the bones surgically.

Etiology

Most cases of osteomyelitis are caused by *Staphylococcus aureus* from a variety of sources both inside and outside the body. Osteomyelitis may also result from various gram-negative bacteria.

Diagnosis

Osteomyelitis is commonly diagnosed because of bone pain found during physical examination, along with a blood test revealing elevated white blood cells. Diagnosis is confirmed by erythrocyte sedimentation rate, x-ray, MRI, or CT. Additionally, the causative organism can be determined through bone, blood, joint flood, or pus samples.

Treatment

Treatment of osteomyelitis involves aggressive intravenous antibiotics, although surgical bone **debridement** may be needed to aid in healing. Surgical hardware, such as screws or plates, is often removed so bones can heal from their effects. If not treated effectively, the condition can become chronic and lead to problems throughout life, including large, open scar tissue and continual drainage from the wound.

The PTA, because it is unlikely the patient will be directly treated for osteomyelitis (unless related to wound care), will most likely treat osteomyelitis patients for underlying issues, debility, and weakness as the result of the infection. The PTA may assist with active range-of-motion exercises to increase flexibility and strength while relieving pain caused by osteomyelitis. Overexertion and possible muscle damage must be avoided. Balance exercises may be used if there is muscle weakness in the legs. Endurance eventually becomes the focus of exercise. Aerobic exercises to increase cardiovascular capacity should be done three to four times per week for 30 minutes each time after the acute phase of the disease is over.

Prognosis

Prognosis is good as long as the condition is acute and antibiotic therapy is sufficient.

Osteoporosis

Osteoporosis is defined as a decrease in bone mass and a porosity of the bone. It leads to major orthopedic problems in nearly one-third of women, beginning usually in middle age, in the United States.

Signs and Symptoms

Early symptoms include compression fractures of the spine and **pathologic** wrist fractures. As the spine is affected, the patient actually decreases in height and has pain in the thoracic and lumbar spine. Over time up to 5 inches of height may be lost. Spine compression fractures can cause the abdomen and thoracic cavity to decrease in size, compressing the organs and causing breathing difficulties. Collapse of vertebral bones may compress the spinal nerve roots that pass through the intervertebral foramina, causing pain to radiate along the course of the compressed nerve (**Figure 16–7**). Patients may complain of being bloated or "full," either after eating only a small amount or persistently. Additional symptoms are kyphosis and a *Dowager's hump* on the upper thoracic spine.

> **RED FLAG**
> Osteoporosis is the most prevalent bone disease throughout the world.

Wrist fractures can occur after only a minor fall when the patient attempts to catch his or her weight before contact, and hip fractures become increasingly likely after falls or other trauma. These types of fractures are often the first symptoms of underlying problems.

Etiology

The pathogenesis of osteoporosis is unclear, but most data suggest an imbalance between bone resorption and formation, meaning that bone resorption exceeds bone formation. Although both factors play a role in most osteoporosis cases, their relative contributions to bone loss may vary based on age, nutritional status, sex, and genetic predisposition. The most common group affected by osteoporosis is women after menopause due to estrogen decline or depletion. These patients are usually osteoporotic due to decreases of both estrogen and calcium as well as lack of exercise.

Diagnosis

Diagnosis of osteoporosis can be confirmed by examination, dual-emission x-ray absorptiometry scans, CT scan, and traditional x-rays.

Treatment

Prevention and early detection of osteoporosis are essential to preventing associated deformities and fractures.

> **RED FLAG**
> An important advance in diagnostic methods used for identifying osteoporosis is the use of bone mineral density assessment.

Regular exercise and adequate calcium intake are also required. Active treatment of osteoporosis uses four types

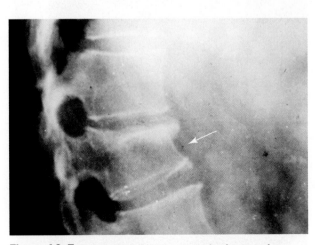

Figure 16–7 Osteoporosis with a compression fracture of vertebral body. Vertebral bodies are less dense than normal, and the front of one vertebral body has collapsed (arrow). Compare the compression fracture in this vertebral body with the vertebra above in which the anterior and posterior surfaces are the same height.

of antiresorptive agents: gonadal hormones (estrogen), calcitonin, fluorides, and biphosphonates. Supplements of calcium and vitamin D are also indicated. Weight-bearing daily exercise is advised. Estrogen and calcium levels should be monitored to avoid breast or gynecologic malignancies and kidney stones.

The role of the PTA is to assist the patient with osteoporosis in performing approved weight-bearing exercises 3 days a week for 25 to 30 minutes each day. Suggested activities are walking and the use of resistance equipment. The patient may also participate in low-impact aerobics, team sports, and racket sports.

Prognosis

Prognosis is based on the severity of osteoporosis when diagnosed and the response to treatment and regular weight-bearing exercise.

Paget's Disease

Paget's disease (osteitis deformans) affects bone formation. It is a chronic metabolic disease characterized by an overgrowth of new bone that occurs more quickly than the breakdown of old bone (**Figure 16–8**). The thicker new bone is actually much weaker than the old bone and has a higher potential for fracture. Its "mosaic" pattern is easily diagnosed via x-rays.

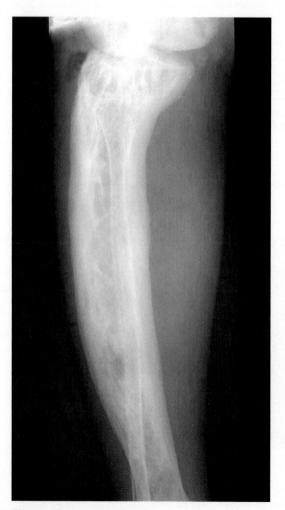

Figure 16–8 Paget's disease.

This disorder primarily affects the pelvis and long leg bones in patients over age 40, worsening with age. Once it becomes symptomatic, bone pain may occur, which intensifies during the night. A spinal curvature or bowed legs may result. Hearing may become impaired because Paget's disease can affect the bones in the ear, and osteosarcoma may develop as a secondary condition.

Signs and Symptoms

Paget's disease manifests with abnormal bone destruction and remodeling, leading to bone deformities. Excessive bone destruction occurs, replaced by fibrous tissue and abnormal bone. The new bone is larger but weaker and filled with new blood vessels. Fragile, misshapen bones result, either in one or two areas or throughout the skeleton. Long bones and the bones of the skull, pelvis, and vertebrae are most often affected. It is more common with increased age. Complications include pathologic fractures, osteoarthritis, heart failure related to hypercalcemia and increased cardiac workload, osteosarcoma, and nerve compression.

Etiology

The exact cause of Paget's disease is unknown, but it is believed to be related to a virus that increases osteoclast activity or because of genetic defects that produce increases in interferon-6.

Diagnosis

Paget's disease is diagnosed via patient history, physical examination, bone scan, x-rays, serum alkaline phosphatase, and serum calcium.

Treatment

Mild cases of Paget's disease require periodic monitoring and no treatment. When needed, treatment is focused on the reduction of fractures and deformities. Medications include bisphosphonates, calcitonin, nonsteroidal anti-inflammatory drugs (NSAIDs), and analgesics. Surgery may be indicated to correct severe bone deformities. The role of the PTA is to assist the patient with exercises that do not put excessive strain on the bones. Physical therapy is essential in maintaining skeletal health, avoiding weight gain, and maintaining joint mobility. The PT should address the patient's joint mobility and ability to benefit from strengthening and low-impact exercises.

Prognosis

Prognosis for Paget's disease is generally good, especially if treatment occurs before serious bone deformities can occur.

Benign Bone Tumors

Most musculoskeletal neoplasms are secondary to tumors from other parts of the body. Benign tumors of the bones are limited within the edges of the bones, have clear edges, and are surrounded by a slight amount of sclerotic bone. The most common benign bone neoplasms include chondroma, osteoma, osteochondroma, and giant cell tumor. A *chondroma* is composed of hyaline cartilage and is common in the bones of the hands and feet. An *osteoma* is small and bony, commonly occurring on long or flat bones or the skull. An *osteochondroma* is the most commonly occurring benign neoplasm of the musculoskeletal system. It occurs while the skeleton is still growing, originating in the epiphyseal cartilage plate. A *giant cell tumor* (*osteoclastoma*) often mimics the growth patterns of malignant bone tumors. It can metastasize through the bloodstream and usually appears in the knee, wrist, or shoulder.

Malignant Bone Tumors

Primary musculoskeletal neoplasms are not common and usually are secondary tumors that metastasize from the breasts, lungs, or prostate. The most common tumor of the bone marrow is myeloma, whereas soft tissue (in immunocompromised patients) tumors include Kaposi's sarcoma. Rhabdomyosarcoma is a rare but malignant skeletal muscle tumor.

Primary malignant tumors appear different from primary benign tumors. They usually have less defined shapes, borders that are not sharp, and may extend beyond the edges of the bones they affect. They occur in all age groups and may appear anywhere in the body. **Table 16–2** lists common types of bone cancers.

> **RED FLAG**
> Metastatic malignant tumors are far more common than primary malignant tumors.

The PTA's role with bone cancer patients must be determined on an individual basis, weighing the potential benefits of therapy versus the potential for fatigue or other possible complications. Mild exercise and stretching is often indicated. Physical therapy is designed to manage pain, increase mobility, improve strength, improve activities of daily living, and improve safety awareness. Resistive or resistance exercises are sometimes avoided because of the potential for bone fractures, with strength training used to improve bone density.

> **RED FLAG**
> Any malignant tumor may spread to the bones. The skeleton is the third most common site of metastasis, following the lungs and liver.

Osteosarcoma

When a primary bone tumor occurs, it is usually an osteosarcoma, affecting the femur, humerus, or tibia (**Figure 16–9**).

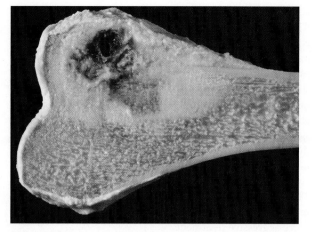

Figure 16–9 Osteosarcoma.

Osteosarcomas are aggressive and highly malignant. They are the most common primary malignant bone tumors and comprise 20 percent of all bone cancers. They often arise near the knee or humerus but can appear in the hands, feet, skull, and jaw. Osteosarcomas are of unknown origin.

Osteosarcoma, also known as *osteogenic sarcoma*, is the sixth most common cancer in children under age 15, with a second peak in incidence occurring in the elderly (often related to Paget's disease, medullary infarct, or prior radiation therapy or x-rays). These tumors grow rapidly and spread to soft tissues, most commonly to the lungs. Patients experience deep, localized pain and swelling that may awaken them during the night.

Treatment requires surgery in combination with a variety of chemotherapy agents. If surgery is indicated, a complete radical surgical en bloc resection is preferred. Amputation may be required but is becoming less common as treatments become more successful. About 90 percent of patients are able to have limb-salvage surgery due to advancements in treatment of osteosarcoma. However, complications such as infection and local tumor recurrence may cause the need for further surgery or amputation.

Ewing's Sarcoma

Ewing's sarcoma is highly malignant and metastasizes rapidly to nearly every body organ. It is the second most common type of primary bone tumor in children and adolescents. It usually appears first in the diaphysis of the femur bone, followed by the pelvis, pubis, sacrum, humerus, vertebrae, ribs, skull, and other flat bones. Ewing's sarcoma commonly causes pain, limited movement, and tenderness as it involves both bones and soft tissues. It often metastasizes to the lungs, bone marrow, and other bones. The diagnostic biopsy is very important because it is not easy to correctly diagnose. Treatment involves chemotherapy, radiation, and surgery. It is considered to be a radiosensitive tumor and, if it has not metastasized, may be highly curable.

> **RED FLAG**
> Ewing's sarcoma most commonly occurs in young people under the age of 20. It may be seen in children as young as 5 months of age. Ewing's sarcoma is uncommon in Black children, affecting mostly White children.

TABLE 16–2	**Types of Primary Bone Cancers**	
Type	**Benign Form**	**Malignant Form**
Bone	Benign osteoblastoma Osteoid osteoma	Parosteal osteogenic sarcoma Osteosarcoma
Bone marrow	—	Multiple myeloma Reticulum cell sarcoma
Cartilage	Chondroblastoma Chondroma Chondromyxoid fibroma Osteochondroma	Chondrosarcoma
Fibrous and fibro-osseous tissue	Fibrous dysplasia	Fibrosarcoma Malignant fibrous histiocytoma
Lipid	Lipoma	Liposarcoma
Miscellaneous	Giant cell tumor	Ewing's sarcoma Malignant giant cell

Chondrosarcoma

Chondrosarcoma affects the cartilage and is the second most common malignant bone tumor. It usually affects men in middle or later life, arising from points of muscle attachment to bones. Common sites of its development include the knee, shoulder, hip, and pelvis (**Figure 16–10**). Chondrosarcomas may be related to benign lesions, including osteochondroma, chondroblastoma, or fibrous dysplasia. Chondrosarcomas are slow growing, tending to be asymptomatic for a long time as they destroy bone and invade soft tissues. Early diagnosis is important because this tumor responds well to early radical surgery. Radiation and chemotherapy are often not helpful. This type of tumor may progress or develop into a highly malignant form (mesenchymal chondrosarcoma), requiring more aggressive treatment.

Multiple Myeloma

Multiple myeloma arises from plasma cells in the bone marrow, resembles leukemia, but usually only affects the bone marrow. Tumors may form that weaken bones and lead to fractures, disability, and pain. In this condition neoplastic cells produce large amounts of protein, increasing blood proteins and viscosity. The protein produced is usually a type of IgG, which can be identified by blood or urine tests. If masses of coagulated myeloma protein accumulate in the tissues, their function may become severely impaired. Often, multiple myeloma results in kidney failure because the produced protein blocks renal tubules. This condition may be treated with thalidomide and its derivatives, which suppress proliferation of blood vessels that help to grow the myeloma cells. Also, localized bone destruction may be treated with radiotherapy.

The role of the PTA with multiple myeloma patients is to help increase strength, flexibility, pain management, and endurance. Stretching exercises may increase range of motion, decrease pain, and improve overall mobility. The patient may also require massage and occupational or speech therapy.

Joint Diseases

The bones of the skeleton are connected by interfaces known as joints. The three types of joints are fibrous joints, cartilaginous joints, and synovial joints. Fibrous joints are found between the bones of the skull. Cartilaginous joints are located between adjacent vertebral bodies in the spine and between the pubic bones of the pelvis. Synovial joints are movable joints (**Figure 16–11**).

Aging usually increases the onset of certain joint diseases. When damage to joints occurs during childhood and adolescence, it often causes no significant pain or impairment until middle age. **Arthritis** is one of the most common (and often) disabling diseases of the skeletal system. **Rheumatism** is defined simply as a condition of stiffness and is an older term that is now usually associated with **rheumatoid arthritis** (RA) or rheumatic fever. Arthritis is very common; for example, a sprained ankle is an arthritic-related condition. Common types of arthritis include **gout**, **osteoarthritis** (degenerative joint disease), and RA.

> **RED FLAG**
>
> Common joint conditions include those related to joint deformity, such as **bunion** (hallux valgus), and other types, such as **temporomandibular joint syndrome**.

Rheumatoid Arthritis

RA is a systemic autoimmune disorder that affects the joints and connective tissues throughout the body. It often causes symptoms of chronic illness by affecting the blood vessels, heart, and lungs. RA most often affects young and middle-aged women, usually involving the small joints of the hands and feet. In the joints RA produces a chronic inflammation and thickening of the synovial membrane (**Figure 16–12**).

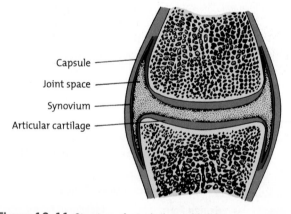

Capsule
Joint space
Synovium
Articular cartilage

Figure 16–11 Structure of a typical movable joint.

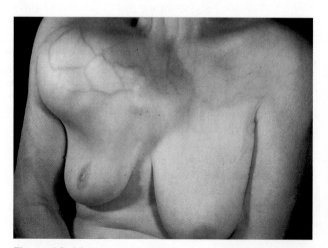

Figure 16–10 A large, well-differentiated cartilaginous tumor (chondrosarcoma) arising from the chest wall.

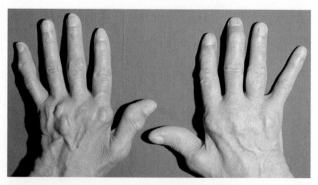

Figure 16–12 Rheumatoid arthritis. Early manifestations, illustrating swelling of knuckle joints (metacarpophalangeal joints) as a result of inflammation and ulnar deviation of fingers.

Signs and Symptoms

RA causes noticeable deformity and destruction in the metacarpophalangeal joints (**Figure 16–13A and B**). Rheumatoid nodules may appear in various areas of the body, including the hands, feet, and elbows, before the joints are fully damaged. Joints initially appear inflamed and feel warm to the touch. Other symptoms related to RA include pleuritis, anemia, valvulitis, lung fibrosis, kidney problems, cardiovascular problems, and glaucoma. When RA affects the neck the spinal cord can be damaged, leading to paralysis or even death.

Patients with RA complain of general fatigue and weight loss, along with symmetric joint swelling, pain, and stiffness. The stiffness is more prominent in the morning and subsides during the day. Patients also show signs of other chronic illness and of body weakness and may experience various, recurring infections. Onset of the disease is highest in women between ages 20 and 40.

Etiology

The exact cause of RA is unknown, but it is related to abnormal antibodies that attack or attach to the body's cells and tissues. RA is believed to be hereditary and may also be triggered by viral infections.

Diagnosis

RA may be diagnosed in part by testing the blood for an antibody called *rheumatoid factor*. Diagnosis is based on family history, physical examination, and laboratory tests (for example, elevated erythrocyte sedimentation rate). Patients are first evaluated for the causes of the arthritic symptoms, including testing for systemic lupus erythematosus, Sjögren's syndrome, polymyositis, scleroderma, cancer, and hormone disorders. Other tests may include complete blood count, synovial fluid analysis, and serum protein electrophoresis. Sometimes RA cannot be diagnosed until the patient is observed over weeks or months.

Treatment

The treatment goals for a person with RA are to manage flare-ups (exacerbations) and pain, minimize stiffness and swelling, maintain mobility, prevent joint deformity, and provide patient education. The treatment plan includes educating about the disease and its treatment, conserving energy, performing therapeutic exercises, and administering medications. Anti-inflammatory medications and analgesics are used for pain management. Corticosteroids are used in the short term for acute attacks. Anti-rheumatic drugs include penicillamine. Also, energy conservation, exercises, and joint protection measures may be used, including orthotics and other devices. Surgical replacement of the joints with artificial joints may be indicated as the disease progresses.

The role of the PTA is to assist the patient with RA in maintaining strength, tone, and overall fitness. Joint function and muscle strength are priorities of treatment. Stretching, flexibility exercises, strength training, low-impact aerobics, and aquatic (water) therapy are all indicated for RA. Heat or ice packs and massage are also used when appropriate (if the condition is exacerbated, heat is not used).

Prognosis

Prognosis may be poor because there is no real way of reversing RA. Although medications and proper management cannot reverse damage from the disease, the goal of treatment is to prevent further damage and manage the disease.

Osteoarthritis

Osteoarthritis is also known as *degenerative joint disease*. In this condition joints simply wear out from use (or "wear and tear"). As part of the normal aging process joints naturally change. With the increased amount of elderly people alive today, osteoarthritis is now the leading cause of disability in the United States. The primary change in osteoarthritis is degeneration of the articular cartilage, making it more rough than normal (**Figure 16–14A, B, and C**).

Signs and Symptoms

Osteoarthritis often affects the weight-bearing joints, such as the hands, hips, knees, and spine (along with the fingers). One of the main differences between osteoarthritis and

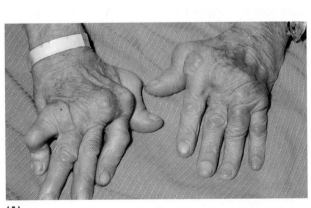

(A)

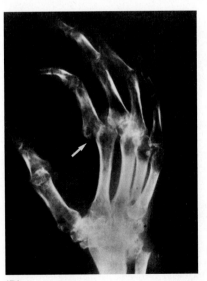

(B)

Figure 16–13 (A) Advanced joint deformities caused by rheumatoid arthritis. (B) Radiograph illustrating destruction of articular surfaces and anterior dislocation of base of index finger (arrow) as a result of joint instability.

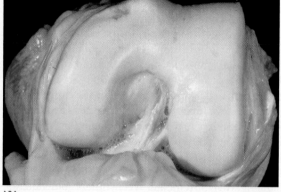

(A)

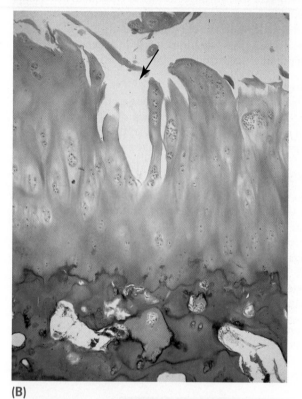

(B)

(C)

Figure 16–14 (A) Knee joint, illustrating smooth articular surface of femoral condyles. (B) Early histologic changes of osteoarthritis, illustrating splitting and fragmentation of articular cartilage (arrow) (original magnification X 160). Compare with normal articular cartilage in Figure 27-2A. C, Advanced osteoarthritis, illustrating loss of articular cartilage (left arrow) and nodular overgrowth of bone (right arrows).

RA is that osteoarthritis often affects these weight-bearing joints. Affected joints in the fingers usually become swollen and painful. The **interphalangeal** joints are often affected and can acquire a "crooked" ("swan neck" or boutonnière) deformity. The **metacarpophalangeal** joints are usually not affected.

When the spine is involved, osteoarthritis can cause chronic back pain. The hips and knees may be affected when the articular cartilage at the end of long bones (such as the femoral head of the hip) is worn away. Raw bone becomes exposed when there is a lack of protective cartilage. New bone forms around and even inside the joint, leading to "bone spurs" that limit joint movement. At this point in the disease process the patient sometimes may require a total hip or knee replacement procedure. Although osteoarthritis can begin in the second decade (depending on lifestyle), it is progressive, with symptoms becoming more evident in a person's fifties and sixties. **Table 16–3** compares osteoarthritis with RA.

> **RED FLAG**
> Even though osteoarthritis symptoms often become more evident during the fifth and sixth decades, nearly 80 percent of people have osteoarthritis symptoms by age 70.

Etiology
Osteoarthritis is of unknown origin, although the amount of wear on the joints, and its severity, leads to the condition occurring at younger ages. Risk factors for development of osteoarthritis include excessive wear or injury to joints, family history, female gender (higher onset), obesity, and increasing age.

Diagnosis
Diagnosis of osteoarthritis is made by patient history and physical examination. X-rays may be helpful but may not always match with the patient's symptoms. Typical changes seen on x-ray are narrowing of joint spaces, subchondral sclerosis and cyst formation, and osteophytes (certain types of bone spurs). In the hands osteoarthritis is diagnosed based on hard tissue enlargement and swelling of certain joints.

Treatment
Treatment for osteoarthritis includes non–weight-bearing exercise (biking or swimming), rest, heat applications (only when symptoms are not flared or exacerbated), and medications such as analgesics and anti-inflammatories. If severe, injections of steroids directly into joint capsules may be required. Surgery to completely replace affected joints may be indicated. Arthroplasty, or joint replacement surgery, is a surgical technique commonly used for osteoarthritis of the hips, knees, shoulders, and other areas of the body. Total replacements of hip, knee, and shoulder joints are becoming more common today. Often, arthroscopic procedures precede these surgeries because of the formation of osteophytes, torn cartilage, and so on. *Arthroscopy* is a minimally invasive surgical procedure in which examination and/or treatment of a joint condition is accomplished. An *arthroscope* is used, which is a type of endoscope inserted into the joint through a small incision.

The role of the PTA in osteoarthritis is to assist patients with general fitness, low-impact aerobics or cardiovascular

TABLE 16-3 Comparison Between Osteoarthritis and Rheumatoid Arthritis

Characteristics	Osteoarthritis	Rheumatoid Arthritis
Development of disease	Often begins gradually, on one side of the body; may be limited to one set of joints (usually fingers or large weight-bearing joints)	Often affects small and large joints on both sides of the body (hands, wrists, elbows, balls of the feet)
Morning stiffness	Lasts less than 1 hour, returns at the end of the day	Lasts longer than 1 hour
Systemic symptoms	None	Frequent fatigue and general feeling of illness
Related symptoms	Symptoms are isolated without being systemic	Frequent fevers, weight loss, or involvement of other organ systems
Severity	Less severe than RA	More severe than osteoarthritis
Disease process	Normal wear and tear on the body	Autoimmune
Gender	Common in both men and women	Affects women more than men
Diagnosis	X-rays	Blood tests: RF, ESR, CRP
Treatment	NSAIDs, possible surgery, such as joint replacement (arthroplasty)	NSAIDs, immunosuppressants, steroids
Age at onset	Usually when elderly	Any time in life
Speed of onset	Slow, over years	Rapid, over weeks to months
Joint symptoms	Painful without swelling	Painful, swollen, and stiff

CRP, C-reactive protein; ESR, erythrocyte sedimentation rate; RF, rheumatoid factor.

exercises, strengthening, and range-of-motion exercises. These may include walking, cycling, swimming, aquatic therapy, weight training, stretching, and strengthening exercises.

Prognosis

Prognosis depends on the age of the patient, reduction of body weight (if required), and degree of joint involvement at diagnosis and the severity of the disease progress.

Ankylosing Spondylitis

Ankylosing spondylitis is a chronic disease that causes inflammation in the joints of the spine that can also affect the pelvis between the spinal joints. Eventually, the condition causes the affected spinal bones to fuse together (**Figure 16–15**). It usually begins between ages 20 and 40, although it may affect children younger than age 10. Males are affected more than females. A related condition is *spondylolisthesis*, which refers to the forward slippage of one vertebral body with respect to the one beneath it.

> **RED FLAG**
> Any vertebral defect is referred to as *spondylolysis*, which is commonly caused by stress fractures.

Signs and Symptoms

Ankylosing spondylitis begins with lower back pain that may develop and disappear spontaneously, with pain usually worsening at night or when inactive, with the potential to disrupt sleep. Activity or exercise usually improves the condition, which often begins between the pelvis and spine, although it may affect the entire spine. Loss of motion or mobility in the lower spine is often seen, as is endurance-type fatigue and an inability to fully expand the chest. Less common signs and symptoms include eye inflammation or uveitis, heel pain, hip pain and stiffness, joint pain in swelling (especially in the shoulders, knees, and ankles), loss of appetite, fever, and weight loss. Although uncommon, ankylosing spondylitis may cause aortic insufficiency, heart rhythm problems, pulmonary fibrosis, or restrictive lung disease.

Etiology

The etiology of ankylosing spondylitis is unknown but may be genetically linked.

Diagnosis

Diagnosis of ankylosing spondylitis is determined by a variety of tests, including complete blood count, erythrocyte sedimentation rate, spinal and pelvic x-rays, and the HLA-B27 blood test, which looks for a specific protein on the surface of white blood cells. The protein is called human leukocyte antigen B27.

Treatment

Treatment includes the use of NSAIDs to reduce pain and inflammation. Corticosteroids and tumor necrosis factor inhibitors also may be used. If these are ineffective, cytotoxic drugs may be used. Severe pain or joint damage may require surgery. The role of the PTA includes assisting with exercises designed to improve posture and breathing. Sleeping may be difficult and uncomfortable until the patient learns individualized positions that cause the least discomfort. The most commonly suggested sleeping position is lying on the back with a pillow placed under the knees.

Prognosis

Prognosis is varied, with symptoms developing and then ceasing spontaneously. Most patients can maintain daily functions unless the hips or spine become severely involved.

Gout

Gout is a clinical syndrome associated with an elevated level of uric acid in the blood and body fluids, leading to precipitation of uric acid as sodium urate crystals in joints and other

NORMAL ANATOMY   ANKYLOSING SPONDYLITIS

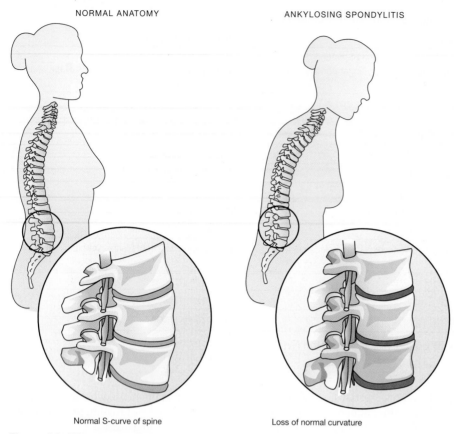

Normal S-curve of spine   Loss of normal curvature

Figure 16–15 Ankylosing spondylitis.

tissues. This condition is sometimes called *primary gout* to distinguish it from the much less common *secondary gout* in which the elevated uric acid is secondary to some other disease or condition.

Signs and Symptoms

Gout primarily affects the **metatarsophalangeal** joint of the great toe, causing the patient to experience episodes of extreme acute pain usually involving (initially) only a single toe. An acute inflammatory response occurs and includes heat, redness, swelling, and pain in the joint. Most patients with gout are men over age 30. If chronic, the uric acid also deposits in the subcutaneous tissue of the great toe, appearing as small, white nodules (**tophi**) (**Figure 16–16A and B**). Other signs are kidney dysfunction and kidney stones.

Etiology

Gout is a disease associated with an inborn error of uric acid metabolism that increases production or interferes with excretion of uric acid. Excess uric acid is converted to sodium urate crystals that precipitate from the blood and become deposited in joints and other tissues.

Diagnosis

Diagnosis of gout is based on arthrocentesis (aspiration of the joint fluid), which is done under local anesthesia. The needle-like uric acid crystals are clearly seen under a microscope.

Treatment

Treatment for gout can include medications such as probenecid and allopurinol, a diet that helps to cause weight loss (if this is needed), and less protein in the diet. In severe

cases surgery to remove the tophi may be required. In untreated patients masses of urate crystals deposited in and around the articular surface of joints cause damage to joint surfaces and adjacent bone. This condition is called "gouty arthritis" (**Figure 16–17**).

The role of the PTA in gout is to assist with exercise to promote weight loss, if indicated, and to increase mobility. Various activities can help increase blood flow to an area, such as strengthening exercises. Combined with medications, this may be helpful in reducing the signs and symptoms of gout.

Prognosis

Although gout cannot be cured, medications can dissolve tophi buildup and reduce inflammation and pain for long-term management. Lowered levels of uric acid will help avoid kidney stones.

Avascular Necrosis

When blood supply to the cartilaginous ends (epiphyses) of bones in children and adolescents experience necrosis and degeneration, the condition is known as *avascular necrosis*. It usually affects the femoral head (**Figure 16–18**), tibial tubercle, articular surface of the femoral condyle, and, sometimes, the small bones of the ankles and feet. This condition may also occur in adults if blood supply to a bone is interrupted (for any reason). Avascular necrosis is also known as *osteonecrosis*.

> **RED FLAG**
>
> A common example of avascular necrosis is interrupted circulation to the femoral head because of a hip fracture or **dislocation**.

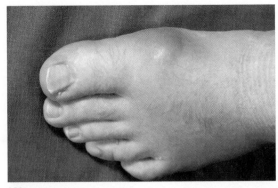

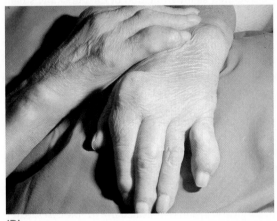

Figure 16–16 (A) Acute gout affecting right great toe. (B) Deformities of hands caused by accumulation of uric acid crystals (tophi) in and around finger joints.

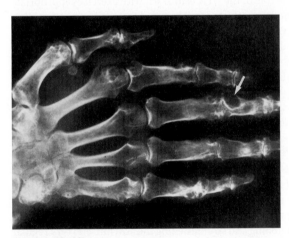

Figure 16–17 Radiograph of right hand of patient with gouty arthritis illustrating area of bone destruction (arrow) caused by masses of uric acid crystals.

Signs and Symptoms

Avascular necrosis causes pain and disability, which are related to the motion of the joint affected.

Etiology

Avascular necrosis sometimes follows an injury but is usually of unknown origin.

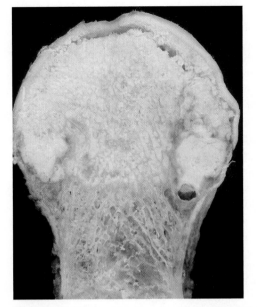

Figure 16–18 Avascular necrosis of femoral head. Articular cartilage has separated from underlying bone, which appears dense and lacks normal structural pattern. In contrast, bone of femoral neck (lower part of photograph) appears normal. Treated by removal of femoral head and replacement with artificial hip joint.

Diagnosis

Diagnosis of avascular necrosis is based on patient history and physical examination, x-rays, MRI, CT scan, and biopsy.

Treatment

Treatments include limiting joint movement, drugs that reduce lipid levels, NSAIDs for pain, use of crutches and other assistive devices to reduce weight bearing on affected bones, range-of-motion exercises, electrical stimulation, and, finally, if all other measures are ineffective, surgery. The role of the PTA is to assist patients with range-of-motion exercises to maintain or improve joint range of motion.

Prognosis

Prognosis is varied, based on what part of the bone or bones become affected, how large the affected area is, and how effectively the bone can rebuild itself with treatment.

Temporomandibular Joint Syndrome

Temporomandibular joint syndrome (TMJ) is an inflammation of the joint that connects the lower jaw to the skull, resulting in severe pain and impairment.

Signs and Symptoms

TMJ may cause severe headaches and pain in the temporomandibular joint, which us aggravated by chewing. Signs of TMJ include a clicking sound made during chewing and a decreased ability to open the mouth fully.

Etiology

TMJ may occur because of overbite, joint tissue lesions, improperly fitted dentures or other dental work, and malocclusion (misalignment of the teeth or dental arches).

Diagnosis

TMJ is diagnosed by physical examination, dental x-rays, CT scan, or MRI.

Treatment

Treatment of TMJ includes correction of the causes of the disorder, bite plates, exercises, and, as a last resort, surgery. The role of the PTA in the treatment of TMJ includes teaching jaw exercises that can greatly reduce the symptoms of the condition. These include exercises related to breathing, relaxation of the jaw, jaw alignment, posture, and muscle strengthening.

Prognosis

Prognosis differs because cases of TMJ sometimes disappear on their own. The use of mouth splints at night may improve prognosis in some patients. Surgery usually reduces pain and other symptoms but has risks that must be considered.

Bunion

Bunion, also known as *hallux valgus*, is a deformity that affects the metatarsophalangeal joint of the great toe (**Figure 16–19**). It is often related to genetics and affects females more often than males. It is aggravated by wearing pointed-toe shoes with high heels. Symptoms of bunion include pain, redness, and swelling near the metatarsophalangeal joint and the inability to wear pointed-toe or high-heeled shoes (or any shoes) due to pain. Most experts believe bunions are inherited but irritated by poor or improper footwear. The deformity progresses over time, with soft tissue and bone building up in the area of the joint.

Bunions are very visible on physical examination and confirmed by x-rays. Mild cases are resolved by only wearing low-heeled, comfortable footwear. For pain, analgesics and anti-inflammatories are given. Severe bunions may require surgical intervention. A *bunionectomy* usually involves removing the soft tissue and bony buildup in the foot to restore normal alignment of the big toe. There are over 100 different types of surgeries for this condition. Prognosis differs based on severity of the condition and whether surgery is required and done successfully. Up to one-third of patients

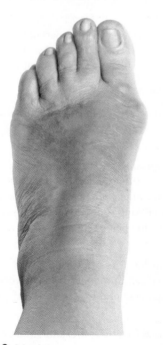

Figure 16–19 A bunion.

who have bunionectomies complain of continued pain and discomfort, although the appearance of the foot is usually much closer to normal. Physical therapy may be indicated for gait training after surgery.

Trauma Affecting the Musculoskeletal System

Most musculoskeletal problems result from trauma. Bones are most commonly injured by fractures. Other trauma-related conditions include **tennis elbow**, sprains, and strains. Lower back pain is one of the most commonly reported musculoskeletal conditions.

Bursitis

Bursitis is defined as inflammation of the bursa, the small, fluid-filled sacs near joints that help reduce friction during joint movement. Symptoms of bursitis include severe pain resulting in limited motion of the joint. Bursitis often results from repetitive motion that irritates the bursa. Bursitis of the shoulder is most common, although any joint can be affected. When bursitis affects the elbow, it is known as *olecranon bursitis*. Bursitis is diagnosed by physical examination to determine the location of the pain and swelling and by which motions cause the pain. X-rays can help to pinpoint the affected area.

Bursitis is usually treated by application of analgesics, anti-inflammatory medications, and rest. If it persists, corticosteroids may be injected or the affected area may be drained. Surgical excision is indicated in extreme cases. After recovery, active range-of-motion exercises are required to reestablish normal joint function. Prognosis is good as long as rest and treatments are adequate. The best prevention of bursitis involves reduction of repetitive movements, exercise, and stretching.

The role of the PTA is to assist with exercises appropriate for the joint affected, such as progressive range-of-motion exercises, walking, and stretching. Warm-up and cool-down periods are essential with this condition. Additional physical therapy includes physical agents appropriate for the stage of inflammation (such as pulsed ultrasound, iontophoresis, and phonophoresis), massage, and hot or cold treatment (depending on the joint involved). In general, most forms of light exercise are approved for bursitis.

Tennis Elbow

Tennis elbow is irritation of the common extensor tendon that affects the elbow joint. Generally, this involves the extensor carpi radialis brevis, but it may involve other tendons. It is best prevented by avoiding overuse or repetitive trauma and by stretching and strengthening the arm muscles on a regular basis. Tennis elbow causes a severe and burning pain on the outside of the elbow that is worsened by pressing the area or by lifting and gripping objects. Tennis elbow is a repetitive motion injury that is not necessarily related to playing tennis. Diagnosis of tennis elbow requires a test in which pressure is placed on the affected area while the patient moves his or her elbow, wrist, and fingers. X-rays are used to rule out fractures or arthritis. Ultrasonography or MRI is sometimes used for diagnosis also, although rarely.

Treatment of tennis elbow is similar to that of bursitis. A large, wide strap (known as a *tennis elbow splint*) is applied just below the elbow to support muscle movement, with the goal being reduction of pain. Prognosis is good if adequate exercise of the arm is accomplished, which reduces future risk of injury.

The role of the PTA is to assist with stretching exercises and light strengthening exercises and to use physical agents appropriate for the stage of inflammation. The use of squeeze balls and resistance grippers are also indicated with supervision, usually when totally pain free. These should be used with extreme caution because they can exacerbate the condition. Other physical therapy components include cortisone cream used with electrical stimulation (phonophoresis) of the elbow. Ultrasound and heat may also be used in lieu of cortisone injections.

Carpal Tunnel Syndrome

Carpal tunnel syndrome is caused by repetitive motion that affects the hands and wrists. It is commonly seen in those who perform repetitive work that involves the fingers, hands, wrists, and lower arms. Examples include computer entry work and manufacturing work. The carpal tunnel ligament (*transverse carpal ligament*) in the wrist area allows blood vessels, nerves, and tendons to pass through to innervate the hands. This ligament forms the roof of the carpal tunnel. Repetitive motions in this area cause the tendons to become inflamed, putting pressure on the medial nerve.

Signs and Symptoms
Symptoms include pain, numbness, clammy skin in the area, swelling, and discoloration of the affected hand and fingers.

Diagnosis
Diagnosis of carpal tunnel syndrome is confirmed by patient history, physical examination, and tests such as the "Phalen's maneuver," which involves flexing the wrist as far as possible and watching for numbness symptoms. If positive, numbness in the median nerve area should occur within 60 seconds after initiation of the maneuver.

Treatment
Treatment of carpal tunnel syndrome includes ceasing the repetitive motion, rest, splints, anti-inflammatory medications, and physical therapy. If unsuccessful, surgery may be indicated, wherein the carpal ligament is separated to enlarge the tunnel and relieve median nerve pressure.

> **RED FLAG**
> Carpal tunnel syndrome often also requires occupational therapy but is an important condition for PTAs to understand.

Prognosis
Prognosis is entirely based on therapy outcomes. Ergonomics and changing job duties help to allow sufficient rest for the affected area.

Dislocations and Subluxations

A *dislocation* is the complete separation of a bone from its normal position within a joint (**Figure 16–20**). A **subluxation** is just a partial separation. Dislocations cause acute pain and deformity of joints that is usually quite obvious. When joint tissue swells rapidly, it is difficult to correct the dislocation. Dislocations are caused by major trauma, such

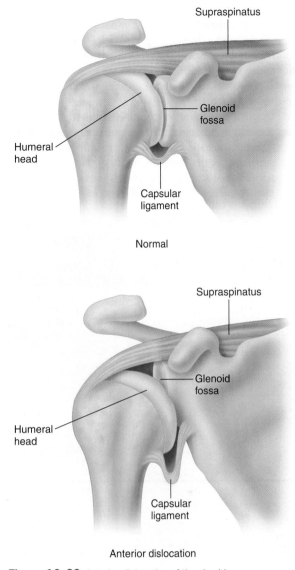

Figure 16–20 Anterior dislocation of the shoulder.

as sports injuries, car accidents, and falls. Joint abnormalities and diseases may also be related, and certain diseases can cause dislocations to occur frequently with no apparent cause. Subluxations are not uncommon with severe cerebrovascular accidents with upper extremity involvement.

Dislocations and subluxations may be diagnosed by patient history and physical examination. X-rays help to determine how serious the injury may be. Due to swelling, dislocated joints should be reduced or repositioned by a qualified healthcare provider immediately. General anesthesia may be indicated due to the intense pain of the procedure. Those who suffer recurrent injuries of this type may be instructed how to reduce the joint themselves. Surgery may be indicated after repeated injuries to tighten the ligaments and support the joint. Prognosis is good with adequate treatment and preventive measures to keep future injuries from happening. Bandages, orthotics, and specialized supportive padding may help to reduce potential injuries.

Fractures

A *fracture* is defined as any discontinuity of a bone. It is synonymous with a "break" (**Figure 16–21A and B**). **Stress fractures** or incomplete fractures may not actually break a bone into two pieces. Fractures can be caused by injury (trauma) or by disease that creates bone weakness (defined as *pathologic* fractures). Types of fractures are as follows:

- **Open fractures**: If the bone has protruded through the skin or an object has punctured the skin to break a bone; also called **compound fractures** as the fracture along with open skin create a "compound" problem; involve a high risk of bone infection and require cleaning and debridement (**Figure 16–22**)

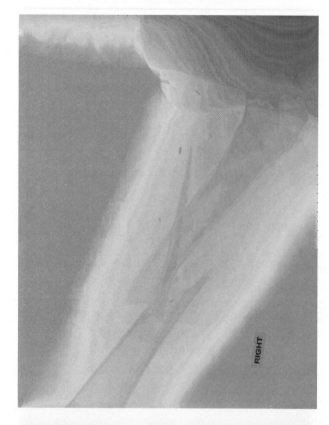

- **Closed fracture**: Also called a **simple fracture**
- **Complete fracture**: One that goes completely through a bone
- **Incomplete fracture**: When the bone is fractured but not in two pieces
- **Greenstick fracture**: Appears as a partial break
- **Displaced fracture**: When bone fragments are out of position
- **Comminuted fracture**: When there are more than two ends or fragments
- **Compression fracture**: When the bone appears to be "mashed" down; often occurs in the vertebrae of the spine
- **Impacted fracture**: Characterized as a bone forced over its other end
- **Avulsion fracture**: Describes a small bone fragment separated from the bone where a tendon or ligament is attached
- **Longitudinal fracture**: Runs the length of a bone
- **Transverse fracture**: Runs across, or at a 90-degree angle, to the bone
- **Oblique fracture**: Runs in a transverse pattern
- **Spiral fracture**: Twists around the bone
- **Stellate fracture**: Forms a star-like pattern

Other descriptive names used to identify the location of a fracture include *intracapsular, extracapsular, intertrochanteric, femoral neck,* and *subcapital* fractures. Some fractures are named for the physicians who first described them, such as *Colles'* or *Pott's* fractures. Fractures are fully described by using several descriptive names that describe their type, position, location, and other pieces of information. Fracture sites vary with age and the common activities of life. **Figure 16–23** shows many types of different fractures.

Signs and Symptoms

Fractures usually cause intense pain, inflammation, discoloration, and, when the skin is punctured, bleeding.

Etiology

Fractures, as discussed above, are usually caused by stress, trauma, or disease.

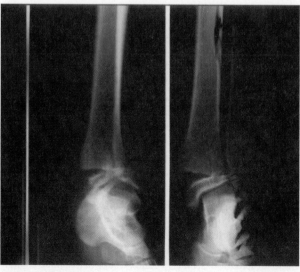

Figure 16–21 Fractures.

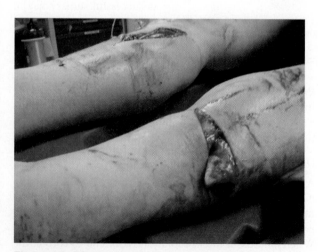

Figure 16–22 Open fracture.

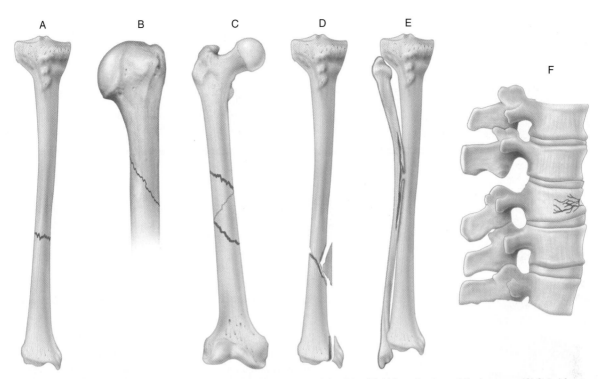

A   B   C   D   E   F

Figure 16–23 Classifications of fractures. (A) Transverse fracture of the tibia. (B) Oblique fracture of the humerus. (C) Spiral fracture of the femur. (D) Comminuted fracture of the tibia. (E) Greenstick fracture of the fibula. (F) Compression fracture of a vertebral body.

Diagnosis

Diagnosis of fractures involves physical examination (see **Figure 16–24**) and radiologic studies.

Treatment

First aid should be administered at the site of the accident or trauma, usually involving splinting the fracture site to immobilize it to prevent further injury. The caregiver should not attempt to realign the bone in any way. Once medical assistance is obtained, the fracture is usually "reduced" by surgical procedures such as "closed reductions," using radiography to determine bone positions.

If the fracture cannot be reduced with internal manipulation, the area is surgically opened for an "open reduction." Devices commonly used for this purpose include pins, plates, rods, or screws. Open reduction, internal fixation, or ORIF, is a method of surgically repairing a fractured bone by using the devices listed above to stabilize injured bones. ORIF is commonly used for fractures of the hips, elbows, ankles, heels, and knees.

Open fractures require cleaning and debridement of the involved tissue with large amounts of cleansing fluids to keep infection and osteomyelitis from developing. Splints or casts may be applied to immobilize the area while the fracture heals, usually over 4 to 8 weeks.

External fixators are devices mounted to injured bones through the skin. They are used when a cast will not allow proper alignment of a fracture. Holes are drilled into uninjured areas of bones around the fracture, and bolts and/or wires are screwed into the holes. Externally, a rod or curved piece of metal utilizes ball-and-socket joints that attach to the bolts to make a rigid support. Because the skin is pierced

when external fixators are applied, it is important to regularly clean the wounds to prevent infection. These devices are usually mounted in an operating room while the patient is under general anesthesia and may be removed in a simple medical office visit.

Traction may be applied to hold fractures in position, reduce muscle **spasms**, allow bone fragment ends to separate, and keep pain and tissue damage at a minimum. Skeletal traction is used over long periods of time or when large muscle groups are involved. This may involve implanting a pin through a bone and then attaching it to ropes, pulleys, and weights. Skin traction is used for short-term therapy or when small muscle groups are involved.

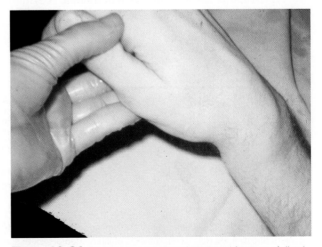

Figure 16–24 Physical examination of displaced fracture of distal radius and ulna.

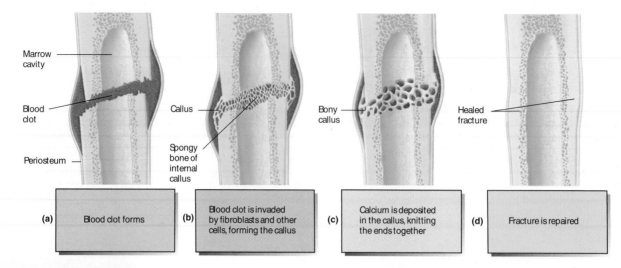

Marrow cavity

Blood clot

Periosteum

Callus

Spongy bone of internal callus

Bony callus

Healed fracture

(a) Blood clot forms

(b) Blood clot is invaded by fibroblasts and other cells, forming the callus

(c) Calcium is deposited in the callus, knitting the ends together

(d) Fracture is repaired

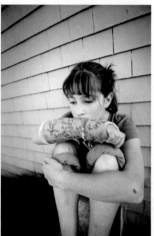

Figure 16–25 Stages of fracture repair.

The role of the PTA in assisting patients to recover from bone fractures is important in slowly increasing activities to avoid further injury. The PTA should educate the patient about movement of the joints not immobilized and may provide gait training with assistive devices or transfer training to maintain the patient's mobility. Once the bone is healed and repaired, it is safe to begin strength training activities.

The muscles initially will be very weak due to atrophy general nonuse.

Prognosis

Prognosis is usually good as long as treatments are initiated correctly and infection or other complications do not develop. Complications can include abnormal or nonhealing of the fracture, avascular necrosis, and osteomyelitis.

Herniated Intervertebral Disk

As part of the normal aging process, the intervertebral disks undergo a progressive "wear-and-tear" degeneration of both the nucleus and the **annulus**. The nucleus is the soft center portion, and the annulus is the tough, fibrous part that surrounds the nucleus. The *nucleus pulposus* acts as a shock absorber and distributes the mechanical stress applied to the spine when the body moves. Physical stress (usually a twisting motion) can tear or rupture the *annulus fibrosus* so the nucleus pulposus herniates into the spinal canal or elsewhere, such as posterolaterally. When this occurs the herniation causes nerve root impingement (irritation) and associated radiculopathy (nerve root pain). A herniated intervertebral disk is shown in **Figure 16–26**. Herniated intervertebral disk is also known as *spinal disk herniation*, *ruptured* or *slipped disk* (an older term), or *herniated nucleus pulposus*.

The nucleus becomes denser because its water content is reduced, and the annulus becomes weakened and thinned. Herniated disks usually occur in adults (men more than women) under age 45. Generally, they occur in the lumbrosacral region of the spine, particularly between the fourth and fifth lumbar vertebrae or between the fifth lumbar vertebrae and sacrum.

Signs and Symptoms

When there is pressure on a spinal nerve root due to a herniated nucleus pulposus, severe lower back pain often occurs, often radiating to the buttocks, legs, and feet (usually unilaterally). This is due to compression of nerve roots supplying these areas. There may be sudden pain and/or sciatic nerve pain after trauma, beginning as a dull pain in the buttocks.

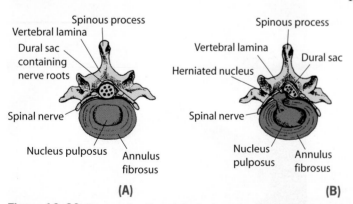

Spinous process
Vertebral lamina
Dural sac containing nerve roots
Spinal nerve
Nucleus pulposus
Annulus fibrosus

(A)

Spinous process
Vertebral lamina
Dural sac
Herniated nucleus
Spinal nerve
Nucleus pulposus
Annulus fibrosus

(B)

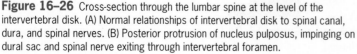

Figure 16–26 Cross-section through the lumbar spine at the level of the intervertebral disk. (A) Normal relationships of intervertebral disk to spinal canal, dura, and spinal nerves. (B) Posterior protrusion of nucleus pulposus, impinging on dural sac and spinal nerve exiting through intervertebral foramen.

Etiology

The three major causes of herniated intervertebral disks are

- Severe trauma or repeated **strain**
- Intervertebral joint degeneration (degenerative disk disease)
- Faulty posture and body function due to years of repetitive poor mechanics

New research suggests that *tumor necrosis factor-alpha* is a central cause of inflammatory spinal pain.

Diagnosis

Herniated intervertebral disks are diagnosed by physical examination and confirmed by MRI, CT scan, or *myelogram* (which involves injecting a contrast dye into the spinal canal and taking x-rays) **(Figure 16–27A, B, and C)**. Myelogram reveals spinal cord and/or spinal nerve compression.

Treatment

Treatment for chronic pain due to disk herniation may include heat application to decrease muscle spasm and aid in pain relief. However, heat should never be put on an acute disk

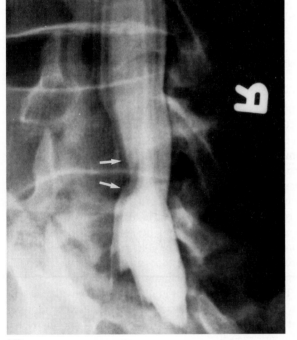

(A)

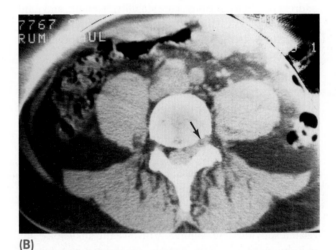

(B)

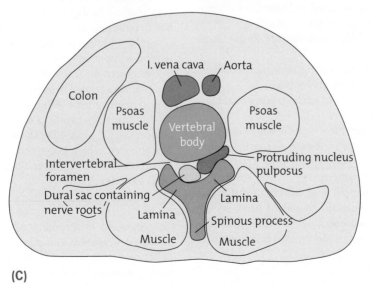

(C)

Figure 16–27 Demonstration of herniated nucleus pulposus ("slipped disk"). (A) X-ray examination obtained after radiopaque contrast material was instilled into dural sac (myelogram). Indentation of dural sac (arrows) results from herniated nucleus pulposus impinging on spinal dura. (B) CT scan of lumbar region. Protruding nucleus pulposus (arrow) is located adjacent to dural sac and fills intervertebral foramen (arrow). Compare with appearance of normal intervertebral foramen on opposite side. (C) Schematic of anatomic structures and lesion as demonstrated on CT scan.

herniation. Exercise programs to strengthen the trunk and core muscles and prevent further deterioration may be helpful. Anti-inflammatory medications such as aspirin, corticosteroids, and NSAIDs are often used. If these measures are not effective, surgery to remove the disk (**diskectomy**) may be indicated. Another type of surgery involves opening the area around the affected spinal nerve (**laminectomy**).

Specific and potent inhibitors of tumor necrosis factor are now available. Targeted anatomic administration of these inhibitors has been shown to be very helpful in treating severe pain caused by disk herniation, bulge, disk tear, or protrusion. Research is showing advancements in the use of stem cells to arrest degeneration or even regenerate intervertebral discs.

The role of the PTA in treating herniated intervertebral disk is very important. Physical therapy often plays a major role in herniated disk recovery. Passive treatments include deep tissue massage, hot and cold therapy, electrical stimulation (transcutaneous electrical nerve stimulation, or TENS), and aquatic therapy. Spinal traction may also be used to reduce the effects of gravity on the spine. Active treatments address flexibility, posture, core stability, strength, and joint movement. Physical therapy may include stretching, flexibility exercises, strength training, and various types of aerobics, including aquatic therapy.

Prognosis

Prognosis is varied based on extent of damage, effectiveness of treatment, and age of the patient.

Sprains

A **sprain** is defined as a traumatic injury to a joint. There may additionally be partial or complete tearing of ligaments. A sprain causes pain, warmth, swelling, and redness as well as potential discoloration (from purple to dark blue) due to blood vessel hemorrhage. Sprains are usually due to sports-related activities and commonly involve the ankle joint due to its biomechanics. Severe sprains involve complete tearing of ligaments. Also, tendons, muscles, and blood vessels may be involved. The following are grades of sprains:

- Grade 1: Slight stretching and damage to the fibrils of a ligament
- Grade 2: Partial ligament tearing; abnormal looseness (laxity) of an affected joint may appear
- Grade 3: Complete ligament tearing; gross instability of an affected joint appears

Usually, a physical examination is sufficient to diagnose a sprain. Additional measures include x-rays, arthroscopy, and MRI. It is important to rule out any bone fractures so treatment is adequate. Treatment depends on severity of the sprain. The "RICE" concepts (rest, ice, compression [via elastic bandages], and evaluation) should be used. As the sprain heals and the pain decreases, light exercise and walking are indicated. Prognosis is good unless bone fracture is detected.

Strains

A *strain* is defined as an overstretching of a muscle that causes injury. Strains are less serious than sprains. Symptoms of a strain include pain, soreness, and tenderness. Strains are simply caused by overusing a muscle so it becomes damaged temporarily. For example, lifting too much weight is a common cause of lumbar strain. Strains are usually diagnosed via patient history and physical examination. There is often swelling and tenderness in the affected area. The grades of a strain are as follows:

- Grade 1: Damage to less than 5 percent of muscle fibers; requires 2 to 3 weeks of rest.
- Grade 2: More extensive muscle damage but not a complete rupture; requires 3 to 6 weeks of rest.
- Grade 3: Complete rupture of a muscle; rehabilitation time is approximately 3 months; if this occurs in a sportsperson, surgery to repair the muscle is usually indicated.

Strains are treated by rest, analgesics, anti-inflammatory medications, and moist heat. As pain decreases physical therapy is indicated to restore flexibility and strength to the affected area. Prognosis is good with adequate rest and treatment.

Tendinitis

Tendinitis is defined as inflammation of a tendon (the connective tissue that attaches muscle to bone). Tendinitis can occur anywhere in the body, with the shoulder being the most common site. It is informally also spelled as "tendonitis." The term *tendinosis* is defined as damage to a tendon at the cellular level, believed to be caused by *microtears* that lead to an increase in tendon repair cells. It is usually brought on by repetitive motion. Chronic tendon degeneration is more common with age, and poor fitness makes sports injuries (commonly seen in tennis or golf) much more common. In chronic tendinosis the body does not repair collagen properly. Tendinosis is often misdiagnosed as *tendinitis*.

Tendinitis causes either gradual pain or pain that is sudden and severe. Tendinitis is commonly caused by motions that are repetitive or by calcium deposits. It may be related to bursitis as well.

Athletes most likely to develop tendinitis are those who play baseball, basketball, or tennis or who swim on a regular basis. Tendinitis is diagnosed by physical examination that reveals tenderness and pain when the muscle to which the tendon is attached is moved or worked against resistance.

Treatment for tendinitis includes rest, application of ice packs (unless related to bursitis), analgesics, and anti-inflammatory medications. After pain decreases, active range-of-motion exercises can help to restore motion. Surgery may be necessary if joint **adhesions** (fibrin that collects to help heal the area, which is not properly reabsorbed afterwards) are present. Prognosis of tendinitis is good unless joint adhesions have developed.

Compartment Syndrome

Compartment syndrome is a serious condition involving increased pressure in a muscle compartment of the body, such as between the two lower leg bones. It can lead to nerve and muscle damage as well as problems with blood flow. Thick layers of tissue (*fascia*) separate groups of muscles in the arms and legs from each other. Inside each layer of fascia is a confined space known as a *compartment*, containing muscle tissue, blood vessels, and nerves. Because fasciae do not expand, any swelling in the compartment leads to increased pressure on the muscle tissue, blood vessels, and nerves. Sufficient pressure can block blood flow completely, leading to sufficient injury that requires immediate emergency attention and surgery to prevent the need for amputation.

Signs and Symptoms

Compartment syndrome is most common between the two bones of the lower leg and forearm. It also occurs in the hand, foot, thigh, and upper arm. The major symptom is severe pain that does not subside when the affected area is raised or when pain medication is taken. Other symptoms include decreased sensation, skin paleness, and weakness.

Etiology

Trauma from car accidents or other occurrences that can result in crushing leads to compartment syndrome. Surgery and complex fractures can also cause the condition. Long-term (chronic) compartment syndrome can also be caused by repetitive activities (such as running). It may also be related to frostbite or other injuries caused by extremely cold temperatures. Poorly fitting casts are a common cause due to compression of the nerve; this is true more often in the lower extremities than in the upper extremities.

Diagnosis

Diagnosis of compartment syndrome is made by physical examination of the affected area. Pain results when the area is squeezed. The skin appears swollen and shiny, and movement of the area causes severe pain. Confirmation is made by measuring the compartment's pressure by inserting a needle attached to a pressure meter. Pressure measurements are performed during and after an activity that causes pain in the compartment.

Treatment

Surgery is used to create long cuts through the fascia to relieve the pressure. The wounds can be left open but covered with a sterile dressing. A second surgery to close the wounds is completed 48 to 72 hours after the initial surgery. Skin grafts may be needed to close the wounds.

Prognosis

Prognosis is excellent as long as prompt diagnosis and treatment occur. Overall prognosis is determined by the type of injury causing compartment syndrome. If diagnosis is delayed, permanent nerve injury and loss of muscle function can occur within only 12 to 24 hours after initial injury.

Muscle and Connective Tissue Diseases

Younger people more commonly experience diseases of the muscles and connective tissues than joint disorders. Some of these diseases have the potential to shorten the life of the patient. These disorders include myositis, polymyositis, muscular atrophy, **muscular dystrophy** (MD), and myasthenia gravis.

Myositis (Myopathy)

The term *myositis* is also known as *idiopathic inflammatory myopathy*. Myositis is defined as inflammation of the skeletal muscles. It may be caused by injury, infection, or autoimmune diseases. Myositis actually describes several different conditions: *dermatomyositis*, *inclusion-body myositis*, juvenile

types of myositis, and *polymyositis*. All these conditions cause swelling and muscle loss. Many cases of myositis are of unknown origin. Aside from muscle weakness and overall fatigue, myositis may also cause a skin rash, which is helpful in diagnosing the condition.

Diagnosis is also based on patient history, blood tests, muscle and skin biopsies, electrodiagnostic tests and antibody testing. Treatment involves a variety of medications (corticosteroids, immunosuppressants, intravenous immune globulin, monoclonal antibodies), protein therapies, and exercise regimens. Vitamin supplements may also be indicated.

> **RED FLAG**
> Several hormonal diseases, autoimmune disorders, and metabolic disorders may cause muscle weakness.

Polymyositis

Polymyositis is a muscle disease involving muscle inflammation near the trunk or torso. It is a chronic condition resulting in severe muscle weakness.

Signs and Symptoms

Polymyositis produces severe muscle weakness resulting in loss of muscle power and atrophy. Other symptoms include difficulty swallowing and moving of the neck muscles, skin inflammation, rash, fatigue, general malaise, and bony prominences of the knuckles, elbows, and knees. About two-thirds of patients with polymyositis are female.

Etiology

Polymyositis is of unknown origin but occurs when white blood cells spontaneously invade muscle tissues.

Diagnosis

Diagnosis is achieved through patient history, physical examination, and intense screening for cancer (because this disorder often accompanies various cancer conditions). Blood analysis is used to search for elevated levels of muscle enzymes. Electromyography shows an abnormal pattern of electrical activity in the inflamed muscles, and a muscle biopsy confirms the diagnosis (**Figure 16–28**).

Treatment

Treatment is directed toward stopping inflammation and inhibiting the overactive immune system. Medications include high doses of steroids and the use of immunosuppressive

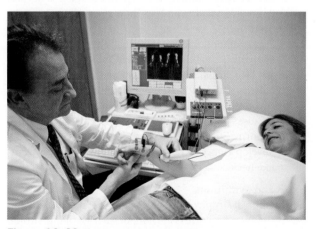

Figure 16–28 An electromyography in progress.

agents (cyclophosphamide and methotrexate). Exercise therapy is added to increase strength and stop muscle atrophy.

The role of the PTA in polymyositis focuses on physical therapy designed to prevent muscle atrophy and regain muscle strength and range of motion. Physical therapy is highly individualized for each patient's needs and abilities. Walking is indicated after all other physical exercise. Low-impact weight training is very useful for therapy for polymyositis. All weight training should be fully supervised.

Prognosis

Prognosis is good as long as medical treatment begins early in the disease's progress. Polymyositis often becomes inactive, and atrophied muscle can be rehabilitated with long-term physical therapy.

Muscular Atrophy

Muscular atrophy may occur when there is a lack of frequent movements against resistance. When the muscles are not used adequately, they shrink in size. Muscle fiber diameter decreases due to a loss of protein filaments. They become weaker (*disuse atrophy*) due to lack of innervation. This condition is commonly seen in debilitated patients who are immobilized. *Denervation atrophy* occurs because of disorders that deprive muscles of their innervation.

When muscle cells die or their axons are destroyed, temporary and spontaneous contractions (*fibrillations*) occur. Contractile proteins are lost and degeneration of the muscles occurs. It is possible for regenerating axons to grow down the connective tissue tube and regenerate muscle cells. If reinnervation occurs after muscle cells have degenerated, no recovery is possible.

Muscular Dystrophy

MD is a term that describes a number of genetic disorders that cause progressive deterioration of skeletal muscles. These conditions develop because of mixed muscle cell hypertrophy, atrophy, and necrosis. As the muscles undergo necrosis, fat and other connective tissue replace muscle fiber. This increases muscle size and results in muscle weakness. MD affects skeletal muscle and is an inherited disorder. *Duchenne's dystrophy* is the most common form, usually affecting boys beginning between ages 2 and 5. Other forms of MD are as follows:

- Becker MD: Similar to Duchenne's but less severe; it involves faulty or less than normal amounts of dystrophin.
- Facioscapulohumeral MD: Usually begins during teenage years, causing progressive muscle weakness in the face, arms, legs, shoulders and chest; it can vary between mild and extremely disabling.
- Myotonic MD: The most common adult form of MD; it causes prolonged muscle spasms, cataracts, cardiac abnormalities, and endocrine disturbances. Patients develop long, thin faces, drooping eyelids, and a swan-like neck.

Signs and Symptoms

Duchenne's dystrophy is usually asymptomatic at birth and during infancy. Early gross movement such as rolling, sitting, and standing occur at the proper age. The postural muscles of the shoulder and hip are usually the first to be affected. Signs of muscle weakness usually become evident starting at 2 to 3 years of age, when frequent falling begins to occur. Other symptoms include leg muscle atrophy and lordosis. Because of weakened pelvic muscles the patient may be unable to get up from a squatting position without using what is known as "Gower's maneuver" (a series of motions including crawling, tripod position, and bracing the body against the floor and walls to stand erect). MD usually causes the patient to become wheelchair-bound by age 9.

Etiology

Duchenne's MD is a sex-linked condition, usually passed from mother to son.

Diagnosis

Diagnosis of MD is based on physical examination, electromyography, and muscle biopsy.

Treatment

Muscular dystrophy is treated with orthopedic devices such as leg braces, physical therapy, and exercise, which help to maintain the patient's mobility. The role of the PTA with muscular dystrophy patients is to assist with weight exercises to strengthen and tone their muscles. Range-of-motion exercises and stretching are very helpful. The PTA should be trained in working with patients who have to wear orthotics or use other medical devices. Aquatic therapy and swimming can also be very beneficial to MD patients.

Prognosis

Prognosis is poor because the muscle wasting of MD usually causes early death.

Myasthenia Gravis

Myasthenia gravis is an autoimmune disorder involving muscle weakness and fatigue that is partially relieved by adequate rest. It occurs as a result of the blocking of acetylcholine neurotransmitters by neuromuscular junction antibodies. See Chapter 10 for a discussion of autoimmune disorders.

Rhabdomyolysis

Rhabdomyolysis is defined as a rapid breakdown of skeletal muscle tissue. It results in a large release of creatine phosphokinase enzymes and other cell byproducts into the bloodstream. As muscle breakdown products accumulate, acute renal failure may result.

Signs and Symptoms

Signs and symptoms of rhabdomyolysis include muscle pain, ranging from mild to severe; urine color changes; massive skeletal muscle necrosis; shock; hyperkalemia, leading to fatal dysrhythmias; and acute renal failure.

Etiology

Rhabdomyolysis may be caused by mechanical, physical, or chemical traumatic injury. Mechanical causes include crushing, burns, compression injuries, and compartment syndrome. Physical causes include prolonged high fever, hyperthermia, electrical or lightning injuries, and excessive physical exertion. Chemical causes include medications, excessive alcohol use, abnormal electrolytes, infections, endocrine disorders, muscle enzyme deficiencies, and, rarely, mushroom poisoning or use of herbal supplements that contain ephedra.

Diagnosis

Diagnosis of rhabdomyolysis is made by patient history and signs and symptoms and is confirmed by laboratory studies revealing abnormal renal function and elevated creatine phosphokinase. A careful medication history is helpful in diagnosing the condition. A urine dipstick test may be positive for blood, although no cells may be seen on microscopic analysis.

Treatment

Treatment of rhabdomyolysis is directed toward rehydration of the patient and correction of electrolyte imbalances via administration of intravenous fluids. If renal failure exists, dialysis may be necessary. In cases of exertional rhabdomyolysis, damage to skeletal muscles usually resolves on its own. Clinically significant rhabdomyolysis is rare but may be life threatening.

The role of the PTA in rhabdomyolysis is often overlooked. Once the patient has been cleared of ongoing pathologic processes, active physical therapy may be initiated. This includes range-of-motion exercises (active and passive), endurance exercises, and gradual resistance training. Most patients can return to training within 4 weeks of onset of rhabdomyolysis.

Prognosis

Prognosis of rhabdomyolysis depends significantly on underlying causes and whether complications have occurred.

SUMMARY

The musculoskeletal system is made up of bones, joints, ligaments, muscles, and tendons. Joints are classified by amount of movement as synarthrotic, amphiarthrotic, or diarthrotic. Contraction and relaxation of muscle fibers controls body movement, as directed by the nervous system. Most muscles in the body are under voluntary control. Pain, disability, and immobility are the most common symptoms of musculoskeletal system disorders.

Diagnosis of musculoskeletal disorders is usually made by physical examination, x-rays, CT scan, and MRI. Fractures are a major type of musculoskeletal system disorder. These disorders may frequently require devices such as crutches, canes, and walkers. Ankylosing spondylitis causes inflammation in the joints between the spinal bones.

Osteoarthritis and RA can be differentiated basically because osteoarthritis often begins on one side of the body, whereas RA affects both sides initially. Compartment syndrome involves pressure in a muscle compartment that can lead to nerve and muscle damage as well as blood flow disorders that may require amputation of affected areas.

REVIEW QUESTIONS

Select the best response to each question.

1. Vitamin D deficiency may cause which of the following conditions?
   a. night blindness
   b. hemorrhage
   c. pernicious anemia
   d. rickets

2. An abnormal lateral curvature of the spine is called
   a. kyphosis
   b. scoliosis
   c. spondylosis
   d. lordosis

3. Most cases of osteomyelitis are caused by which microorganism?
   a. *Staphylococcus aureus*
   b. *Klebsiella pneumoniae*
   c. *Escherichia coli*
   d. *Mycobacterium tuberculosis*

4. The pathogenesis of osteoporosis is which of the following?
   a. deficiency of vitamins D and K
   b. deficiency of estrogen and progesterone
   c. obesity
   d. unknown etiology

5. The most common malignant tumor of bone is which of the following?
   a. Ewing's sarcoma
   b. chondrosarcoma
   c. osteosarcoma
   d. Kaposi's sarcoma

6. Deposition of uric acid in joints may cause which condition?
   a. gout
   b. avascular necrosis
   c. rheumatoid arthritis
   d. osteoarthritis

7. Which of the following is a possible cause of compartment syndrome?
   a. crushing injuries
   b. frostbite
   c. gout
   d. both A and B

8. Which of the following disorders occurs as a result of the blocking of acetylcholine neurotransmitters in the neuromuscular junction?
   a. tetanus
   b. myasthenia gravis
   c. myositis
   d. bursitis

9. Bone cells responsible for resorption of bone and removing mineral content are known as
   a. osteocytes
   b. osteoblasts
   c. osteoclasts
   d. periosteum

10. A painful condition in which the medial nerve becomes pressed at the wrist is called
    a. carpal tunnel syndrome
    b. arthritis
    c. bursitis
    d. ganglion cyst

CASE STUDIES

Karen Coupe, PT, DPT, MSEd

Case 1

A 75-year-old woman was referred to physical therapy for general strengthening and gait training after a three-level thoracic kyphoplasty. Patient medical history: Spinal osteoporosis, bilateral hip osteopenia, hypertension controlled by medication, alcoholic from ages 55 to 68, gastric bypass surgery 10 years ago.

1. Compare and contrast osteoporosis with osteopenia.
2. What is the primary diagnostic test for both pathologies, and what determines one diagnosis over the other?
3. What are the risk factors for osteoporosis? Looking at the patient's past medical history, are there additional risk factors for this patient?
4. What is the purpose of a kyphoplasty? How is the procedure different from a vertebroplasty?
5. The physician referral is for general strengthening and gait training. What precautions and/or contraindications should the PTA heed for a patient with osteopenia and/or osteoporosis?

Case 2

A 44-year-old man was referred to physical therapy with a diagnosis of a posterolateral L4–5 disk herniation with radiculopathy. Occupational history: Car mechanic since age 18. Patient medical history: Early stages of lumbar spondylosis. Previous level of function: Independent in all activities. Current level of function: Ambulates with decreased cadence and lack of arm swing, unable to sit beyond 5 minutes secondary to increased s/s, unable to work. Plan of care includes mechanical lumbar traction, therapeutic exercise, and instruction in body mechanics and positioning.

1. Explain the components of a disk and what occurs with a disk herniation.
2. Explain radiculopathy and why this could occur with a disk herniation. Could a patient have a herniation without radiculopathy?
3. What are the most common causes of disk herniation? Is the patient's occupation a potential risk factor? Why or why not.
4. The plan of care includes mechanical lumbar traction and body mechanics. Explain the effects of traction on a herniated disk. What educational material on body mechanics is important for this patient?
5. List and briefly explain the potential surgical procedures for a disk herniation.

WEBSITES

http://orthoinfo.aaos.org/topic.cfm?topic=a00420

http://www.healthcentral.com/channel/408/1278.html

http://www.mayoclinic.com/health/herniated-disk/ds00893

http://www.merck.com/mmhe/sec05/ch058/ch058g.html

http://www.ninds.nih.gov/disorders/carpal_tunnel/detail_carpal_tunnel.htm

http://www.nlm.nih.gov/medlineplus/bonediseases.html

http://www.peoples-health.com/joint_dislocation.htm

http://www.webmd.com/a-to-z-guides/understanding-fractures-basic-information

http://www.wrongdiagnosis.com/sym/joint_disease.htm

Respiratory System Disorders

LEARNING OBJECTIVES

After completion of this chapter the reader should be able to

1. Explain the structures and functions of the respiratory system.
2. Describe the causes and clinical effects of chronic bronchitis.
3. Define hemothorax and pleural effusion.
4. Differentiate between bronchitis and bronchiectasis.
5. Describe the clinical manifestations and treatment of chronic obstructive pulmonary disease.
6. Describe the cause and manifestations of bronchial asthma and respiratory distress syndrome.
7. Explain the cause and effects of pulmonary embolism.
8. Describe the risk factors for lung cancer and the principles of treatment.

KEY TERMS

Acini: Clusters of cells with a "berry-like" appearance, such as the alveoli of the lungs.

Acute bronchitis: Inflammation of the large bronchi, usually caused by viruses or bacteria, that lasts for several days or weeks.

Acute rhinitis: Acute inflammation of the nose and nasal membranes.

Adult respiratory distress syndrome (ARDS): A serious reaction to various types of injuries to the lung.

Anthracosis: Any lung disease related to inhalation of coal or carbon.

Apnea: Suspension of external breathing.

Arterial blood gases: Blood tests performed by using blood from an artery; the tests are used to determine blood pH, partial pressure of carbon dioxide and oxygen, and bicarbonate levels.

Asbestosis: A chronic inflammatory, fibrotic condition that affects the lungs due to inhalation and retention of asbestos fibers.

Asthma: A common chronic inflammatory disease of the airways characterized by variable, recurring airflow obstruction and bronchospasm.

Atelectasis: The lack of gas exchange within alveoli, due to alveolar collapse or fluid consolidation.

Bronchiectasis: Localized, irreversible dilation of part of the bronchial tree.

Bronchoscopy: A method of visualizing the inside of the airways by inserting a bronchoscope through the mouth or nose and, sometimes, via a tracheostomy.

Chronic bronchitis: A chronic inflammation of the bronchi in the lungs defined as a persistent cough that produces sputum and mucus lasting between 3 months and 2 years.

Chronic obstructive pulmonary disease: A condition that refers to both chronic bronchitis and emphysema in which the airways become narrowed.

KEY TERMS CONTINUED

Clubbing: A deformity of (usually) the fingers and fingernails usually related to various conditions of the lungs and heart.

Cyanosis: A blue coloration of the skin and mucous membranes due to higher than normal levels of deoxygenated hemoglobin in blood vessels near the skin surface.

Dysphonia: An impaired ability to produce normal vocal sounds.

Dyspnea: Shortness of breath.

Emphysema: Long-term, progressive lung disease that primarily causes shortness of breath; it causes the airways to become unable to hold their functional shape when exhaling.

Empyema: A collection of pus within an anatomic cavity.

Hemoptysis: Coughing up of blood or blood-stained sputum from the bronchi, larynx, trachea, or lungs.

Hypoxemia: Decreased partial pressure of oxygen in the blood.

Hypoxia: A deprivation of adequate oxygen supply.

Induration: An area of soft tissue or organ hardening.

Influenza: The "flu"; a viral infection that causes chills, fever, muscle pains, sore throat, coughing, severe headache, weakness, fatigue, and general malaise.

Laryngitis: Inflammation of the larynx.

Orthopnea: Shortness of breath that occurs when the patient is lying flat.

Pharyngitis: Inflammation of the throat or pharynx.

Pleural effusion: Excess fluid that accumulates in the pleural spaces that surround the lungs.

Pleurisy: Inflammation of the pleura; it causes sharp pain when breathing in.

Pneumoconioses: Occupational, restrictive lung diseases caused by inhalation of various types of dust.

Pneumothorax: A collection of air or gas in the pleural cavity between the lung and chest wall.

Productive cough: A cough that produces phlegm.

Pulmonary abscess: A collection of pus inside lung tissue.

Pulmonary edema: Fluid accumulation in the lungs.

Pulmonary embolism: A blockage of the main artery of the lung, or one of its branches, by a thrombus (blood clot) from elsewhere in the body.

Rales: Clicking, crackling, or rattling noises of the lungs when breathing in.

Rhinorrhea: "Runny nose"; a discharge or flow of nasal fluids.

Rhonchi: Harsh, rattling sounds usually caused by bronchial secretions.

Silicosis: A type of occupational lung disease caused by inhalation of crystalline silica dust; it is a type of pneumoconiosis.

Sinusitis: Inflammation of the paranasal sinuses.

Sputum: Secretions expelled from the respiratory tract, such as mucus or phlegm (mixed with saliva).

Status asthmaticus: An acute exacerbation of asthma that is resistant to standard bronchodilators and steroid treatments.

Tachypnea: Rapid breathing.

Wheezing: Continuous, harsh whistling sound produced during exhalation.

Overview

The respiratory system provides the mechanisms for transporting oxygen from the air into the blood and for removing carbon dioxide from the blood. Oxygen is vital for cell metabolism. Carbon dioxide is a waste material that results from cell metabolism, which influences the acid-base balance in body fluids. Breathing is a complex process that involves the neurologic, circulatory, and respiratory systems. The circulatory system transports oxygen and carbon dioxide in the bloodstream.

In working with patients who have respiratory conditions, the physical therapist assistant (PTA) will have to work around various types of accessory devices:

- Continuous positive airway pressure devices keep the airway open so the user does not stop breathing while asleep.
- Ventilators provide a mechanism of breathing for people who cannot breathe on their own.
- Pocket face masks safely deliver rescue breaths during cardiac or respiratory arrest.

- Bag valve masks provide positive pressure ventilation to patients who are not breathing or who are breathing inadequately.
- Nasal cannulas deliver supplemental oxygen or airflow to patients needing respiratory help.
- Non-rebreather masks are used for patients in emergencies who require oxygen therapy at higher concentrations.
- Flow-restricted, oxygen-powered ventilation devices are manually triggered to assist with ventilation for apneic or hypoventilating patients and to provide supplemental oxygen for breathing patients.
- Inhalers are used to deliver medications into the body via the lungs, primarily to treat asthma or chronic obstructive pulmonary disease (COPD).
- Airway adjuncts are devices used to assist with breathing by use of either an oropharyngeal or nasopharyngeal tube.

Anatomy and Physiology of the Respiratory System

The respiratory system consists of the upper and lower respiratory tracts. The organs of the *upper respiratory tract* include the nose, nasal cavity, paranasal sinuses, and pharynx (**Figure 17–1**). The organs of the *lower respiratory tract* include the larynx, trachea, bronchial tree, and lungs (**Figure 17–2**).

The *nose* is supported by both bone and cartilage and has two openings (*nostrils*) that allow air to enter and leave the nasal cavity. Internal hairs prevent large air particles from entering the nasal cavity. The *nasal cavity* is actually a hollow space behind the nose that is divided into right and left portions by the *nasal septum*. The bones and bone processes that curl outward from the lateral walls of the nasal cavity are known as the *nasal conchae*. The mucous membranes contain many goblet cells, which secrete mucus, and networks of blood vessels. Heat from these blood vessels warms incoming air so it becomes closer to body temperature. Incoming air is also moistened by water that evaporates from the mucous membranes. Mucus is secreted to trap dust and small particles that enter along with the air. Entrapped particles are pushed by the cilia of the epithelial lining toward the pharynx, where they are swallowed. Upon reaching the stomach, gastric juices destroy any microorganisms contained in the mucus.

The *paranasal sinuses* are air-filled spaces located inside the maxillary, frontal, ethmoid, and sphenoid bones of the skull. They open into the nasal cavity and also contain mucous membranes. The paranasal sinuses serve to act as resonant chambers, which affect the quality of the voice, and to reduce the weight of the skull.

The *pharynx* (throat) is located behind the oral cavity, nasal cavity, and larynx. It allows food to pass from the oral cavity to the esophagus and also allows air to pass from the nasal cavity to the larynx. The pharynx also helps to produce the vocal sounds needed for speech and is subdivided into the nasopharynx, oropharynx, and laryngopharynx.

The *larynx* is located in the airway above the trachea and below the pharynx. It allows air in and out of the trachea while preventing foreign objects from entering. It contains the *vocal cords* and is made up of muscles and cartilages bound by elastic tissue. The primary cartilages of the larynx are the *thyroid* (Adam's apple), *cricoid*, and *epiglottic cartilages*. Two pairs of horizontal *vocal folds* extend inward. The upper folds (*false vocal cords*) help to close the airway during swallowing but do not produce vocal sounds. The lower folds (*true vocal cords*) vibrate from side to side because of air forced between them (**Figure 17–3A, B, and C**). This generates sound waves that are the basis for vocal sounds. The pharynx and oral cavity change shape, working with the tongue and lips to produce words. Increasing tension on the vocal cords raises the pitch, whereas relaxing tension lowers it. Stronger blasts of air in the vocal cords produce more volume.

During normal breathing the vocal cords are relaxed, and the *glottis* between them is shaped like a triangular slit. When food or liquids are swallowed, muscles inside the false vocal cords close the glottis to prevent them from entering the trachea. Cartilage supports a flap-like *epiglottis*, which usually stands upright to allow air inside the larynx. When swallowing, the larynx rises and the epiglottis presses downward, partially covering the opening of the larynx. This keeps foods and liquids from entering the air passages.

The *trachea* (windpipe) is a flexible tube about 12.5 centimeters in length, extending downward to the esophagus. It continues into the thoracic cavity, splitting into the right and left bronchi. Inside the walls of the trachea are approximately 20 C-shaped pieces of hyaline cartilage. Each piece has an open end toward the back of the trachea, with smooth muscle and connective tissues filling the gaps. The rings keep the trachea from collapsing and blocking the airway. The soft tissues in the back of each ring allow the esophagus to expand as food moves through.

The *bronchial tree* leads from the trachea to the alveoli (microscopic air sacs in the lungs). The branches of the bronchial tree begin with the right and left *primary bronchi*, arising from the trachea near the fifth thoracic vertebra. Each primary bronchus soon divides into secondary bronchi, branching into tertiary bronchi, and then smaller and smaller tubes, including the *bronchioles*. These smaller tubes divide into terminal and respiratory bronchioles, alveolar ducts, and end in thin-walled alveolar sacs. These sacs lead to the microscopic *alveoli* inside capillary networks.

The tubes that branch from each bronchus have less cartilage than the trachea, with more smooth muscle. The alveolar ducts have only a few muscle fibers in comparison. The mucous membranes of the bronchial tree branches filter

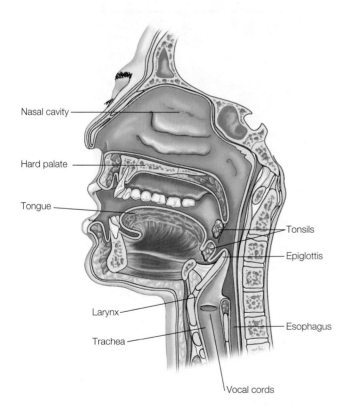

Nasal cavity

Hard palate

Tongue

Tonsils

Epiglottis

Larynx

Esophagus

Trachea

Vocal cords

Figure 17–1 The upper respiratory tract.

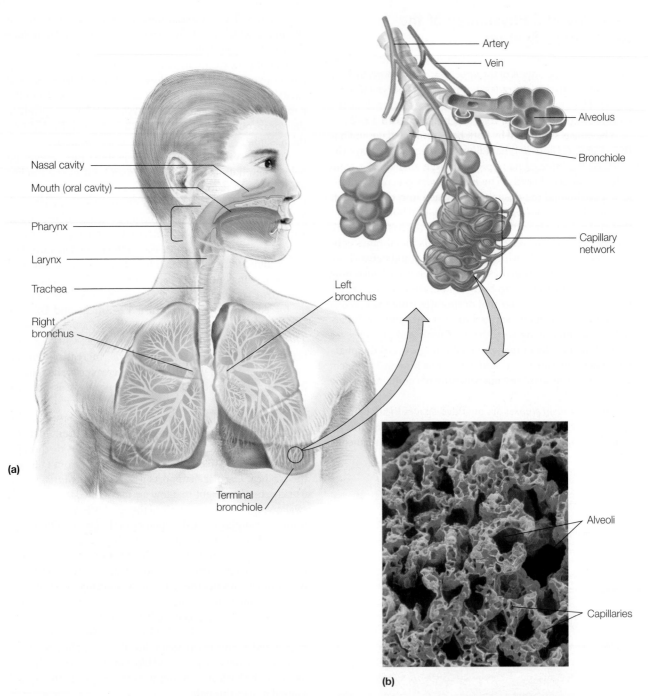

Figure 17–2 The respiratory system. (A) This illustration shows the air-conducting portion and the gas-exchange portion of the human respiratory system. The insert shows a higher magnification of the alveoli where oxygen and carbon dioxide exchange occurs. (B) A scanning electron micrograph of the alveoli, showing the rich capillary network surrounding them.

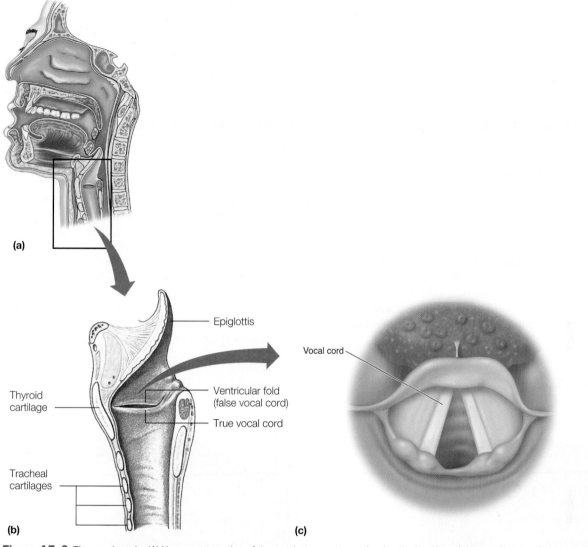

(a)

Epiglottis

Thyroid
cartilage

Ventricular fold
(false vocal cord)

True vocal cord

Tracheal
cartilages

(b)

Vocal cord

(c)

Figure 17–3 The vocal cords. (A) Uppermost portion of the respiratory system, showing the location of the vocal cords. (B) Longitudinal section of the larynx showing the location of the vocal cords. Note the presence of the false vocal cord, so named because it does not function in phonation. (C) View into the larynx of a patient showing the true vocal cords from above.

incoming air and distribute it to the alveoli of the lungs. The alveoli provide a large surface area of squamous epithelial cells where gas exchange can easily occur. Oxygen moves from the alveoli into the nearby capillary blood, and carbon dioxide moves from this blood into the alveoli.

The lungs are spongy and differ in size from each other. The right lung has three lobes, but the left lung has only two because it must also accommodate the heart in its side of the chest (**Figure 17–4A and B**). The lungs are found in the pleural cavity, which is lined with the membranous *pleura* in the thorax. A second pleura covers the lungs. Between the two pleural membranes is a liquid that lubricates them and prevents friction from occurring during the breathing process.

The airways of the respiratory system are basically divided into two parts: the upper and lower respiratory systems. The upper respiratory system includes the nose, nasal cavities, mouth, sinuses, pharynx, and larynx. The lower respiratory system includes the trachea, bronchi, and bronchioles. At the distal end of the terminal bronchioles the alveoli (grape-like clusters of tiny air sacs) are surrounded by capillaries (**Figure 17–5**). At this point the exchange of carbon dioxide and oxygen occurs in the lungs.

Respiration has two functions: ventilation and gas exchange. *Ventilation* is defined as movement of air into and out of the respiratory system. The rate varies with the patient's age and health condition. Ventilation is also called *breathing. Gas exchange* occurs between alveolar air and pulmonary capillaries. Chemosensory receptors in spinal fluid control ventilation via arterial carbon dioxide tension as well as deficiency of oxygen in the aortic and carotid arteries. When decreases or increases in carbon dioxide and/or oxygen are sensed, ventilation increases or decreases accordingly. The respiratory control center in the medulla of the brain controls respiration but may be altered by either respiratory or neurologic disease.

At the tissue level the exchange of gases occurs in the lungs and throughout the body. Inside the lungs the capillary beds release carbon dioxide into the alveolar spaces by a process known as *diffusion*. Similarly, oxygen is moved from the air spaces into the capillaries so it can be transported to the tissues. At the tissue level, throughout the body, this process is reversed. Oxygen is moved from the bloodstream into the tissues, whereas carbon dioxide moves from the tissues into the blood. It is then transported to the lungs and removed from the body (**Figure 17–6**).

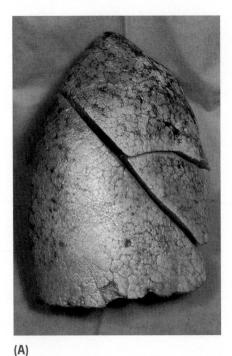

(A)

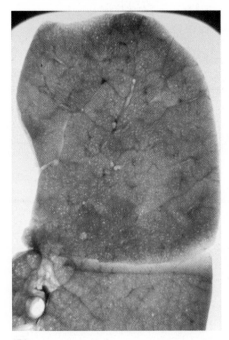

(B)

Figure 17–4 Normal lung that has been inflated and air dried so that the structure of the lobes and lobules can be visualized and the fine structure of the alveoli can be studied. (A) External surface illustrating lobes and fissues. The faint cobblestonelike pattern of the pleural surface defines the individual lung lobules. (B) A backlighted section of lung illustrating the fine, spongelike pattern produced by the respiratory units where gas exchange occurs.

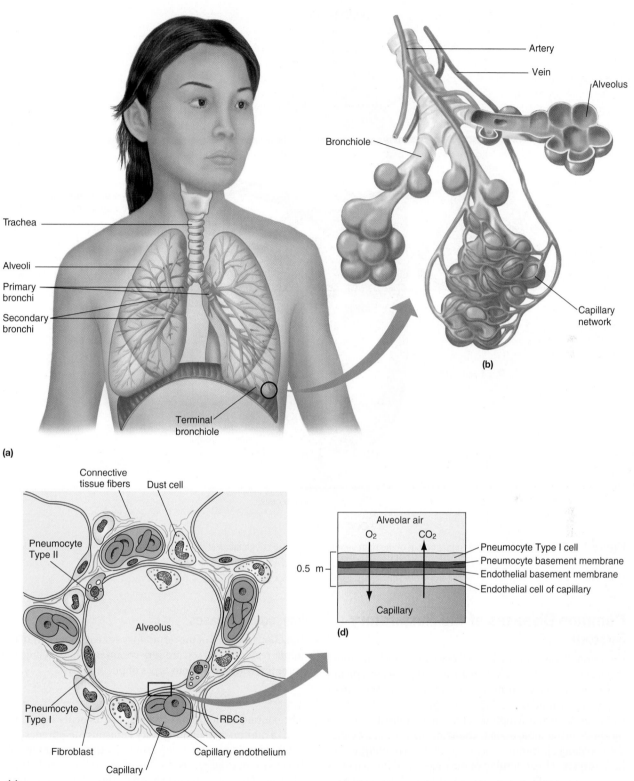

Figure 17–5 The trachea (A) conveys air from the larynx to the bronchi, which distribute air throughout the lungs. The alveolar wall (B) includes pneumocyte type I and II cells (C), dust cells and the endothelial cells of the alveolar capillaries. Gases must cross a thin membrane (D), composed of pneumocyte type I cells and their basement membrane, and endothelial cells and their basement membrane to diffuse between the blood and the alveolar air.

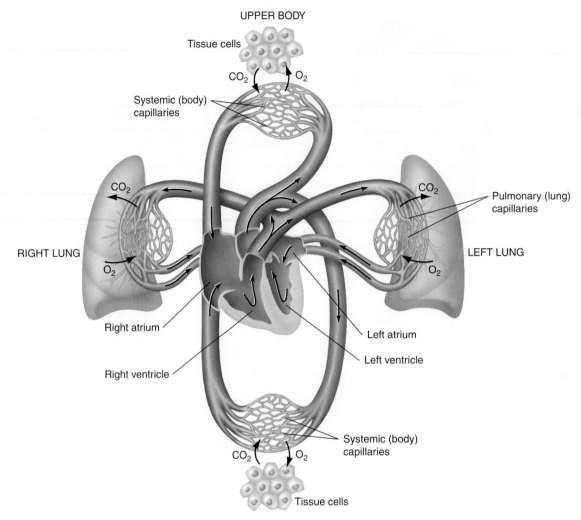

UPPER BODY

Tissue cells

CO_2 O_2

Systemic (body)
capillaries

CO_2 Pulmonary (lung)
capillaries

RIGHT LUNG   LEFT LUNG

O_2 O_2

Right atrium   Left atrium

Left ventricle

Right ventricle

Systemic (body)
capillaries

CO_2 O_2

Tissue cells

LOWER BODY

Figure 17–6 The lungs receive the entire output of the right ventricle. Following oxygenation in the lungs, this blood returns to the left side of the heart.

Common Diseases of the Respiratory System

Common diseases of the respiratory system include upper respiratory tract diseases, bronchi and lung diseases, pleura and chest diseases, cardiovascular-related diseases, pneumothorax, hemothorax, and those that cause suffocation. Common signs and symptoms of respiratory disease include **dyspnea, orthopnea, apnea, wheezing, hypoxemia, cyanosis**, coughing up **sputum** (meaning **productive cough**), and **hemoptysis**. Also, **clubbing** of the fingers and fingernails is a condition usually related to poor distal circulation of oxygenated blood (**Figure 17–7**).

Diagnostic tests for respiratory conditions may look for **tachypnea**, **rales**, and **rhonchi**. Tissue biopsy may be obtained during a **bronchoscopy**. Chest x-rays are used routinely for most respiratory disorders. Lung function is most accurately assessed by measuring the amounts of carbon dioxide and oxygen in the blood. This requires arterial blood samples, and the tests are known as **arterial blood gases** (ABGs).

Infectious Diseases

Infectious diseases of the respiratory system, especially of the upper respiratory tract, are very common. They include the common cold and various types of pneumonia.

The Common Cold

The common cold (**acute rhinitis**) causes acute inflammation of the upper respiratory tract's mucous membranes. It is nearly impossible to develop immunity to the common cold because it may be caused by one of several hundred strains of virus. Thorough, regular hand washing helps to prevent catching a cold from another person.

Signs and Symptoms
The common cold causes **rhinorrhea** (runny nose), stuffy head (swollen, congested nasal passages), watery eyes, sneezing, sore throat, and fever.

Etiology
The cold is easily passed to others via physical touch and from air droplets via sneezing and coughing. A person's resistance

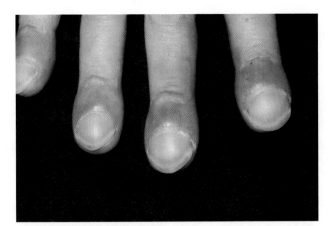

Figure 17–7 Clubbed fingers.

may be lowered by getting wet or chilled, but these factors do not *cause* the cold itself. Because of lowered immunity children, older adults, and those in poor health are at increased risk of catching a cold.

Diagnosis

Diagnosis of a cold is based on physical examination and present signs and symptoms.

Treatment

Treatment involves providing comfort to the patient: rest, increasing fluid intake to prevent dehydration, and the use of antipyretics and analgesics, either over the counter or, if severe, by prescription.

Prognosis

Prognosis is usually good, with the cold resolving itself in 10 days or less.

Sinusitis

Sinusitis is the inflammation of the mucous membrane lining the sinuses. These are air-filled cavities in the bones of the head, with membranes that extend into them from the nose. Sinusitis may be less likely to occur when patients use humidifiers and avoid smoking and air pollution, alcohol (because it swells the nasal membranes), and swimming too often in chlorinated swimming pools.

Signs and Symptoms

Sinusitis causes pain in the affected area of the sinus, headaches after sleeping, tiredness, coughing during the night, nasal congestion, runny nose, and sore throat.

Etiology

Sinusitis is often a result of acute rhinitis. Most cases of sinusitis are of viral origin, including rhinovirus, influenza A and B, and respiratory syncytial virus. Sinusitis also may be caused by bacteria such as *Streptococcus pneumoniae* and *Haemophilus influenzae*. Blowing the nose too hard may spread infection into the sinuses. The drainage system of the sinuses becomes blocked as mucous membranes become swollen. Mucus then accumulates in the sinuses. Pressure increases as a result, causing the symptoms and, sometimes, dizziness and difficulty breathing. Sinusitis may also result from air pollution, nasal deformity, and tooth infections.

Diagnosis

Sinusitis is diagnosed via patient history, physical examination, computed tomography (CT) scan, magnetic resonance imaging (MRI), and various laboratory tests. The most sensitive test for detecting maxillary sinusitis is the CT scan.

Treatment

Sinusitis is often treated with antibiotics and decongestants. Treatment should be as aggressive as possible to avoid the condition from leading to encephalitis, mastoiditis, and other serious infections.

> **RED FLAG**
> When bacterial infection is present, patients recover somewhat more quickly with antibiotics, but most recover with symptomatic treatment alone.

Prognosis

Prognosis is good with aggressive treatment.

Epiglottitis

Epiglottitis is an acute infection, with inflammation, usually caused by the bacterium *H. influenzae* type b. Usually seen in children between 3 and 7 years of age, it causes swelling of the larynx, upper glottic area, and epiglottis.

> **RED FLAG**
> Epiglottitis has decreased dramatically since the introduction of the *H. influenzae* type b vaccine in the middle 1980s.

This causes airway obstruction that is rapid, with fever and sore throat accompanying the symptoms. The child may refuse to swallow due to the pain, and drooling as well as inspiratory stridor (a high-pitched sound) may occur. The child will struggle to breathe and be both pale and very anxious. Immediate treatment is required, using oxygen and antimicrobial therapy. Intubation or tracheotomy may also be required.

Laryngitis

Laryngitis is inflammation of the larynx and vocal cords.

Signs and Symptoms

Laryngitis causes the voice to become hoarse (**dysphonia**), difficulty swallowing (dysphagia), a sore throat, and fever. Dysphonia can also be seen in patients suffering from laryngeal cancer, and it manifests as the only symptom of that disease.

Etiology

Laryngitis can be of viral or bacterial origin or because of irritants (including chemical fumes, smoke, and very hot or very cold air). This condition may follow the common cold, pharyngitis, and sinusitis. Overuse of the voice for an extended time (such as experienced by singers) may cause laryngitis.

Diagnosis

Diagnosis of laryngitis is made based on recent upper respiratory tract infections or influenza and physical examination to listen for wheezing from the throat. A laryngoscope is used to view the vocal cords and airway for other signs of inflammation.

Treatment

Laryngitis is treated by resting the voice, analgesics, increasing fluid intake, using throat lozenges, and keeping away from irritants and people with viral or bacterial infections.

Prognosis

Prognosis is good with proper rest and treatment.

Pharyngitis

Pharyngitis is an inflammation of the throat, also known as *sore throat*.

Signs and Symptoms

Symptoms of pharyngitis include sore throat, fever, headache, pain while swallowing, and swollen lymph glands in the neck area.

Etiology

Pharyngitis is usually caused by a viral infection, although in children a bacterial infection (usually *streptococcus*) may occur. Other causes of pharyngitis include breathing chemical fumes, smoke, and very hot or cold air.

Diagnosis

Pharyngitis is diagnosed by physical examination of the pharynx (throat), eyes, lymph nodes, and skin. If a streptococcal ("strep") infection is suspected, a throat swab culture may be taken.

Treatment

Pharyngitis is treated based on the cause. If viral, the patient is kept comfortable and given throat lozenges, and is told to gargle with antiseptic or saltwater mixtures, and to take analgesics. Bacterial infections (such as strep throat) also require antibiotics. If pharyngitis is chronic, usually due to adenoiditis or tonsillitis, the adenoids or tonsils may be surgically removed.

Prognosis

Prognosis is good with adequate rest and treatment. After the pharyngitis resolves, it is wise to get a new toothbrush to avoid reinfection.

Acute Bronchitis

Acute bronchitis is the inflammation of the mucous membrane lining the bronchus. When this condition involves the trachea, it is called *tracheobronchitis*. To help avoid this condition, patients should use thorough hand washing techniques, avoid smoke and second-hand smoke, avoid allergens, avoid sharing eating utensils, and maintain a healthy lifestyle.

Signs and Symptoms

Symptoms of acute bronchitis include chest tightness, fever, and coughing that progresses from dry (and nonproductive) to productive.

Etiology

Acute bronchitis often follows an upper respiratory tract infection and usually only lasts for a short time. Other causes include inhaling cold air, dust, fumes, smoke, and other irritants.

Diagnosis

Acute bronchitis is usually diagnosed by patient history, physical examination, and x-rays.

Treatment

Acute bronchitis is treated with increased fluid intake, cough syrup, rest, analgesics, and antipyretics. If secondary bacterial infection occurs, antibiotics are prescribed. The role of the PTA is to implement the physical therapist's program of light exercise for patients with acute bronchitis, as approved by their physician.

Prognosis

Prognosis is usually good; however, infants and small children can become very ill due to the size of their bronchioles, which can easily become obstructed. Also, older adults and chronically ill patients have increased risk of secondary bacterial infections such as pneumonia.

Influenza

Influenza (commonly referred to as the "flu") is a very contagious, acute respiratory tract infection that is responsible for over 36,000 deaths in the United States every year. Those most at risk include young children, older adults, pregnant women, and people with certain other diseases or conditions.

> **RED FLAG**
> Recent evidence of excess mortality in two previous influenza pandemics supports vaccinating women in any trimester during a pandemic.

Signs and Symptoms

Influenza usually causes sudden fever, chills, back muscle pain, headache, cough, runny nose, sneezing, sore throat, hoarseness, nausea, vomiting, and diarrhea.

Etiology

Influenza is of viral origin, usually spread by the coughing of respiratory secretions. There are many different strains of influenza, including A, B, and C, with subtypes such as H_1N_1 and others. Avian (bird) flu, a type A strain of influenza, has been attributed to deaths outside of the United States. Because the flu virus has so many genetic varieties, it is able to cause yearly epidemics, most often in the winter and early spring. An individual may develop influenza an unlimited number of times because immunity to a specific viral strain does not provide immunity to another.

Diagnosis

It is difficult to diagnose influenza from the common cold and bacterial infections. Diagnosis involves patient history and physical examination. The sudden onset of flu symptoms is indicative of the disease. The influenza virus may be rapidly diagnosed, in less than 30 minutes, by currently available blood tests.

Treatment

Treatment of influenza is based on symptoms and includes bed rest, analgesics, antipyretics, antivirals (such as oseltamivir and zanamivir), and antibiotics (only if secondary bacterial infections occur). Antivirals must be started within 2 days of symptoms appearing to be effective.

Prognosis

Prognosis is entirely based on severity of infection and whether treatment is started quickly enough. Although most cases resolve, the potential for additional serious infections makes prognosis uncertain.

Pneumonia

Pneumonia is an inflammation of the bronchioles and alveoli because of bacterial, viral, or other pathogenic infections.

Bacterial pneumonias are usually the most serious, whereas viral pneumonias are the most common. If inflammation of the bronchioles and alveoli occur without infection, it is termed *pneumonitis*, which is usually caused by hypersensitivities to chemicals and dusts. Types of pneumonia include pneumococcal, aspiration, and tuberculosis (TB). It may also be described by the location in the lungs, such as *lobar*, *bilateral*, and *double*. The location and cause of the pneumonia are often used together to describe the condition, for example, *lobar pneumococcal pneumonia*. Pneumonia ranges from mild to life threatening.

Signs and Symptoms

Pneumonia symptoms are related to the area and amount of tissue involved. They include dyspnea, weakness, chills, fever, chest pain, and cough.

Etiology

Pneumonia is commonly caused by pathogens that invade lung tissue. Smoking, general anesthesia, immobility, and endotracheal intubation are actions that compromise the respiratory system's protective functions, allowing pathogens to enter. Septicemia also may allow pathogens to invade lung tissue. When the alveoli become inflamed, blood, fluid, and white cells pour out of the capillaries into the tissues to fill the alveoli. Hypoxia results, and this inflammation and infection of the lungs together is called pneumonia.

Diagnosis

Diagnosis of pneumonia requires patient history, physical examination, arterial blood gas, complete blood count, sputum culture, chest x-rays, chest CT, and bronchoscopy. The role of the PTA is to assist pneumonia patients with whatever light exercise is authorized by the physician.

Treatment

Treatment is based on the cause of pneumonia. For bacterial pneumonia antibiotics are used. Other treatments for all types of pneumonia include rest, analgesics, increased fluid intake, high-calorie diets, and oxygen therapy.

> **RED FLAG**
> Oxygen therapy uses oxygen saturation or dissolved oxygen, which is a relative measure of the amount of oxygen contained in a given medium, usually water.

Prognosis

Prognosis is based on severity of disease and response to treatment. Pneumonia is more likely to cause death in older adults, the chronically ill, and immunocompromised patients.

Pulmonary Abscess

Pulmonary abscess (lung abscess) is a collection of infectious material contained within a capsule in the lung.

Signs and Symptoms

Symptoms of pulmonary abscess include chills, fever, chest pain, and coughing. Another indication of this condition is the coughing of bloody or foul-smelling sputum. The breath of the patient may be similarly foul smelling.

> **RED FLAG**
> The most important preventative measure to avoid pulmonary abscess is preventing aspiration.

Etiology

Lung abscess may be related to diseases such as pneumonia, lung cancer, and TB. It can also be caused by aspiration of foreign objects or food.

Diagnosis

Diagnosis of pulmonary abscess is made by patient history, physical examination, chest x-rays, and sputum cultures.

Treatment

Lung abscesses are usually treated with antibiotics as long-term therapy, although surgical resection may be used if unsuccessful or if the abscess is large.

Prognosis

Prognosis is generally good with antibiotic therapy or surgery.

Pulmonary Tuberculosis

Pulmonary tuberculosis is a special type of pneumonia. It is a contagious bacterial infection of the lungs that can also spread to organs such as the bones, brain, and kidneys. Nearly one-third of people throughout the world have been affected by TB.

Signs and Symptoms

TB may be asymptomatic, so testing is required to determine its presence. Visible signs may include loss of appetite, energy, and weight. Once the disease progresses, signs may include a chronic productive cough, dyspnea, fever, and night sweats.

Etiology

Pulmonary TB is caused by the acid-fast bacterium known as *Mycobacterium tuberculosis*. This condition is acquired by breathing air infected with the bacteria. It is spread by coughing and sneezing. The bacterium has a strong coating that protects it outside of the body for a long time, meaning it may be transferred long after it has been ejected from an infected person's body. Risk factors for TB include poor sanitation, infected travelers, immunocompromised individuals, and drug resistance of the bacterium to medication. A primary lesion begins in the lungs, and immune cells begin producing antibodies that "wall off" the infection into granulomas called *tubercles*.

The tubercles eventually change by fibrosing and calcifying, and the disease can be rendered inactive for a long period of time (**Figure 17–8**). These lesions are referred to as Ghon complexes. The individual may, at any time, become symptomatic with progressive primary TB. Antibodies develop in the patient's blood that continue to attack TB bacteria for the rest of his or her life. These antibodies are what a TB skin test is based on. A secondary form of TB may occur when the disease reinfects an individual or the primary form is reactivated due to decreased resistance. In secondary TB the tubercle masses may become liquefied and coughed up, which leaves cavities in the lung tissue. This causes ruptures and the spitting up,

> **RED FLAG**
> Unexpectedly low oxygen saturation levels are found in a wide variety of lung diseases. Oxygen levels below 90 percent are unsafe.

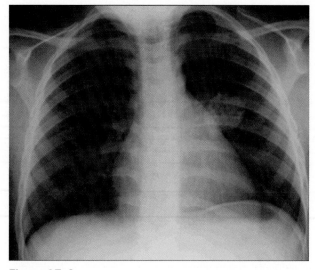

Figure 17–8 Ghon complexes.

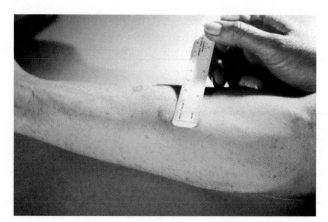

Figure 17–9 Positive TB skin test.

or coughing up, of infected blood, which may further spread the disease.

The lungs then cannot oxygenate blood as well as before. The individual develops signs of being "consumed" by the disease, hence its previous common term, *consumption*. These include dyspnea, a cachetic appearance (meaning loss of weight with muscle atrophy), and other signs. TB has killed many people over time because of the previous lack of effective medications.

Diagnosis

Chest x-rays reveal nodular lesions, patchy infiltrates (mainly in the upper lobes), cavity formation, scar tissue, and calcium deposits. Tuberculin skin may be done, which consists of an injection of a small amount of purified protein derivative tuberculin into the dermis. If the person has been infected by the bacilli, a local reaction (**induration**) occurs (**Figure 17–9**). A history of the bacillus Calmette-Guérin vaccination will produce a false-positive reaction. The sputum of the patient can be stained and cultured. CT or MRI scans allow evaluation of lung damage and can aid in confirming diagnosis when it is difficult to do so otherwise. Bronchoscopy shows inflammation and altered lung tissue and may also be performed to obtain sputum if the patient cannot produce an adequate sputum specimen.

> **RED FLAG**
> Children with compromised immune systems (such as by AIDS or cancer) may not generate enough of a response to test positive for TB.

Treatment

TB requires extended treatment with antibiotics over time. These include isoniazid, rifampin, pyrazinamide, and ethambutol. Precautions when working with TB patients include isolation of the patient and the wearing of protective masks, gloves, and gowns when in close proximity to the patient. The role of the PTA is based on the physician's determination about when the patient is able to tolerate exercise. Gait training and exercises are often provided to maximize the return

of function. Deep breathing exercises are usually avoided in pneumonia patients entirely.

Prognosis

Prognosis is based on severity of the disease state, which determines effectiveness of treatment.

Fungal Diseases

The inhalation of an airborne fungus may cause a fungal disease of the lungs. These fungi cause lesions that form granulomatous inflammations (such as seen in TB). The fungus can spread to cause acute illness, with fever and dyspnea. Treatment requires rest and antifungal medications. The two forms of fungal disease of the lungs include *coccidioidomycosis* ("desert fever" or "valley fever"), which produces windborne spores in hot, dry areas such as in the southwestern United States, and *histoplasmosis*, found in bird or bat droppings, which occurs mostly in the midwestern United States.

Legionnaires' Disease

This bacterial disease was named because of a 1976 outbreak at an American Legion convention in Philadelphia. Legionnaires' disease is caused by the bacterium *Legionella pneumophila* that lives in water storage tanks and air conditioning (cooling) systems. The condition represents one of the atypical infectious diseases, mostly affecting immunocompromised patients, diabetics, smokers, patients with renal disease, and those with chronic lung disease. It primarily affects middle-aged or elderly men.

The *Legionella* bacteria are found in water supplies, air conditioners, showers, condensers, and aerosol nebulizers. Transmission occurs by inhalation and aerosolized bacteria. Symptoms include a nonproductive cough that becomes productive, high fevers, with relative bradycardia, pleuritic chest pain, diarrhea, and visible signs of toxicity. The treatment of choice is typically oral erythromycin or similar macrolide antibiotics.

Obstructive Lung Disease

Obstructive lung disease is the term that describes any disease characterized by airway obstruction. This includes asthma, emphysema, bronchitis, COPD, and, sometimes, cystic fibrosis.

Asthma

Asthma is a disease that involves periodic episodes of severe but reversible bronchial obstruction in patients who have hypersensitive or hyperresponsive airways. Frequent, repeated attacks of acute asthma may lead to irreversible lung damage and the development of chronic asthma (chronic obstructive lung disease). Acute asthma attacks may continue to exist during a chronic asthmatic condition. Asthma affects up to 10 percent of children and is the leading cause of chronic childhood illness. Before puberty more boys are diagnosed with asthma, but after puberty the disorder is more evenly distributed by males and females.

> **RED FLAG**
> Nearly 23 million people in the United States, including 7 million children, have asthma. The condition is more prevalent in lower income families.

Signs and Symptoms

Asthma exhibits episodes of dyspnea and wheezing on exhalation, which result from *bronchospasm* (**Figure 17–10**). Other symptoms include extreme shortness of breath and mild to severe anxiety. Coughing during the attack starts as dry and nonproductive, progressing to large amounts of mucus. The skin is pale and moist if the attack is mild, and hypoxia may develop. In severe attacks the lips and nail beds may be cyanotic. Breathing is slightly easier if the patient sits and leans forward with the hands resting on the knees, because this position helps all the respiratory muscles to be used. The primary respiratory muscles are the diaphragm, intercostal muscles, and abdominal muscles. The secondary respiratory muscles are the sternocleidomastoids and trapezius muscles.

Severe attacks lasting for days are referred to as **status asthmaticus,** which is more common in the elderly. These attacks are life-threatening medical emergencies. Respiratory acidosis develops over time because of trapped air. Marked fatigue causes decreased respiratory effort with a weak cough. This condition may be aggravated by developing metabolic acidosis due to hypoxia and from metabolic acid accumulating from increased metabolic activity and dehydration.

Etiology

Asthma is commonly related to a family history of hay fever, asthma, and eczema. Viral upper respiratory tract infections frequently precipitate attacks. Causative allergens include dust, pollen, pet dander, smoke, or a variety of fumes. Other contributing factors include stress, infections, temperature and humidity changes, and exercise.

Diagnosis

Diagnosis of asthma is made after patient history, physical examination, and lung function tests. A medication is then ordered on a trial basis; if it is successful, diagnosis is usually confirmed.

Treatment

Treatment of asthma includes avoiding allergens, desensitization, medications, and education about the condition. Deep breathing techniques, relaxation techniques, and proper posture of the body are encouraged. Bronchodilators are used to relax and open the bronchi, and mucolytics are used to thin excessive mucus. In addition, glucocorticoids may be

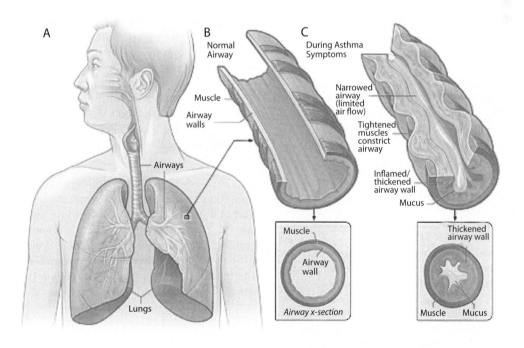

Figure 17–10 Asthma. (A) Location of the lungs and airways in the body. (B) Cross-section of a normal airway. (C) Cross-section of an airway during asthma symptoms. COPD Learn More Breathe Better® Campaign, National Heart, Lung, and Blood Institute.

administered by inhalation but are more effective in reducing the second state of inflammation in the airways. These drugs may be useful when chronic inflammation develops.

For status asthmaticus hospital care is essential when patients do not respond to bronchodilators. For prophylaxis and treatment of chronic asthma, leukotriene receptor antagonists such as zafirlukast (Accolate) and montelukast (Singulair) block inflammatory responses when stimuli are present. Cromolyn sodium is a prophylactic medication that is administered by inhalation on a regular daily basis.

The role of the PTA in implementing a program for asthma patients focuses on teaching deep breathing techniques, relaxation, and posture activities and exercises. Short, intermittent activities such as volleyball, gymnastics, and baseball are acceptable. Activities that require longer periods of exertion, such as long-distance running, should be avoided. Ideally, the asthma patient should get 30 minutes of exercise four to five times per week.

Prognosis

Prognosis is varied based on severity of attacks, other disease states, age of the patient, and compliance with treatment.

Cystic Fibrosis

Cystic fibrosis is caused by an exocrine gland dysfunction and affects a variety of organ systems besides the lungs. All secretory organs are affected by cystic fibrosis. It is the most common fatal genetic disease in White children. This disease causes many complications.

RED FLAG
About 1 in every 20 Americans is an unaffected carrier of the abnormal *CF* gene.

Signs and Symptoms

Signs and symptoms of cystic fibrosis include chronic airway infection, thick respiratory secretions, bronchiectasis, bronchiolectasis, pancreatic insufficiency, intestinal dysfunction, sweat gland dysfunction, and reproductive dysfunction.

Etiology

Cystic fibrosis is caused by a chromosomal disorder, causing decreased regulation of chloride and sodium transport across epithelial membranes.

Diagnosis

Diagnosis of cystic fibrosis involves double sweat tests to detect elevated levels of sodium chloride, chest x-rays, stool samples to detect absence of trypsin, and family history of the disease.

Treatment

Treatment is focused on helping to maintain as normal a lifestyle as possible and depends on the organ systems involved. Treatments include hypertonic radiocontrast materials, breathing exercises, antibiotics, mucolytics, beta-adrenergic agonists, pancreatic enzyme replacement, sodium-channel blockers, uridine triphosphate, salt supplements, dornase alfa, recombinant alpha-antitrypsin, gene therapy, and, ultimately, lung or heart transplantation.

Exercise plays an important role in the treatment of cystic fibrosis. The role of the PTA is to implement a program of exercises that can increase lung capacity, strength, energy, endurance, life expectancy, airway clearance, and bone density. The PTA may also educate parents or the patient on positioning for lung drainage and chest percussion techniques to mobilize secretions. In general, cystic fibrosis patients should have 20 to 30 minutes of aerobic exercise at least three times per week.

Prognosis

Prognosis is varied based on severity of the disease, although most patients do not live past 32 years of age.

Chronic Obstructive Pulmonary Disease

Chronic obstructive pulmonary disease (COPD) actually describes two diseases, chronic bronchitis and emphysema, characterized by difficulty breathing (**Figure 17–11**). Because these two diseases often coexist, they are usually collectively called COPD. Both disorders cause excessive inflammation and permanently obstructed airflow.

RED FLAG
COPD is the fourth most significant cause of death in the United States.

Individuals with COPD have high levels of carbon dioxide in their blood but cannot increase breathing to remove it. Therefore, the respiratory system adapts to the condition and begins responding to the secondary stimulus of low blood oxygen. Because high oxygenation removes their stimulus to breathe, giving oxygen to these individuals can be fatal.

Stages of COPD are as follows:

- Stage 1 (mild): Often minimal shortness of breath, with or without cough and/or sputum; abnormal lung function is usually unrecognized.
- Stage 2 (moderate): Often moderate to severe shortness of breath upon exertion, with or without cough, sputum, or dyspnea; medical attention is often sought for the first time at this stage because of chronic symptoms or exacerbation.
- Stage 3 (severe): More severe shortness of breath, with or without cough, sputum, or dyspnea; repeated exacerbations may affect quality of life.
- Stage 4 (very severe): Shortness of breath greatly impairs quality of life, exacerbations may become life threatening.

Signs and Symptoms

Lung damage causes COPD. Smokers often develop COPD after 40 or 50 years, and symptoms can occur many years after quitting. With aging, smokers lose lung function at a rate that is about five times faster than nonsmokers. Once smoking has destroyed a large amount of the lungs, COPD symptoms appear as the individual ages and continues to lose lung function as result of the passage of time. Common symptoms of COPD include dyspnea, chronic coughing, wheezing, hemoptysis, cyanosis, weight loss, pursed-lip breathing, and a bulging, rounded chest ("barrel chest").

Etiology

COPD is caused by cigarette smoking 90 percent of the time. The other 10 percent of COPD patients develop the condition because of air pollution, industrial pollutants, or chronic respiratory tract infections.

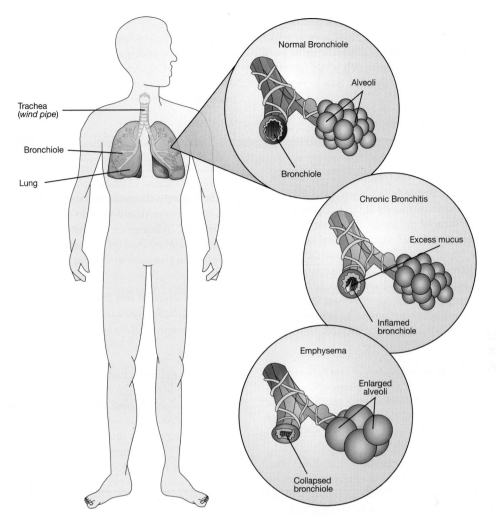

Figure 17–11 Chronic obstructive pulmonary disease (COPD) is often one of or a mixture of two diseases—chronic bronchitis and emphysema.

Diagnosis

COPD is diagnosed by patient history, physical examination, and by ruling out other diseases. The retention of carbon dioxide is important in the diagnosis of COPD. Simply increasing supplemental oxygen can cause more damage due to inability of the patient to exhale properly. This can actually cause retention of carbon dioxide. Diagnostic tests include chest x-rays, pulmonary function tests, and ABGs.

> **RED FLAG**
>
> It is important to remember that COPD patients may require oxygen during exercise. If the patient is in *hypoxic drive* (the use of oxygen instead of carbon dioxide receptors to regulate respiration), oxygen must be used with caution.

Treatment

COPD is treated based on present symptoms. Treatments include bronchodilators, inhalers, cough medications, and mucolytics. COPD patients may experience aggravated symptoms if they are exposed to individuals with respiratory tract infections. COPD patients should also be vaccinated against influenza. Smoking cessation can slow or reverse early stages of the disease and ease later symptoms.

The role of the PTA in treating COPD patients includes techniques to help clear the respiratory passages of heavy secretions. Postural drainage, chest compressions, and percussion are indicated.

Flexibility and stretching exercises are indicated. Walking, cycling, or swimming help to build endurance. Strength training with weights may also be beneficial.

Prognosis

Prognosis for end-stage COPD is poor because there is no cure, and debilitation usually occurs. Pulmonary function deteriorates, leading to respiratory failure and death.

Emphysema

Emphysema is a form of COPD characterized by abnormal, permanent enlargement of the **acini**, accompanied by destruction of the alveolar walls (**Figure 17–12**). Obstruction results from tissue changes rather than mucous production, which occurs with asthma and chronic bronchitis. Emphysema is characterized by airflow limitation due to lack of elastic recoil in the lungs.

Signs and Symptoms

Signs and symptoms of emphysema include coughing, dyspnea, tachypnea, and wheezing. The over-distention and over-inflation of the lungs cause the chest to assume a "barrel" shape. There are decreased breath sounds caused by air trapped in the alveoli and alveolar wall destruction. *Clubbed fingers* and toes are seen in emphysema, which is related to chronic hypoxic changes. Additionally, pursing the lips helps to hold the alveoli open while forcefully exhaling. The face and skin may redden due to the extra pressure required.

Etiology
Emphysema is usually caused by *alpha₁-antitrypsin* deficiency and cigarette smoking.

Diagnosis
Chest x-rays in advanced emphysema show a flattened diaphragm, reduced vascular markings at the periphery of the lungs, and over-aeration of the lungs. Pulmonary function tests indicate increased residual volume and total lung capacity. ABG analysis usually reveals reduced partial pressure of arterial oxygen and a normal partial pressure of arterial carbon dioxide (until late in the disease process). A complete blood count usually reveals an increased hemoglobin level late in the disease, when the patient has persistent and severe hypoxia.

Treatment
Bronchodilators such as beta-adrenergic blockers are used to reverse bronchospasms and promote mucociliary clearance. Antibiotics may be indicated to treat respiratory tract infection. Adequate amounts of fluids are required to liquefy and mobilize secretions. Hypoxia may be corrected by using low settings of oxygen therapy.

The role of the PTA includes educating the patient about the types of exercise that are used for emphysema patients, including breathing and posture exercises, walking, and general strengthening. Exercise needs to be started with very low impact techniques and progress slowly to more rigorous activities. Cycling and weight training are used based on the severity of the condition.

Prognosis
Prognosis for emphysema is poor, with irreversible destruction of the alveolar walls.

Chronic Bronchitis

Chronic bronchitis involves inflammation of the bronchi caused by irritants or infection.

Signs and Symptoms
Chronic bronchitis causes increased mucous production, productive cough, hypertrophy of the mucous-secreting glands, thickening of the mucous membrane, and *bronchiectasis* (a chronic dilation of the bronchus). This latter condition allows the pooling of mucus, which produces a foul-smelling cough (known as "smoker's cough") during morning hours. Bronchial obstruction worsens during disease progression, and breathing becomes more difficult. Coughing, dyspnea, and **hypoxia** with cyanosis occur.

Etiology
Common causes of chronic bronchitis include cigarette smoking, exposure to irritants or noxious gases, genetic predisposition, exposure to inorganic or organic dusts, and respiratory tract infection.

Diagnosis
Chest x-rays may show hyperinflation and increased bronchovascular markings. Pulmonary function studies indicate increased residual volume, forced expiratory flow, and decreased vital capacity. Analysis of sputum may reveal many microorganisms and neutrophils.

Treatment
For treatment, patients should avoid smoke from tobacco products (or stop smoking), air pollutants, and second-hand smoke. Recurrent infections are treated with antibiotics and the administration of bronchodilators. Oxygen therapy may also be required if blood oxygen saturation is low. Occasionally, corticosteroids are used to combat inflammation. The role of the PTA in chronic bronchitis is similar to that of acute bronchitis and is based on the therapy plan of care outlined by the physical therapist according to the physician's orders.

Prognosis
Prognosis is poor if this condition progresses so that symptoms are continuous. Lung damage occurs, the individual becomes debilitated, and death ensues.

Bronchiectasis

Sometimes the bronchial walls in areas of the lung become weakened due to severe inflammation or other factors. The affected bronchi become markedly dilated. This condition is called **bronchiectasis**, which is usually a secondary problem rather than a primary one. It develops in patients with cystic fibrosis or COPD. It may result from childhood infections, aspiration of foreign bodies, or congenital weakness of the bronchial wall. Based on the cause, bronchiectasis may be localized in one lung or (more commonly) diffused in both lungs.

The significant signs of bronchiectasis are chronic cough and production of copious amounts of purulent sputum. Other signs include *rales* and *rhonchi* in the lungs, dyspnea, hemoptysis, weight loss, anemia, and fatigue. Bronchiectasis

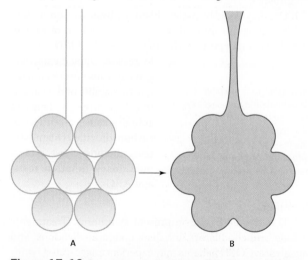

Figure 17–12 Derangement of pulmonary function resulting from enlargement of air spaces and reduction of pulmonary capillary bed. (A) Normal structure, illustrating schematically a cluster of alveoli surrounded by a rich capillary bed connected to normal bronchiole. (B) Emphysema, illustrating coalescence of air spaces to form a large cystic space with greatly reduced capillary bed and narrowed bronchiole.

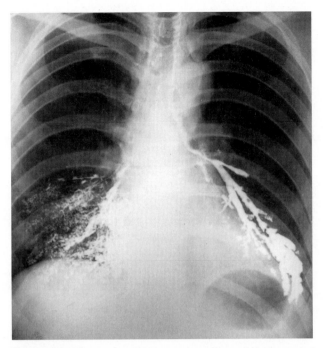

Figure 17–13 Chest x-ray illustrating bronchiectasis demonstrated by bronchogram. Right lower lobe bronchi (left) appear normal. Bronchi on the opposite side exhibit saclike and fusiform dilatation, as outlined by radiopaque contrast material within dilated bronchi.

may be diagnosed by a specific radiologic examination called a *bronchogram*, which reveals abnormal, dilated bronchi (**Figure 17–13**).

Pneumoconioses

Pneumoconioses are a group of environmentally induced diseases causing progressive, chronic inflammation and infection. These diseases are frequently caused by inhaling small dust particles of different types and can take from between a few years up to 30 years to develop. Types of pneumoconioses include **asbestosis** (the most common type, related to insulating and fireproofing), **anthracosis** (from carbon and coal; often called "black lung" or "coal miner's disease"), and **silicosis** (from silicone; often affects glass cutters, sand blasters, and stone masons).

Vascular Disorders

Pulmonary vascular disorders are those that affect the pulmonary circulation. They include pulmonary embolism, pulmonary arterial hypertension, pulmonary edema, and pulmonary hemorrhage. The most common of these disorders are discussed below.

Pulmonary Embolism

Pulmonary embolism is a sudden pulmonary artery blockage by an embolism. Prevention includes ambulation, anti-embolic stockings, and leg exercises.

Signs and Symptoms

Symptoms of this disorder are varied, based on size of the clot and which area of the respiratory system is affected. Symptoms include coughing, dyspnea, apprehension, and chest pain.

Etiology

Pulmonary embolism can be caused by any floating material that blocks a pulmonary artery. This includes blood clots, pieces of tissue, and globules of fat. Often, a blood clot (thrombus) develops in the veins of the pelvis, lower legs, or thighs. The clot then breaks loose and becomes wedged in a pulmonary artery, resulting in a pulmonary embolism. Factors contributing to pulmonary embolism are prolonged bed rest, obesity, and fracture or trauma to the pelvis or legs.

Diagnosis

Pulmonary embolism can be confirmed with x-rays, lung scans, MRI, or pulmonary angiography.

Treatment

Treatment involves administering oxygen and anticoagulation medications so that cardiopulmonary function can be maintained. The role of the PTA is to implement a program of moderate exercise with the goal of eventual activity totaling approximately 30 minutes per day.

Prognosis

Prognosis is based on severity of the condition, which can lead to cyanosis, shock, and death.

Pulmonary Edema

Pulmonary edema refers to fluid collecting in the alveoli and interstitial tissue. It may be a life-threatening medical emergency. Many conditions can lead to the development of pulmonary edema. The accumulation of fluid reduces the amount of oxygen diffusing into the blood and interferes with lung expansion. It also reduces oxygenation of the blood.

Signs and Symptoms

Pulmonary edema causes coughing, orthopnea (difficulty breathing when lying down), and rales. As congestion increases, hemoptysis often occurs. Sputum becomes frothy due to air mixed with the secretions. Breathing becomes difficult, and the patient feels as if he or she is drowning. Hypoxemia increases and cyanosis develops in the advanced stage.

Etiology

Cardiovascular disease is a common cause of pulmonary edema. With left-sided congestive heart failure, backup of blood from the failing left ventricle causes high pressure in the pulmonary circulation. This condition may be chronic or acute. However, any disease that affects blood pressure, blood fluid levels, or heart function can lead to pulmonary edema. These include hypertension and pulmonary embolism. Pulmonary edema also results from hypoproteinemia due to kidney or liver disease, in which serum albumin levels are low.

Diagnosis

Diagnosis of pulmonary edema may be determined by ABGs and chest x-rays. ABGs reveal increased carbon dioxide levels, with x-rays revealing increased opacity (which appear as a white area on the image).

Treatment

The causative factors of pulmonary edema must be treated with supportive care, including oxygen administration. In severe cases positive-pressure mechanical ventilation may

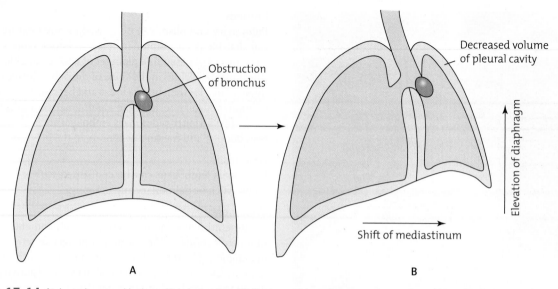

Figure 17–14 Atelectasis caused by bronchial obstruction. (A) Blockage of bronchus prevents aeration of lung supplied by obstructed bronchus. (B) Absorption of air causes collapse of the lung and a corresponding reduction in size of the pleural cavity. The diaphragm rises, and the mediastinum shifts toward the affected side.

be necessary. Medications include diuretics, cardiogenics, and morphine.

Prognosis

Prognosis is entirely based on severity of symptoms and treatment of the underlying cause.

Expansion Disorders

Expansion disorders occur when the lungs become under- or over-inflated or collapsed. They include atelectasis, pleural effusion, empyema, hemothorax, pneumothorax, pleurisy, and flail chest.

Atelectasis

Atelectasis is defined as the collapse of part or all of a lung. It may also be defined as an airless state of a lung (**Figure 17–14 and 17–15A and B**). It usually affects only a small section of a lung.

Signs and Symptoms

Atelectasis causes cyanosis, dyspnea, anxiety, tachypnea, tachycardia, signs of hypoxemia, reduced chest expansion, absence of breath sounds, and intercostal retractions. Additional symptoms may include fever, other signs of infection, and signs of respiratory distress.

Etiology

Atelectasis often occurs because of inadequate breathing patterns due to pain. Common causes of these breathing patterns include pain from surgery or fractured ribs and airway blockage by mucous plugs.

Diagnosis

Atelectasis is diagnosed by physical examination and a positive chest x-ray.

Treatment

Atelectasis is treated by walking (ambulation), frequent deep breathing and coughing, and analgesics. Focus of treatment is on opening airways and expanding alveoli. Deep breathing

exercises are indicated, and the role of the PTA is to assist with educating the patient about correct breathing techniques and helping to implement walking regimens.

Prognosis

Prognosis is good if complications such as pneumonia do not occur.

Pleural Effusion

Pleural effusion, also known as *hydrothorax*, is an excessive collection of fluid in the pleural cavity. Normally, a very small amount (approximately 5 mL) of fluid is present in the pleural cavity for lubrication. Excessive fluid compresses the lungs and causes limited expansion ability during inhalation. Fluid accumulation can create various effusions, such as blood (due to trauma), exudates (due to inflammation), transudate (due to increased hydrostatic pressure), or pus (due to infection). Excess fluids may cause the pleural membranes to separate (**Figure 17–16**).

Signs and Symptoms

Pleural effusion can be asymptomatic, or the affected patient may have dyspnea, chest pain, tachypnea, tachycardia, and pleural friction rub (pleurisy).

Etiology

Hydrothorax may be caused by congestive heart failure, pneumonia, or TB.

Diagnosis

Diagnosis of hydrothorax includes patient history, physical examination, x-rays, CT, complete blood count, and thoracentesis (needle aspiration of chest fluid). **Figure 17–17** illustrates an x-ray showing pleural effusion.

Treatment

Treatment of pleural effusion involves treating the causative conditions, with thoracentesis if required. Deep breathing exercises are indicated for pleural effusion, which the PTA may assist the patient in implementing.

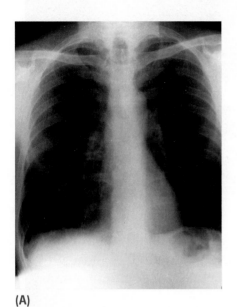

(A)

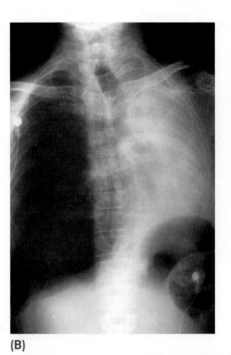

(B)

Figure 17–15 Complete atelectasis of the left lung caused by obstruction of left main bronchus. (A) Chest x-ray before development of atelectasis. (B) Atelectasis of entire left lung. The collapsed lung appears dense because the air has been absorbed. The left half of diaphragm is elevated. Trachea and mediastinal structures are shifted toward the side of the collapse.

Prognosis

Prognosis is generally good if the underlying condition is successfully treated.

Empyema

Empyema is a collection of pus in the chest cavity. It can be prevented by rapid and appropriate treatment of underlying conditions.

Signs and Symptoms

Symptoms of empyema include coughing, chest pain on the affected side, and dyspnea.

Etiology

Empyema can result from an ulcerated tumor or a rupture of a lung abscess. Today, it is not as common because better antibiotics are available.

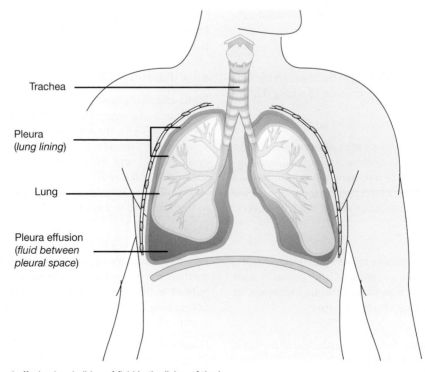

Trachea

Pleura
(*lung lining*)

Lung

Pleura effusion
(*fluid between pleural space*)

Figure 17–16 Pleural effusion is a buildup of fluid in the lining of the lungs.

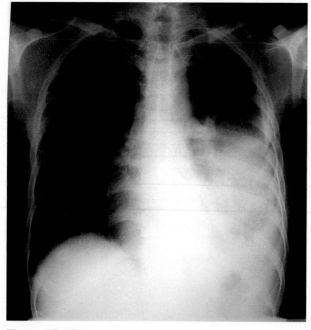

Figure 17–17 X-ray of pleural effusion.

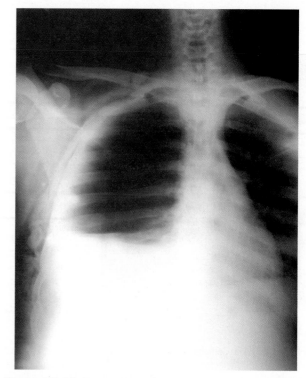

Figure 17–18 Hemothorax.

Diagnosis

Diagnosis of empyema is via x-rays and *thoracentesis* (the removal of fluid from between the pleura and chest wall). The fluid is then analyzed to determine the infective organism.

Treatment

Empyema, because it is of bacterial origin, is treated with antibiotics. The role of the PTA in empyema is to assist with light exercise and educate the patient about its benefits over such other treatments as spirometry.

Prognosis

Prognosis is based on symptoms and effective antibiotic therapy.

Hemothorax

Hemothorax is a collection of blood in the chest cavity. This may cause a partial or complete collapse of a lung (**Figure 17–18**).

Signs and Symptoms

Symptoms of hemothorax include lung collapse, severe chest pain, severe dyspnea, shock, shallow respirations, "sucking" breath sounds (in the case of traumatic wounds), increased air pressure, and a shifting of the mediastinum toward the affected side. If the mediastinum shifts, it is a true medical emergency.

Etiology

Common causes of hemothorax include pulmonary disease, a tear of pulmonary tissue, or tumors. Other causes include wounds to the chest such as from gunshot, stabbings, or crushing. Rib fracture may also be causative.

Diagnosis

Diagnosis of hemothorax includes auscultation of the chest to listen for decreased or absent breath sounds. It is confirmed by chest x-rays.

Treatment

Treatment involves monitoring blood pressure and blood loss, thoracentesis (if necessary), oxygen therapy, and analgesics.

Prognosis

Prognosis is based on success of treating any lung collapse or bleeding.

Pneumothorax

Pneumothorax is a collection of air in the pleural cavity that often results in partial or complete lung collapse on the affected side. It may occur when air leaks into the pleural space (**Figure 17–19**).

Signs and Symptoms

Symptoms of pneumothorax are related to the severity of the lung collapse. If complete, the collapse causes sudden, severe chest pain, severe dyspnea, and shock. Respirations become weak and shallow. If there is a traumatic wound, sucking breath sounds may be heard. On the affected side increased air pressure may cause a shift of the mediastinum to that side, and this is a medical emergency.

Etiology

Common causes of pneumothorax include a tear of pulmonary tissue, tumors, or pulmonary disease. Traumatic pneumothorax is defined as air entering the pleural cavity from outside of the chest, as often caused by gunshot, stabbing, or crushing wounds. Rib fractures may also cause traumatic pneumothorax.

Diagnosis

Diagnosis of pneumothorax involves auscultation of the chest, confirmed by x-rays.

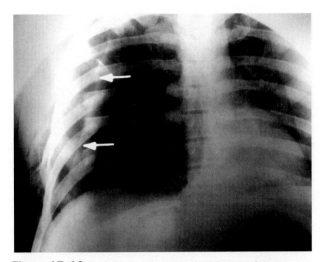

Figure 17–19 X-ray illustrating pneumothorax secondary to multiple rib fractures in which broken ends of fractured ribs have torn through the pleura and torn underlying lung. The arrows indicate the surface of lung that is no longer in contact with chest wall.

Treatment

For a mediastinum shift emergency treatment includes placing clean hands, an occlusive dressing, or a plastic material over the sucking chest wound to prevent additional air from entering. If not an emergency, treatment may include thoracentesis (inserting a chest tube to withdraw air) so that the lung can reexpand, oxygen therapy, and analgesics.

Prognosis

Prognosis is based on the reason for the lung collapse or air in the pleural cavity and how it is treated.

Pleurisy

Pleurisy, also known as *pleuritis*, is the inflammation of the membranes covering the lung (visceral pleura) and lining the chest cavity (parietal pleura).

Signs and Symptoms

Pleurisy mostly causes a sharp pain in the chest that worsens with coughing and inspiration. The pain may be so severe that movement in the affected area is limited.

Etiology

Pleurisy may be cause by a bacterial infection of the pleura, and secondary pleurisy usually follows pneumonia, trauma, neoplasms, or TB.

Diagnosis

Diagnosis is based on the distinctive chest pain as well as auscultation, which reveals a characteristic friction rub or a "squeaky" sound upon inspiration. To identify the cause of pleurisy, procedures include chest x-rays, CT scans, biopsy, and/or analysis of fluid in the pleural space.

Treatment

Treatment of pleurisy is aimed at the symptoms, using analgesics, application of heat, and taping the chest to restrict pain from excessive movement. The role of the PTA is to implement a program of light exercise after pleurisy treatments

have occurred, based on the amount of pain caused by breathing, per the therapy plan of care and the physical therapist's direction.

Prognosis

Prognosis is based on treating the underlying condition.

Flail Chest

Flail chest is a loss of chest structure due to multiple chest fractures. Flail chest occurs from fractures of the thorax, ribs, and/or sternum, as are commonly caused by car accidents and falls (**Figure 17–20**). These injuries often cause contusions with edema and bleeding inside lung tissue. Atelectasis may occur if a broken rib punctures the pleura.

The main component of flail chest is the loss of chest wall rigidity, which causes opposite movements during inspiration and expiration. Pressure changes affect ventilation and oxygen level. Inward movement of the ribs during inspiration prevents the affected lung from expanding. During expiration the unstable part of the chest is pushed outward, altering airflow. In general, air gets pushed up into the bronchus and into the opposite lungs during both inspiration and expiration. The mediastinum gets pushed back and forth, resulting in reduction of cardiac output and oxygen supplies to cells. Stale air is shunted between the lungs, lowering oxygen content and decreasing venous return.

Treatment for flail chest is aimed at protecting the lungs and preventing the onset of pneumonia. One hundred–percent oxygen is given to every patient with this condition. Intubation or the insertion of a chest tube may be indicated. Mechanical ventilation is used to achieve chest cavity stabilization. The need for corrective surgery is assessed on a case-by-case basis. Analgesic pain medications help provide relief.

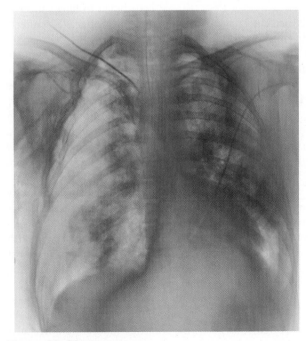

Figure 17–20 Flail chest.

Laryngeal Cancer

Laryngeal cancer is the most common upper respiratory tract malignancy. Most involve squamous cell carcinomas. Approximately one-third of all newly diagnosed cases result in patient death. If confined to the true vocal cords (glottis), growth is slow and metastasis occurs slowly. However, if the supraglottis (false vocal cords) and subglottis are involved, metastasis is early to the lymph nodes in the neck. Laryngeal cancer is primarily linked to prolonged use of alcohol and tobacco, although genetics may also play a part. It is much more common in men than women and usually occurs between the ages of 50 and 70.

Laryngeal cancer manifests with hoarseness, shortness of breath, and pain during speaking. Throat irritation may occur, which lasts for longer than 2 weeks, with a change in vocal quality. Lumps may be found upon palpation, and nodes may be tender before they can be palpated. The mouth and tongue may display sores, lumps, or nodules. Treatment involves surgery, laser vaporization of abnormal cell layers, radiation, partial or total laryngectomy, chemotherapy, and insertion of a permanent tracheostomy stoma.

The role of the PTA concerns physical therapy to improve back and neck flexibility after surgery and other treatments. The PTA may also educate the patient about the use of various devices to amplify the sounds of the vocal cords if a total laryngectomy is performed. Additional treatments include occupational and speech therapy.

Lung Cancer

Lung cancer is the most common cause of death of all cancers, in both genders, in the United States. The most common type of lung tumor is bronchogenic carcinoma, which arises from the bronchial epithelium. The percentage of all cancer deaths attributed to lung cancer is 28 percent. Lung cancer is most prevalent after age 70, affecting men more than women.

> **RED FLAG**
> In the United States lung cancer kills more people every year than breast, colon, and prostate cancers *combined*.

Unfortunately, only 16 percent of lung cancers are found in the early stages, while it still remains localized. The two major types are small cell and non–small cell lung cancers (**Figure 17–21**). Small cell lung cancer is almost always caused by smoking and is usually in the neuroendocrine cells of the lung bronchoepithelium. It multiplies quickly into large tumors, spreading to the lymph nodes and other organs. Usually, by the time it is diagnosed small cell lung cancer has spread, often to the brain.

Non–small cell lung cancer actually makes up the majority of all lung cancers and is divided into *squamous cell carcinoma*, *adenocarcinoma*, and *large cell undifferentiated carcinoma*. Squamous cell carcinoma is also associated with smoking. Of the three types adenocarcinoma occurs most often, accounting for 40 percent of all non–small cell lung cancers.

Most lung cancer appears in the hilus of the lung, near the larger divisions of the bronchi. The growth of cancer cells into carcinomas makes the bronchial lining become irregular and uneven. Sometimes, tumors penetrate into surrounding

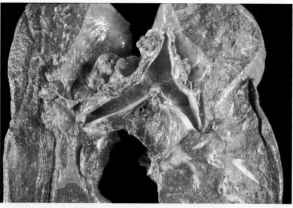

(A)

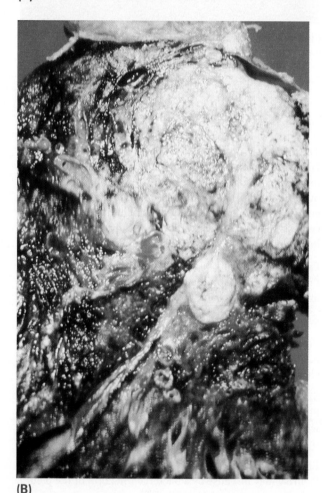

(B)

Figure 17–21 The normal (A) and cancerous (B) lung.

tissue or grow into the bronchial openings. More than 50 percent of patients have tumor metastasis into lymph nodes and other organs. Systemic effects are primarily seen in the endocrine, hematologic, dermatologic, and neuromuscular systems.

Signs and Symptoms

Onset of lung cancer is often misperceived because, frequently, by the time symptoms are noticed, the cancer has metastasized to other sites. Early signs include persistent productive cough, dyspnea, wheezing, pneumonia, hemoptysis, chest pain, hoarseness, headache, facial or arm edema, dysphagia, and atelectasis. Other symptoms include weight loss, anemia, fatigue, paraneoplastic syndrome, and signs of metastasis such as bone pain or pathologic fracture. Complications include bronchial obstruction, emphysema, pulmonary abscesses, bronchitis, pleuritis, and compression on the vena cava.

Etiology
Cigarette smoking and second-hand smoke are the primary causes of lung cancer. Lung cancer is 10 times more common in smokers than in nonsmokers. Genetics and family history may also play a role. Gene mutations may be related as well. Lung tumors may develop as a result of COPD. Exposure to carcinogens is also a major cause of lung cancer, as is any long-term exposure to respiratory irritants, such as asbestos, coal dust, arsenic, radon, silica, or vinyl chloride.

Diagnosis
Diagnosis is made via chest x-rays, CT scans, MRI, bronchoscopy, and biopsy. Also, mediastinoscopy aids in checking lymph nodes, and bone scans detect metastasis to bones. Pulmonary function tests clarify the effects of tumors on airflow.

Treatment
For localized lesions surgical resection or lobectomy may be performed. Chemotherapy and radiation may be used but are frequently not highly effective on many lung tumors. Photodynamic therapy may be used, wherein a chemical is injected that migrates to the tumor cells, where activation by laser light causes it to destroy them.

The role of the PTA includes assessing changes in sputum color; decreased breath sounds, rales, or rhonchi; abnormal breathing patterns; pleural effusion; and altered vital signs. Treatment is focused on airway management, reduction of anxiety, oxygen therapy, airway stabilization, cough enhancement, mechanical ventilation, positioning, and respiratory monitoring. PTAs may assist patients who have lung cancer with supervised exercises to help improve their overall health and functional abilities. Walking and yoga are two extremely well-tolerated exercises for lung cancer patients. Range-of-motion and light resistance training is indicated. Massage is also beneficial.

Prognosis
Prognosis for lung cancer is poor unless the tumors are in the very early stage of development. The 5-year survival rate for lung cancer is only 15 percent. Advancements in cancer research have not improved the survival rate.

Infant Respiratory Distress Syndrome

Infant respiratory distress syndrome causes neonatal death, commonly in premature infants. The mortality rate has decreased with improved testing and therapies. Surfactant, which reduces surface tension in the lung alveoli and promotes expansion, is not produced in sufficient quantities as a result of this disease. Without enough surfactant the first breaths an infant

> **RED FLAG**
> Severe hypoxia may lead to brain damage.

takes become very difficult because the lungs totally collapse during each expiration. Inadequate blood and oxygen supplies cause continually low levels of surfactant to be produced. This results in atelectasis, pulmonary vasoconstriction, and severe hypoxia. Increased alveolar capillary permeability develops, further impairing lung expansion. Acidosis may then develop, leading to anaerobic metabolism and increased lactic acid.

Signs and Symptoms
Upon delivery, or shortly thereafter, respiratory difficulty may become evident. Signs include respiratory rate of over 60 breaths per minute, nasal flaring, low body temperature, chest retractions, and rales. Frothy sputum and grunting upon expiration develop, followed by falling blood pressure, cyanosis, and peripheral edema. Severe hypoxemia is signified by decreased responsiveness, irregular respirations with apnea, and decreased breath sounds.

Etiology
Infant respiratory distress syndrome is usually caused by premature birth, occurring more often in boys and after cesarean delivery. Also, infants born to diabetic women are predisposed to this condition.

Diagnosis
Diagnosis is based on arterial blood gas analysis and chest x-rays.

Treatment
Women in premature labor may be given glucocorticoids, which increase the maturation process of the infant. Immediately after birth (and sometimes continuing thereafter), synthetic surfactant (colfosceril) may be administered to the neonate. Mechanical ventilation and oxygen therapy may be used with constant monitoring. If oxygen concentrations are too high, the infant may develop pulmonary damage as well as varying degrees of eye damage. The intake of adequate fluids and nutrition must be monitored.

Prognosis
Prognosis varies based on the age of the premature infant and the severity of the other related factors. Most infant deaths occur between days 2 and 7 after birth, with prognosis improving slowly but steadily after day 7.

Adult Respiratory Distress Syndrome

Adult respiratory distress syndrome (ARDS), also referred to as "shock lung," is a sudden and life-threatening failure of a lung or both lungs. It is actually a syndrome that may develop 24 to 48 hours after the occurrence of a major injury or illness. To avoid ARDS from developing after another disorder, lung damage must be prevented. Only low levels of oxygen should be used, and infections should be promptly treated.

Signs and Symptoms
ARDS develops suddenly with symptoms of extreme dyspnea, severe hypoxemia, cyanosis, tachypnea, and pulmonary hypertension (defined as high blood pressure in the pulmonary arteries).

Etiology

About one-third of ARDS cases are caused by sepsis (a serious blood infection), with other causes including inhalation of smoke or fumes, severe chest trauma, fat emboli, near-drownings, aspiration pneumonia, major burns, acute pancreatitis, and massive blood transfusions. ARDS is characterized by fluid that escapes the vascular system and fills the alveoli. This results in acute respiratory failure.

Diagnosis

ARDS is diagnosed based on patient history, physical examination, chest x-rays, and arterial blood gases.

Treatment

ARDS is treated with mechanical ventilation

Prognosis

Prognosis is not good for ARDS. Even with proper treatment there is a high mortality rate. Two-thirds of ARDS patients die within a few weeks, usually because of pneumonia and/or heart failure. The one-third of patients that recover often have permanent respiratory damage.

Acute Respiratory Failure

Acute respiratory failure often occurs as a result of many pulmonary conditions. It is indicated after severe hypoxemia, hypercapnia, and/or increased serum pH. *Respiratory insufficiency* describes an interim state where blood gases are abnormal but cell function is able to continue. *Respiratory arrest* describes the cessation of respiratory activity.

Manifestations of acute respiratory failure are rapid, shallow, and labored respirations. The condition may result from acute or chronic conditions such as emphysema, pneumonia, pneumothorax, central nervous system depression, chest trauma, pulmonary embolism, acute asthma, myasthenia gravis, amyotrophic lateral sclerosis, or muscular dystrophy. The primary cause must be resolved initially, with supportive treatment given to maintain respiratory functioning.

SUMMARY

The intake of oxygen and the removal of carbon dioxide is the chief function of the respiratory system. All other body systems may be compromised by decreased respiratory function because they need oxygen to operate effectively. Respiratory diseases may be diagnosed by physical examination, chest x-rays, ABGs, and pulmonary function tests. These diseases are responsible for high rates of disability and death, with the common cold, pneumonia, and influenza affecting all age groups.

Most chronic respiratory diseases are found in older adults. Smoking is the single greatest factor that contributes to chronic respiratory disease and is responsible for 90 percent of lung cancers. COPD has four stages, ranging from mild to very severe. Exercise is important for the treatment of most respiratory conditions. Normal oxygen saturation is greater than 99 percent, whereas levels below 90 percent are unsafe. The role of the PTA in treating respiratory diseases involves specific precautions that must be taken (with conditions such as TB) and the ability to work around respiratory accessory devices the patient may need to wear.

REVIEW QUESTIONS

Select the best response to each question.

1. An abnormal decrease in depth and rate of respiration is known as
   a. dyspnea
   b. apnea
   c. hypoxia
   d. hypopnea

2. Which of the following is the primary symptom of laryngeal cancer?
   a. dysphonia
   b. aphasia
   c. apnea
   d. cephalgia

3. In which part of the lung does the exchange of gases take place?
   a. larynx
   b. alveoli
   c. trachea
   d. bronchioles

4. Which of the following is the medication of choice for the treatment of Legionnaire's disease?
   a. gentamycin
   b. penicillin
   c. erythromycin
   d. cefuorxime

5. Which of the following tests is most sensitive for detecting maxillary sinusitis?
   a. tomography
   b. ultrasound
   c. plain radiograph
   d. CT scan

6. The definition of chronic bronchitis is which of the following?
   a. condition associated with the destruction of lung tissue
   b. chronic productive cough of at least 3 months' duration that occurs for 2 consecutive years
   c. reduction in lung compliance by 30 percent or more
   d. chronic productive cough that fails to respond to antibiotics

7. Which of the following tests is used in the initial evaluation of persistent hemoptysis?
   a. bronchoscopy
   b. MRI of the chest
   c. chest radiograph
   d. CT scan of the chest

8. Exposure to radon gas has been associated with the development of what disease?
   a. renal cell carcinoma
   b. lung cancer
   c. pancreatic cancer
   d. bladder cancer

9. Clubbing is thought to be a result of
   a. chronic hypoxemia
   b. chronic hypercarbia
   c. malignancy
   d. protein storage disease

10. Which of the following is a common inherited lung disorder?
   a. cystic fibrosis
   b. pneumonconiosis
   c. pulmonary embolism
   d. asthma

CASE STUDIES

Karen Coupe, PT, DPT, MSEd

Case 1

A 45-year-old man went to the emergency department complaining of chest pain, pain with breathing, and reports of coughing up blood and weight loss. Diagnostic testing revealed pulmonary TB. Patient medical history: HIV positive, type 1 diabetes. During hospitalization the patient developed a pulmonary abscess that was treated with antibiotics. Prior level of function: Independent in all activities. Patient evaluation: Current level of function: Bed mobility w/minimum × 1, transfers w/mod × 1, ambulation × 10 ft with front-wheeled rolling walker and mod × 1 secondary to weakness and dyspnea. Plan of care includes therapeutic exercise, bed mobility, transfer training, and gait training.

1. What are the etiology, pathogenesis, and clinical manifestations of pulmonary TB?
2. Does the past medical history put the patient at greater risk for TB? Why or why not?
3. What is the method of transmission for this pathology? What standard precautions need to be followed by the PTA?
4. The patient developed a pulmonary abscess. Explain this development.
5. What is dyspnea? Why could a patient with this pathology have this issue? How does it affect the plan of care and as a PTA what strategies will you use?

Case 2

A 54-year-old man went to the emergency department complaining of shortness of breath. Diagnostic testing revealed stage 3 COPD with an FEV_1 of 40 percent. Occupational and social history: Over the road truck driver, three-pack-a-day smoker for 40 years, 40 lbs overweight. Prior level of function: Independent in all activities with limited walking distances of 20 ft before rest due to shortness of breath and six steps before shortness of breath. PT evaluation current level of function: Supplemental O_2 nasal cannula at 3 LPM. Resting vital signs: blood pressure 140/85, heart rate 105, resting rate 20, O_2 saturation rate 92. Independent bed mobility, transfers with min x1 secondary to LOB, ambulation × 10 ft w/min × 1 secondary to LOB × 3, O_2 saturation rate of 86 with 45-second recovery to 90. Two-minute post vital signs: blood pressure 145/88, heart rate 115, resting rate 28, O_2 saturation rate 90; 5-minute post: blood pressure 141/85, heart rate 107, resting rate 21, O_2 saturation rate 92. Plan of care includes functional transfer and gait training, therapeutic exercises, and breathing exercises.

1. What are the etiology, pathogenesis, and clinical presentation of COPD? Does this patient have any risk and/or complicating factors for COPD?
2. Define the stages of COPD. Explain the FEV_1 and how this relates to staging.
3. Compare and contrast the resting vital signs and O_2 sat rates with the 2- and 5-minute post-evaluation vital signs and O_2 saturation rates. What are considered normal vital signs for a patient without pathology? Why would this patient present with vital signs in the range as noted above?
4. The PTA is working on gait training with the patient while the patient is on a portable O_2 tank set at 3 LPM. The patient becomes short of breath, O_2 saturation rate is 86. How should the PTA react to this situation? Can a PTA increase the portable O_2 LPM to 4 or 5?
5. Explain what muscles the patient would use during normal, deep, and forced inhalation. Based on this patient's presentation of staging and vital signs, what type of inhalation would you expect to see?

WEBSITES

http://emedicine.medscape.com/article/759765-overview

http://library.thinkquest.org/15401/resp_quiz.html

http://people.eku.edu/ritchisong/301notes6.htm

http://www.cdc.gov/flu/

http://www.emedicinehealth.com/bronchitis/article_em.htm

http://www.getbodysmart.com/ap/respiratorysystem/menu/menu.html

http://www.lib.uiowa.edu/hardin/md/resp.html

http://www.lungcancer.org/

http://www.mayoclinic.com/health/common-cold/ds00056

http://www.webmd.com/lung/tc/pneumonia-topic-overview

http://www.wrongdiagnosis.com/sym/respiratory_symptoms.htm

Digestive System Disorders

LEARNING OBJECTIVES

After completion of this chapter the reader should be able to

1. Describe the structures and functions of the stomach, small intestine, and large intestine.
2. Explain the major functions of the liver.
3. Describe the causes of esophageal varices and reflux esophagitis.
4. Describe the etiology and early signs of gastric cancer.
5. Differentiate between cirrhosis of the liver and cholecystitis.
6. Explain malabsorption syndrome and its etiology.
7. Describe pancreatic cancer and its common signs and symptoms.
8. Compare diverticulosis with diverticulitis, and explain the most common diagnostic test.

KEY TERMS

Abdominocentesis: Surgical puncture of the abdomen with a needle to withdraw fluid.
Achalasia: A disorder of the esophagus that prevents normal swallowing.
Achlorhydria: Absence of hydrochloric acid in the stomach's gastric secretions.
Adenocarcinoma: A cancer of the epithelia originating in glandular tissue.
Adhesions: Conditions of body tissues that are normally separate growing together.
Amylase: An enzyme that breaks starch down into sugar.
Anastomoses: Surgical or pathologic connections between several vessels or tubular structures.
Appendicitis: Inflammation of the appendix.
Ascites: Accumulation of fluid in the peritoneal cavity.
Autodigestion: Digestion of the body's own tissue by its enzymes.
Caput medusae: Distended, engorged pariumbilical veins, radiating from the umbilicus across the abdomen, to join the systemic veins.
Cholecystectomy: Surgical removal of the gallbladder.
Cholecystitis: Inflammation of the gallbladder.
Cholelithiasis: Formation of gallstones due to hardening of bile components.
Cirrhosis: A result of chronic liver disease characterized by replacement of liver tissue by fibrosis, scar tissue, or regenerative nodules.
Colorectal: Referring to the colon and rectum.
Constipation: A symptom of infrequent, hard to pass bowel movements.
Defecate: Eliminate feces from the digestive tract via the anus.
Delirium tremens: An acute episode of delirium usually caused by withdrawal from alcohol.
Dental caries: Tooth decay or "cavities."
Dental plaque: A natural biofilm that may develop on teeth, becoming hardened and discolored; it often leads to dental caries.
Diverticulitis: Inflammation of one or more of the pouches (diverticula) that form because of diverticulosis.

KEY TERMS CONTINUED

Diverticulosis: A common digestive disease, usually in the large intestine, wherein pouches form on the outside of the colon.

Dysentery: An inflammatory condition of (usually) the large intestine that consists of severe diarrhea containing mucus and/or blood, fever, and abdominal pain; untreated dysentery may lead to death.

Dysphagia: Difficulty swallowing.

Edema: Swelling of body tissues because of fluid accumulation.

Enamel: The hard white substance covering the crown of a tooth.

Enteritis: Inflammation of the small intestine.

Esophageal varices: Extremely dilated submucosal veins in the lower esophagus.

Exacerbation: Irritation; generally refers to a worsening of any condition.

Fulminant: Occurring quickly, with extreme severity.

Gastritis: Inflammation of the lining of the stomach.

Gastroenteritis: An inflammation of the gastrointestinal tract, involving the stomach and small intestine, that results in extreme diarrhea.

GI hemorrhage: Bleeding in the gastrointestinal tract.

Gilbert's syndrome: The most common hereditarily linked cause of raised bilirubin levels, resulting in jaundice.

Gingivitis: Inflammation of the gum tissue.

Gluten-induced enteropathy: A pathologic intestinal condition brought about by a reaction to the proteins *gliadin* and *glutenin* (which collectively form *gluten*).

Gynecomastia: Development of abnormally large mammary glands in males, causing breast enlargement.

Hematemesis: Vomiting of blood.

Hematochezia: Passage of a maroon-colored stool.

Hemochromatosis: An iron overload from a hereditary or primary cause.

Hemorrhoids: Normal structures in the anal canal that may become pathologic when swollen or inflamed.

Hepatic encephalopathy: A condition caused by liver failure wherein the patient exhibits confusion, altered levels of consciousness, followed by coma, and, potentially, death.

Hepatitis: Inflammation of the liver.

Hepatomegaly: An enlarged liver.

Hiatal hernia: Protrusion of the upper stomach into the thorax through a weakness or tear in the diaphragm.

Ileus: A disruption of normal, propulsive gastrointestinal activity due to nonmechanical causes.

Inguinal hernia: A protrusion of the abdominal cavity contents through the inguinal canal.

Intestinal obstruction: Bowel obstruction that may be mechanical or functional; it can occur in any section and is a medical emergency.

Intestinal polyps: Abnormal growths of intestinal tissue.

Intrinsic factor: A glycoprotein produced in the stomach that is required for the absorption of vitamin B_{12}.

Intussusception: A condition wherein part of the intestine has folded into another section of the intestine.

Irritable bowel syndrome: Spastic colon; a functional bowel disorder characterized by abdominal pain, discomfort, bloating, and altered bowel function.

Islets of Langerhans: Regions of the pancreas that contain its endocrine cells.

Jaundice: A yellowish discoloration of the skin, sclera, and mucous membranes due to various liver conditions.

Malabsorption syndrome: A condition that arises from abnormality in absorption of food nutrients across the gastrointestinal tract.

Malaise: A feeling of general discomfort or uneasiness.

Melena: Black, "tarry" feces associated with gastrointestinal hemorrhage.

Motility: Ability to move spontaneously and actively, which requires energy.

Occult blood: Blood that is present but not visibly apparent.

Palmar erythema: Reddening of the palms.

Pancreatitis: Inflammation of the pancreas, which may be acute or chronic.

Paralytic obstruction: Paralytic ileus; obstruction of the intestine due to paralysis of the intestinal muscles.

Peptic ulcer: An ulcer of the gastrointestinal tract that is usually acidic and extremely painful.

Perforation: A small hole or tear.

Periodontal disease: Any condition involving bacterial plaque, the gums, teeth, and the immunoinflammatory mechanisms of the patient.

Peristalsis: A symmetric contraction of muscles that moves substances through a body structure, such as food through the intestines.

Peritonitis: Inflammation of the peritoneum (the mucous membrane that lines the abdominal cavity and viscera).

Polyp: A fleshy growth.

Portal hypertension: High blood pressure in the portal vein and its tributaries.

Reflux esophagitis: Inflammation of the esophagus caused by abnormal "reflux" of stomach acid into the esophagus, causing heartburn.

Regional enteritis: Crohn's disease; an inflammatory disease of the intestines that may affect any part of the gastrointestinal tract, causing pain, vomiting, diarrhea, weight loss, and other symptoms.

Remission: The state of absence of disease activity in patients with a known, incurable chronic illness.

Septicemia: Pathogenic microorganisms in the bloodstream, leading to sepsis.

Spider angiomas: Central reddish spots with spider-like reddish extensions on the skin; they consist of dilated blood vessels and may indicate liver disease.

Splenomegaly: Enlargement of the spleen.

Testicular atrophy: Diminished size of the testicles of the male, sometimes accompanied by loss of function.

Ulcerative colitis: A form of inflammatory bowel disease that includes ulcers in the colon.

Varicosities: Enlarged varicose veins.

Volvulus: A bowel obstruction in which a loop of the bowel has twisted upon itself.

Overview

Nutrients reach the structures of the body after being processed by the digestive system. This involves the processes of ingestion, digestion, and absorption. Wastes are eliminated by the digestive system. Digestive disorders are among the most common medical problems. These disorders may affect one person very differently from another. Digestive problems are usually caused by diseases, poor nutrition, or structural abnormalities.

Anatomy and Physiology of the Digestive System

The two main purposes of the digestive system are to break down food into simpler substances for absorption into the blood and body cells and to eliminate wastes from the body. The alimentary canal begins with the mouth and runs through the head, neck, thorax, and abdomen to end at the anus. The accessory organs of digestion are the tongue, teeth, salivary glands, gallbladder, pancreas, and liver.

The *gastrointestinal (GI) tract* (**Figure 18–1**) actually refers to the stomach and intestines but is used interchangeably with the alimentary canal. The length of the canal, if uncoiled, is about 30 feet. The organs of the abdomen and walls of the abdominal cavity are covered by a serous membrane that secretes a lubricating fluid. In the mouth the teeth begin the digestive process by breaking food into smaller pieces. The tongue moves food around in the mouth as the salivary glands secrete *saliva*, which moistens the food for digestion. After chewing, swallowed food passes through the pharynx into the esophagus.

The *salivary glands* have two types of secretory cells: *serous* and *mucous* cells. The amounts of these cells vary in different types of salivary glands. Serous cells produce a watery fluid containing the digestive enzyme *salivary amylase*, which breaks down starch and glycogen into disaccharides. Mucous cells secrete a thick liquid called *mucus*, which binds food particles together and lubricates food while swallowing. The major salivary glands are as follows:

- *Parotid glands*: The largest in size, they lie between the skin of the cheek and the masseter muscle, anterior and slightly inferior to each ear; they secrete a clear, watery fluid rich in amylase.
- *Submandibular glands*: Located in the floor of the mouth, on the inside surface of the lower jaw; they secrete a more viscous fluid than the parotid glands because their secretory cells are about equally mucus and serous.
- *Sublingual glands*: The smallest in size, they lie on the floor of the mouth, inferior to the tongue; containing mostly mucous cells, their secretions are thick and stringy.

Figure 18–2 shows the various types of salivary glands.

The esophagus is a tube that is approximately 9 inches in length and extends from the pharynx to the stomach. Its muscular walls contract to move food into the stomach in a process known as **peristalsis** (**Figure 18–3**). The stomach lies just below the diaphragm in the upper abdomen, connected to the esophagus at the cardiac orifice, an opening surrounded by a thick ring of smooth muscle called the *gastroesophageal*

sphincter (also known as the cardiac sphincter). The stomach is subdivided into the following sections:

- Fundus: Food begins to be broken down by the actions of the enzyme *pepsin* and hydrochloric acid.
- Body: Stomach contractions mix food with these chemicals, and a substance called **intrinsic factor** is secreted, which is required for the absorption of vitamin B_{12}.
- Pylorus: Connects to the *duodenum*, the first part of the small intestine, via the *pyloric orifice*, which is surrounded by the *pyloric sphincter*

The *pancreas* is both an endocrine and exocrine gland. Its exocrine function is to secrete digestive *pancreatic juice*. This organ is closely associated with the small intestine, extending horizontally across the posterior abdominal wall in the C-shaped curve of the duodenum. *Pancreatic acinar cells* produce pancreatic juice and are clustered around tiny tubes that receive their secretions. Pancreatic juice contains enzymes that are able to digest carbohydrates (*pancreatic amylase*), fats (*pancreatic lipase*), nucleic acids (*nucleases*), and proteins (*trypsin, chymotrypsin,* and *carboxypeptidase*). Pancreatic juice release is regulated by the nervous and endocrine systems. When parasympathetic impulses stimulate the secretion of gastric juice, other impulses stimulate the pancreas to release digestive enzymes. As acidic chyme enters the duodenum, the peptide hormone *secretin* is released by the duodenal mucous membrane. Secretin stimulates secretion of pancreatic juice with a high concentration of bicarbonate ions that neutralize the acid of the chyme.

The *liver* lies in the upper right quadrant of the abdominal cavity, slightly inferior to the diaphragm. It is surrounded partially by the ribs and extends from the fifth intercostal space to the lower margin of the ribs. The liver is reddish-brown in color and extremely well supplied with blood vessels. It is enclosed in a fibrous capsule and is divided into a larger *right lobe* and a smaller *left lobe*. Each lobe contains many tiny *hepatic lobules*, the functional units of the liver, that consist of many hepatic cells, a *central vein*, and vascular channels called *hepatic sinusoids*. Blood from the digestive tract is carried in the *hepatic portal vein*.

The liver is vital for a variety of metabolic activities, helping to maintain concentration of blood glucose, oxidizing fatty acids, and synthesizing lipoproteins, phospholipids, and cholesterol. It also converts parts of carbohydrates and proteins into fat molecules, storing fats in the adipose tissue. The most important liver functions concern protein metabolism. It also stores many substances, including vitamins (A, D, and B_{12}), iron, and glycogen. *Bile* is a yellow-green liquid secreted continuously by the liver. It contains bile salts and pigments, cholesterol, and electrolytes.

The *gallbladder* is a pear-shaped, sac-like organ that lies in a depression on the liver's inferior surface. It is connected to the *cystic duct*, which joins the *common hepatic duct*. The gallbladder stores bile between meals, contracts to release bile into the small intestine, and reabsorbs water to concentrate bile. As bile collects in the *common bile duct*, it backs up into the cystic duct, flowing into the gallbladder for storage. Bile salts aid digestive enzymes and break down fat globules into smaller droplets (*emulsification*). This increases the total surface area of the fatty substance, with the droplets mixing

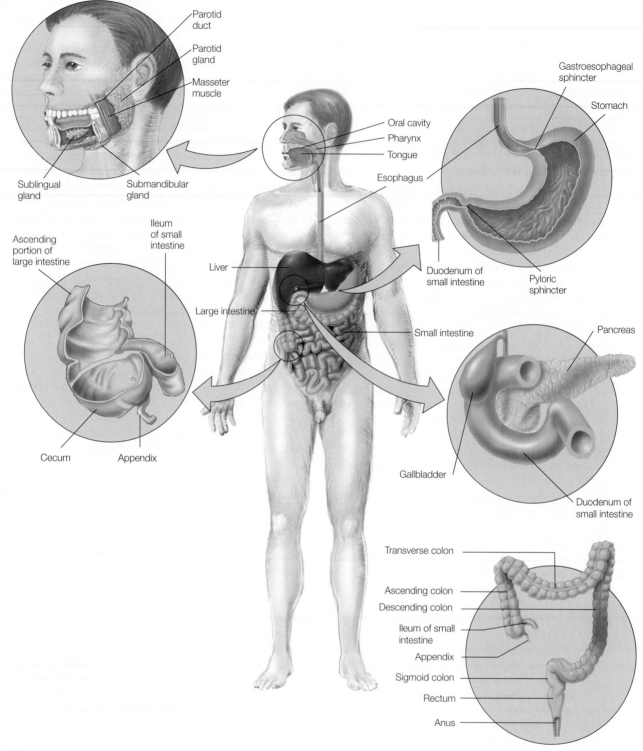

Figure 18–1 The human digestive system.

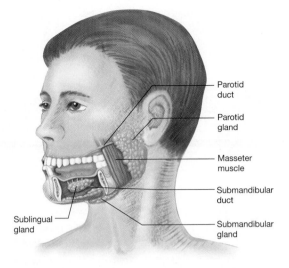

Figure 18–2 Salivary glands.

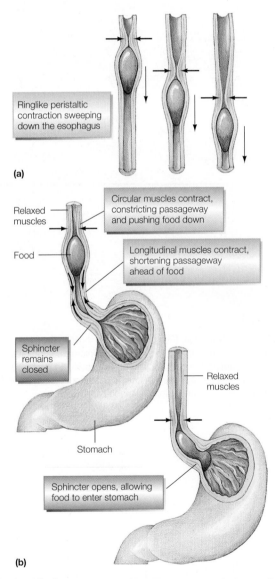

Figure 18–3 Peristalsis. (A) Peristaltic contractions in the esophagus propel food into the stomach. (B) When food reaches the stomach, the gastroesophageal sphincter opens, allowing food to enter.

with water so that lipases can digest them more effectively. Lack of bile salts causes poor absorption of lipids and vitamin deficiencies. **Figure 18–4** shows the liver, gallbladder, and pancreas.

The small intestine extends to the *ileocecal valve*, which is where the large intestine begins. The small intestine, in most adults, is between 4 and 7 meters in length, which is much longer than the large intestine. The names of each part of the intestine are based on their thicknesses, not lengths. The sections of the small intestine are as follows:

- Duodenum: Receives bile from the liver and pancreatic juices from the pancreas
- Jejunum: Located on the left side of the upper abdomen; coiled throughout the abdomen
- Ileum: Where most of the absorption of nutrients takes place

Material is moved through the small intestine via peristalsis. On its inside surface small, finger-like projections (*villi*) are found, which contain lymph vessels and blood capillaries. Smaller *microvilli* cover the villi to form a soft surface that increases the surface area of the small intestine, enhancing nutrient absorption (**Figure 18–5**). Nutrients pass through these capillaries and are delivered to the cells of the body.

The large intestine, or *colon*, is subdivided into these sections:

- Cecum: Located in the lower-right quadrant
- Ascending colon: Located in the midlevel area of the abdomen, it rises to the next section
- Transverse colon: Crosses the abdomen at the umbilicus level
- Descending colon: Descends on the left side into the pelvic cavity

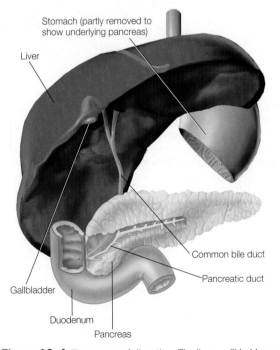

Figure 18–4 The organs of digestion. The liver, gallbladder, and pancreas all play key roles in digestion. All empty by the common bile duct into the small intestine, in which digestion takes place.

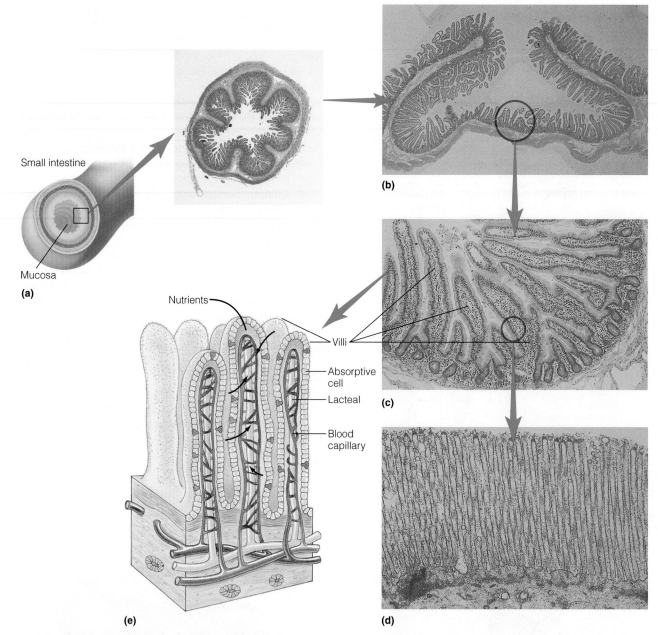

Figure 18–5 The small intestine. The small intestine is uniquely "designed" to increase absorption. (A) A cross section showing the folds. LN means lymph nodules (aggregation of lymphocytes); V means villi; PC means plica circulares (circular fold). (B) A light micrograph of folds and villi. (C) Higher magnification of villi. (D) An electron micrograph of the surface of the absorptive cells showing the microvilli. (E) Each villus contains a loose core of connective tissue; a lacteal, or lymph, capillary; and a network of blood capillaries. Nutrients pass from the lumen of the small intestine through the epithelium and into the interior of the villi, where they are picked up by the lymph and blood capillaries.

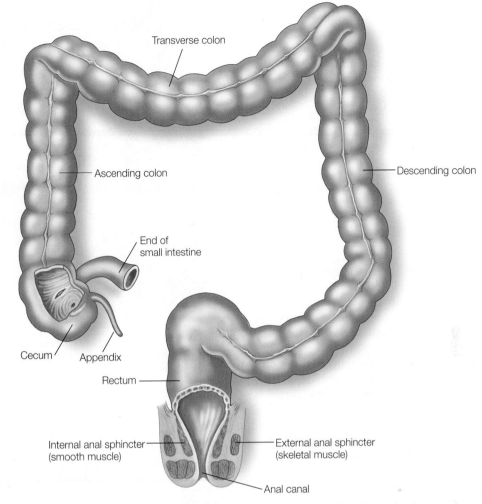

Figure 18–6 The large intestine. This organ consists of four basic parts: the cecum, appendix, colon, and rectum.

- Sigmoid colon: Forms an S-shaped tube that extends into the lower pelvis, ending at the rectum and anus (**Figure 18–6**)

Although absorption and digestion continue in the large intestine, which is about 5 feet long, its most important function is the absorption of water and electrolytes. It also eliminates *feces* (the material not absorbed by the intestines).

Common Diseases of the Digestive System

Digestive system disorders often cause symptoms such as various severities of hemorrhage, altered **motility** (movement) of materials inside the digestive passages, and **perforation**. Terms used to describe hemorrhage include **hematemesis**, **hematochezia**, and **melena** (dark, tarry *stool*). If the digestive tract becomes perforated, the condition may become life threatening because contents may spill into the abdominal cavity, contaminating it. **Peritonitis**, with potentially severe pain, is a common result. As the contents of the digestive tract are acidic, they are corrosive to abdominal organs and contain large amounts of bacteria. If infection results from this spillage, it can lead to **septicemia**. Perforations are com-

monly caused by peptic ulcer, untreated appendicitis, and wounds (such as from gunshots or stabbings).

When motility is altered and food cannot move normally through the digestive tract, signs and symptoms may include nausea, vomiting, constipation, or diarrhea (frequent, watery stools). When the intestinal lining is irritated, peristalsis becomes hyperactive, moving watery contents in the small intestine rapidly through the large intestine. Therefore, the water cannot be absorbed normally by the large intestine, resulting in diarrhea. This massive loss of fluids can lead to dehydration. Diarrhea is commonly caused by bacterial or viral infection, food poisoning, stress, and nervous conditions.

The opposite of diarrhea is **constipation**, with the stool remaining in the colon for too long a period of time. Because more water is absorbed, the stool becomes harder and drier and cannot pass through easily. Constipation is often due to a poor diet and poor elimination habits. Avoiding the urge to **defecate** increases the amount of time the stool remains in the colon and increases constipation.

Common tests used for digestive system disorders include x-rays, endoscopy (using a lighted scope to look inside the digestive tract), upper GI series (swallowing of barium for x-rays), lower GI series (instilling an enema of barium for x-rays), and other procedures. A new technique involves swallowing a capsule that holds a tiny video camera that transmits video images to a special belt worn by the patient. The images are then transferred to a computer. Fecal examination is also available for evaluating patients with GI bleeding, obstruction, parasites, dysentery, or colitis. This procedure is called **occult blood** screening.

Disorders of the Oral Cavity

The mouth's main digestive function is to break down food into smaller particles. Common diseases of the oral cavity include oral cancer, **dental caries**, and **periodontal disease**, such as **gingivitis**. Dental caries is linked to the formation of **dental plaque**.

Infections

Infections of the mouth and throat may be seen as a result of fungal, viral, or bacterial development. Herpes simplex (cold sores) is a recurrent viral infection that affects the skin and mucous membranes. Herpes simplex blisters can develop on the lips and inside the mouth, causing painful ulcers. The vesicles are caused by the herpes simplex virus type 1 and are common.

Thrush is a fungal infection in the mouth and throat producing sore, creamy white, slightly raised "curd-like" patches on the tongue and other oral mucosal surfaces. Thrush is caused by *Candida albicans* and is common in infants or people who are debilitated, immunosuppressed, or receiving long-term antibiotic, corticosteroid, and antineoplastic therapy. Treatment consists of an antifungal medication for 2 weeks.

Oral Leukoplakia

Leukoplakia is hyperkeratosis or epidermal thickening of the buccal mucosa, palate, or lower lip. Oral leukoplakia is a precancerous lesion or lesions occurring anywhere in the mouth. It appears as gray-white or yellow-white leathery surfaced lesions with clearly defined borders. Oral leukoplakia may be caused by chronic oral mucosal irritation, usually because of the use of tobacco and alcohol.

Cancer of the Oral Cavity

Although tumors can occur on the inner cheeks as well as the gums, lips, palate, or tongue, the most common *oral cancer* is squamous cell carcinoma of the lips, which may be localized or invasive (**Figure 18–7**). In the past three decades cases of oral cancer have slightly decreased. Men are more susceptible than women to developing oral cancers.

Signs and Symptoms
Oral cancer includes squamous cell carcinoma or **adenocarcinoma** of the lips, cheek mucosa, anterior tongue, floor of the mouth, and hard palate. It usually causes a small lump on the affected area that is pale in color and painless.

Etiology
The cause of malignant oral tumors is unknown, although certain risk factors such as tobacco use seem to affect the development of these tumors. The risk of oral cancer may also be increased by alcohol consumption. Viral infections (especially

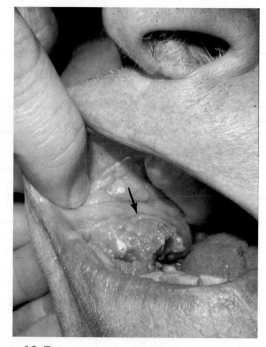

Figure 18–7 Squamous cell carcinoma of oral mucosa (arrow), which appears as an irregular overgrowth of tissue arising from the mucosa of the cheek.

the human papillomavirus), chronic irritation (such as from dentures), inadequate nutrition, poor dental hygiene, and immunodeficiencies are additional risk factors.

Diagnosis
Oral cancers are most effectively diagnosed via tissue biopsy.

Treatment
Treatment for oral cancer is usually very effective, including radiation therapy and surgical removal (excision). Depending on the location of the cancer, surgery may be difficult. Speech therapy is often required after treatment to improve chewing, speech, and swallowing.

Prognosis
Prognosis is generally good for oral cancers unless not treated early.

Esophagus Diseases

Throat and esophagus diseases range widely in severity and duration. Common diseases of this type include esophageal varices, hiatal hernia, and reflux esophagitis.

Esophageal Varices

Esophageal varices are dilated varicose veins in the esophagus. Treating or preventing liver disease can prevent them from developing.

Signs and Symptoms
Symptoms of esophageal varices include vomiting of blood and black stools. When an endoscope is used to examine the esophagus, the blood vessels appear dilated.

Etiology

Esophageal varices are caused by unusually high pressure in the veins of the esophagus, causing them to greatly enlarge. This is caused by blockage or reduced blood flow into the liver, which causes poor venous return from the esophagus. This condition is usually related to cirrhosis of the liver. Excessive alcohol consumption is the most common cause of cirrhosis. When the varices hemorrhage, it may be life threatening.

Diagnosis

With esophageal varices physical examination reveals bloody stools, low blood pressure, and symptoms of chronic liver disease. An *esophagogastroduodenoscopy* (EGD) confirms diagnosis.

Treatment

Treatment of esophageal varices is aimed at decreasing venous pressure. Treatment may require blood pressure medications, portal vein bypass surgery, changing the diet to only soft, nonirritating foods, and the use of stool softeners to prevent straining. If bleeding from the vessels is chronic, a sclerosing agent may be used to harden or destroy the vessel. For acute bleeding, cold saline may be instilled to cleanse the area and pressure may be applied via a nasogastric tube. Sometimes, both procedures are used together.

Prognosis

Prognosis is varied based on the extent of the underlying liver disease.

Hiatal Hernia

Hiatal hernia is a sliding of part of the stomach into the chest cavity through the hole in the diaphragm where the esophagus passes to the stomach. Risks for hiatal hernia may be reduced by maintaining a healthy weight and avoiding smoking and heavy lifting.

Signs and Symptoms

Many hiatal hernias are asymptomatic. When they do cause discomfort, symptoms are usually related to esophageal reflux.

Etiology

Hiatal hernia is caused more often in older individuals due to weakening of the cardiac sphincter.

Diagnosis

Hiatal hernias are diagnosed via upper GI x-rays.

Treatment

Treatment of hiatal hernia is usually the same as for reflux esophagitis: medications that block acid production, medications to treat infections, pain medications, corticosteroids, intravenous nutrition, endoscopy, and surgery. Precautions that should be considered when treating patients with hiatal hernia are education about not consuming water with meals and about eating small meals only of nonirritating foods. Additional precautions include avoiding any exercise activities that may pull or stretch the affected area and aggravate the herniation.

The role of the physical therapist assistant (PTA) in hiatal hernia involves an awareness of the exercise precautions

noted above, scheduling the patient for therapy at least 30 minutes after the completion of a meal, and allowing the patient to receive treatment with the head elevated if lying flat aggravates the condition. Exercises that may be discussed or monitored as a part of therapy include minitrampoline jumping, walking, jogging, martial arts, yoga, aerobics, gymnastics, stretching, and weight lifting. Other exercises indicated for this condition include swimming and dancing. Patients should be cautioned not to exercise until exhausted and not to exercise on a full stomach (except for walking).

Prognosis

Prognosis is good with effective treatment.

Reflux Esophagitis

Reflux esophagitis, commonly called *gastroesophageal reflux disease (GERD)*, is an inflammation of tissue at the lower end of the esophagus. Controlling weight, avoiding smoking, and limiting caffeine, carbonated beverages, chocolate, high-fat foods, and late-night meals are indicated.

Signs and Symptoms

GERD causes a burning sensation in the mid-chest (epigastric) area (also called "heartburn"). Long-term GERD can cause bleeding, scarring of the esophagus, and ulceration. Scarring can lead to difficulty swallowing.

Etiology

Reflux esophagitis is caused by reflux (backflow) of stomach acid through the cardiac sphincter. This acid then moves into the esophagus, burning its tissues.

Diagnosis

Diagnosis of reflux esophagitis requires an upper GI series, which involves swallowing barium and then undergoing x-rays. If required, an EGD with biopsy is performed.

Treatment

Treatments include avoiding large meals, spicy foods, caffeine, and tight clothing. Medications to treat reflux esophagitis include laxatives, stool softeners, and antacids. Both prescription and over-the-counter drugs are designed for acid reflux specifically. Sleeping with the head portion of the bed raised may be helpful. Surgery is only used in extreme reflux conditions.

The role of the PTA in reflux esophagitis is to educate the patient about physical therapies designed to improve postures that exacerbate symptoms. Exercises are designed to keep the body as straight as possible. Positions that should be avoided include slouching, postures that increase root nerve compression, hunching over due to stomach pain, forward neck posture, and tightening of the abdominal muscles. Precautions noted in hiatal hernia are relevant in this condition as well.

Prognosis

Prognosis is usually good with adequate dietary and lifestyle modifications as well as proper medication.

Esophageal Cancer

Esophageal cancer is more prevalent in the elderly and accounts for nearly 6 percent of all GI cancers. It is more frequently seen in men than women and is the seventh leading cause of cancer death among men (with higher incidence in

Black men). The two types of esophageal cancer are *squamous cell carcinoma* and *adenocarcinoma*. Most squamous cell esophageal carcinomas are related to alcohol and tobacco use. They usually occur in the middle or lower third of the esophagus. Esophageal adenocarcinomas are on the increase in the United States and usually develop in the distal esophagus, invading the upper part of the stomach. Esophageal cancer is linked to **achalasia** when obstructions are not adequately relieved.

The most frequent complaint signifying esophageal cancer is **dysphagia**, first occurring when bulky food is ingested. It worsens, occurring even when soft foods and then liquids are ingested. Unfortunately, dysphagia is a late manifestation of the disease, with other symptoms including anorexia, fatigue, weight loss, and pain during swallowing. Treatment is based on tumor stage. Surgical resection may cure early stage tumors but is done on a palliative basis when they are late stage. Other treatments include radiation and chemotherapy. Prognosis is poor but seems to be improving. By the time diagnosis is made, the disease has usually metastasized, limiting long-term survival chances.

> **RED FLAG**
> A stricture is a narrowing of the esophagus caused by a scar. Reflux esophagitis with ulceration and scarring may lead to a stricture.

Stomach Diseases

Stomach diseases often cause pain, especially after eating. The incidence of diseases of the stomach increases with age, ranging from mild gastritis to peptic ulcer to cancer of the stomach.

Gastritis

Gastritis is an inflammation of the stomach that may be acute or chronic.

Signs and Symptoms

Gastritis usually causes abdominal pain and may also cause belching, nausea, and vomiting. Patients in whom acute gastritis is associated with mucosal ulceration often have more pronounced signs and symptoms. Ulcerated areas may bleed profusely.

Etiology

Gastritis may be caused by nonsteroidal anti-inflammatory medications, alcohol consumption, smoking, and bacterial infections (such as *Helicobacter pylori*). More than 50 percent of Americans over age 60 have *H. pylori* infections. Chronic gastritis may be caused when this bacterium weakens the mucous lining of the stomach and stomach acid contacts the stomach tissues below it. This may lead to pain and ulceration. *H. pylori* gastritis is believed to be a major factor in gastric ulcer formation. Gastritis increases with age, and **achlorhydria** (atrophic gastritis) may result when there is not enough hydrochloric acid in the stomach to kill bacteria that is ingested. Achlorhydria causes loss of *intrinsic factor*, leading to pernicious anemia.

> **RED FLAG**
> *Helicobacter pylori* produce an enzyme called *urease* that decomposes urea. This decomposition of urea yields ammonia, which neutralizes gastric acid.

Diagnosis

Diagnosis of gastritis is determined by a blood test that checks for anemia, a stool test to detect the presence of blood and *H. pylori* in the stool, and either an upper GI endoscopy or EGD for visual confirmation.

Treatment

Gastritis is treated with medications to reduce stomach acid. For *H. pylori*, treatment with antibiotics is indicated. Healthy changes include avoiding irritating foods and medications, reducing alcohol consumption, and smoking cessation. Gastritis is usually resolved when the underlying cause is successfully treated. The role of the PTA with gastritis patients is to educate them about exercises and activities designed to relax the abdominal muscles. This leads to healthy digestion and lessened tension, both of which exacerbate symptoms of gastritis.

Prognosis

Prognosis is good with proper treatment and the following of suggested guidelines.

Peptic Ulcer

An *ulcer* is an area of tissue that has eroded, leaving a crater-like appearance. A **peptic ulcer** is a chronic form of ulcer that is found in the stomach or duodenum (**Figure 18–8A and B**). It may be caused by the action of pepsin (a digestive enzyme). Peptic ulcers are further described to designate their locations in the stomach (gastric ulcer) or duodenum (duodenal ulcer).

Signs and Symptoms

Pain from peptic ulcer comes from hydrochloric acid irritating the ulcerated area. Complications may include massive bleeding (hemorrhage), obstruction, and perforation.

Etiology

Most peptic ulcers are associated with *H. pylori*, although other factors include heavy intake of drugs or alcohol, smoking, and severe stress.

Diagnosis

Diagnosis of peptic ulcer is based on symptoms and gastroscopy (visual examination of the inside of the stomach).

Treatment

Treatment of peptic ulcer includes reduction of gastric acidity, antibiotics (if caused by *H. pylori*), reducing potential causes of the ulcer, using antacids, and, in severe cases, surgery. Severe cases include those that may cause extreme pain, hemorrhage, obstruction, or perforation. The role of the PTA in peptic ulcer is to educate patients about exercises and activities designed to relax the muscles of the affected areas. Physical therapy is aimed at relaxation in this condition and not increasing muscle tone.

Prognosis

Prognosis is good as long as treatment is adequate.

Cancer of the Stomach

Cancer of the stomach is much more common in countries outside of the United States (mostly in Japan, central Europe, the Scandinavian countries, and South and Central America).

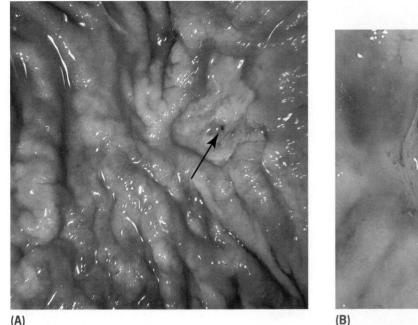

(A)

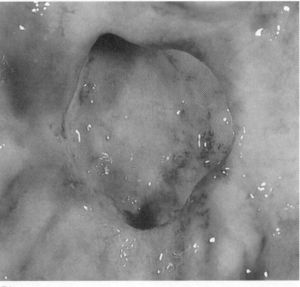

(B)

Figure 18–8 Peptic ulcers. (A) Gastric ulcer, which eroded a blood vessel in the base of the ulcer (arrow) and bled profusely. (B) Large chronic duodenal ulcer.

It is the major cause of cancer death worldwide. Stomach cancer often metastasizes to organs such as the esophagus, intestine, or pancreas. Other metastasis sites include the liver, lungs, and lymph nodes. Unfortunately, it is often undiagnosed until metastasis has already occurred.

Signs and Symptoms

Stomach cancers are often asymptomatic until late in their course of development. When symptoms do occur, they are usually vague, including chronic dyspepsia and epigastric discomfort that is linked to tumor growth, weight loss, feelings of fullness after eating, anemia, fatigue, and loss of appetite. Blood in the stool due to erosion of the gastric mucosa by tumors is also seen.

Etiology

Stomach cancer is of unknown origin, although it may be related to food additives and foods that are pickled, salted, or smoked. Cigarette smoking is another risk factor. Infection with *H. pylori* appears to serve as a cofactor in some types of gastric carcinomas. Men are diagnosed with stomach cancer more than women.

Diagnosis

Diagnosis of stomach cancer includes endoscopy, barium x-ray studies, biopsy, and cytologic studies of gastric secretions. Cytologic studies can be extremely useful as routing screening tests for patients with atrophic gastritis or gastric polyps. Computed tomography (CT) scan and endoscopic ultrasonography are often used to observe the spread of a diagnosed stomach cancer.

Treatment

Treatment of stomach cancer includes resection of a large part of the stomach together with the surrounding tissues and the draining of the lymph nodes (**Figure 18–9**). Other treatments include chemotherapy and radiation. The role of the PTA is to implement a program of simple overall exercises that help to stimulate endorphins, which help to strengthen the body's ability to fight disease. Physical therapy should focus on helping to relieve pain, fatigue, and guarded posture while addressing mobility issues, abdominal discomfort, breathing problems, and normal daily living requirements. Light resistance exercises and range-of-motion training are usually helpful. The patient should be taught to practice abdominal breathing, weight distribution techniques, and simplification of movements to enhance work effectiveness. Edema can be reduced by special massage techniques, gentle stretching exercises, the use of compression garments, and pumps designed to reduce swelling.

Prognosis

Prognosis is good if discovered early, but this is rarely the case. Unfortunately, the cancer is in an advanced state by the time it causes symptoms. Therefore, prognosis is relatively poor.

Lower Gastrointestinal Diseases

Disorders of the lower GI tract often cause pain to radiate across the abdomen, intestinal upset, and ulcers. These diseases include gastroenteritis, inguinal hernia, malabsorption syndrome, and regional enteritis (Crohn's disease).

Gastroenteritis

Gastroenteritis is an inflammation of the stomach and intestines. The term "**enteritis**" is used to describe inflammation of the small intestine.

Signs and Symptoms

Symptoms of gastroenteritis may occur very quickly and violently. They include nausea, vomiting, abdominal cramping,

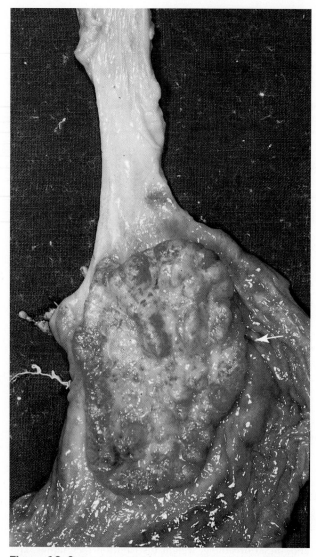

Figure 18–9 Carcinoma of the stomach. The stomach has been opened, revealing a large ulcerated neoplasm arising from gastric mucosa (arrow) and extending upward to gastroesophageal junction. Esophagus is seen in upper part of photograph.

and diarrhea that lead to fluid and electrolyte loss. Additional symptoms may include **malaise** and stomach "rumbling."

Etiology
Gastroenteritis can be caused by bacteria (or their toxins), parasites, or viruses as well as ingestion of tainted food, allergic reactions to food or drugs, stress, and lactose intolerance. They are generally of short duration.

Diagnosis
Gastroenteritis may be diagnosed via stool samples to determine the cause of the condition.

Treatment
Treatment is based on the present symptoms and can include medications to treat nausea, antidiarrheals, antibiotics, fluids to support hydration, nutritional support, and the management of stress. The role of the PTA is to implement a light, tolerable exercise program that helps to relieve stress.

Prognosis
Prognosis is usually good for gastroenteritis once the causative factor is treated.

Inguinal Hernia

An **inguinal hernia** is a pouching of the small intestine and peritoneum into the groin. It is more common in males than females. Preventive measures include losing weight, avoiding smoking, lifting properly, and avoiding constipation because it leads to straining (and potential hernia). The small intestine may herniate through a variety of body openings, including the femoral canal or umbilicus.

Signs and Symptoms
Symptoms of inguinal hernia include a bulge in the groin or scrotum, with pain that worsens with lifting or bending but is relieved by lying down. If the hernia has become "strangulated" (pressurized so that blood flow is restricted, a potentially life-threatening condition), there will be sudden pain, nausea, and vomiting.

Etiology
Inguinal hernia may be caused by congenital conditions or weakness in the abdominal wall.

Diagnosis
Inguinal hernia is diagnosed via patient history, physical examination, ultrasound, and CT scan.

Treatment
Inguinal hernia can be repaired surgically so tissue death of the affected area does not occur. The role of the PTA in inguinal hernia is to assist with exercises designed to relieve pain. Exercises are tailored to the individual and the severity of the hernia. Commonly used exercises focus on the legs, hips, shoulders, and abdomen.

Prognosis
Prognosis is good with proper treatment. Surgery is usually very effective.

Malabsorption Syndrome

Malabsorption syndrome occurs when the small intestine cannot adequately absorb nutrients (especially lipids) and minerals into the blood.

Signs and Symptoms
Symptoms of malabsorption syndrome include anemia, diarrhea, edema, muscle cramping, weight loss, heart arrhythmias (due to lack of potassium), and blood clotting disorders (due to lack of vitamin K absorption). If this condition develops in children, their normal growth pattern may be affected. The condition may be inherited.

Etiology
Causes of malabsorption syndrome include cystic fibrosis, diabetes mellitus, lactose intolerance, pancreatic deficiencies, and gluten enteropathy. This condition can range from mild intestinal upset to chronic ulcers or enteritis.

Diagnosis
Diagnosis of malabsorption syndrome requires a variety of different tests that measure abnormalities of the GI tract, including patient history, physical examination, various blood

tests, x-rays, endoscopies, stool samples, ultrasound, CT scans, and magnetic resonance imaging.

Treatment

Malabsorption syndrome is usually treated with strict dietary changes and avoiding certain foods that may worsen the condition.

Prognosis

Prognosis is usually good with adequate diet.

Regional Enteritis

Also known as "Crohn's disease," **regional enteritis** is a chronic inflammatory disease characterized by periods of **remission** and **exacerbation** that affect the intestinal wall. Crohn's disease is also characterized by inflammation and ulceration of the bowel mucosa with marked thickening and scarring of the bowel wall (**Figure 18–10**). Until complete diagnosis is made, regional enteritis is usually classified as *inflammatory bowel disease (IBD)*. As it progresses the intestinal wall thickens, resulting in its lumen becoming narrowed.

Signs and Symptoms

Symptoms of regional enteritis include anorexia, abdominal pain, flatulence, constipation, and diarrhea. The condition appears to worsen during times of stress, emotional upset, or depression, with young girls most often affected.

Etiology

The cause of regional enteritis is not yet determined, although it appears to be genetically linked, infectious, immunologic, and related to stress.

Diagnosis

Regional enteritis is diagnosed via blood tests, upper GI series, CT scans, and colonoscopy. A new technique used for this condition is "video capsule endoscopy."

Treatment

Treatment is designed to support the health of the patient and often involves diet and medications to control the symptoms. If perforation or obstruction occurs, surgical resection is indicated. The role of the PTA in regional enteritis is

to implement a program of exercises designed to maintain overall health and reduce stress. Patients should be advised to drink water when exercising and to avoid temperature extremes.

Prognosis

Prognosis is generally good with healthy diet and stress reduction.

Gluten-Induced Enteropathy

Gluten-induced enteropathy is an immune disorder that causes sensitivity to gluten proteins. It is also known as *celiac (nontropical) sprue disease*. Gluten proteins are found in products made of rye, wheat, barley, and oats. The condition causes impaired absorption of related proteins, fats, carbohydrates, and vitamins. Treatment involves the restriction of all foods containing glutens.

Intestinal Polyps

Intestinal polyps are noncancerous (benign) tumors of the intestinal linings. They are often removed via surgery because they can increase the risk of cancer.

Appendicitis

Appendicitis is inflammation of the *vermiform appendix*, a primarily lymphoid structure located near the point where the small and large intestines join. The term "vermiform" means "worm-like," and the appendix indeed does resemble a worm. Although not preventable, appendicitis may be avoided by eating a diet that includes proper amounts of fruits and vegetables.

Signs and Symptoms

Appendicitis pain begins throughout the abdomen but shifts to the lower right quadrant. Appendicitis also causes nausea, vomiting, fever, and leukocytosis. If the appendix ruptures the pain may decrease, but a condition known as *peritonitis* may develop. Peritonitis can be fatal if not treated with antibiotics. Other signs include inflammation in the area of the appendix and potential gangrene.

Etiology

Appendicitis is usually caused by infection or obstruction caused by bacteria-laden fecal contents. Because of an obstruction, secretions that are normally produced by the epithelial cells lining the appendix drain poorly from the area distal to the blockage. As the secretions accumulate, they create pressure within the lumen of the appendix, compressing blood vessels in the mucosa and impairing its viability (**Figure 18–11A and B**).

Diagnosis

Proper diagnosis is essential as appendicitis can mimic the symptoms of kidney stones, pelvic inflammatory disease, and pancreatitis.

Treatment

Appendicitis is treated by surgical removal of the appendix, ideally before a rupture occurs. The role of the PTA is to implement a program, after surgery, of low-impact muscle stretching and strengthening to assist the patient in returning to prior functional level.

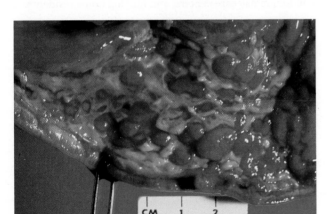

Figure 18–10 Crohn's Disease (regional enteritis). Mucosa is ulcerated and covered by inflammatory exudate.

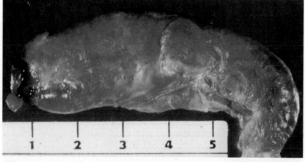

(A)

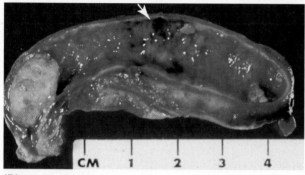

(B)

Figure 18–11 Acute appendicitis. (A) Exterior of appendix is swollen, congested, and covered with inflammatory exudate. (B) Appendix bisected to reveal interior. Pus within lumen has been removed. Mucosa is congested and ulcerated (arrow). The base of the appendix (left side of photograph) is plugged by a firm mass of fecal material.

Prognosis

Prognosis is usually good with prompt surgery and antibiotics to prevent infection.

Colon Polyps

A colon **polyp** is an inward projection of its mucosal lining. Although not preventable, their occurrence may be lessened with a healthy diet that is low in fat, limited use of alcohol, avoiding smoking, a healthy body weight, and exercise.

Signs and Symptoms

Colon polyps may cause rectal bleeding but are usually asymptomatic.

Etiology

Colon polyps can be the result of an inflammatory reaction or can be caused by either benign or malignant neoplasms.

Diagnosis

Routing colonoscopy or sigmoidoscopy examinations often reveal colon polyps.

Treatment

Treatment of colon polyps includes biopsy, excision, or surgical resection based on the amount and type of polyps discovered.

Prognosis

Prognosis varies based on the type of polyps, their amount, and the stage of development.

Diverticulosis and Diverticulitis

Diverticulosis is a condition wherein small pouches (diverticula) develop in the colon (often, the sigmoid portion of the colon). Diverticulosis may be asymptomatic until the pouches are packed with fecal material, causing irritation (**Figure 18–12A, B, and C**). Once they become inflamed, the condition is called **diverticulitis**.

Signs and Symptoms

Diverticulitis causes cramping and low abdominal pain. The inflammation caused by this disorder can lead to hemorrhage, narrowing of the lumen of the colon (and obstruction), or perforation.

Etiology

Diverticulitis occurs more with increased age and is linked to lack of physical activity, poor bowel habits, and poor dietary habits.

Diagnosis

Diagnosis of diverticulosis and diverticulitis is made via colonoscopy to examine the diverticula of the colon. The role of the PTA is to assist patients with these conditions with low impact exercises to improve overall fitness. No specific exercises are indicated. The PTA does not work with this condition specifically, because it is usually present with other problems.

Treatment

This condition is treated primarily by increasing the amount of dietary fiber, which includes fruits, vegetables, beans, potatoes, cereals, and rice. If acute diverticulitis develops, antibiotics may be required.

Prognosis

Prognosis is usually good with dietary modifications. It is poorer when hemorrhage, narrowing, obstruction, or perforation occur and requires aggressive treatment.

Dysentery

Dysentery is a term that describes various GI disorders that cause acute inflammation. It is common in underdeveloped countries because of poor sanitation. When dysentery does occur in the United States, it is usually seen in immigrants, inner-city housing residents, frequent international travelers, children in day care centers, and nursing home residents.

Signs and Symptoms

Dysentery causes severe abdominal pain, cramping, and large amounts of bloody or watery diarrhea.

Etiology

Dysentery is caused by microorganisms that invade the colon's lining, usually because of contaminated food or water.

Diagnosis

Dysentery is diagnosed by examining stool samples for causative microorganisms.

Treatment

Treatment of dysentery is based on the causative microorganism. If bacterial in origin, antibiotics are usually effective. Antivirals may also be used if of viral origin.

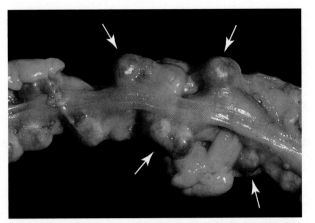

(A)

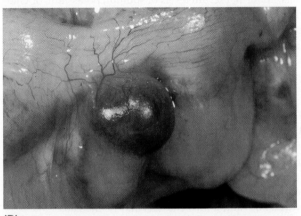

(B)

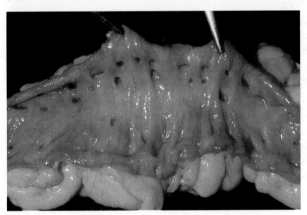

(C)

Figure 18–12 Diverticulosis of colon. (A) Exterior of colon illustrating several diverticula projecting through wall of colon (arrows). (B) A closer view of diverticulum. (C) Interior of colon, illustrating openings of multiple diverticula. Several of the openings are well demonstrated in the mucosa just below the clamps.

Prognosis

Prognosis is generally good with prompt treatment. Methods to reduce transmission of dysentery include regular hand washing, avoiding the sharing of eating utensils or straws, avoiding tap water and ice cubes when in a foreign country, and avoiding salads, fresh fruit, and fresh vegetables when in a foreign country.

Hemorrhoids

Hemorrhoids are internal or external varicose veins that develop in the rectum. If Internal hemorrhoids are located on the rectal wall and can be viewed by using a *proctoscope*. External hemorrhoids are located in the lower anal canal and develop when internal hemorrhoids emerge through the anal opening. External hemorrhoids can be viewed around the anus, are slightly bluish in color, and may bleed during bowel movements if the patient strains. Preventive measures include stool softeners, good bowel habits, adequate fluid intake, increased dietary fiber, exercise, and avoiding the use of laxatives.

Signs and Symptoms

Hemorrhoids commonly cause bleeding with bowel movements, itching, and rectal pain.

Etiology

Hemorrhoids are caused by pressure, as from straining during bowel movements, chronic constipation, prolonged standing or sitting, pregnancy, and childbirth. Other causes include loss of muscle tone and heredity.

Diagnosis

External hemorrhoids are easily diagnosed by digital rectal examination. Internal hemorrhoids may require visual inspection with either an *anoscope* (used to view the anus) or *proctoscope* (used to view the rectum). The role of the PTA for patients with hemorrhoids is to educate them on how to exercise the muscles of the buttocks to strengthen the affected area. The PTA should be aware that these patients may not tolerate the usual positions for traditional physical therapy and should work to find positions that make the patient more comfortable.

Treatment

Hemorrhoids can be treated with a variety of medications, soaking in a warm bath for between 20 and 30 minutes on a regular basis, surgical reduction, cryosurgery, and hemorrhoidectomy.

Prognosis

Prognosis varies based on the severity of the condition.

Intestinal Obstruction

Intestinal obstruction may be either a disease or a symptom of another disease process. It is defined as an inability to move intestinal contents through the bowel.

Signs and Symptoms

Symptoms of intestinal obstruction include nausea, vomiting, and mild to severe abdominal pain and distention.

Etiology

An intestinal obstruction can be due to a blockage, a disease, or **ileus** (absence of peristalsis). Blockage can be caused by **adhesions**, hernias, or twisting of the colon (**volvulus**). If the colon twists enough to "telescope" back on itself, the condition may develop into a blockage called **intussusception**. When peristalsis slows or stops, causing an obstruction, this is classified as a **paralytic obstruction**. This may be caused by peritonitis or a postoperative complication.

Adhesions are defined as *adhesive bands of connective tissue*, which may form within the abdominal cavity (often because of surgery). **Figure 18–13** shows an example of an adhesion. *Hernias* are protrusions of a loop of the bowel through a small opening, often in the abdominal wall. The herniated loop will push out the peritoneum to form a hernia sac (**Figure 18–14**). A *volvulus* is a rotary twisting of the bowel on the fold of the peritoneum that suspends it from the posterior abdominal wall (the *mesentery*). When one segment of bowel telescopes into an adjacent segment, it is called an *intussusception* (**Figure 18–15**).

Diagnosis

Intestinal obstruction is diagnosed via abdominal x-rays, abdominal CT scan, or upper or lower GI series.

Treatment

Treatment usually involves surgery, although suctioning of the intestine via a nasogastric tube is also used. The role of the PTA is to educate patients about the Wurn technique, a massage form of therapy that may help to reduce or eliminate adhesions.

Prognosis

Prognosis depends on the severity of the obstruction, damage to the intestine, and other conditions that may exist.

Peritonitis

Peritonitis is inflammation of the peritoneum. It can be local or generalized and acute or chronic. A patient who displays sudden severe, diffuse abdominal pain, fever, weakness, nausea, and vomiting requires emergency medical attention.

Signs and Symptoms

When the peritoneum becomes irritated or infected, fluid accumulates in the peritoneal space, causing *hyperemic* and *edematous* states. Resulting inflammation may cause the formation of abscesses and adhesions in the abdominal cavity. Signs and symptoms may include abdominal pain, nausea, vomiting, profuse sweating, and weakness. Pain may become so severe the patient is immobilized. Other symptoms include fever, abdominal tenderness and distension, and paralytic ileus. If the peritonitis fulminates, the body absorbs the toxic *exudate*, causing septicemia, shock, and even death.

Etiology

Peritonitis may be a primary infection caused by organisms from the blood or genital tract. If secondary in nature, it may be contaminated by GI secretions from perforations of the GI tract or nearby organs. Causes include bacterial invasion after surgery or because of a breakdown of **anastomoses**. This allows contaminated secretions from the intestines to spill into the abdominal cavity. Other causes include penetrating abdominal wounds and systemic lupus erythematosus. Additional causes include noninfective secretions (such as bile from the gallbladder) or invasions by *Escherichia coli*, anaerobic streptococci, or *Pseudomonas aeruginosa*.

Diagnosis

Diagnosis of peritonitis is based on elevated white blood cells; abnormal serum levels of sodium, potassium, or chloride; and radiographic abdominal examination that shows gaseous bowel distention. Radiography may also show perforation of an organ or air in the abdominal cavity. Aspirated peritoneal fluid will appear cloudy. The causative microorganism is identified by a culture and sensitivity study of the peritoneal fluid.

Treatment

The treatment of peritonitis involves broad-spectrum antibiotics, antiemetics, and analgesics. Fluids and electrolytes are usually replaced parenterally. A perforation requires surgery to correct the source of infection and drain any spilled contents. To eliminate the infection continuous peritoneal lavage with saline–antibiotic solutions may be indicated.

Prognosis

Peritonitis is life threatening without prompt, aggressive medical intervention. Many of its underlying causes cannot be easily predicted.

Irritable Bowel Syndrome

Irritable bowel syndrome is actually the most common disorder of the intestines and is often confused with *inflammatory bowel disease (IBD)*. Irritable bowel syndrome is also known as *spastic colon*, which is a functional disorder of motility in the intestine. It does not involve inflammation or lesions, both of which are commonly seen in IBD.

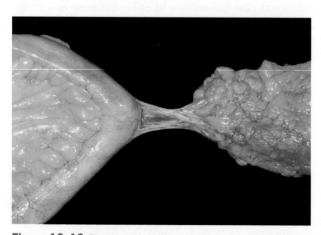

Figure 18–13 Fibrous adhesion between loop of small intestine (left side of photograph) and omentum.

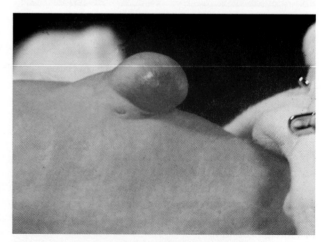

Figure 18–14 A large umbilical hernia in an infant.

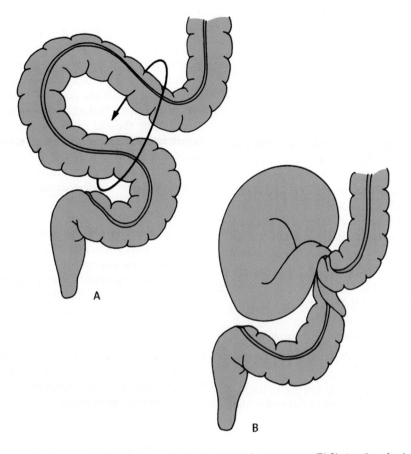

Figure 18–15 Pathogenesis of volvulus. (A) Rotary twist of sigmoid colon on its mesentery. (B) Obstruction of colon and interruption of its blood supply caused by volvulus.

Signs and Symptoms

Irritable bowel syndrome can cause abdominal pain, altered motility, constipation, and diarrhea.

Etiology

The cause of irritable bowel syndrome is unknown but is related to stress, spicy food, alcohol, caffeine, and certain food seasonings. Irritable bowel syndrome is a chronic condition that usually begins in early adulthood, recurring frequently throughout life.

Diagnosis

Irritable bowel syndrome is diagnosed via stool samples, blood tests, endoscopy, and x-rays. A colonoscopy is very effective in confirming diagnosis.

Treatment

Irritable bowel syndrome is treated by avoiding stress and dietary causes to allow normal intestinal motility to return. Stress reduction techniques include biofeedback, counseling, regular exercise, meditation, deep breathing, hypnosis, and yoga. The role of the PTA in irritable bowel syndrome is to educate patients about pelvic floor exercises, such as Kegel exercises, which may help lessen the symptoms by strengthening the muscles of the pelvic floor.

Prognosis

Prognosis is based on avoiding the causative factors.

Ulcerative Colitis

Ulcerative colitis is a chronic inflammation of the colon.

Signs and Symptoms

Ulcerative colitis causes inflammation and ulcers in the lining of the colon and rectum. It is also generally referred to as IBD until actual diagnosis is confirmed. This condition causes multiple ulcerations leading to abdominal pain, bloody stools, anemia, and diarrhea.

Etiology

Ulcerative colitis is of unknown origin, but it appears to be related to stress, autoimmune disorders, diet, and heredity. Ulcerative colitis may increase the risk of developing colon cancer.

Diagnosis

Ulcerative colitis is diagnosed by blood tests (to search for anemia), stool samples, CT scan, and colonoscopy (which is the preferred method of diagnosis).

Treatment

Ulcerative colitis can be treated with a limited diet, mild sedatives, anti-inflammatory medications, and stress reduction. Surgery may be indicated if other treatments fail and often involves a temporary or permanent colostomy. The role of the PTA is to implement an exercise program designed to relieve stress, which contributes to ulcerative colitis.

Indicated exercises include low-impact aerobics and breathing exercises.

Prognosis

Prognosis is based on severity of the disease and whether surgery is required.

Cancer of the Colon and Rectum

Colorectal cancer describes cancer of the colon and/or rectum. The most common type of colorectal tumor is an adenocarcinoma that arises from the mucosal lining. This type of cancer affects both sexes. At age 50 all people should have annual stool examinations to check for colorectal cancer. Adenocarcinomas tend to grow slowly but may become large enough to obstruct the lumen and spread through the wall of the colon. It can then metastasize to the lymphatic and vascular systems, spreading throughout the body (but usually to the liver).

Signs and Symptoms

Symptoms of colorectal cancer differ based on the location of the malignancy but usually include constipation or diarrhea, blood in the stool, pencil-sized stool, anemia, abdominal discomfort, and obstruction.

Etiology

Although of unknown origin, it may be linked to familial history of colon polyps, ulcerative colitis, and a diet that is high in red meat and low in fiber.

Diagnosis

Colorectal cancer may be diagnosed by stool examinations for occult blood, a barium enema procedure, or colonoscopy. Certain rectal tumors can be palpated by digital examination.

Treatment

Colorectal cancer is curable via surgical resection if discovered early. In this operation some or all of the colon is removed, with the two healthy ends of the bowel joined together (*anastomosis*). If a larger amount of the colon must be removed, a permanent or temporary opening (*colostomy*) may be required. In this procedure the end of the colon is brought through an opening in the abdominal wall, leaving a pink opening (*stoma*) through which fecal matter will pass. It is covered by a colostomy bag that must be emptied several times a day.

Sometimes after bowel surgery the colostomy procedure is done as a temporary procedure that allows the bowel to heal. Then, another surgery is performed to reconnect the colon together. Other treatments for colorectal cancer include radiation and chemotherapy. The role of the PTA is to implement a low-impact exercise program designed to improve overall body health, strength, and condition. The lessening of fatigue symptoms with exercise is indicated. Other goals of physical therapy are to improve bowel function, boost the immune system, and reduce anxiety and depression. Additional therapies include electrical stimulation, acupuncture, and techniques designed to reduce edema.

Prognosis

Prognosis is good if the carcinoma is detected before metastasis but poor if metastasis has already occurred.

Imperforate Anus

Imperforate anus is defined as a congenital abnormality in which the colon does not develop a normal anal opening (**Figure 18–16**). A rare condition, imperforate anus has two major types: (1) a normally formed rectum and anus but no anal orifice through the skin or (2) the entire distal rectum has not developed. In the first type a small fistula (tract) often extends from the anal canal and terminates in the urethra, vagina, or surface of the skin. This is easily treated by excising the covering tissue. In the second type there are often other urogenital and skeletal abnormalities, and surgical repair is difficult with less satisfactory outcomes.

Liver Diseases

The liver is the largest solid body organ and plays a role in digestion, absorption, metabolism, blood clotting, synthesis of chemicals, and storage of nutrients. It consists of two lobes and lies in the right upper quadrant of the abdomen. It produces and secretes bile, which is used to digest fats. The liver also produces cholesterol, fibrinogen, and prothrombin. It oxidates fatty acids and glycerol to provide the body with energy. Carbohydrates, fats, and proteins are metabolized by the liver. It converts glucose to glycogen for storage and reverses the process for energy needs. The liver also synthesizes amino acids, detoxifies drugs and other toxins, and stores vitamins and minerals.

An obvious symptom of liver disease is *jaundice*, a yellowish discoloration of the skin and sclera of the eyes. Jaundice is caused by high levels of *bilirubin* in the blood. Bilirubin is created by the breakdown of heme (the main component of hemoglobin in red blood cells). Bilirubin is normally filtered

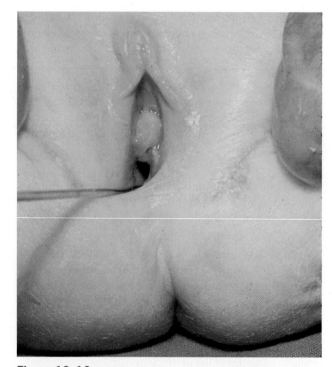

Figure 18–16 Imperforate anus in newborn infant. Metal probe has been placed in vagina.

by the liver and excreted in bile. It is also filtered by the kidneys, causing the urine to appear dark brown. The most common hereditarily linked cause of raised bilirubin levels is **Gilbert's syndrome**.

Liver function tests use blood samples to measure levels of albumin (blood protein), bilirubin, and alkaline phosphatase (an enzyme). Ultrasound, x-rays, CT scans, and biopsies are also used to diagnose various conditions. Liver (as well as gallbladder) diseases affect over 25 million people in the United States. Common liver diseases include cirrhosis, hepatitis, and liver cancer.

Hemochromatosis

Hemochromatosis causes the body to absorb and store excessive iron and is the most common inherited disease. Liver damage is likely, and this condition is diagnosed by blood tests for iron levels. Treatment requires up to 2 units of blood to be moved weekly until iron levels return to normal. This procedure must occur every 4 months throughout life.

Cirrhosis

Cirrhosis is a chronic, degenerative disease that is irreversible. It is also known as *end-stage liver disease*. Cirrhosis causes normal liver cells to be replaced with fibrous, nonfunctioning scar tissue (**Figure 18–17**). The cirrhotic liver appears to be covered in nodules. At this point the liver has impaired blood flow and altered functionality. Exposure to all types of hepatitis (as well as being vaccinated against hepatitis A and B) reduce occurrence of cirrhosis that is not caused by alcohol or congestive heart failure.

Signs and Symptoms

Severe cirrhosis causes the following complications:

- **Varicosities**: Varicose veins, usually in the esophagus; when occurring across the front of the abdomen (a condition called **caput medusae**) they are very unattractive in appearance.
- **Splenomegaly**: Enlarged spleen; leads to increased destruction of blood cells, anemia, leucopenia, and thrombocytopenia.

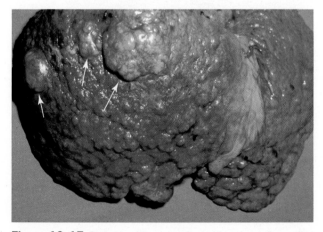

Figure 18–17 Cirrhosis of liver complicated by primary liver cell carcinoma (arrows).

- **GI hemorrhage**: Caused by thrombocytopenia and the liver's inability to secrete blood proteins needed for clotting; *hematemesis* is often the first sign of severe cirrhosis.
- **Ascites**: An accumulation of fluid in the abdominal cavity due to liver failure and portal hypertension; excessive fluid can be drained by piercing the abdominal wall (**abdominocentesis**).
- **Edema**: Swelling of (commonly) the ankles and feet due to liver failure; normally, the liver produces *albumin* to control the osmotic pressure of blood. Without this the blood fluid leaks into the tissues and accumulates there.
- **Jaundice**: Yellowish discoloration resulting from bile duct obstruction due to cirrhosis.
- Altered sex hormone metabolism: A cirrhotic liver cannot inactivate estrogen (as it normally does), and males may develop characteristics related to excessive estrogen (**gynecomastia**, **palmar erythema**, **spider angiomas**, *female hair distribution*, and **testicular atrophy**).
- **Hepatic encephalopathy**: Due to the cirrhotic liver's increased inability to detoxify the blood, nitrogenous waste products can circulate in the blood to affect the brain; symptoms include mental confusion, stupor, shaking, tremor, and hallucinations (when shaking and hallucinations occur simultaneously, it is known as **delirium tremens**).

Etiology

Cirrhosis of the liver is usually caused by chronic alcoholism. It is more common in men and can also be of idiopathic origin (or due to chronic hepatitis or congestive heart failure). Cirrhosis usually develops over years and is asymptomatic until serious damage to the liver tissue has occurred. Sometimes symptoms such as loss of appetite, indigestion, weakness, weight loss, and nausea occur as the disease progresses. Blood may back up in the hepatic portal vein due to the scar tissue in the liver altering blood flow. Detoxification of the body therefore decreases. Alcoholism causes the liver to be unable to detoxify the blood, and blood alcohol levels rise. When the portal system backs up with blood, pressure in the portal vein increases (**portal hypertension**).

Diagnosis

Cirrhosis is diagnosed by physical examination, blood tests (searching for elevated liver enzymes and bilirubin, and low serum albumin), x-rays, and liver biopsy.

Treatment

Cirrhosis is treated with attempts designed to prevent further damage to the liver. The patient must stop all consumption of alcohol to have a chance of survival. Rest and nutrition must be monitored, and the diet is supplemented with vitamins and minerals. Edema and ascites may be reduced with diuretics. The role of the PTA is to implement an exercise program designed to improve overall fitness. Exercise has been shown to help the cirrhosis patient develop increased energy and to reduce the cravings for alcohol due to stimulation of the brain via endorphins and other substances.

Prognosis

Prognosis is unfavorable. Most individuals survive only 10 to 15 years after diagnosis with cirrhosis. Once ascites appears most individuals only survive for up to 5 years. Death is usually caused by hepatic encephalopathy, various metabolic disorders, or massive hemorrhage caused by esophageal varices.

Fatty Liver

Fatty liver is defined as the accumulation of fat in the liver cells (**Figure 18–18A**). This may occur because of metabolic disruptions, causing fat globules to accumulate within the cytoplasm of liver cells (**Figure 18–18B**). The most common cause of fatty liver is excessive alcohol consumption. Alcoholic fatty liver is the mildest form of *alcoholic liver disease* and is reversible once alcohol consumption ceases. Other causes of fatty liver include drugs, chemicals, poisons, and volatile solvents. Fatty liver is seen more often in obese and diabetic patients. It is also a characteristic of Reye's syndrome. Although heavy infiltration of fat in the liver impairs the organ's function, this may be reversed, with liver cells returning to normal once the causative agent is removed.

Hepatitis

Hepatitis is the inflammation of the liver, leading to abnormal function and other disease states. There are six main types of viral hepatitis:

- Hepatitis A
  - The least serious form of hepatitis.
  - Ninety-eight percent of patients recover.
  - It is spread by the fecal–oral route and never leads to chronic hepatitis or cirrhosis.
  - Hepatitis A vaccine should be received by those living or traveling in areas of poor sanitation and overcrowding.
- Hepatitis B (HBV)
  - Known as *serum hepatitis*, its particles are composed of an inner core and an outer coat.

- Incubation period varies from 6 weeks to months.
- Much more surface antigen is produced within infected cells than is required to coat virus particles, and a large excess is released into the bloodstream, making this HBsAg-positive blood infectious.
- The corresponding antibody (anti-HBe) often appears with the surface antigen (anti-HBs) during recovery (**Figure 18–19**).
- It may be spread by contact with saliva, feces, urine, semen, or across the placenta from mother to infant.
- HBV is considered a sexually transmitted disease.
- It is 100 times more infectious than *HIV*.
- This type of hepatitis can be carried by an individual throughout a lifetime.
- It may lead to chronic hepatitis and cirrhosis via attacking the DNA of cells.
- Ten percent of infected patients become chronic carriers of the virus.
- High-risk individuals include drug addicts, homosexuals with multiple partners, blood transfusion recipients, and health care workers.
- More than 350 million people are infected worldwide, with about 1 million dying each year due to complications of HBV.
- The HBV vaccine is 95 percent effective in preventing the disease.
- Hepatitis C (HCV)
  - This form is spread in a similar fashion to HBV but attacks the RNA of cells instead of the DNA.
  - It causes most "post-transfusion" cases of hepatitis.
  - It is most likely to cause chronic hepatitis and cirrhosis of all the various forms.
  - If exposed to HCV, there are no agents (such as gamma globulins) that can protect the patient from the disease.
  - There is no available immunizing agent against HCV.

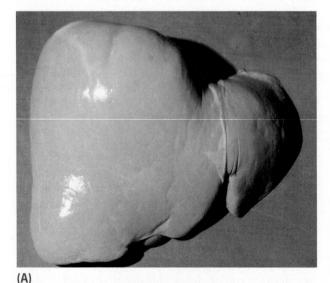

(A)

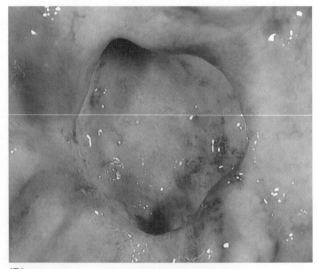

(B)

Figure 18–18 Fatty liver. (A) The liver appears yellow because of a large amount of fat within liver cells, but otherwise appears normal. (B) A section of liver that appears normal except for the yellow color caused by the fat.

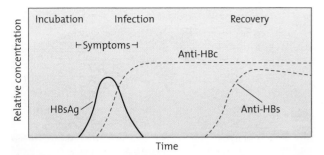

Figure 18–19 Acute HBV infection and recovery, illustrating serial changes of major antigens and antibodies used to aid in the diagnosis of HBV infection and monitor its course. Serial changes in HBeAg and anti-HBe are not shown. HBeAg rises along with HBsAg during active infection, and anti-HBe appears along with anti-HBc during recovery.

- All HCV-positive persons should be referred for further medical evaluation and treated with drugs that inhibit viral multiplication (usually *ribavirin*).
- Nearly 3 percent of the world population is infected with HCV.
- Those at highest risk include illegal drug users, anyone who received antihemophilic globulin or other clotting factors before 1987, those who received blood transfusions before 1992, health-care workers who have been exposed to blood or body fluids, and children born to HCV-infected mothers.
- Hepatitis D
  - Also known as *delta virus.*
  - This form requires HBV to be present to replicate.
  - HBV and hepatitis D together can cause worsened symptoms and increase the risk of developing chronic hepatitis with sudden, severe signs.
- Hepatitis E
  - This form is also spread through the fecal–oral route, often because of contaminated water.
  - Although hepatitis E does not result in chronic hepatitis, it can be fatal to pregnant women.
- Hepatitis G
  - This newly discovered form has been caused by transfused blood.

- It is possible to be transferred by pregnancy and through sexual intercourse.
- Often, patients with hepatitis G also have either HBV or HCV as well.
- When diagnosed, hepatitis G usually causes mild symptoms and is of short duration.
- It has the potential to be carried throughout life.

Table 18–1 summarizes the features of the three major types of viral hepatitis (A, B, and C).

Signs and Symptoms

Common signs of symptoms of liver conditions including hepatitis are jaundice, anorexia, malaise, fever, myalgia, and abdominal pain. Should they develop, chronic or fulminant hepatitis causes high fever, skin and mucous membrane hemorrhage, confusion, stupor, coma, and death.

Etiology

Hepatitis may be caused by viruses, drugs, toxic substances, and chronic alcoholism. *Viral hepatitis* is the form of hepatitis most often thought of when this condition is described. It is the most prevalent liver disease in the world. Once symptoms occur, they may be very vague, and misdiagnosis is common.

Diagnosis

Blood tests confirm hepatitis virus antibodies, and physical examination may reveal **hepatomegaly**. Urine may be checked for a darker-than-normal color, and the stools should be sampled to see if they are clay-colored or light-colored, which indicates the inability of the liver to form normal bile.

Treatment

For viral hepatitis, treatment is symptomatic, involving adequate rest and good nutrition. Nearly 85 percent of patients recover within 6 weeks. The most serious complications are development of chronic hepatitis and **fulminant** hepatitis. Chronic hepatitis develops in one-fourth of patients and often causes cirrhosis of the liver, whereas fulminant hepatitis is acute, causing extensive liver necrosis. Precautions when treating patients with hepatitis include the use of personal protective equipment to protect the health-care

---

TABLE 18–1	Features of Hepatitis A, B, and C		
Feature	**Hepatitis A**	**Hepatitis B**	**Hepatitis C**
Antigen-antibody test results	Anti-HAV (confers immunity)	Those infected are HbsAg positive and lack anti-HBs Immune persons lack HbsAg and have anti-HBs	HCV RNA in blood indicates virus in blood and active infection Anti-HCV indicates infection (does not confer immunity)
Complications	No carriers or chronic liver disease	Ten percent of patients become chronic carriers and may develop chronic liver disease	Seventy-five percent of patients become carriers and many develop chronic liver disease
Immunization available	Yes	Yes	No
Incubation period	2–6 wk	6 wk to 4 mo	3–12 weeks
Method of transmission	Fecal–oral (contaminated food or water)	Blood or body fluids	Blood or body fluids
Prevention of disease after exposure	Gamma globulin	Hepatitis B immune globulin	None

provider from contracting the disease. The role of the PTA is to implement an overall low-impact exercise program designed to improve body health. No specific exercises are indicated. The PTA should be aware that personal protective equipment may be required during treatment.

Prognosis

Prognosis is based on severity of disease and effectiveness of treatment. Fulminant hepatitis is 90 percent fatal even with adequate, prompt care.

Liver Cancer

Primary cancers of the liver are uncommon and very rare in the United States. However, *liver cancer* is a common type of malignant tumor in Asian and African countries. In the United States a primary liver carcinoma is more often seen in relation to HBV and chronic liver disease. Chronic HCV infections also cause higher incidence of cirrhosis and liver cancer. Usually, tumors in the liver have metastasized from other cancers (most commonly, breast, lung, and digestive system cancers). **Figure 18–20** shows a cross-section of the liver containing multiple nodules of metastatic carcinoma.

Signs and Symptoms

Unfortunately, liver cancer is usually discovered when it is already at late or end stage. Symptoms include anorexia, abdominal discomfort, and weight loss.

Etiology

The cause of liver cancer is not fully understood. Metastatic carcinoma may spread to the liver via the portal venous blood. The tumors also are carried in the blood delivered to the liver from the hepatic artery.

Diagnosis

Various diagnostic procedures can be used to identify liver tumors. Diagnosis of liver cancer is confirmed by needle or open biopsy. Alpha-fetoprotein levels will be elevated, as will various liver enzymes. CT scans are very effective in detecting liver cysts and tumors (**Figure 18–21**).

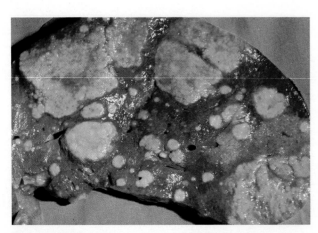

Figure 18–20 A cross-section of liver containing multiple nodules of metastatic carcinoma.

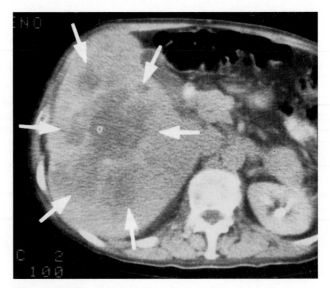

Figure 18–21 A CT scan of the upper abdomen illustrating liver and upper abdominal organs. A large irregular area in the liver (arrows) is caused by deposit of metastatic carcinoma.

Treatment

Treatment of liver cancer involves chemotherapy, radiation, and surgery. The role of the PTA is to implement a low-impact exercise program designed to improve overall body fitness. Range-of-motion and resistance training, as well as stretching, may be indicated.

Prognosis

Even with aggressive treatment the prognosis of liver cancer is very poor. Only 10 percent of patients live for 5 years after diagnosis.

Gallbladder Diseases

The gallbladder is a small organ positioned just below the liver. It is pear-shaped and stores excess bile until it is needed by the intestine for the digestive process. Bile travels to the duodenum of the intestine via the cystic duct and common bile duct.

Common symptoms of gallbladder disease include right-sided abdominal pain that occurs after a meal containing fat. Other symptoms include nausea, pain, and excessive gas. Gallbladder diseases are diagnosed by ultrasound, x-rays (cholecystogram and cholangiogram), and CT scans. Common gallbladder diseases include cholecystitis and cholelithiasis.

Cholecystitis

Cholecystitis is inflammation of the gallbladder. It may be prevented by maintaining a healthy body weight and eating a high-fiber diet, including fruits and vegetables.

Signs and Symptoms

Cholecystitis causes the gallbladder to become inflamed and then contract, creating pain in the upper right abdomen. It may be accompanied by nausea and vomiting after eating a meal. Complications of cholecystitis include rupture of the gallbladder and potential peritonitis, bile backup into the liver, and, potentially, liver damage and cirrhosis.

Etiology

Cholecystitis is most often caused by a gallstone obstructing bile flow. The bile becomes highly concentrated, irritating the gallbladder's lining and causing inflammation. A fatty meal causes the gallbladder to contract and release bile.

Diagnosis

Cholecystitis is confirmed by ultrasound and cholecystogram (the procedure of swallowing a dye that the liver absorbs and excretes into the bile). X-rays can confirm the presence of gallstones.

Treatment

To treat cholecystitis caused by gallstones, the preferred treatment is **cholecystectomy** (surgical removal of the gallbladder). This is accomplished by either abdominal incision or laparoscopy. A *laparoscopic cholecystectomy* is performed by passing a thin, tubular scope through a small cut made below the umbilicus (navel). The laparoscope allows the gallbladder to be viewed during surgery, and three other small incisions are made in the abdomen so surgical tools may be inserted.

Removal of the gallbladder in this manner reduces pain drastically, with recovery time much shorter than by surgery accomplished with a large abdominal incision. After this procedure bile from the liver flows from the common bile duct into the duodenum. Fatty foods should be avoided for the most part so there is enough bile to break down any consumed fat, allowing for normal digestion. The role of the PTA is to implement an exercise program designed to reduce stress, as well as activities and exercises that will return the patient to prior functional status.

Prognosis

Prognosis is generally good after cholecystecomy.

Cholelithiasis

Cholelithiasis is the presence of gallstones in the gallbladder or bile ducts (**Figure 18–22**). Gallstones affect women more than men, and nearly 600,000 people in the United States undergo surgical removal of gallstones each year. Decreasing dietary fat will not help stones to dissolve but may help in preventing their development.

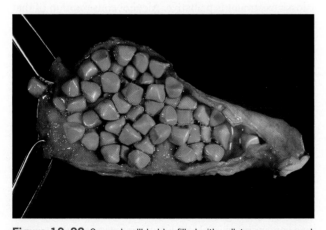

Figure 18–22 Opened gallbladder filled with gallstones composed of cholesterol.

Signs and Symptoms

Gallstones are often asymptomatic, but when they do cause symptoms it is usually because they are blocking the outflow of the gallbladder or its ducts. Symptoms include nausea, vomiting, and upper right abdominal pain after fatty meals. Complications include cholecystitis and jaundice.

Etiology

Gallstones are formed from cholesterol and bile salts. They can vary in size and shape and in composition, color, and number. Cholesterol stones are the most common type, formed when the composition of bile changes. The "five Fs of cholelithiasis" are as follows:

- Female gender
- Fair complexion
- Fat or obese body state
- Fertile state or having already had children
- Forty years of age or older

Diagnosis

Cholelithiasis is confirmed via patient history, ultrasound, and a cholecystogram.

Treatment

Cholelithiasis is treated with *extracorporeal shockwave lithotripsy*, which breaks up stones so they can be passed. If not effective or if it is not indicated for a patient, a cholecystectomy is performed. The role of the PTA focuses on assisting patients with physical activities to make the digestive system work more rapidly. Regular exercise has been shown to reduce prevalence of gallstones by nearly 33 percent.

Prognosis

Prognosis is generally good with prompt, adequate treatment.

Pancreatic Diseases

The pancreas lies behind the stomach between the duodenum and spleen and has exocrine and endocrine functions. It secretes most of the body's digestive enzymes and also secretes hormones. The pancreas secretes intestinal juices that contain chymotrypsin, trypsin, amylase, and lipase, all with separate functions related to the breakdown of proteins, carbohydrates, and fats. Pancreatic juices flow out of the pancreatic duct into the duodenum. The endocrine tissue of the pancreas is made up of multiple small clusters of cells that are scattered throughout the gland. These clusters are called the pancreatic islets or **islets of Langerhans**. They secrete hormones directly into the bloodstream. The two main types are alpha cells and beta cells. Alpha cells produce the hormone called glucagon and beta cells secrete insulin (**Figure 18–23A and B**).

Pancreatitis causes acute abdominal pain. Blood tests used to measure pancreatic function include those that test for serum amylase (which breaks down carbohydrates) and serum lipase (which breaks down fats). Unfortunately, pancreatic diseases are often very advanced by the time symptoms appear. They may be related to alcoholism. When the pancreas is not functioning properly or has been surgically removed, pancreatic enzymes and insulin may need to be administered. Other important pancreatic disorders include

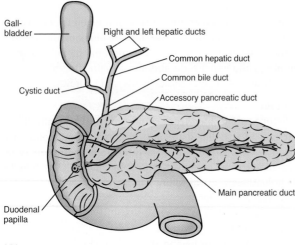

(A)

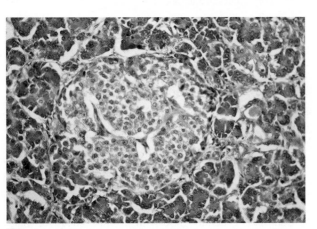

(B)

Figure 18–23 (A) Duct system of pancreas. The main pancreatic duct usually joins the common bile duct to form a common channel that enters the duodenum by a single opening at the apex of a nipple-like projection called the duodenal papilla (ampulla of Vater). A much smaller accessory pancreatic duct, illustrated in the diagram, is frequently present and opens into the duodenum by a separate opening proximal to the duodenal papilla. (B) A photomicrograph of pancreatic islet surrounded by exocrine pancreatic tissue.

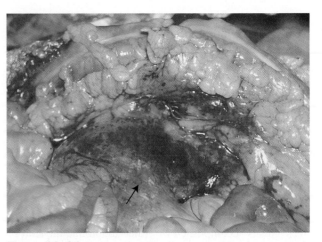

Figure 18–24 Acute pancreatitis. Transverse colon (upper part of photograph) has been elevated to reveal pancreas (arrow) which is inflamed and contains large areas of hemorrhage.

Signs and Symptoms

An acute pancreatitis attack causes radiating pain that may be slightly relieved by bringing the knees up toward the abdomen. It may also cause nausea, vomiting, sweating, and tachycardia. Chronic pancreatitis may cause constant back pain and similar symptoms to those seen in an acute attack. Disease progression causes fibrous tissue to replace pancreatic tissue, losing pancreatic function. Diabetes mellitus–like symptoms then occur, and digestive disorders such as malabsorption occur as exocrine function slows.

Etiology

Pancreatitis is often caused by alcoholism. It can also be caused by gallstones blocking the pancreatic ducts. However, many causes are idiopathic.

Diagnosis

Pancreatitis is diagnosed based on patient history and blood tests. A high blood **amylase** is indicative of pancreatitis.

Treatment

Treatment of pancreatitis is based on the causative factor. Removal of the gallbladder and stones is usually successful if the pancreatitis was caused by the gallstones. For other causes treatment is palliative. Alcohol consumption (if that is the cause) must be ceased, and analgesics and nutritional support implemented. Cigarette smoking should be stopped, and a low-fat diet should be implemented.

Prognosis

Prognosis for alcohol-related and idiopathic pancreatitis is poor, but those cases caused by gallstones usually respond well to surgery.

Pancreatic Cancer

Pancreatic cancer is usually diagnosed as an adenocarcinoma in the head of the pancreas that spreads very rapidly. It has no proven prevention, but its likelihood may be reduced by avoiding smoking, maintaining a healthy diet, avoiding excessive consumption of alcohol, and exercising regularly.

diabetes mellitus and hypoglycemia, which are discussed in Chapter 20.

Pancreatitis

Pancreatitis is inflammation of the pancreas, which has the potential to cause death. The pancreas becomes inflamed, edematous, hemorrhagic, and necrotic (**Figure 18–24**). Powerful digestive enzymes from the pancreas may escape its cells and ducts to cause the pancreas to be digested (**autodigestion**) by the body. The surrounding tissues may likewise be digested. If this process reaches the blood vessels, hemorrhaging occurs, leading to severe pain and shock. An alcohol binge may cause the acute hemorrhagic pancreatitis to occur, leading to death regardless of medical attention.

Signs and Symptoms

Symptoms usually occur only after metastasis has already occurred. Destruction of pancreatic tissue can cause abdominal and back pain, nausea, vomiting, loss of appetite, jaundice, fatigue, and weakness.

Etiology

Although of unknown origin, carcinogens that may influence the development of pancreatic cancer include high coffee consumption, cigarette smoking, exposure to chemicals, and a high-fat diet.

Diagnosis

Pancreatic cancer is diagnosed via ultrasound, CT scan, magnetic resonance imaging, and biopsy.

Treatment

Treatment of pancreatic cancer includes chemotherapy, radiation, and surgical resection. This type of cancer usually responds very poorly to any type of treatment. Treatment is supportive, including nutritional support and pain management. The role of the PTA in pancreatic cancer is to implement a low impact exercise program designed to improve strength and endurance. These are individualized programs based on the stage of the disease, per the physical therapy plan of care and physical therapist instructions.

Prognosis

Prognosis is poor because of the speed at which this cancer spreads. Pancreatic cancer is a leading cause of cancer deaths.

SUMMARY

The digestive system consists of a long, hollow tube beginning at the mouth and ending at the anus. Digestive functions include ingestion, digestion, absorption of fluids and nutrients, and elimination of wastes. Digestive organs include the mouth, pharynx, esophagus, stomach, gallbladder, pancreas, liver, intestines, rectum, and anus. There are many common digestive disorders, including infections, inflammation, ulcers, and various cancers. Older adults have a higher risk of digestive disorders due to decreased activity and other lifestyle or physiologic changes.

The liver, when diseased, may cause a variety of other conditions to develop in the body. Should the liver fail completely, a transplant must occur. Hepatitis is the most common liver disorder, and viral hepatitis is the most common form. Cirrhosis is a chronic, progressive disease of the liver usually linked to alcohol consumption. Gallbladder disease affects thousands of people on an annual basis, and pancreatic disorders are often only diagnosed when they are too late to reverse. Older adults are at higher risk for liver, gallbladder, and pancreas disorders.

REVIEW QUESTIONS

Select the best response to each question.

1. Diverticulosis occurs particularly in which of the following structures?
   a. lungs
   b. cecum
   c. ileum
   d. colon
2. A 46-year-old woman comes to the emergency room complaining of nausea, vomiting, and pain in the upper abdomen. She also appears to have mild jaundice. These symptoms are most characteristic of what condition?
   a. diabetes insipidus
   b. cholelithiasis
   c. stomach cancer
   d. hyperinsulinism
3. Esophageal varices are usually related to what condition?
   a. chronic pancreatitis
   b. diabetes mellitus
   c. peptic ulcer
   d. cirrhosis of the liver
4. *Helicobacter pylori* may cause which of the following problems?
   a. intestinal obstruction
   b. diverticulitis
   c. gastritis
   d. oral leukoplakia
5. Gluten-induced enteropathy is a(n)
   a. endocrine disorder
   b. immune disorder
   c. reproductive disorder
   d. kidney disorder
6. A large amount of bloody or watery diarrhea may be a symptom of what condition?
   a. dysentery
   b. stomach cancer
   c. inguinal hernia
   d. esophageal varices
7. The risk of developing colon cancer may be associated with what condition?
   a. gastroenteritis
   b. inguinal hernia
   c. ulcerative colitis
   d. pancreatitis
8. When the body absorbs and stores excessive iron, the condition is called
   a. hemochromatosis
   b. hematopoiesis
   c. pneumoconiosis
   d. poikilocytosis
9. Complications of severe cirrhosis of the liver include all the following *except*
   a. splenomegaly
   b. peptic ulcer
   c. varicosis
   d. jaundice
10. When a part of the intestine has folded into another section, the condition is called
    a. volvulus
    b. hematochezia

   c. intussusception
   d. inguinal hernia

CASE STUDIES

Karen Coupe, PT, DPT, MSEd

Case 1

A 28-year-old woman is attending outpatient physical therapy for a 2-week s/p right anterior cruciate ligament (ACL) repair. Patient medical history: GERD, irritable bowel syndrome, and bouts of gastritis. Previous level of function: Independent in all activities. Current level of function: Independent ambulation weight bearing as tolerated with axillary crutches, requires assistance with carrying secondary to crutches. Plan of care includes therapeutic exercise and neuromuscular electrical stimulation.

1. What is GERD? What signs and symptoms could the patient have during treatment that may indicate GERD?
2. During a treatment session the PTA will likely put the patient in a variety of positions on the treatment table and will have the patient go through various therapeutic activities. Which positions and/or activities could bring on the symptoms of GERD and therefore may need to be avoided?
3. Explain the etiology and clinical manifestation of irritable bowel syndrome.
4. How could irritable bowel syndrome affect treatment sessions?
5. This patient has bouts of gastritis. If this occurred during a treatment session, what signs and symptoms would be noted by the PTA?

Case 2

A 68-year-old man is referred to outpatient physical therapy secondary to an 8-week post left humeral neck fracture. Patient medical history: Colon cancer with colostomy 2 weeks post, currently undergoing chemotherapy, previous history of ulcerative colitis. PT evaluation reveals decreased range of motion and strength of the left shoulder. Plan of care includes therapeutic exercise, functional training, and modalities as needed.

1. Explain the etiology and clinical manifestations of colon cancer. Did the patient have any risk factors?
2. This patient has recently undergone a colostomy and has a colostomy bag just to the left of the umbilicus. Why is this a necessary procedure with a patient who has colon cancer? What positions could be uncomfortable for this patient during physical therapy treatment?
3. What effects could the chemotherapy treatments have on the plan of care?
4. The patient had a previous history of ulcerative colitis. Explain the etiology and clinical manifestations.
5. The plan of care includes modalities as needed. What modalities are contraindicated with this patient based on his medical history?

WEBSITES

http://alcoholism.about.com/

http://digestive.niddk.nih.gov/ddiseases/topics/diagnostic.asp

http://digestive.niddk.nih.gov/ddiseases/topics/stomach.asp

http://www.gi.org/patients/gihealth/diverticular.asp

http://www.gicare.com/Diseases/Pancreatic-Disease.aspx

http://www.medicinenet.com/inflammatory_bowel_disease_intestinal_problems/article.htm

http://www.netdoctor.co.uk/diseases/facts/gallbladderdisease.htm

http://www.netwellness.org/healthtopics/mouthdiseases/

http://www.nlm.nih.gov/medlineplus/analandrectaldiseases.html

http://www.nlm.nih.gov/medlineplus/liverdiseases.html

http://www.vivo.colostate.edu/hbooks/pathphys/digestion/basics/index.html

http://www.wrongdiagnosis.com/e/esophagus_diseases/intro.htm

http://www.wrongdiagnosis.com/sym/digestive_symptoms.htm

Urinary System Disorders

OUTLINE

LEARNING OBJECTIVES

After completion of this chapter the reader should be able to

1. Describe the structure and functions of the kidneys.
2. Describe the clinical manifestations of glomerulonephritis and nephrosclerosis.
3. Explain the manifestations of urinary tract obstruction.
4. List the signs and symptoms of pyelonephritis.
5. Describe methods used in the diagnosis and treatment of kidney stones.
6. Explain the manifestations of the nephrotic syndrome.
7. Describe the causes, signs, and symptoms of renal failure.
8. Describe the principles and techniques of hemodialysis.

KEY TERMS

Albuminuria: Presence of albumin in the urine.

Anuria: Complete suppression of urine formation and excretion.

Blood urea nitrogen (BUN): Amount of nitrogen in the blood in the form of urea, which is used to test renal function.

Bowman's capsule: Glomerular capsule; a cup-shaped structure around the glomerulus of each nephron in the kidneys that serves as a filter.

Catheterization: Inserting a tube into a body cavity, duct, or vessel.

Creatinine clearance test: A test that gauges the volume of blood plasma that is cleared of creatinine over a unit of time; it helps to determine the glomerular filtration rate.

Cystitis: Inflammation of the urinary bladder.

Cystogram: A visualization of the urinary bladder with the use of a catheter, radiocontrast agent, and x-rays.

Cystoscopy: Endoscopy of the urinary bladder via the urethra.

Dialysis: Provision of an artificial replacement for lost kidney function in people who have renal failure.

Dysuria: Painful urination.

Encephalopathy: Any disorder or disease of the brain.

Erythropoiesis: Process by which red blood cells (erythrocytes) are produced.

Frequency: Need to urinate more often than usual.

Glomerulonephritis: Inflammation of the glomeruli (small blood vessels) in the kidneys.

Hematuria: Presence of red blood cells in the urine.

Hydronephrosis: Distention and dilation of the renal pelvis and calices of the kidney.

Hypervolemia: Fluid overload; a condition of too much fluid in the blood.

In and out catheterization: A temporary procedure wherein a catheter is removed as soon as urine is drained from the urinary bladder.

KEY TERMS CONTINUED

Indwelling catheter: A catheter placed into the urinary bladder for longer periods of time.

Interstitial cystitis: A urinary bladder disease characterized by pain during urination, urinary frequency, urgency, and pressure in the bladder and/or pelvis.

Intravenous pyelogram (IVP): A radiologic procedure used to visualize abnormalities of the urinary system.

Kidneys-ureter-bladder (KUB): A diagnostic medical imaging technique of the abdomen.

Lipoid nephrosis: Earliest stage of childhood nephrotic syndrome.

Lithotripsy: Use of shock waves to break up stones in the urinary system.

Nephrectomy: Removal of a kidney.

Nephrons: Filtering units of the kidneys.

Neurogenic bladder: Dysfunction of the urinary bladder due to a nervous system disease that relates to the control of urination.

Nocturia: The need to urinate during the night, interrupting sleep.

Oliguria: Decreased production of urine.

Polycystic kidney disease: A genetic kidney disorder wherein multiple, fluid-filled cysts form, greatly enlarging kidney size.

Proteinuria: Presence of excess serum proteins in the urine.

Pyelitis: Inflammation of the renal pelvis of the kidney.

Pyelonephritis: An ascending urinary tract infection that has reached the renal pelvis of the kidney.

Pyuria: Pus in the urine.

Radical cystectomy: Surgical removal of all or part of the urinary bladder.

Renal calculi: Kidney stones.

Renal failure: Failure of the kidneys to adequately filter toxins and waste products from the blood.

Suprapubic catheter: A catheter used to drain urine from the bladder by insertion through the abdominal wall just above the pubic bone.

Transurethral resection: Passage of a cystoscope into the bladder through the urethra and a resectoscope that removes tissue for biopsy and burns away any existing cancer cells.

Urgency: A sudden, compelling urge to urinate.

Urinalysis: A variety of tests performed on the urine to test a variety of substance levels.

Urinary incontinence: Involuntary excretion of urine.

Urine culture and sensitivity test: A test used to diagnose urinary tract infections; it usually takes between 24 and 48 hours to culture any bacteria that are present.

Overview

The urinary system excretes urine and reabsorbs electrolytes, water, and various compounds. In these ways it helps to maintain homeostasis. Disturbances to the circulatory or nervous systems may also affect the urinary system. Common urinary disorders include a variety of infections and kidney or bladder disorders.

Anatomy and Physiology of the Urinary System

The urinary system is made up of two kidneys, two ureters, one bladder, and one urethra (**Figure 19–1**). The kidneys lie retroperitoneally (behind the peritoneum) in the lumbar area and are about the size of an adult male's fist.

Each kidney contains 1 million microscopic filtering units, or **nephrons**. Each nephron consists of a **Bowman's capsule** or glomerular capsule, proximal convoluted tubule, loop of Henle, distal convoluted tubule, and collecting duct (**Figure 19–2**). Each section is responsible for excreting or reabsorbing certain substances.

The kidneys excrete urine to maintain homeostasis. They regulate the volume, electrolyte concentration, and acid-base balance of body fluids. The kidneys also detoxify the blood and eliminate wastes, regulate blood pressure, and support red blood cell production (**erythropoiesis**). They produce an active type of vitamin D (calciferol or vitamin D_3) used for bone strengthening.

The two ureters are tubules running from the kidneys to the bladder, transporting urine from the renal pelvis. The bladder is muscular, able to expand and contract, and can hold up to 500 mL of urine. Its ability to hold urine is affected by diseases, disorders, and actual bladder tone. The process of voiding (emptying) the bladder is known as *micturition*

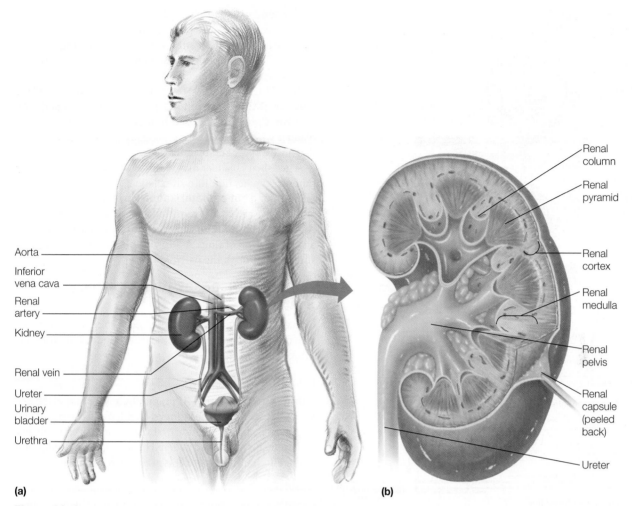

Figure 19-1 The urinary system. (A) Anterior view showing the relationship of the kidneys, ureters, urinary bladder, and urethra. (B) A cross-section of the human kidney showing the cortex, medulla, and renal pelvis.

(urination). The pelvic nerves usually stimulate the bladder to urinate.

The hollow urethra runs from the bladder to the external opening (meatus) for excretion and is much longer in males than in females. In females only urine passes through the urethra, whereas in males both urine and semen are conducted. Urine is usually clear and slightly yellow to almost gold in color. The color of urine can be changed by certain drugs or foods. There is a distinct odor to urine, but this is usually not foul smelling unless disease is present. The normal specific gravity of urine is between 1.005 and 1.030, with a pH of about 6. A disease may be indicated by changes in these values.

Signs of urinary abnormalities are as follows:

- **Anuria**: No urine output
- **Dysuria**: Difficulty or pain when urinating
- **Frequency**: Urinating frequently
- **Hematuria**: Blood in the urine
- **Nocturia**: Increased voiding during the night
- **Oliguria**: Decreased urine output

TABLE 19-1 Normal and Abnormal Urinalysis Findings

Urinalysis Test	Normal	Abnormal
Acetone	Negative	Ketonuria
Albumin (protein)	Negative	Albuminuria
Bacteria	Negative	Present
Bilirubin	Negative	Bilirubinuria
Casts	Rare	Present (several to many)
Color	Clear amber	Very light or dark; cloudy
Glucose	Negative	Glycosuria
Odor	Aromatic but pleasant	Unpleasant or offensive
pH	4.6–8.0	Higher or lower than normal
Red blood cells	2–3 per HPF	Hematuria
Specific gravity	1.005–1.030	Higher or lower than normal
White blood cells	4–5 per HPF	White, cloudy urine

HPF, high powered field.

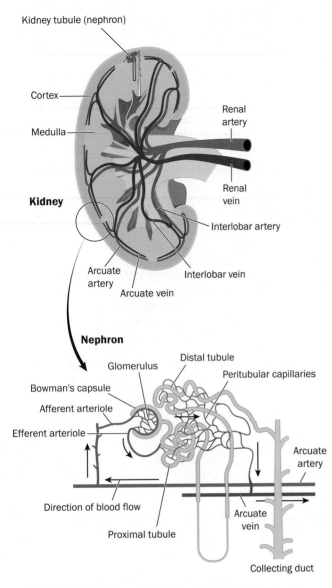

Figure 19–2 Nephrons of the kidney. Part of the nephron is located in the cortex, and part is located in the medulla. The electron micrograph to the left of the illustration is of a glomerulus from a human nephron.

- **Proteinuria**: Protein in the urine; when albumin is identified, the condition is called **albuminuria**
- **Pyuria**: Pus in the urine
- **Urgency**: Need to urinate immediately

There are a few common tests used to diagnose urinary conditions:

- **Urinalysis**: Checks for pH, specific gravity, and the presence of protein, glucose, sugar, or blood (**Table 19–1**).
- **Urine culture and sensitivity test**: After urinalysis, this may be used to detect an abnormal number of white cells or bacteria in the urine.

- **Blood urea nitrogen (BUN)**: Determines levels of urea nitrogen or waste product in the blood.
- **Creatinine clearance test**: Determines the ability of the renal glomeruli to filter creatinine out of the blood after it is ingested.

Radiologic urinary tests include **kidneys-ureter-bladder (KUB)**, **intravenous pyelogram (IVP)**, and **cystogram**. **Cytoscopy** is used to look inside the urethra and bladder with a lighted scope. Biopsies may be performed to diagnose kidney and bladder diseases.

The urinary bladder may require **catheterization** to instill fluids or medication into the bladder or for the removal of urine. **In and out catheterization** is a temporary procedure wherein the catheter is removed as soon as urine is drained. An **indwelling catheter** is placed into the urinary bladder for a longer period of time. A **suprapubic catheter** is inserted surgically through the pelvic wall.

Common Diseases of the Urinary System

Urinary tract infections are the most common urinary disorders. Other common diseases include kidney diseases and bladder diseases.

Urinary Tract Infection

A urinary tract infection (UTI) may be any disease of the urinary tract, including the kidneys, bladder, and urethra. Common forms of UTIs include cystitis, pyelitis, pyelonephritis, and urethritis, discussed in detail below. Signs and symptoms of the different forms of UTIs are relatively similar.

Cystitis

Cystitis is more commonly referred to as a "bladder infection." It may be caused by a bacterial infection, calculus, or tumor. Cystitis is characterized by pain, urgency and frequency of urination, and hematuria. Diagnosis by culture is not always necessary, but when done, it requires demonstration of significant bacteriuria in properly collected urine. It is usually treated with antibiotics and antispasmodic medications to decrease bladder spasms. A follow-up urinalysis and culture is important to make sure all bacteria have been eliminated. Recurrent cystitis is common.

> **RED FLAG**
> UTIs are most often caused by *Escherichia coli*, which is part of the normal intestinal flora.

Pyelitis

Pyelitis primarily affects younger girls and is usually the result of an ascending infection from the bladder, although it can also be a hematogenous infection. Signs and symptoms include pain and tenderness in the loins, irritability of the bladder, bloody or purulent urine, and pain when flexing the thigh. Diagnosis is via urinalysis, which will reveal many pus cells, and occasionally, erythrocytes. This condition requires rapid diagnosis and treatment to keep it from causing pyelonephritis. The drugs of choice for pyelitis are usually sulfonamides. Antibiotics and urinary antiseptics may also be used.

Pyelonephritis

Pyelonephritis is inflammation of the nephrons of the kidneys and can be caused by either an ascending or hematogenous infection. Risks are increased by obstruction or urine flow blockage. *E. coli* is the most influential bacterial cause. Causative factors include pregnancy, prostate enlargement, stones, or tumors. Pyelonephritis can be acute or chronic. Usually, abscesses form and rupture inside one or both kidneys, causing pus to form, leading to pyuria. Other symptoms include fever, chills, flank pain, and hematuria. Diagnostic procedures for pyelonephritis include patient history, physical examination, urinalysis, urine and blood cultures, complete blood count, IVP, renal ultrasound, computed tomography (CT) scan, cystoscopy, and biopsy. Treatment includes antibiotics, but repeat occurrence leads to kidney scarring, uremia, and kidney failure.

> **RED FLAG**
> Pyelonephritis is more common in females, probably because of a shorter urethra and the short distance from the urinary meatus to the vagina and the rectum.

Kidney Diseases

Kidney diseases affect the body's ability to filter itself and can lead to serious effects on all other body systems. Symptoms may appear initially in the affected body system before they appear in the urinary system. For example, hypertension may appear first, actually having been caused by inappropriate reabsorption of sodium and water. Common kidney diseases include adenocarcinoma of the kidney, glomerulonephritis (acute or chronic), hydronephrosis, polycystic disease, renal calculi, and renal failure.

> **RED FLAG**
> Patients with chronic pyelonephritis may have a childhood history of unexplained fevers or bed-wetting.

Nephrotic Syndrome

Nephrotic syndrome results from antibody-antigen complexes lodging in the glomerular membrane. It is actually a group of conditions that result from increased glomerular permeability to plasma proteins. These conditions can be primary or secondary to diseases such as diabetes mellitus, hepatitis B, amyloidosis, and systemic lupus erythematosus. Primary glomerular changes that can lead to nephrotic syndrome include lipoid nephrosis (minimal change disease), membranous glomerulonephritis, and focal segmental glomerulosclerosis. In children under age 15 nephrotic syndrome is usually of primary origin but is usually secondary to another disease in adults. It is more common in boys than in girls.

> **RED FLAG**
> Age plays no part in the progression or prognosis of nephrotic syndrome. Primary nephrotic syndrome is found predominantly in the preschool-age child.

Nephrotic syndrome is characterized by massive proteinuria and lipiduria, hypoalbuminemia, general edema, and hyperlipidemia. This condition originates from a change in glomerular membranes that cause increased permeability to plasma proteins. This allows protein to escape from the plasma into the glomerular filtrate.

The general edema that may occur results from sodium and water retention and a loss of serum albumin. It usually appears first in the lower extremities, becoming more generalized as nephrotic syndrome progresses. Pulmonary edema, dyspnea, pleural effusions, ascites, and problems with the respiratory diaphragm may result.

Albumin is lost in great quantities, but globulins are also diminished, making the patient more susceptible to infections. Because many binding proteins are also lost, the plasma levels of iron, copper, zinc, thyroid hormones, and sex hormones may be lower than normal. Drugs taken during this state may have increased effects as the number of available protein-binding sites has been reduced.

> **RED FLAG**
> Lipid nephrosis is the main cause of nephrotic syndrome in children younger than age 8.

> **RED FLAG**
> Nephrotic syndrome causes marked proteinuria, hyperlipidemia, hypoalbuminemia, and edema.

Additionally, a loss of coagulation and anticoagulation factors may occur, causing thrombotic complications, which may include deep vein thrombosis and pulmonary emboli. Elevated levels of triglycerides and low-density lipoproteins occur, although high-density lipoproteins are usually normal. Therefore, people with nephrotic syndrome are at higher risk for developing atherosclerosis.

Acute Tubular Necrosis

Acute tubular necrosis accounts for most cases of acute renal failure. It damages the tubular segment of the nephrons, with mortality ranging between 40 and 70 percent. Acute tubular necrosis may result from diseases of the tubular epithelium, obstruction of urine flow, and ischemic injuries.

Acute tubular necrosis results from ischemic or nephrotoxic injury. It is seen most commonly in debilitated patients such as those who have undergone extensive surgery. In ischemic injury, blood flow to the kidneys is disrupted because of circulatory collapse, severe hypotension, hemorrhage, trauma, cardiogenic or septic shock, dehydration, anesthetics, surgery, or reactions to blood transfusions. This disorder is usually difficult to diagnose because primary disease states may mask its signs and symptoms. It is signified, however, by decreased urine output, hyperkalemia, uremic syndrome with oliguria and confusion, dry mucous membranes and skin, and lethargy, twitching, or seizures.

Complications of acute tubular necrosis may include heart failure, uremic pericarditis, pulmonary edema, uremic lung conditions, anemia, anorexia, vomiting, and poor wound healing. Fever and chills may signify an onset of infection, which is the leading cause of death from acute tubular necrosis. Diagnosis is unfortunately not usually made until the disease has progressed to an advanced stage. Urinary sediment tests reveal red blood cells and casts, with a dilute urine of low specific gravity. BUN and serum creatinine are elevated, and an electrocardiogram may reveal arrhythmias due to electrolyte imbalances.

Treatment includes the restoration of normal kidney function, diuretics, fluids to flush tubules, and, for long-term needs, the following:

- Daily replacement of fluid losses
- Transfusions of packed red blood cells and epoetin alfa
- Administration of antibiotics
- Emergency intravenous administration of 50 percent glucose, regular insulin, and sodium bicarbonate
- Sodium polystyrene sulfonate with sorbitol
- Peritoneal dialysis or hemodialysis

Acute Glomerulonephritis

Acute **glomerulonephritis** is an inflammation of the glomerulus (filtering unit) of the kidney and is the most common form of kidney disease.

Signs and Symptoms

Signs and symptoms of acute glomerulonephritis include fever, flank pain, loss of appetite, and malaise. Swelling of the ankles and around the eyes may appear, and hematuria or oliguria may be present. Albuminuria and casts (proteins that "mold" to the kidney tubules' shapes) may be present. Smoky or coffee-colored urine may result because of dyspnea, hematuria, and orthopnea from pulmonary edema related to **hypervolemia**.

> **RED FLAG**
> The presenting features of glomerulonephritis in children may include **encephalopathy** with seizures and local neurologic deficits.

Etiology

Acute glomerulonephritis usually affects children (especially boys) between the ages of 3 and 7 years within 4 weeks after a streptococcal infection of the respiratory tract. Other causes include impetigo, scarlet fever, or **lipoid nephrosis**. This disorder is a type of allergic or immune disease caused by an antigen-antibody reaction. An antigen is produced that causes antibodies to develop that stick to the antigen, producing large "complexes" that circulate until they are trapped in the glomeruli capillaries. Pressure, irritation, and inflammation result. Blood flow is decreased to the glomeruli, which weakens and allows red blood cells and plasma proteins to leak into Bowman's capsules and appear in the urine.

Diagnosis

Urinalysis will show red blood cells, white blood cells, and increased protein (which indicates nephron damage). Increased electrolytes, creatinine, or urea nitrogen in the blood and decreased serum protein levels also help to diagnose this condition. Confirmation may be through ultrasound, x-rays, CT scan, or renal biopsy.

> **RED FLAG**
> Significant proteinuria is not a common finding in elderly patients.

Treatment

Acute glomerulonephritis is treated with loop diuretics such as furosemide to reduce extracellular fluid overload. Vasodilators (hydralazine, nifedipine) decrease hypertension. Antibiotics are administered for 7 to 10 days to treat infections that may contribute to the ongoing antigen-antibody response.

Bed rest will reduce metabolic demands. Fluids should be restricted to decrease edema, and sodium should be restricted to prevent fluid retention. Correction of electrolyte imbalances is essential. The diet may be changed to restrict salt, fluids, and proteins.

Prognosis

Prognosis is generally good as long as the condition does not become chronic. Streptococcal and other bacterial infections should be treated properly so they do not influence development of glomerulonephritis. Prognosis is better for children than adults.

Chronic Glomerulonephritis

Chronic glomerulonephritis occurs because of progressive glomeruli destruction. It can often lead to chronic kidney failure, end-stage kidney disease, and chronic hypertension.

Signs and Symptoms

The symptoms of chronic glomerulonephritis are similar to the acute form and may also include uremia and kidney failure as the disease progresses.

Etiology

The chronic form may occur because of repeat attacks of the acute form of this disease. As the glomeruli are continually destroyed the kidney cannot produce urine, leading to edema, increased fluid volume in the blood, salt retention, and hypertension. This disease usually strikes individuals with a history of kidney disease, but in 25 percent of patients it is of unknown origin, possibly related to an immune abnormality.

Diagnosis

Diagnosis is via urinalysis, complete blood count, BUN, and creatinine. Symptoms of anemia and uremia are helpful in diagnosing the disease. CT scan, ultrasound, and biopsy may also be used.

Treatment

Control of hypertension influences successful treatment of chronic glomerulonephritis. Diet and fluid restrictions may be used to prevent kidney failure. Some forms of this disease are treated with immunosuppressants and steroids. Once end-stage disease occurs, hemodialysis or kidney transplant may be needed.

Prognosis

Prognosis is based on severity of disease and success of treatments, and prompt treatment improves prognosis.

Nephrosclerosis

Nephrosclerosis is similar to arteriosclerosis but occurs in the kidneys. Excessive vascular changes cause the walls of the arterioles and small arteries to harden and then to narrow or occlude the lumina of the blood vessels. This reduces blood supply to the kidney, causing atrophy, ischemia, increased renin secretion, and increased blood pressure. If ischemia continues, renal tissue is destroyed and ultimately fails. Damage is often asymptomatic until in an advanced stage.

Nephrosclerosis may be primary in the kidney or secondary to essential hypertension, nephropathy, diabetes mellitus, or other conditions. The cycle of nephrosclerosis and hypertension must be stopped to prevent renal failure or other complications (such as congestive heart failure). Treatment involves antihypertensive agents, diuretics, beta-blockers, and angiotensin-converting enzyme inhibitors. Sodium intake should also be reduced.

Hydronephrosis

Hydronephrosis is defined as a collection of urine in the renal pelvis because of an obstruction. The pelvis becomes dilated and distended as a result (**Figure 19–3A and B**).

Signs and Symptoms

Based on either acute or chronic obstructions, symptoms vary. One or both kidneys may be affected, and when the condition affects both kidneys it is easier to detect. Regardless of the location of the obstruction, flank pain or loin pain occur. Anuria or uremia may develop if both kidneys are affected.

Etiology

Hydronephrosis may occur because of congenital urinary defects, kidney stones, enlarged prostate, tumors, or UTIs. Permanent damage can occur if the obstruction is not removed, with the renal pelvis becoming nonfunctioning. Obstruction may be bilateral hydronephrosis or hydroureter (swelling in the ureters). Both these conditions are unilateral

if the obstruction is located low in the ureter (caused by an obstructing calculus). If it is located at the junction of the renal pelvis and ureter (which can occur due to ureter scarring), a unilateral hydronephrosis develops (**Figure 19–4**).

Diagnosis

Physical examination may reveal an enlarged kidney or kidneys. Blood tests may indicate electrolyte imbalance and elevated creatinine, with a pyelogram confirming diagnosis.

Treatment

Treatment of hydronephrosis involves surgical intervention to immediately drain the renal pelvis and relieve the obstruction.

Prognosis

Prognosis is based on speed of treatment. Although not preventable, prompt treatment of causative conditions can reduce its incidence.

Polycystic Kidney Disease

Polycystic kidney disease (PKD) is an inherited disorder characterized by multiple, bilateral, grape-like clusters of fluid-filled cysts

> **RED FLAG**
> Renal deterioration is more gradual in adults than in infants. However, in both age groups the disease progresses relentlessly, to fatal uremia.

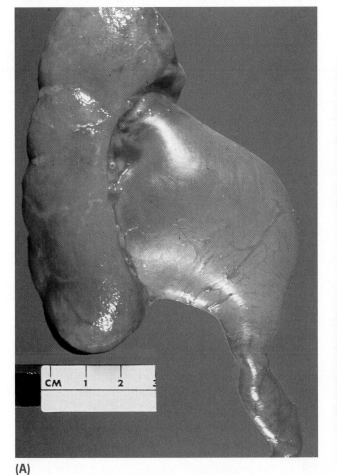

(A)

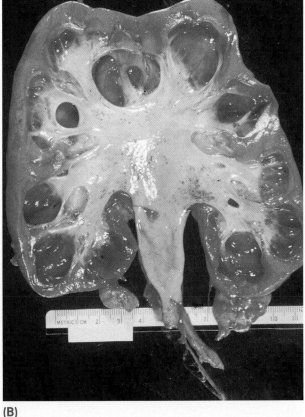

(B)

Figure 19–3 (A) Marked hydronephrosis and hydroureter. (B) Bisected hydronephrotic kidney, illustrating enlargement of calyces with atrophy of the renal parenchyma caused by the increased pressure exerted by the urine within the distended renal pelvis and calyces.

A   B   C

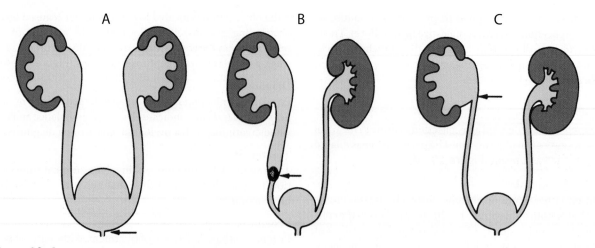

Figure 19–4 Possible locations and results of urinary tract obstruction. The arrows indicate sites of obstruction. (A) Bilateral hydronephrosis and hydroureter with distention of the bladder caused by urethral obstruction. (B) Unilateral hydroureter and hydronephrosis caused by obstruction of the distal ureter. (C) Unilateral hydronephrosis caused by obstruction at the ureteropelvic junction.

that enlarge the kidneys, compressing and eventually replacing functioning renal tissue (**Figure 19–5A and B**). The kidneys may increase to a weight of up to 30 pounds, with the disease slowly progressing. It usually begins in teenagers and younger adults, leading to renal failure by ages 30 to 40. PKD appears in males and females equally.

Signs and Symptoms
Kidney tissue is damaged, and function decreases as this disease progresses. Symptoms include hypertension, hematuria, lumbar pain, and recurrent UTIs.

Etiology
PKD is inherited. A parent with the disease has a 50 percent chance of passing the gene to the child. There are two forms of PKD: autosomal dominant trait (the adult type) and autosomal recessive trait (the infantile type). The adult form has an insidious onset but usually becomes obvious between ages 30 and 50.

Diagnosis
Diagnosis of PKD is made via family and clinical history. Retrograde urography shows enlarged kidneys with elongation of the renal pelvis, flattening of the calices, and indentations in the kidneys caused by cysts. Ultrasonography, tomography, and radioisotope scans show kidney enlargement and cysts. Magnetic resonance imaging shows multiple areas of cystic damage.

Treatment
PKD is treated by antibiotics for infections and adequate hydration to maintain fluid balance. Dialysis or kidney transplantation for progressive renal failure is also required. The role of the physical therapist assistant (PTA) is to assist the patients with exercises designed to reduce low back pain. Treatments may include ice massage, heating pads, whirlpool, and the Alexander technique.

> **RED FLAG**
> A few infants with PKD survive for 2 years and then die of hepatic complications or renal, heart, or respiratory failure.

Prognosis
Prognosis is poor because the disease usually progresses to renal failure.

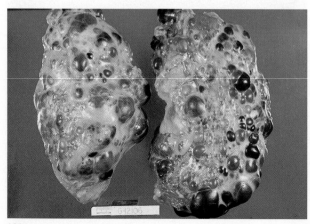

(A)

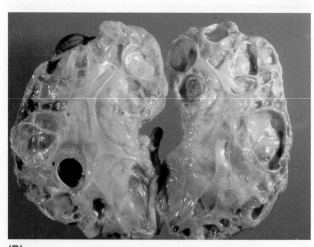

(B)

Figure 19–5 (A) Greatly enlarged abnormal kidneys characteristic of congenital polycystic kidney disease. (B) Cut surfaces of diseased kidneys, illustrating multiple large cysts. No normal renal tissue remains.

Renal Calculi

Renal calculi are commonly known as "kidney stones." They are often made of calcium salts, although other substances may be involved, and can vary in location, number, and size (**Figure 19–6**). They commonly occur between ages 30 and 50, rarely occurring in children, and affect men more than women. Calcium calculi generally occur in middle-aged men with a familial history of calculus formation.

Signs and Symptoms

Kidney stones usually cause hematuria and colic (renal or urinary). Colic is an extreme and spasmodic flank pain caused when an obstructed ureter contracts. It may be very severe and sharp. Symptoms are nausea and vomiting, fever and chills from infection, and anuria from obstruction (either bilateral or unilateral).

Etiology

The etiology of kidney stones is unknown, but the known risk factors are chronic UTIs, dehydration, and immobility (or prolonged bed rest). Kidney stones can sometimes result from gout, hyperparathyroidism, or severe bone disease. A prevalent type, *staghorn calculi*, forms in the renal pelvis and can enlarge to fill the pelvis. Although calculi usually form in the kidney, they may also form in the bladder. When this occurs there is difficulty emptying the bladder, causing frequent infections. Once stones become caught in the ureters or block the urinary tract, symptoms arise.

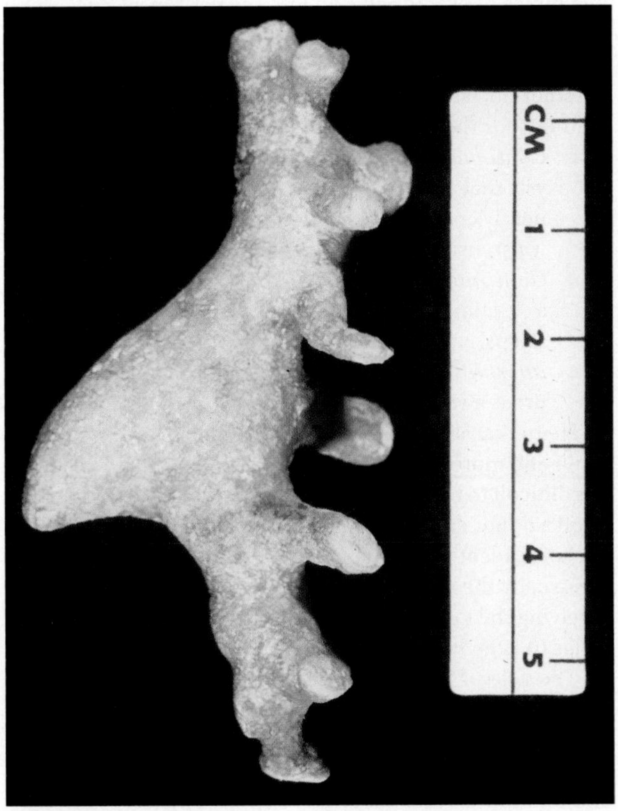

Figure 19–6 Large staghorn calculus of kidney.

Diagnosis

Renal calculi are diagnosed via an IVP, KUB radiography, or renal ultrasonography, which can detect obstructive changes (such as unilateral or bilateral hydronephrosis). Urine culture may show pyuria, a sign of UTI. A 24-hour urine collection can determine calcium oxalate, phosphorus, and uric acid excretion levels.

Treatment

Treatment of renal calculi includes pain medication and increased fluid intake to help pass the stone(s) in the urine. The urine may be strained by using a filter to catch the stone so its type can be identified. If totally obstructed, emergency surgery is required to prevent hydronephrosis and kidney damage. A "retrieval" instrument may be passed through the urethra, bladder, and ureter to remove stones. Another procedure called **lithotripsy** may be used to break up the stone(s). This involves placing the patient in a tub of water and using external shock waves to shatter the hard stones.

Prognosis

Prognosis is based on the severity of the stones and whether adequate treatment is given before the development of other conditions.

Renal Failure

Renal failure is defined as the kidneys' inability to cleanse the blood of wastes. Normally, urea forms in the liver, with the kidneys filtering it out of the blood for excretion in the urine. When the kidneys fail, urea remains in the blood, with high levels causing uremia. Urea is converted to ammonia, which has toxic effects on the entire body.

Signs and Symptoms

Symptoms are unseen in renal failure until the kidneys have been approximately three-fourths destroyed. Symptoms then include drowsiness, mental confusion, visual disturbances, convulsion, urine smell of the breath, nausea, vomiting, diarrhea, glycosuria, hematuria, pyuria, dryness of the skin, pruritus, rash, infertility, impotence, bone weakness, and coma.

Etiology

Renal failure may be acute or chronic. The acute form is usually caused by embolism, hemorrhagic or surgical shock, dehydration, congestive heart failure, stones, tumors, or enlarged prostate. Acute renal failure may be treated with success by treating the cause, changing the diet per a physician's recommendations, or via dialysis. Chronic renal failure occurs slowly, usually because of glomerulonephritis, pyelonephritis, PKD, renal hypertension, substance abuse, alcoholism, and diabetes.

Diagnosis

Patient history, physical examination, and blood tests assist in diagnosing renal failure. It is indicated by elevated blood creatinine and elevated BUN.

Treatment

Treatment is first aimed at the causative factors. Protein and sodium should be limited in the diet, and fluid intake as well as urine output should be monitored. Medications include antihypertensives, diuretics, and antibiotics. Long-term treatments may include dialysis and kidney transplantation.

Dialysis is a process that cleanses the blood of waste products. There are two types of dialysis, both of which use a semipermeable membrane along with a washing solution to basically perform the same functions as healthy kidneys. *Hemodialysis* is the most common type. The patient's blood is routed out of (usually) the brachial or radial artery through the *hemodialyzer* and put back into a vein.

To maintain access to the arteries and veins, usually an arteriovenous shunt is made by placing catheters in the required vessels (**Figure 19–7**). These are connected (shunted) to silicone rubber tubes. These sites must be kept clean to prevent infection and clots from occurring.

The second type of dialysis is *peritoneal dialysis*, which involves performing a *paracentesis* procedure. This requires

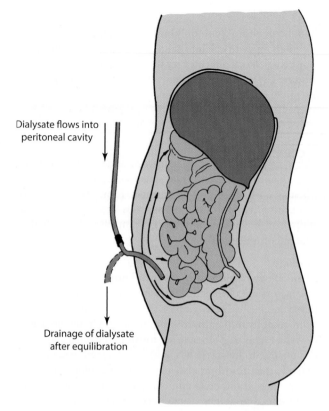

Figure 19–8 Principle of peritoneal dialysis. Dialysate fills peritoneal cavity. Waste products diffuse (arrows) from blood vessels beneath peritoneum into dialysate. Fluid is drained after equilibration.

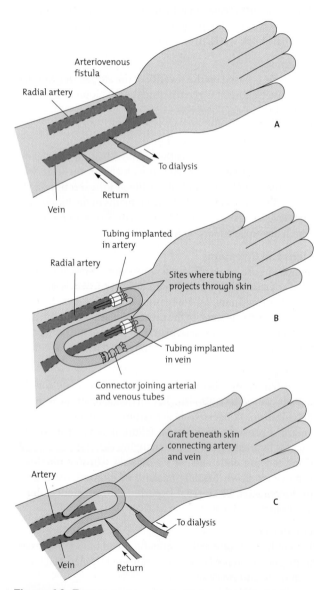

Figure 19–7 Procedures used to facilitate access to patient's circulatory system for hemodialysis. (A) Arteriovenous fistula created between radial artery and adjacent vein. (B) Permanently implanted tubes in radial artery and vein project through skin and are interconnected between dialysis treatments. (C) Graft of synthetic material or bovine artery connects patient's artery and vein.

instilling a dialyzing solution into the peritoneal cavity for a predetermined length of time (**Figure 19–8**). Waste products diffuse out of the peritoneal capillaries into the dialyzing solution, which is drained and discarded. There are three methods for this procedure:

- *Continuous ambulatory peritoneal dialysis*: Self-dialysis that uses gravity to drain fluid through a permanently connected catheter into a bag worn around the waist; usually must occur several times per day.
- *Continuous cycling peritoneal dialysis*: Requires a "cycling" machine that works while the patient sleeps.
- *Intermittent peritoneal dialysis*: Performed several times a week in a medical clinic.

Hemodialysis is the preferred type of dialysis because it is faster and more efficient. However, it is also more expensive. It is difficult to match a donor kidney with those of a recipient, but if a donor can be found renal transplant is the treatment of choice. Identical twins or other immediate family members are usually the most compatible kidney donors. The patient receiving the kidney may need lifelong immunosuppressant drugs to keep his or her body from rejecting the organ.

The role of the PTA in renal failure is important. Progressive exercise has been shown to be very helpful to many patients with renal failure. The PTA should monitor the patient's vital signs, including pulse rate, respiration rate, and blood pressure. Suggested exercises include stationary

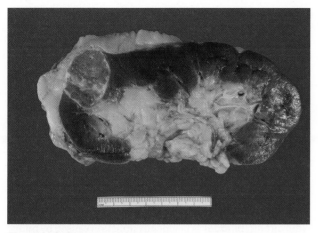

Figure 19–9 Renal cell carcinoma.

cycling, activities of daily living, strengthening exercises, and walking.

Prognosis

Prognosis is based on the severity of the renal failure and how the patient responds to treatment. Kidney failure may be prevented by controlling risk factors and maintaining a healthy diet and lifestyle.

Renal Cancer

Relatively uncommon, renal cancer usually affects men over age 55. The most common types are renal cell adenocarcinoma or renal cell carcinoma (**Figure 19–9**).

Signs and Symptoms

Renal cell carcinoma is typically asymptomatic in early stages. As it progresses, clinical manifestations include hematuria without pain, palpable mass, weight loss, anemia, hypertension, and fever. Renal cancer is known to metastasize to the brain, bones, or liver before symptoms become apparent.

Etiology

The cause of renal cancer is unknown. Tobacco is the most significant risk factor. Cigarette smokers have twice the incidence of renal cancer, and pipe and cigar smokers are also more susceptible. Additional risk factors include obesity (particularly in women), hypertension, estrogen therapy without progesterone, and exposure to asbestos, petroleum products, and heavy metals. There is also an increased incidence in patients with chronic renal failure.

Diagnosis

Diagnosis is confirmed via patient history, physical examination, urinalysis, IVP, CT scan, KUB x-ray, magnetic resonance imaging, cystoscopy, renal arteriogram, and biopsy.

Treatment

Treatment of kidney cancer involves **nephrectomy** (excision or removal of the cancerous kidney). If metastasis has occurred, additional treatments include chemotherapy and radiation. The role of the PTA is to assist patients with exercises designed to increase stamina and regain strength. Physical therapy is individualized based on the staging of the cancer and the patient's ability to tolerate various forms of exercise.

Prognosis

Prognosis varies because, without metastasis, the nephrectomy may completely cure the patient. Once metastasis has occurred, prognosis is poor.

Bladder Diseases

Obstructive disorders of the lower urinary tract are primarily related to storage of urine in the bladder or emptying of urine through the bladder outlet. The cause of the obstruction may include neurogenic and anatomic alteration or, in some instances, a combination of both. Incontinence is a common symptom of the bladder obstruction.

Urinary Incontinence

Urinary incontinence is defined as the loss of control of urine flow. It affects females much more than males. Nearly 40 percent of women aged 60 or older are affected.

Signs and Symptoms

Urinary incontinence is a very troublesome disorder, affecting sleep, exercise, travel, and sexual activity. There are several types:

- Overflow incontinence: The bladder does not properly empty and leaks when overfilled.
- Stress incontinence: The urine cannot be held when coughing, laughing, or sneezing.
- Urge incontinence: There is a sudden uncontrollable urge to empty the bladder.

Etiology

Female incontinence may be caused by childbirth, pregnancy, hysterectomy, and menopause. When incontinence does affect males, it is usually due to an enlarged prostate or as an effect of prostate surgery. Other causative factors include stroke, UTI, and certain medications.

Diagnosis

Urinary incontinence is diagnosed via a medical history, physical examination, and keeping a "voiding" diary, which records how often the patient urinates or experiences incontinence. Testing includes urinalysis and complete blood count to check for underlying infections. The status of the bladder and urethra may be measured via cystometry. A catheter may be placed into the bladder to determine how much urine remains inside after voiding. Cystoscopy may be used to find cysts, foreign bodies, or tumors of the bladder.

Treatment

Treatment of incontinence may involve wearing incontinence pads, menstrual pads, adult diapers, or waterproof underwear. Males may be able to wear external appliances to catch urine. Stress incontinence may be treated by frequently voiding. It may also be treated by strengthening the pelvic muscles and external sphincter by performing "Kegel exercises," which involves the tightening or contracting of these muscles. Kegel exercises, if performed several times a day, may greatly reduce or even eliminate stress-related urinary incontinence.

Pelvic floor biofeedback therapy helps patients to learn to strengthen and relax the pelvic floor muscles. Biofeedback uses electrical and mechanical instruments to measure the activity of the pelvic floor muscles and provides feedback to the patient about how the muscles and exercises are working. There are usually six to eight sessions during initial treatment. The role of the PTA is to assist with these therapies as directed by the physical therapist.

Other treatments are injecting collagen near the external sphincter to narrow the urethra, laparoscopic bladder suspension, a Marshall-Marchetti-Krantz procedure to suspend the bladder neck and urethra, and (for women) estrogen therapy. Overflow incontinence is treated with medications, self-catheterization, and surgery. Urge incontinence is treated with bladder training, Kegel exercises, and surgery. After prostate surgery, men must exercise the pelvic floor muscles to prevent incontinence. In more severe cases collagen injections or the implanting of an artificial sphincter may be indicated.

Prognosis

Prognosis is based on the type of incontinence, age, reduction of causative factors, and response to treatment.

Bladder Cancer

Malignant tumors of the urinary bladder commonly arise from the transitional epithelium that lines the bladder in the trigone area. This type of cancer often develops as multiple tumors and tends to recur. *Bladder cancer* is the most common urinary system cancer, usually occurring in men after age 60. It is actually three times more common in males than females.

Signs and Symptoms

The early sign of bladder cancer is hematuria, either gross or microscopic. Dysuria, nocturia, or frequency may develop, and infection is common. Unfortunately, symptoms do not usually appear until the disease has progressed extensively.

> **RED FLAG**
> Bladder cancer commonly metastasizes to the lungs, liver, and bones.

Etiology

Bladder cancer is of unknown origin but may be linked to cigarette, pipe, or cigar smoking. It has a higher incidence in individuals who work with chemicals and other potentially harmful substances, commonly dyes, rubber, and aluminum. Other predisposing factors are bladder infections and long-term overuse of analgesics.

Diagnosis

Bladder cancer is diagnosed by urine cytology (malignant cells in the urine) and biopsy.

Treatment

Treatment of bladder cancer is based on the stage of the disease. A **transurethral resection** may be used to remove part of the bladder, although the more common treatment is a **radical cystectomy**, or total removal of the bladder. Radiation and chemotherapy are indicated if metastasis has occurred.

The role of the PTA in bladder cancer patients is to promote physical therapy to increase overall body strength and mobility skills. Occupational therapy may also be indicated.

Prognosis

Prognosis is poor because the disease is usually discovered in its latter stages. Any cases of cystitis should be treated promptly to prevent development of cancer.

Trauma

Common types of trauma that affect the urinary system include neurogenic bladder and straddle injuries.

Neurogenic Bladder

Neurogenic bladder is bladder dysfunction caused by injury to a part of the nervous system controlling the bladder or urinary tract. Other names for this disorder include neuromuscular dysfunction of the lower urinary tract, neurologic bladder dysfunction, and neuropathic bladder.

Signs and Symptoms

Symptoms of neurogenic bladder vary based on the involved nerves. Patients may complain of having no feeling of the need to void or having it constantly. Additional symptoms include mild to severe urinary incontinence, inability or difficulty in emptying the bladder, and spasms of the bladder.

> **RED FLAG**
> Neurogenic bladder may result in incontinence, UTI, calculus formation, and renal failure.

Etiology

Many factors can interrupt bladder innervation. A spinal cord injury is related to the development of neurogenic bladder. Other types of trauma include cerebrovascular accidents, herniated lumbar disks, and tumors. Conditions that may cause this disorder include dementia, diabetes, Parkinson's disease, multiple sclerosis, and brain tumor. Cervical spondylosis, poliomyelitis, spina bifida, acute infectious diseases (such as Guillain-Barré syndrome), heavy metal toxicity, chronic alcoholism, and lupus erythematosus are other risk factors.

Diagnosis

Neurogenic bladder is not easy to diagnose. Diagnosis is accomplished with patient history, physical examination, neurologic examination, and a variety of urologic studies.

Treatment

Treatment of neurogenic bladder involves prevention of UTIs, control of incontinence (usually with indwelling urinary catheters), and intermittent self-catheterization. The role of the PTA is to assist with pelvic floor exercises, which can help the patient control bladder function. Certain weight training may also be beneficial, as directed by the physician.

Prognosis

Prognosis depends on the possibility of reversing any nerve damage. If related to herniated lumbar disks, disk repair usually restores bladder function. However, permanent nerve damage that causes neurogenic bladder means the condition will be lifelong.

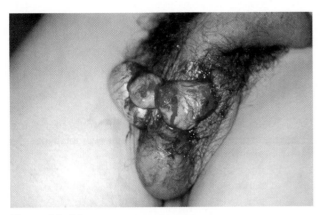

Figure 19–10 Straddle Injury.

Straddle Injuries

Straddle injuries usually occur when an individual falls while in a straddling position and often cause damage to the urethra. These injuries usually affect males more than females.

Signs and Symptoms

Signs and symptoms are similar to other bladder conditions.

Etiology

Straddle injuries often occur due to falling from a fence, roof beam, horse, or motorcycle. Any fall that occurs while the legs are in a "straddling" position may damage the urethra (**Figure 19–10**).

Diagnosis

Diagnosis basically requires physical examination and patient history.

Treatment

Treatment varies depending on the severity of the injury and is similar to treatments for other urinary conditions. The role of the PTA is to assist the patient with a straddle injury in light exercises designed to strengthen the muscles involved with the injury.

Prognosis

Prognosis is good, depending on the severity of the injury.

Rare Diseases

Rare urinary diseases discussed here are Goodpasture's syndrome and interstitial cystitis.

Goodpasture's Syndrome

Goodpasture's syndrome is an autoimmune disorder wherein the body's own antibodies attack the kidney membranes as well as the lungs.

Signs and Symptoms

This condition may result in glomerulonephritis and pulmonary hemorrhage. Other symptoms include hemoptysis, chest pain, dyspnea, and anemia.

Etiology

This syndrome may be triggered by a respiratory infection of viral origin or by inhaling hydrocarbon solvents. Men are eight times more likely to develop the syndrome than women, and it usually occurs in early adulthood.

Diagnosis

Diagnosis is based on patient history, physical examination, auscultation, urinalysis, blood tests, x-rays, and kidney or lung biopsy.

Treatment

Treatment involves *plasmapheresis* (the removal of antibodies from the blood). Medications include corticosteroids, antihypertensives, angiotensin-converting enzyme inhibitors, and angiotensin receptor blockers. Dialysis or kidney transplant may be indicated for severe cases.

Prognosis

Prognosis is poor because this syndrome usually results in renal failure and death.

Interstitial Cystitis

Interstitial cystitis is a chronic, nonbacterial condition involving inflammation of the inner lining of the bladder. It usually affects young women.

Signs and Symptoms

Symptoms include inflammation and swelling in the bladder, which decreases its capacity. The patient will need to urinate frequently and may experience hematuria due to ulceration of the bladder lining. Pain above the pubic area and lower abdomen, bladder fullness, and urgency to void may also occur.

Etiology

Interstitial cystitis is believed to be caused by an autoimmune disorder.

Diagnosis

Diagnosis is based on patient history and physical examination. Diagnostic tests include urinalysis, urine culture, biopsy, cystoscopy, and distention of the bladder while the patient is under anesthesia.

Treatment

Treatment may last for up to 12 weeks and involves instillation of liquid medications into the bladder. This distends the bladder and allows it to heal. The role of the PTA is to assist with pelvic floor exercises and biofeedback to allow the patient to understand how these exercises can improve the condition.

Prognosis

Prognosis is good because the available treatment methods are usually effective.

SUMMARY

The urinary system consists of the kidneys, ureters, bladder, and urethra. The main function of the kidneys is regulation of body fluids and electrolytes, controlling body temperature, and removing waste materials. There are numerous disorders of the urinary system, including UTIs such as cystitis and pyelonephritis. Common disorders of the kidneys include nephrotic syndrome, glomerulonephritis, hydronephrosis, renal calculi, and renal failure. Rarer diseases include acute tubular necrosis, nephrosclerosis, polycystic kidney disease, and renal cancer. Bladder cancer is one of the most common urinary system disorders. Bladder disorders that are more common in elderly people are urinary incontinence and trauma to the spinal cord or brain, which may cause neurogenic bladder.

REVIEW QUESTIONS

Select the best response to each question.

1. The disease that encompasses a group of symptoms and is referred to as "the kidneys losing protein" is which of the following?
   a. polycystic kidney disease
   b. acute glomerulonephritis
   c. nephrotic syndrome
   d. hydronephrosis
2. The cause of neurogenic bladder, a bladder control dysfunction, is
   a. hydronephrosis
   b. acute renal failure
   c. renal calculi
   d. damage to the spinal cord supplying the lower urinary tract
3. The term that describes decreased urine output is
   a. pyuria
   b. oliguria
   c. anuria
   d. nocturia
4. The following factors are causes of pyelonephritis *except*
   a. hydronephrosis
   b. pregnancy
   c. prostate enlargement
   d. ascending infection
5. Polycystic kidney disease usually leads to which of the following conditions?
   a. renal failure
   b. kidney stones
   c. renal cancer
   d. stroke
6. The following factors are causes of acute renal failure *except*
   a. dehydration
   b. prostatitis
   c. hemorrhagic shock
   d. congestive heart failure
7. Lipoid nephrosis is also known as
   a. Goodpasture's syndrome
   b. acute glomerulonephritis
   c. urinary bladder disease
   d. minimal change disease
8. The early sign of bladder cancer is which of the following?
   a. polyuria
   b. glycosuria
   c. hematuria
   d. albuminuria
9. When the urine cannot be held during coughing, laughing, or sneezing, it is called
   a. stress incontinence
   b. overflow incontinence
   c. urge incontinence
   d. voiding
10. Which of the following renal disorders may cause glomerulonephritis and pulmonary hemorrhage?
    a. nephrotic syndrome
    b. polycystic kidney disease
    c. nephrosclerosis
    d. Goodpasture's syndrome

CASE STUDIES

Karen Coupe, PT, DPT, MSEd

Case 1

A PTA is working in a rehabilitation facility equipped with a 25-chair dialysis center. The physical therapy department has recently started working directly with patients who are undergoing dialysis. Each patient is evaluated by the PT to determine any functional issues and to determine the appropriate exercise intensity. The PTA is currently seeing a 32-year-old woman undergoing hemodialysis secondary to end-stage renal failure caused by chronic glomerulonephritis. Plan of care is for low intensity treadmill training to improve ambulation distance and endurance.

1. Explain the etiology and clinical manifestations of glomerulonephritis.
2. Why is controlling hypertension important with this pathology? What other secondary pathologies could occur if hypertension were uncontrolled?
3. Explain what occurs to the kidneys with renal failure. How does this affect the body?
4. This patient is undergoing hemodialysis. Explain this procedure and how it is beneficial to the patient.
5. Research physical therapy and hemodialysis. Besides functional improvement, what are other evidence-based benefits for patients undergoing hemodialysis?

Case 2

A PTA is working in an outpatient facility equipped with a pool. The facility treats a number of patients with osteoarthritis and fibromyalgia using aquatic therapy. During the course of treating patients with the above pathologies the PTA comes across the following situations:

1. A 42-year-old woman who is currently undergoing aquatic therapy for fibromyalgia advises the PTA she is currently being treated for a UTI with antibiotics. Explain the etiology and clinical manifestations of a UTI. Who should be advised of the change in status? Is it okay for the patient to continue with aquatic therapy?
2. A 64-year-old woman with a right total hip replacement admits to the PTA that she suffers from urinary incontinence. What are common causes of urinary

incontinence? Is it okay for the patient to continue with aquatic therapy?

3. Urinary incontinence can be treated with physical therapy. Research physical therapy and urinary incontinence. What are some methods used to assist patients who have this issue?

4. A 72-year-old man with osteoarthritis advises the PTA that due to renal failure he will start peritoneal dialysis next week. What is peritoneal dialysis? Who should be advised of the change in status? Is it okay for the patient to continue with aquatic therapy?

5. A 47-year-old man reports to the PTA that he was just diagnosed with pyelonephritis. Explain the etiology and clinical manifestations of pyelonephritis. Who should be advised of the change in status? Is it okay for the patient to continue with aquatic therapy?

WEBSITES

http://health.nih.gov/topic/BladderDiseases

http://www.aahf.info/sec_exercise/section/urinary.htm

http://www.cancer.gov/cancertopics/types/bladder

http://www.childrenshospital.org/az/Site1117/mainpageS1117P0.html

http://www.kidney.org/atoz/content/dialysisinfo.cfm

http://www.mayoclinic.com/health/urinary-tract-infection/DS00286

http://www.medicinenet.com/kidney_failure/article.htm

http://www.merck.com/mmhe/sec11/ch144/ch144b.html

http://www.nlm.nih.gov/medlineplus/kidneydiseases.html

http://www.wrongdiagnosis.com/u/urinary_disorders/intro.htm

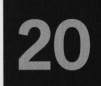

Endocrine System Disorders

LEARNING OBJECTIVES

After completion of the chapter the reader should be able to

1. Describe the role of the hypothalamus in regulating pituitary control of endocrine function.
2. State the major difference between positive and negative feedback control mechanisms.
3. Describe the mechanisms of endocrine hypofunction and hyperfunction.
4. State the effects of a deficiency in growth hormone.
5. Relate the functions of thyroid hormone to hypothyroidism and hyperthyroidism.
6. Relate the functions of the adrenal cortical hormones to Addison's disease and Cushing's syndrome.
7. Compare the three types of diabetes and their etiology.
8. Define dwarfism, diabetes insipidus, simple goiter, and Hashimoto's disease.

KEY TERMS

Acromegaly: Abnormal, continued growth of parts of the body that begins after puberty.

Aldosterone: A hormone that increases reabsorption of water and sodium and the release of potassium in the kidneys.

Asphyxiation: Suffocation; the inability to breathe normally.

Cretinism: Severely stunted physical and mental growth due to untreated congenital hypothyroidism.

Diabetes insipidus: A condition of excessive thirst and secretion of large amounts of severely diluted urine, most commonly caused by a deficiency of antidiuretic hormone.

Diabetes mellitus: Commonly known as "diabetes"; a condition of abnormally high blood sugar, either due to the inability of the body to produce enough insulin or because body cells do not respond to the insulin produced.

Diabetic ketosis: A condition wherein, as a result of diabetes, the body has elevated levels of ketone bodies in the blood; these bodies are formed when glycogen stores in the liver are depleted.

Dwarfism: Abnormally short stature due to a variety of conditions, most commonly abnormally low amounts of human growth hormone.

Euphoria: A profound sense of well-being.

Exophthalmos: An outward protrusion of the eyeballs.

Gigantism: Abnormal, continued growth of parts of the body that begins before puberty.

Glycosuria: Presence of glucose in the urine.

Graves' disease: An autoimmune disorder involving overactivity of the thyroid; excessive production of thyroid hormones results in hyperthyroidism and thyrotoxicosis.

KEY TERMS CONTINUED

Hashimoto's thyroiditis: An autoimmune disease in which the thyroid gland is destroyed by various immune processes; it often results in either hypo- or hyperthyroidism.

Hirsutism: Excessive hair growth on parts of the body that usually only experience minimal or complete lack of hair growth.

Hypercortisolism: High levels of cortisol in the blood, leading to Cushing's syndrome.

Hypoglycemia: Lower than normal levels of blood glucose.

Hyperparathyroidism: Overactivity of the parathyroid glands, resulting in excess parathyroid hormone.

Hypoparathyroidism: Underactivity of the parathyroid glands, resulting in lower than normal levels of parathyroid hormone.

Myxedema: A specific type of cutaneous and dermal edema secondary to increased deposition of connective tissue components; related to hypothyroidism and Graves' disease.

Nephrogenic: Originating in the kidneys.

Polyuria: Excessive elimination of urine.

Simple goiter: A goiter, defined as a swelling in the thyroid, that has spread through the entire thyroid.

Thyroid cancer: A malignant neoplasm that can be treated with radioactive iodine or by surgical resection; in fewer cases chemotherapy or radiotherapy are used.

Tropic: Targeting endocrine glands, such as in "tropic hormone" from the anterior pituitary gland.

Overview

The endocrine system is made up of glands, clusters of specialized cells, hormones, and target tissues. It is responsible for the secretion of hormones and chemical transmitters, which respond to nervous system (and other types of) stimulation. The endocrine system works with the nervous system to regulate and integrate metabolic activities and to maintain internal homeostasis. Target tissues have receptors for certain hormones. When these hormones connect with them, a hormone–receptor complex triggers the response of the target cell. The immune system is also extensively regulated by hormones such as the adrenal corticosteroid hormones. Therefore, the endocrine system affects many body functions, such as growth, development, energy metabolism, muscle and adipose tissue distribution, sexual development, fluid and electrolyte balance, inflammation, and the immune response.

Anatomy and Physiology of the Endocrine System

The human endocrine system consists of several small glands scattered throughout the body (**Figure 20–1**). The glands of the endocrine system secrete hormones into the bloodstream that are responsible for many unique functions in the body.

The levels of many hormones in the body are regulated by negative feedback mechanisms. This type of system functions similarly to that of a thermostat in a heating system. Sensors detect a change in hormone levels and adjust hormone secretion so that normal body levels are maintained within an appropriate range. Although most hormone levels are regulated by negative feedback mechanisms, a few are under positive feedback control. In this situation rising hormone levels cause another gland to release a hormone that is stimulating to the first hormone. Levels of each hormone in the bloodstream trigger the amount needed to be secreted. Secretion

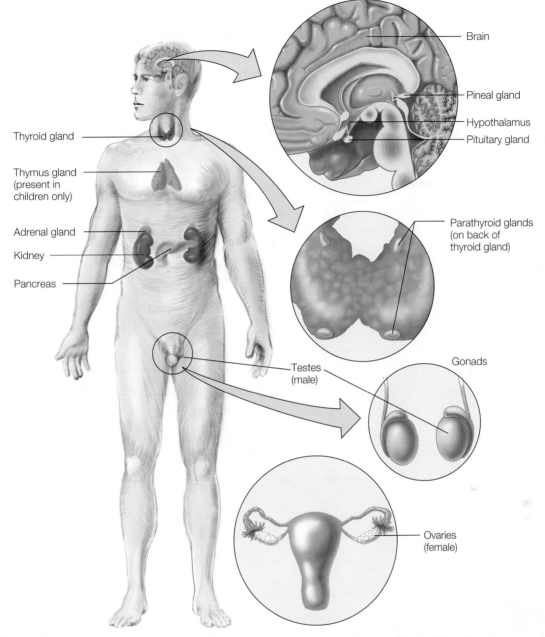

Figure 20–1 The human endocrine system. The endocrine system consists of a scattered group of glands that produce hormones: chemicals that regulate growth and development, homeostasis, reproduction, energy metabolism, and behavior.

of hormones is controlled by the hypothalamus, located in the third ventricle of the brain. Its hypothalamic hormones regulate the functions of the anterior pituitary gland (**Figure 20–2A and B**). The hypothalamus itself produces antidiuretic hormone (ADH) and oxytocin, which are stored in the posterior pituitary gland (neurohypophysis). **Table 20–1** lists the structures of the endocrine system and the functions of the hormones they secrete.

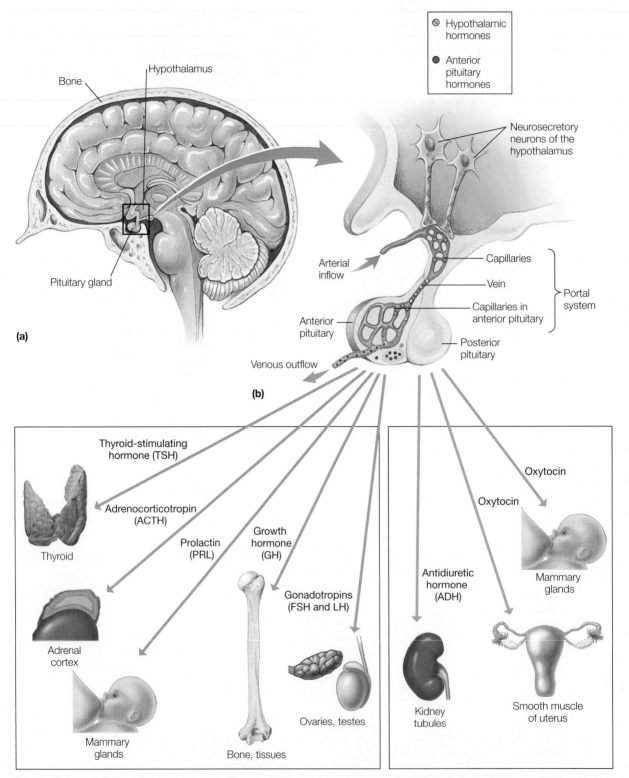

Figure 20–2 The pituitary gland. (A) A cross-section of the brain showing the location of the pituitary and hypothalamus. (B) The structure of the pituitary gland. Releasing and inhibiting hormones travel via the portal system from the hypothalamus to the anterior pituitary, where they affect hormone secretion.

TABLE 20–1   Endocrine Structures, Functions, and Hormones

Structure	Location	Hormone(s)	Function
Hypothalamus	Beneath the thalamus in the third ventricle of the brain	Inhibiting and releasing hormones	To control hormone release from the anterior pituitary
Hypophysis (pituitary) Anterior (adenohypophysis)	Base of the brain	Adrenocorticotropic hormone (ACTH)	Stimulates release of adrenal cortex hormones
		Thyroid-stimulating hormone (TSH)	Stimulates release of thyroid gland hormones
Posterior (neurohypophysis)		Somatotropin hormone (STH, also known as growth hormone [GH])	Stimulates growth
		Melanocyte-stimulating hormone (MSH)	Stimulates melanin production
		Prolactin	Stimulates mammary glands and lactation
		Follicle-stimulating hormone (FSH) and luteinizing hormone (LH)	Induces ovulation (females) and testosterone secretion (males)
		ADH	Increases reabsorption of water in kidneys
		Oxytocin	Stimulates uterine contraction and initiation of breast milk flow (females) and increases sperm ejection into seminal fluid (males)
Pineal	Behind the midbrain	Melatonin	Affects circadian rhythms
Thymus	Mediastinal cavity, under the sternum	Thymopoietin	Causes immune response development (newborns) and maintains it (adults)
Thyroid	In the anterior neck, on each side of the trachea	Triiodothyronine (T_3) Thyroxine (T_4)	Stimulates growth and development, regulates metabolism
		Calcitonin	Increases calcium deposits into bones
Parathyroids (four)	In the posterior part of the thyroid	Parathyroid hormone (PTH)	Regulates calcium and phosphate levels, increase calcium reabsorption from bones
Adrenals (two)—first portion: Adrenal cortex	One on top of each kidney	Glucocorticoids	Affects sodium and water reabsorption
		Mineralocorticoids	Promotes sodium and water reabsorption
		Sex hormones	Develops secondary sex characteristics
second portion: Adrenal medulla		Epinephrine	Fight or flight response, increases blood pressure and metabolism
		Norepinephrine	Causes vasoconstriction, increases blood pressure
Pancreatic islets Alpha cells	Embedded in the pancreas	Glucagon	Increases blood glucose levels and opposes insulin
Beta cells		Insulin	Regulates protein, carbohydrate, and fat metabolism
Delta cells		Somatostatin	Opposes insulin, glucagon, and somatotropin (STH)
Ovaries	On each side of the uterus	Estrogen Progesterone	Regulates growth, development, maturation, secondary sex characteristics, and the female reproductive cycle
Testes	In each side of the scrotum	Testosterone	Regulates growth, development, maturation, secondary sex characteristics, and the male reproductive system

Common Signs and Symptoms

Many endocrine disorders are caused by either hyposecretion or hypersecretion from certain glands. Diagnosis of endocrine conditions is complicated by the difficulty in linking the signs and symptoms to the cause. The pituitary gland is known as the "master gland" because its secretions control the actions of many other glands. Signs and symptoms that may initially appear to be related to another gland may actually be related to the pituitary gland. Common signs and symptoms of endocrine disorders include lethargy, fatigue, mental disorders, and eventual muscle atrophy.

Diagnostic Tests

Several tests are available for assessing endocrine function and hormone levels. One test measures the effect of a hormone on body function. For example, measurement of blood glucose reflects insulin levels and is an indirect method of assessing insulin availability. The most common method is to measure hormone levels directly via blood tests, urine tests, stimulation and suppression tests (via administration of hormones), genetic tests and imaging (magnetic resonance imaging, computed tomography scan, ultrasound), and biopsy.

Common Diseases of the Endocrine System

Common diseases of the endocrine system include pituitary gland diseases, thyroid gland diseases, parathyroid gland diseases, adrenal gland diseases, endocrine dysfunction of the pancreas, and precocious puberty. Abnormalities of any of these glands may be the result of injury from surgery, trauma, infection, radiation, or unknown causes.

Pituitary Gland Diseases

Pituitary gland diseases include hyperpituitarism (gigantism and acromegaly), hypopituitarism, dwarfism, and diabetes insipidus.

Hyperpituitarism (Gigantism and Acromegaly)

Hypersecretion of the pituitary produces **gigantism** (if it begins before puberty) or **acromegaly** (if it begins after puberty) (**Figures 20–3** and **20–4**). Hyperpituitarism is an abnormal increase in hormone production by the pituitary, especially affecting the production of growth hormone (or somatotropin). This leads to excessive growth of bones and tissues.

Signs and Symptoms

Gigantism is signified by increased rates of growth: sometimes up to 6 inches in a year in children with this disorder. Other signs include slowed sexual development and slowed mental development. Acromegaly is signified by enlargement of the small bones of the hands, feet, and face. In the face, jaw enlargement, wider than normal spacing of teeth, tongue enlargement, large forehead, and toughened, oily skin

with pigmentation changes are seen. Females may experience excessive hair growth.

Etiology

Hyperpituitarism is usually caused by benign pituitary tumors, which cause excessive secretion of adenohypophyseal trophic hormones. It may also be caused by carcinoid tumors. Hyperpituitarism may also cause changes in other hormone secretion rates, including thyroid hormones and prolactin.

Diagnosis

Physical examination is the first step in diagnosing hyperpituitarism to document abnormal or excessive growth. Blood tests may reveal high levels of growth hormone, thyroid hormone, and prolactin. A pituitary tumor can be revealed via MRI.

Treatment

In children, the growth process can be slowed by microsurgical removal of the pituitary tumor, radiation, and drug

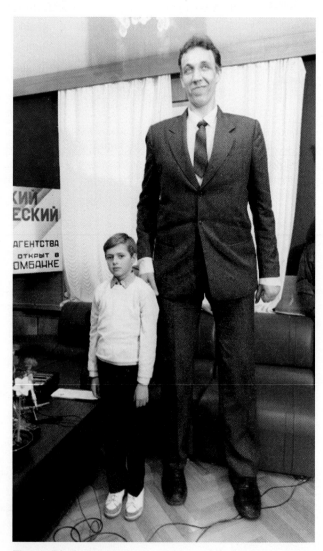

Figure 20–3 Pituitary giant.

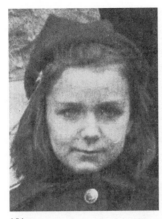
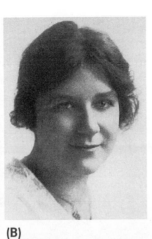

(A)   **(B)**

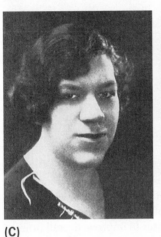

(C)   **(D)**

Figure 20–4 Acromegaly. Hypersecretion of growth hormone in adults results in a gradual thickening of the bone, which is especially noticeable in the face, hands, and feet. There is no sign of the disorder at age 9 (A) or age 16 (B). Symptoms are evident at age 33 (C) and age 52 (D).

Source: Reproduced from Am. J. Med., vol. 20, Mendelhoff, A. I., and Smith, D. E., Acromegaly, diabeties, hypermetabolism..., pp. 133-144. Copyright 1956, with permission from Elsevier.

therapy (**Figure 20–5**). In adults, surgical removal of a pituitary tumor often leads to hypopituitarism, with reoccurrence of pituitary tumors common. The role of the physical therapist assistant (PTA) is to assist patients with developmental exercises that will not cause excessive strain on their bodies. Moderate aerobic exercise is usually indicated. In adults the program addresses functional deficits.

Prognosis

Prognosis for gigantism is usually good with early diagnosis and treatment, based on signs and symptoms of the patient. However, the prognosis for acromegaly differs. Acromegaly often shortens life expectancy and may lead to congestive heart failure, respiratory disease, and cerebrovascular disease.

Hypopituitarism (Dwarfism)

Hypopituitarism is an abnormal decrease in pituitary activity, which leads to a deficiency or absence of some or all **tropic** hormones. A decrease in growth hormone leads to impaired growth of the entire body, and severe deficiencies cause **dwarfism** (**Figure 20–6**). Children affected by dwarfism are proportionately small, may be underdeveloped sexually, and may have mental impairments. Lack of gonadotropins such as follicle-stimulating hormone and luteinizing hormone can cause abnormal development or absence of secondary sexual characteristics.

Signs and Symptoms

Hypopituitarism commonly causes deficiencies of growth hormone and gonadotropin. In adult women amenorrhea or infertility may be seen. Males may show lowered testosterone levels, decreased libido, abnormal loss of facial and body hair, and metabolic disorders. Dwarfism causes extremely short stature and proportional body size reduction. There may be

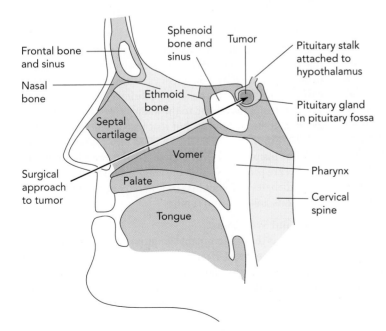

Frontal bone and sinus

Nasal bone

Sphenoid bone and sinus

Tumor

Pituitary stalk attached to hypothalamus

Ethmoid bone

Septal cartilage

Pituitary gland in pituitary fossa

Vomer

Palate

Pharynx

Surgical approach to tumor

Tongue

Cervical spine

Figure 20–5 Transsphenoidal resection of a pituitary tumor.

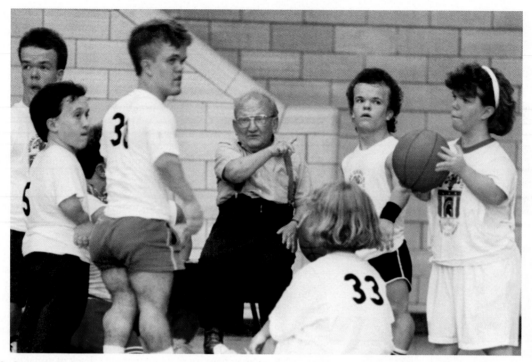

Figure 20–6 Pituitary dwarves.

varying degrees of mental retardation. In children, secondary tooth eruption may be delayed, and fatty deposits may occur in the lower trunk of the body.

Etiology

A primary benign pituitary tumor is commonly the cause of hypopituitarism. As the tumor grows it interferes with hormone production. Other causes that can potentially damage the pituitary gland are radiation, head injury, stroke, brain surgery, brain tumor, and infection. Dwarfism can be congenital or caused by a cranial hemorrhage after birth. Sometimes the cause is unknown. Deficiency of growth hormone-releasing hormone from the hypothalamus is called "secondary hypopituitarism" and occurs due to head trauma, infection, or a tumor.

Diagnosis

Clinical history and blood tests confirm diagnosis. Specific blood hormone tests of the levels of tropic hormones determine pituitary function. Target organ function can be assessed by checking the blood levels of triiodothyronine (T_3), thyroxine (T_4), estrogen, progesterone, testosterone, and cortisol. For dwarfism, physical examination determines growth rates that are below normal. Although general health is usually normal, the signs and symptoms mentioned above may indicate the condition. Persistently low serum growth hormone levels can be found by blood tests. A computed tomography scan may reveal a cranial tumor.

Treatment

Treatment of hypopituitarism involves hormone replacement therapy and monitoring and adjusting hormone levels. For dwarfism, somatotropin (human growth hormone) may be administered until the child reaches 5 feet in height.

Replacement of thyroid and adrenal hormones may also be necessary. As puberty approaches, sex hormones may need to be administered. The role of the PTA is to assist the patient with moderate aerobic exercises to improve overall fitness.

Prognosis

Prognosis is good unless the pituitary gland becomes nonfunctional or destroyed. In this case *panhypopituitarism* exists, which can lead to all the previously mentioned disorders and potentially be fatal. For dwarfism, prognosis is good as long as growth hormone replacement therapy is started early during the child's development. Hormone replacement is necessary to help children with dwarfism to reach normal adult height.

Diabetes Insipidus

Diabetes insipidus is a disturbance of water metabolism that results in extreme thirst and excessive secretion of dilute urine. It is caused by a deficiency in the release of ADH (or vasopressin) from the posterior pituitary gland. A type of diabetes insipidus related to the kidneys is termed "**nephrogenic** diabetes insipidus," but its cause is due to a defect in kidney response to ADH. It is a good idea for patients with diabetes insipidus to wear a medical alert bracelet to notify health care providers about the condition. The risk of developing diabetes insipidus may be lowered by promptly treating infections, injuries, and tumors.

Signs and Symptoms

Polyuria is the predominant symptom. The patient may urinate between 2 and 15 gallons of nearly colorless urine in a single day. Excessive polydipsia (thirst) is produced because the body needs to avoid dehydration. Other symptoms include constipation, dizziness, and hypotension.

Etiology

Diabetes insipidus is caused by a decrease of ADH release, usually because of damage to the pituitary gland by a tumor, surgery, trauma, or infection. This is known as "primary" or "central" diabetes insipidus. Another type is nephrogenic diabetes insipidus, which is caused by kidney disorders.

Diagnosis

Diabetes insipidus is diagnosed by urinalysis and a water restriction test. Urinalysis shows urine lacking in color with a very low specific gravity. Water restriction involves limiting intake for several hours while measuring urine output and concentration as well as blood pressure. Then, vasopressin is administered. If urine output decreases and urine concentration increases, diabetes insipidus is confirmed. An MRI of the pituitary and kidneys aids in diagnosis.

Treatment

Primary diabetes insipidus can be treated with vasopressin in either tablet or nasal spray form. Nephrogenic diabetes insipidus is treated with increased fluid intake and medications that decrease urine output. It is important to also treat the underlying kidney condition. The role of the PTA is to educate patients with diabetes insipidus about staying hydrated before, during, and after exercise. The PTA should alert the PT concerning any increases in physical therapy and exercise. If any signs of dehydration occur, such as thirst, dry mouth, dry skin, skin flushing, fatigue or weakness, and chills, exercise should cease immediately.

Prognosis

Prognosis is generally good.

Thyroid Gland Diseases

Thyroid gland diseases include simple goiter, Hashimoto's disease, hyperthyroidism (Graves' disease), hypothyroidism (cretinism and myxedema), and thyroid cancer.

Simple Goiter

Simple goiter involves an enlarged thyroid gland caused by attempted production of T_4 in adequate amounts (**Figure 20–7**). Adequate intake of dietary iodine can prevent the development of goiters.

Signs and Symptoms

Simple goiter is more prevalent in females and may be asymptomatic until the thyroid gland enlarges enough to be seen or felt. The front of the neck appears to "bulge," with extreme cases causing pressure on the trachea and esophagus, which can lead to dyspnea and dysphagia. A goiter can range from a small nodule to a large neck lump.

Etiology

Causes of simple goiter include a family history, eating large amounts of foods that inhibit production of thyroid hormone (such as soy, peanuts, peaches, spinach, turnips, cabbage, Brussels sprouts, etc.), regular use of certain medications that affect thyroid hormone production (such as lithium and propylthiouracil), and iodine deficiency. Iodine deficiency is rare in the United States because iodized table salt is commonly used and readily available.

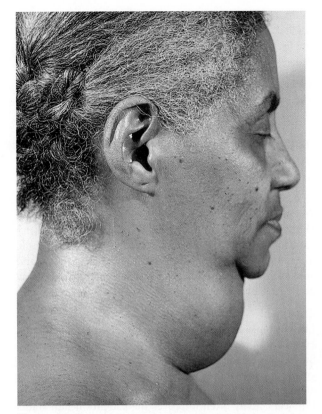

Figure 20–7 Goiter. An enlargement of the thyroid gland most often results from a lack of iodine in the diet.

Diagnosis

Physical examination confirms enlargement of the thyroid gland. Other diagnostic methods include measurement of T_3 and T_4 in the blood, ultrasound of the thyroid gland, and fine-needle biopsy of the thyroid.

Treatment

Initial treatment includes administration of potassium iodide. If the goiter is due to iodine deficiency, the patient should increase iodized salt in the diet. Goitrogenic foods, if the causative agent, should be removed from the diet or limited to only very small amounts. A goiter that is unresponsive to these treatments may require surgery to reduce the size of the thyroid gland.

Prognosis

Prognosis is good as long as the goiter size does not restrict breathing or swallowing.

Hashimoto's Thyroiditis

Chronic autoimmune thyroiditis is also called chronic lymphocytic thyroiditis, which occurs when autoantibodies destroy thyroid gland tissue. Chronic autoimmune thyroiditis associated with goiter is called **Hashimoto's thyroiditis**, which is a chronic disease of the immune system that attacks the thyroid gland.

Signs and Symptoms

Hashimoto's thyroiditis primarily affects women between 45 and 65 years of age. It is the leading cause of non–simple goiter and hypothyroidism. Thyroid gland enlargement is gradual and painless. Other symptoms include weakness, fatigue, forgetfulness, sensitivity to cold, mental apathy, unexplained weight gain, and constipation.

Etiology

The cause of Hashimoto's thyroiditis is unknown but is believed to have a genetic component. It is characterized by the production of antibodies in response to thyroid antigens and the replacement of normal thyroid structures with lymphocytes. As it enlarges, the thyroid is infiltrated by many lymphocytes and plasma cells, with glandular tissue being replaced by fibrous tissue.

Diagnosis

Diagnosis of Hashimoto's thyroiditis involves history, physical examination, a radioimmunoassay uptake test, checking for serum thyroid-stimulating hormone (TSH) elevation and autoantibodies in the blood. Needle biopsy of the thyroid may also be used to confirm the diagnosis.

Treatment

Lifelong replacement of thyroid hormone is indicated to treat Hashimoto's thyroiditis and prevent further goiter growth. Surgical excision, chemotherapy, or radiation is also indicated. The role of the PTA is to assist patients with moderate exercise to reduce weight and improve overall fitness. Physical activity often improves the patient's health status and may combat the symptoms of this condition and may help to reduce cholesterol levels.

Prognosis

Mild hypothyroidism is common, and prognosis is good with lifelong thyroid hormone–replacement therapy.

Hyperthyroidism (Graves' Disease)

Hyperthyroidism is defined as excessive secretion of T_4 by the thyroid gland. It is also known as *thyrotoxicosis*. **Graves' disease** is a condition of primary hyperthyroidism. It occurs when the thyroid gland is hypertrophied completely, resulting in a diffuse goiter. The onset usually occurs between the ages of 20 and 40 years, with women being five times more likely to develop the disease than men.

Signs and Symptoms

Signs and symptoms of Graves' disease include increased metabolic changes resulting in tachycardia, hypertension, palpitation, nervousness, excitability, insomnia, weight loss even with excessive appetite, profuse perspiration, warm and moist skin, heat intolerance, excessive thirst, nausea, vomiting, muscle weakness, dermopathy, hyperactivity, tremor, and hair loss. Advanced Graves' disease causes **exophthalmos (Figure 20–8A and B)**. If symptoms are suddenly exacerbated, *thyroid storm* may be occurring, which can be life threatening.

Etiology

Graves' disease is believed to be an autoimmune disorder characterized by abnormal stimulation of the thyroid gland by thyroid-stimulating antibodies (thyroid-stimulating immunoglobulins). These immunoglobulins act through the normal TSH receptors. The condition may be associated with other autoimmune disorders such as myasthenia gravis

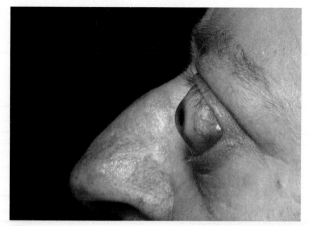

(A)

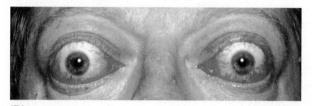

(B)

Figure 20–8 Exophthalmos.

and pernicious anemia. It is also believed to be genetically linked.

Diagnosis

A thorough patient history is obtained, and serum levels of T_3 and T_4 are evaluated. Blood tests may also reveal elevated antithyroid immunoglobulins. A thyroid scan is undertaken to show increased uptake of radioiodine.

Treatment

Treatment is aimed at reducing formation and secretion of thyroid hormone by administering propylthiouracil or methimazole. If present, tachycardia and hypertension are treated by beta-blockers. If the patient does not respond to these treatments or the disease is severe, radioactive iodine therapy or surgery is used to reduce thyroid gland activity. Thyroid hormone levels must be continually monitored throughout life. Additional treatment may focus on reducing anxiety and physical discomfort caused by the disease. Even with treatment, exophthalmos usually remains. Helpful strategies associated with exophthalmos include cool compresses, wearing sunglasses, using eye lubricants, and elevating the head of the bed.

The role of the PTA is to assist patients with moderate exercise, following the PT's plan of care, to improve overall fitness. However, because too much exercise can increase undesired cardiovascular responses, careful monitoring of vital signs is essential.

Prognosis

Prognosis is good as medical therapies usually restore balance to the body. Difficult cases may cause complications, and some cases reoccur spontaneously.

Hypothyroidism (Cretinism and Myxedema)

Hypothyroidism is common in iodine-deficient areas of the world and may result in mental deficiency. **Cretinism** is a form of hypothyroidism that develops during infancy or early childhood (**Figure 20–9**). **Myxedema** is a form of hypothyroidism that develops in older children or adults and may be severe (**Figure 20–10**).

Signs and Symptoms

Because the thyroid gland is absent or nonfunctional, cretinism leads to mental and growth deficiencies. Children with cretinism are short and stocky, with a protruding abdomen. Cretinism causes the sex organs to fail to develop and difficulty standing or walking due to lack of muscle tone. Facial characteristics include a broad nose, short forehead, small wide-set eyes, puffy eyelids, widely opened mouth with a thick and protruding tongue, dry skin, and lack of expression.

Myxedema causes menorrhagia in females, dry skin, reduced sweating, bloating of the face, thickening of the tongue, puffy eyelids, muscle weakness, fatigue, weight gain, hair loss, constipation, cold intolerance, slurred speech, mental apathy, diminished physical ability, and, in severe cases, coma and death.

Etiology

Cretinism may be caused by failure of the thyroid gland to develop or function normally. There also may be a congenital absence of an enzyme required to synthesize T_3 and T_4. A fetus may develop cretinism because of thyroid deficiency in the mother or as a result of the mother taking antithyroid drugs. Myxedema develops from impaired T_4 synthesis, destruction of the thyroid gland, removal of the thyroid without replacement therapy, or failure of the gland to function. Myxedema may also be caused by failure of the pituitary to produce thyrotropin.

Diagnosis

Cretinism is indicated by blood tests that show an absence or reduction of T_4 with elevated levels of thyrotropin. A thyroid scan shows reduced iodine uptake levels. If cretinism is not detected during the neonatal period, the infant will not respond readily in response to stimuli and development is delayed. Myxedema is diagnosed by blood tests that show abnormally low levels of T_4 and/or thyrotropin (TSH). The absence of response to thyrotropin may be indicated by radioactive iodine uptake tests.

Treatment

Thyroid hormone therapy may promote physical growth but will not stop mental retardation that develops in cretinism. Lifelong thyroid replacement therapy will be required. For myxedema, levothyroxine sodium (Synthroid) is administered to achieve normal thyroid function. The role of the PTA is to assist patients with low impact exercises (such as walking, strengthening exercises, posture retraining) that can greatly help to promote

> **RED FLAG**
> Elderly patients with hypothyroidism should initially be given a very low dose of T_4 to prevent cardiac problems. TSH levels determine gradual increases in dosage.

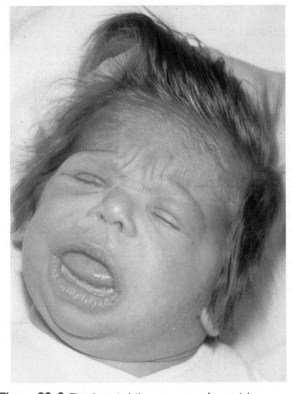

Figure 20–9 The characteristic appearance of neonatal hypothyroidism (cretinism) as a result of a congenital absence of thyroid gland. Treatment with thyroid hormone reversed manifestations of hypothyroidism.

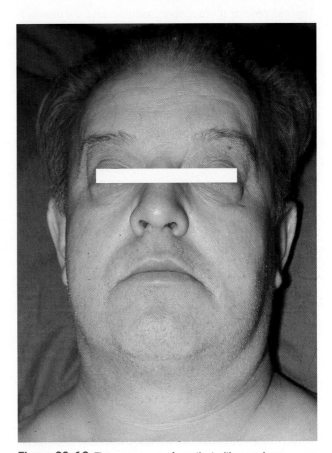

Figure 20–10 The appearance of a patient with myxedema.

general fitness. The patient may also perform cycling, swimming, volleyball, and aerobics.

Prognosis

If cretinism is discovered early in life and thryoxine replacement begins, prognosis is good. Skeletal abnormalities may be reversed with prompt and continuing treatment. For myxedema, prognosis with treatment is usually good, and symptoms improve. However, untreated myxedema affects almost every body system.

Thyroid Storm

Thyroid storm, also known as "thyroid crisis," is a life-threatening form of thyrotoxicosis. Although it occurs rarely, it is most often seen in patients with hyperthyroidism who have either never been diagnosed or have not been properly treated. Thyroid storm often follows stressful events such as diabetic ketoacidosis, respiratory (or other) infections, trauma, or manipulation of the thyroid during a thyroidectomy. It causes extremely high fever, congestive heart failure, tachycardia, angina, agitation, delirium, and restlessness. Thyroid storm often causes the death of the patient. Immediate treatment must occur, including the application of cold packs (yet while preventing shivering), fluid and electrolyte replacement, glucose administration, beta-adrenergic blockers, glucocorticoids, thyroid-blocking agents, and radioiodides. Aspirin must be avoided because it increases the level of free thyroid hormones.

Thyroid Cancer

Thyroid cancer is often asymptomatic until the disease is advanced. Patients who complain of persistent hoarseness, difficulty swallowing (dysphagia), or a painless and/or hard nodule in the neck should be screened for thyroid cancer as early as possible. The four main types of thyroid cancer are papillary, follicular, medullary, and anaplastic.

Signs and Symptoms

Signs and symptoms include those listed above as well as vocal cord paralysis, throat obstruction, cervical-lymph adenopathy, diarrhea, facial flushing, and Cushing's syndrome.

Etiology

Thyroid cancer is not common, accounting for 6 percent of thyroid nodules. Women are affected by this disease three times more than men. It is also genetically linked or may be caused by exposure to radiation. Papillary and follicular carcinomas grow slowly in people under age 45, and survival rates are high. Medullary carcinomas are usually inherited, and anaplastic tumors, although rare, typically do not respond to treatment.

Diagnosis

Thyroid cancer is usually discovered by the patient or through radiologic examination for another condition. Confirmation is through fine-needle aspiration and histologic examination of the nodule tissue. Additionally, abnormal levels of calcitonin and carcinoembryonic antigen may indicate thyroid cancer.

Treatment

Surgery is primarily used for papillary, follicular, and medullary thyroid cancers. Usually, the entire thyroid and nearby lymph nodes are removed. Radioiodine is then given to destroy any remaining tissue or tumors. T_4 therapy is also used to prevent additional tumor growth and hypothyroidism. Anaplastic tumors are treated primarily with radiotherapy and/or chemotherapy. The role of the PTA is to assist with walking and exercises to maintain strength. When surgery has been performed, the PTA may be required to assist with neck exercises. A speech therapist may be needed to assist with vocal retraining.

Prognosis

Prognosis is good based on age at diagnosis, size of primary tumor, and presence of tissue invasion or metastases. Approximately 95 percent of patients under age 40 survive 5 or more years after diagnosis. However, survival after diagnosis for patients over age 40 is only 65 percent. Anaplastic tumors have a very poor 5-year survival rate, with death linked to local cancer in the neck only months after diagnosis.

Parathyroid Gland Diseases

Parathyroid gland diseases include hyperparathyroidism and hypoparathyroidism.

Hyperparathyroidism

Hyperparathyroidism results from overproduction of the parathyroid hormone (PTH) by one or several of the parathyroid glands and is classified as primary or secondary. Primary hyperparathyroidism is more common in women, usually after menopause. Because postmenopausal women are at higher risk for developing osteoporosis, the effects of increased levels of PTH on bone disease can significantly worsen osteoporosis.

Signs and Symptoms

Hyperparathyroidism causes calcium to be released from the bones, causing weakness and fractures. Additional signs and symptoms are kidney stones, hypercalcemia, abdominal pain, vomiting, constipation, and arrhythmias.

Etiology

This disease is usually caused by a parathyroid tumor or idiopathic hyperplasia of one of the glands.

Diagnosis

Hyperparathyroidism is generally diagnosed by eliminating all other possible causes of hypercalcemia. Correct diagnosis requires at least a 6-month history of symptoms associated with hypercalcemia. These include hypophosphatemia, kidney stones, and increased urinary calcium levels. Tests used to document hyperparathyroidism include measurement of serum calcium, magnesium, phosphorus, and pH as well as x-rays of the bones and radioimmunoassays.

> **RED FLAG**
> After a parathyroidectomy, calcium gluconate or calcium chloride IV should be readily available at the bedside for emergency administration if tetany occurs.

Treatment

Treatment involves removal of the parathyroid tumor or the glands themselves. Normal PTH levels can be maintained by even one-half of a single parathyroid gland. Additional treatments include diuretics and limited dietary intake of calcium.

The role of the PTA is to assist patients with regular exercise, including strength training and weight-bearing activities, to maintain strong bones. The physical therapist should evaluate and develop an individualized physical therapy program based on the patient's overall condition and health.

Prognosis

Prognosis is usually good as long as treatment is adequate. However, severe hyperparathyroidism can cause cardiac arrest.

Hypoparathyroidism

Hypoparathyroidism is defined as a decrease in the normal amount of PTH, leading to abnormally low blood calcium levels.

Signs and Symptoms

Symptoms associated with hypoparathyroidism are mostly those of hypocalcemia. A lowered threshold for nerve and muscle excitation causes muscle spasms, clonic-tonic convulsions, laryngeal spasms, and, in severe cases, death by **asphyxiation**. Other symptoms include dry skin and scalp, hair loss, hypoplasia of developing teeth, cataracts, and bone deformities such as bowing of long bones.

Etiology

Hypoparathyroidism usually results from surgical removal of all parathyroid glands, or after a thyroidectomy. The incidence of the irreversible acquired form is greatest in adults who have undergone surgery for hyperthyroidism or other head and neck conditions.

> **RED FLAG**
> The incidence of the idiopathic and reversible forms of hypoparathyroidism is greatest in children.

Diagnosis

Hypoparathyroidism is diagnosed by physical examination and blood tests to check for low blood calcium and low PTH. Physical exam includes checking for Chvostek's and Trousseau signs. Chvostek's test involves tapping over the facial nerve to cause a facial muscle spasm. The Trousseau test involves applying pressure to the upper arm, resulting in muscle spasms. X-rays or bone scans can also be used to reveal weak bone structure due to low calcium levels.

Treatment

Treatment is directed toward alleviation of the hypocalcemia. When acute, this requires parenteral administration of calcium. Maintenance doses require vitamin D and oral calcium. The role of the PTA is to assist the patient with regular exercise, including weight-bearing exercises, to strengthen the bones. These exercises also improve balance, helping to reduce the risks of falling and bone fractures.

Prognosis

Prognosis is good with calcium and vitamin D treatment.

Adrenal Gland Diseases

Adrenal gland diseases include Cushing's syndrome and Addison's disease.

Cushing's Syndrome

The term *Cushing's syndrome* refers to the manifestation of **hypercortisolism** due to any cause. Two forms of this syndrome result from excess glucocorticoid production by the body. The pituitary form (Cushing's disease) results from excessive adrenocorticotropic hormone (ACTH) production by a tumor of the pituitary gland. The second form is the adrenal form (Cushing's syndrome), caused by a benign or malignant adrenal tumor.

Signs and Symptoms

The major manifestations of Cushing's syndrome are a rounded or "moon-shaped" face and a "buffalo hump" on the upper back (**Figure 20–11**). Symptoms include fatigue, poor wound healing, rounded abdomen, very thin arms and

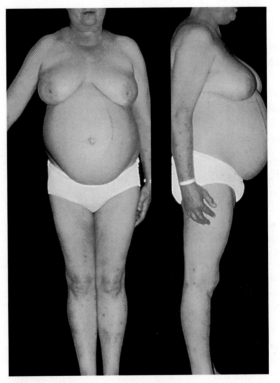

(A)

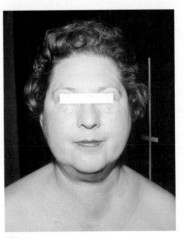

(B)

Figure 20–11 Cushing's syndrome. (A) Body manifestations of Cushing's syndrome. (B) Facial manifestations of Cushing's syndrome.

legs, weakness, hypertension, and stretch marks (striae) on the skin. Osteoporosis may develop due to destruction of bone proteins and alterations in calcium metabolism, which can lead to back pain, compression fractures of the vertebrae, and rib fractures. As calcium is mobilized from the bones, renal calculi may also develop.

Cortisol increases gastric acid secretion, which may provoke gastric ulceration and bleeding. Increased androgen levels cause **hirsutism**, mild acne, and, in women, menstrual irregularities. Excess glucocorticoids may cause extreme emotional changes, ranging from mild **euphoria** and lack of normal fatigue states to wildly psychotic behavior.

Etiology
Cushing's syndrome may be caused by a pituitary gland or adrenal cortex tumor. It can also develop after prolonged doses of cortisone.

Diagnosis
Diagnosis of Cushing's syndrome depends on hypersecretion of cortisol. The determination of 24-hour excretion of cortisol in the urine provides a reliable and practical index of cortical secretion. Other tests include the measurement of the plasma levels of ACTH. MRI or computed tomography scans can locate or confirm adrenal or pituitary tumors.

Treatment
Cushing's syndrome may be treated by surgical removal of the pituitary or adrenal cortex tumor, followed by lifetime hormone therapy. The role of the PTA is to educate the patient about exercises such as water aerobics, walking, and cycling. Physical activity should start slowly and increase slowly, based on the patient's tolerance.

Prognosis
Prognosis is good with surgery and hormone therapy.

Addison's Disease

Adrenal hypofunction is classified as either primary or secondary. Primary adrenal hypofunction or insufficiency is known as Addison's disease. It originates inside the adrenal gland and is characterized by decreased secretion of mineralocorticoids, glucocorticoids, and androgens. The secondary type is caused by a disorder outside the adrenal gland, such as impaired pituitary secretion of corticotropin (ACTH). It is characterized by decreased glucocorticoid secretion. Usually, the secretion of **aldosterone** (the major mineralocorticoid) is unaffected.

Signs and Symptoms
Clinical features vary between the two types of adrenal hypofunction. Signs and symptoms of Addison's disease include fatigue, weakness, anorexia, weight loss, and gastrointestinal complications. Conspicuous bronze discoloration of the skin may occur, especially in the creases of the hands, elbows, and knees (**Figure 20–12**). Primary hypofunction is associated with cardiovascular abnormalities such as irregular pulse, reduced cardiac output, and postural hypotension. Primary hypofunction also causes anxiety, depression, and emotional distress. The patient may not be able to retain salt and water. Addison's disease becomes life threatening when dehydration, electrolyte imbalance, and hyperkalemia occur.

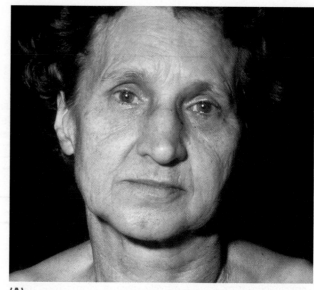

(A)

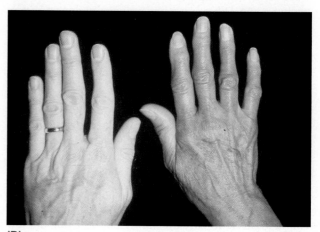

(B)

Figure 20–12 Patient with Addison's disease. (A) Appearance of face illustrating increased skin pigmentation. (B) Appearance of hand (right side of photograph) compared with hand of normal subject.

Etiology
Addison's disease is relatively uncommon. It can occur at any age and in both sexes but is more common in White females. Onset is usually gradual, with adrenal destruction caused by an autoimmune condition, hemorrhage, tuberculosis, fungal infections, neoplasms, or surgical removal. Addison's disease may be genetically linked, and the condition may also be secondary to hypopituitarism.

Diagnosis
Addison's disease is diagnosed by low blood and urine cortisol levels as well as low serum sodium and fasting glucose levels. Additionally, blood urea nitrogen, serum potassium, lymphocyte, eosinophil, and hematocrit levels will be elevated. The heart may be smaller than normal, and radiographic studies will indicate calcification of the adrenal glands.

Treatment
With early diagnosis and adequate replacement therapy, the disease is treated with glucocorticoid and mineralocorticoid

drugs, control of salt and potassium intake, increased fluid intake, and eating larger amounts of carbohydrates and proteins. Hormone replacement therapy must continue throughout life. Stress and infections should be well managed. A life-threatening emergency called *Addisonian crisis* may occur because of a sudden decrease in adrenocortical hormone levels. Symptoms of this crisis are increased heart and respiratory rate, nausea, headache, dehydration, and confusion.

The role of the PTA is to educate patients about weight-bearing exercises, such as running and weight lifting, and non–weight-bearing exercise, such as swimming. The PTA may assist the patient with general strengthening activities to promote fitness. Close monitoring of the patient's blood pressure, pulse, and other vital signs should occur because of the potential for Addisonian crisis.

Prognosis

Prognosis for both primary and secondary adrenal hypofunction is good with treatment.

Endocrine Dysfunction of the Pancreas

Endocrine dysfunction of the pancreas includes diabetes mellitus, gestational diabetes, and hypoglycemia.

Diabetes Mellitus

Diabetes mellitus is a chronic metabolic disorder characterized by hyperglycemia (elevated glucose level), which results from lack or decrease of insulin, a lack of the normal effects of insulin, or both. There are three general classifications:

- Type 1: Absolute insulin insufficiency
- Type 2: Insulin resistance with varying degrees of insulin secretory defects
- Gestational diabetes: Emerges during pregnancy

Onset of type 1 diabetes mellitus usually occurs primarily in children and young adults. Affected patients are prone to develop a condition called **diabetic ketosis** caused by a lack of insulin. Patients appear thin, requiring exogenous insulin and dietary management to control the disease. In contrast, type 2 diabetes mellitus usually occurs in obese adults after age 40.

> **RED FLAG**
> Ketosis does not usually occur as a complication of type 2 diabetes.

Gestational diabetes mellitus occurs when a previously nondiabetic woman shows glucose intolerance during pregnancy. This may occur if placental hormones counteract insulin, which causes insulin resistance. Gestational diabetes mellitus is a significant risk factor for future occurrence of type 2 diabetes mellitus.

Signs and Symptoms

Diabetes mellitus causes polyuria, polydipsia, polyphagia, **glycosuria**, hyperglycemia, and formation of ketones in the blood and urine. Other signs and symptoms include weight loss, headache, fatigue, weakness, and reduced energy levels. School or work performance may be impaired because of low intercellular glucose levels. Electrolyte imbalances may cause muscle cramps, irritability, and emotional instability. Neural tissue damage may result in numbness and tingling.

Type 1 diabetes, formerly known as insulin-dependent diabetes mellitus or juvenile-onset diabetes, is the most serious form. Although it is possible to develop type 1 diabetes as an adult, it is very uncommon. Additional signs include slower than normal breathing and a sweet, fruity odor of the breath. Signs of insulin shock include sweating, light-headedness, and trembling. Long-term complications include atherosclerosis, myocardial infarction, cerebrovascular accidents (strokes), peripheral vascular disease, diabetic retinopathy, blindness, and kidney failure.

Type 2 diabetes, formerly known as non–insulin-dependent diabetes mellitus or adult-onset diabetes, is the more common form. It mostly affects overweight adults, although the trend is changing, with overweight younger adults and even children developing this form of the disease. Type 2 diabetes is usually controllable through diet, exercise, and oral medications that stimulate the secretion of insulin.

> **RED FLAG**
> Type 1 diabetes usually has a rapid onset, typically with polydipsia, polyuria, weakness, weight loss, dry skin, and ketoacidosis.

Etiology

Diabetes mellitus is a chronic condition that affects the metabolism of carbohydrates because of inadequate insulin production by the pancreatic islets of Langerhans. Evidence indicates that diabetes mellitus has diverse causes, such as heredity, environment (infection, diet, toxins, stress), pregnancy, and lifestyle changes in people who are genetically susceptible to the disease.

> **RED FLAG**
> Type 2 diabetes is typically slow and insidious in onset and usually unaccompanied by symptoms.

Diagnosis

In adult men and nonpregnant women, diabetes mellitus is diagnosed by two criteria, which are obtained at least 24 hours apart. Diagnosis involves using the same test twice or any combination of the following tests:

> **RED FLAG**
> Type 2 diabetes is by far the more common type and is a more complex metabolic defect.

- Fasting plasma glucose level of 126 mg/dL or more on at least two occasions
- Typical symptoms of uncontrolled diabetes and random blood glucose level of 200 mg/dL or more
- Blood glucose level of 200 mg/dL or more 2 hours after ingesting 75 grams of oral dextrose

Diagnosis may also be based on diabetic retinopathy on ophthalmologic examination as well as urinalysis, which checks for the presence of acetone. A special "Hb_{A1C}" test should be given every 3 to 6 months to measure glycosylated hemoglobin in the blood. This test is a great indicator of the effectiveness of diabetes management.

Treatment

Effective treatment of type 1 and type 2 diabetes optimizes blood glucose control and decreases complications. Treatment for all types of diabetes involves management via patient education and lifelong attention to diet, medication, and exercise. Long-term complications may be avoided by frequent monitoring of blood glucose levels and using medications to regulate them.

When a diabetic patient requires physical therapy for another condition, the role of the PTA focuses on educating the patient about aerobic exercises, such as walking, jogging, cycling, and dancing. Swimming, rowing, and chair exercises are also indicated. The diabetic patient should always warm up and cool down before and after regular exercise. The PTA may also be involved in gait training, wound care and education of the patient about skin care, proper shoe selection, and detecting signs of blood sugar fluctuations secondary to exercise, diet, and nutrition.

Prognosis

Prognosis for type 2 diabetes is good based on the patient following treatment guidelines. Prognosis for type 1 diabetes is often poorer due to the many complications this disease can cause and lack of patient compliance. However, proper disease management may allow these patients to live relatively normal lives.

Hypoglycemia

Hypoglycemia is defined as abnormally low blood sugar, with levels of blood glucose below 60 mg/dL. Symptoms may occur at varying levels, however, based on each individual's tolerance to them. Hypoglycemia is much more dangerous than hyperglycemia, because the brain cannot store glucose and constantly requires it to function. Severe hypoglycemia results in brain damage.

Signs and Symptoms

Symptoms of hypoglycemia include light-headedness, diaphoresis (sweating), and trembling. Untreated hypoglycemia can lead to mental confusion, coma, and possible death. Most people have experienced this condition at least once in their lives. Diabetic ketoacidosis is a related condition, wherein the body uses fat instead of sugar as a fuel source. Byproducts of fat breakdown, called ketones, build up in the body. The major signs and symptoms of diabetic ketoacidosis are deep and rapid breathing, dry skin and mouth, flushed face, a fruity odor of the breath, nausea, vomiting, and stomach pain.

Etiology

Common causes of hypoglycemia include excessive exercise, fasting, and skipping regular meals. It may also be caused by over-administration of insulin, pancreatic adenoma, gastrointestinal disorders, and certain hereditary conditions.

Diagnosis

Hypoglycemia may be diagnosed by observing the classic symptoms and testing blood glucose levels. Diagnosis is confirmed if blood glucose levels are below normal when blood is tested and if relief occurs after eating.

RED FLAG

The PTA must recognize the effects of hypoglycemia on the central nervous system. This event is an emergency situation that must be treated properly to avoid syncope, various injuries, cardiovascular shock, and brain damage.

Treatment

When hypoglycemia occurs in a diabetic patient, he or she should consume glucose tablets, orange juice, or candy. It is recommended that diabetics carry these items with them on a regular basis. If the hypoglycemic attack is acute, immediate emergency attention should be given via intravenous glucose administration. Exercise levels are important in managing hypoglycemia. The role of the PTA is to assist patients with moderate exercises, based on the therapy plan of care.

Prognosis

Prognosis is good as long as measures are in place to avoid hypoglycemia. These include a well-balanced diet, eating smaller meals more often, having snacks available, avoiding sugar-rich foods on an empty stomach, avoiding alcoholic beverages on an empty stomach, maintaining a healthy body weight, avoiding smoking, and regular exercise.

SUMMARY

The endocrine system is made up of many glands located throughout the body, each with unique functions and hormones. It helps to regulate growth and metabolism in normal conditions. However, over- or underproduction of hormones from the body's glands may cause dysfunction of other body systems. Endocrine disorders include gigantism, acromegaly, dwarfism, diabetes insipidus, hyperparathyroidism, hypoparathyroidism, Cushing's syndrome, Addison's disease, and diabetes mellitus. Type 1 diabetes mellitus usually begins in childhood and type 2 usually begins in adulthood. Type 2 diabetes is beginning to affect younger people, partially because of increased obesity. With the aging process, endocrine disorders greatly increase the risk for other systemic problems to develop. As aging increases, endocrine secretions are reduced.

REVIEW QUESTIONS

Select the best response to each question.

1. What condition is caused by hypersecretion of growth hormone before puberty?
   a. myxedema
   b. acromegaly
   c. dwarfism
   d. gigantism
2. Diabetes insipidus results from the lack or deficiency of which of the following hormones?
   a. insulin
   b. aldosterone
   c. antidiuretic hormone
   d. thyroxine
3. Which of the following glands regulates the level of calcium in the blood?
   a. pituitary
   b. parathyroid
   c. pancreas
   d. thymus
4. Iodine deficiency may cause what condition?
   a. impaired growth
   b. renal hypertrophy
   c. anemia
   d. goiter

5. Hashimoto's disease is a condition involving what structure?
   a. thyroid gland
   b. thymus gland
   c. pancreas
   d. adrenal cortex
6. Cushing's syndrome is defined as which of the following?
   a. inflammation of the pericardium
   b. a tick-borne disease characterized by skin lesions, malaise, fatigue, and facial palsy
   c. hyperactivity of the adrenal cortical gland that develops from an excess of the glucocorticoid hormone
   d. an inflammatory autoimmune disease that attacks the thyroid gland
7. Conspicuous bronze discoloration of the skin may occur in which of the following conditions?
   a. thyroid storm
   b. Addison's disease
   c. Hashimoto's thyroiditis
   d. acromegaly
8. Which of the following thyroid disorders is also known as thyrotoxicosis?
   a. Graves' disease
   b. Hashimoto's thyroiditis
   c. simple goiter
   d. myxedema
9. Which of the following conditions, if severe, may cause asphyxia and death?
   a. hyperthyroidism
   b. hypothyroidism
   c. hypoparathyroidism
   d. hyperparathyroidism
10. Which type of diabetes mellitus was formerly known as insulin-dependent diabetes mellitus?
   a. type 1
   b. type 2
   c. gestational diabetes
   d. insipidus diabetes

CASE STUDIES

Karen Coupe, PT, DPT, MSEd

Case 1

A 40-year-old man was involved in a motor vehicle accident and suffered multiple lower extremity fractures and rib fractures with subsequent pneumothorax. Patient medical history: Type 1 diabetes diagnosed at age 20 with resultant LE peripheral neuropathy. Prior level of function: Independent in all activities of daily living. The patient is 7 weeks post-injury and was referred to outpatient physical therapy. The PT evaluation reveals LE muscle weakness, independent ambulation with a front-wheeled rolling walker for 15 feet before fatigue, decreased cardiopulmonary endurance, and LE neuropathy. Plan of care includes progressive strengthening, cardiopulmonary endurance activities, patient education

in skin and footwear, and progression of ambulation from a walker to a cane.

1. What is the difference between type 1 and type 2 diabetes?
2. How does exercise affect a patient's blood sugar levels? Would you educate your patient about this issue?
3. Before each treatment the patient tests his blood sugar. What blood sugar level is considered too high to begin treatment? Too low?
4. During a treatment session the patient complains of a headache and the PTA notes diaphoresis, trembling, weakness, and decreased coordination. What is the patient demonstrating? How should the PTA react to this situation?
5. How would LE peripheral neuropathy affect the patient during treatment? The plan of care includes patient education in foot care. How is this related to the neuropathy? What are some important skin and footwear instructions for this patient?

Case 2

A 32-year-old woman is referred to outpatient physical therapy secondary to chronic back pain. Patient medical history: Diagnosed with Graves' disease 1 week ago. Current level of function: Ambulates independently distances up to 20 feet, requires assistance with household chores secondary to back pain. PT evaluation reveals a hyperlordotic postural dysfunction, abdominal and gluteal weakness, and poor cardiopulmonary endurance. Plan of care is for modalities, postural correction through strengthening/stretching, lumbar stabilization, aerobic activity, and instruction in back care and body mechanics.

1. Explain the etiology and clinical manifestations of Graves' disease.
2. How could Graves' disease affect the patient when the PTA is working on aerobic activities? How would the PTA monitor these concerns?
3. The plan of care includes modalities. For a patient with Graves' disease, which modalities may not be tolerated?
4. How will the environmental temperature of the facility affect a patient with Graves' disease?
5. What is the medical treatment for Graves' disease? Sometimes the treatment puts the patient on the other spectrum, hypothyroidism. If this occurred, what signs and symptoms would alert the PTA to this change? How could this affect the plan of care?

WEBSITES

http://parathyroid.com/

http://www.emedicinehealth.com/anatomy_of_the_endocrine_system/article_em.htm

http://www.endocrineweb.com/thyroid.html

http://www.healthsystem.virginia.edu/uvahealth/adult_endocrin/pithub.cfm

http://www.mayoclinic.com/health/precocious-puberty/ds00883

http://www.medicinenet.com/diabetes_mellitus/article
  .htm
http://www.nlm.nih.gov/medlineplus/adrenalglanddisorders
  .html
http://www.nlm.nih.gov/medlineplus/ency/imagepages/
  1093.htm

Male Reproductive System Disorders

LEARNING OBJECTIVES

After completion of the chapter the reader should be able to

1. Name the anatomic structures of the male reproductive system.
2. Discuss the causes of male infertility.
3. Describe common congenital abnormalities in males.
4. Explain cryptorchidism and its treatment.
5. Differentiate benign prostatic hypertrophy from cancer of the prostate.
6. Explain various hormones of the male reproductive system.
7. Compare epididymitis and orchitis.
8. Describe the signs and symptoms of testicular cancer.

KEY TERMS

Bulbourethral glands: Mucous glands at the base of the penis that secrete into the penile urethra.

Cryptorchidism: Failure of one or both testicles to descend into the scrotum.

Differentiation: Increased specialization of cells for certain functions.

Ductus deferens: Duct that carries sperm from the epididymis to the ejaculatory duct.

Epididymis: A coiled structure in the testis for the storage and transport of sperm to the vas deferens.

Epispadias: An abnormal urethral opening on the upper surface of the penis.

Exogenous: Originating from outside the body.

Gynecomastia: Abnormal enlargement of breast tissue in men.

Hydrocele: A fluid-filled cavity or duct that may occur in the scrotum.

Meatus: External urethral orifice.

Orchiopexy: Surgical descent of the testes into their normal position within the scrotum.

Scrotum: Pouch of skin comprising the part of the male external genitalia that contains the testes.

Seminal vesicles: A pair of sac-like glandular structures that lay posterolateral to the urinary bladder in the male and function as part of the reproductive system.

Seminiferous tubules: Tubules in the testes where the sperm cells form.

Spermatic cord: Collectively, the spermatic vessels, nerves, lymphatic vessels, and ductus deferens, extending between the testes and proximal end of the inguinal canal.

Spermatogenesis: Formation and development of spermatozoa.

KEY TERMS CONTINUED

Testosterone: Primary male hormone; it is produced mainly in the testes and is secreted into the blood.

Tunica vaginalis: Serous membrane surrounding the testis and epididymis.

Varicocele: Distended or swollen veins in the spermatic cord of males.

Overview

The male gonads are called the testes, which produce sperm cells and hormones required for the reproductive process. The male reproductive system is designed to transfer sperm cells into the female to fertilize an ovum, producing an embryo and then fetus. Sperm is transported through various ducts, including the epididymis, ductus deferens, and ejaculatory ducts. The accessory organs of reproduction in males include the seminal vesicles, prostate gland, bulbourethral glands, and penis. Many conditions that affect the male reproductive system have the potential to result in sterility, although early treatment can usually prevent this from occurring.

Anatomy and Physiology of the Male Reproductive System

The primary structures of the male reproductive system are the gonads (*testes*), which are suspended in the **scrotum**, which is a sac outside of the abdominal cavity. The complete structures of the male reproductive system are shown in **Figure 21–1A and B**. The testes produce sperm and the sex hormone called **testosterone**.

The scrotum, or *scrotal sac*, is made up of a skin layer that is continuous with the perineal skin layer, plus an inner layer of fascia and muscle. This skin layer is a loose, fleshy pouch that encloses the testes of the male. Inside the scrotum the two testes are separated by a septum made of connective tissue. The **tunica vaginalis** encloses each testis and its attached epididymis. The tunica vaginalis has two walls and a small amount of fluid between its layers. Arteries, lymphatics, and veins are contained in the **spermatic cord**.

The testes are located outside of the abdominal cavity to have an adequate temperature for sperm production, which is 2 to 3 degrees Fahrenheit below normal body temperature. The testes are drawn in closer to the body by the scrotal muscle when environmental temperatures drop, with the function reversed in warmer temperatures. Sperm production or infertility may result when higher temperatures affect the testes, such as when excessively tight clothing is worn or in males with **cryptorchidism**. In the fetus the testes normally descend from the abdominal cavity through the inguinal canal into the scrotum (**Figure 21–2**). This occurs during the third trimester of pregnancy, followed by the closing of the inguinal canal.

The testes mature and begin to produce sperm and testosterone during puberty. This is controlled by gonadotropins secreted by the adenohypophysis. Additional male reproductive structures include accessory glands and those that form and transport semen, including the **ductus deferens**, **epididymis**, and **seminiferous tubules**.

Spermatogenesis is the continual production of spermatozoa. This process takes between 60 and 70 days to complete. **Table 21–1** lists the steps involved in spermatogenesis.

At the time of emission *semen* is formed, which contains many substances from various accessory structures, as follows:

- The **seminal vesicles** behind the bladder provide a secretion that includes *fructose*, which nourishes sperm.
- The *prostate gland*, surrounding the urethra at the base of the bladder, secretes an alkaline fluid providing the desired pH of 6 for fertilization (without this secretion, fertilization is not likely to occur because both male and female secretions are normally acidic).
- The **bulbourethral glands** (*Cowper's glands*), near the base of the penis, secrete an alkaline mucus that helps neutralize any residual urine in the male urethra.

The amount of semen ejaculated at one time is between 2 and 5 mL. It mostly consists of fluid but contains between 1 and 2 hundred million sperm.

Male Hormones

The adenohypophysis (anterior pituitary gland) releases many gonadotropic hormones: follicle-stimulating hormone, which initiates spermatogenesis, and luteinizing hormone, also known as *interstitial cell-stimulating hormone*, which stimulates the production of testosterone by the interstitial "Leydig" cells of the testes (**Figure 21–3**).

TABLE 21–1   Steps of Spermatogenesis

Structure	Description or Function
Testes, which consist of many lobules containing the seminiferous tubules	"Sperm factories" of the body
Efferent ducts	Conduct sperm into the *epididymis*, where they mature
Epididymis	Peristaltic movements assist the sperm to move into the *ductus deferens* (*vas deferens*) and then to the *ampulla*
Ampulla	Motile sperm may be stored here for several weeks until ejaculation occurs (Note: *Vasectomy* involves cutting or obstructing the vas deferens to block sperm passage)

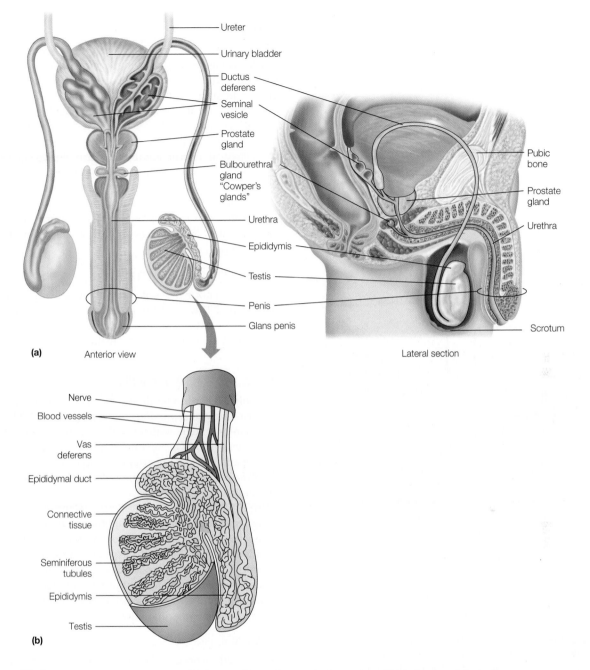

Figure 21–1 The male reproductive system. (A) Organs of the male reproduction system. (B) Interior view of the testis.

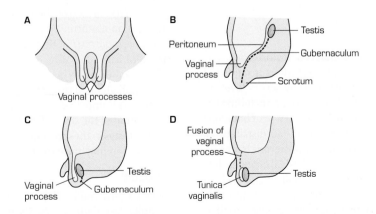

Figure 21–2 Descent of the testes. (A) Anterior view, illustrating vaginal processes extending into scrotum. (B) Lateral view prior to testicular descent, illustrating the gubernaculum extending from the testis into the scrotum posterior to the vaginal process. (C) Testis descends into scrotum posterior to vaginal process. (D) Proximal part of vaginal process obliterated; distal part persists as tunica vaginalis.

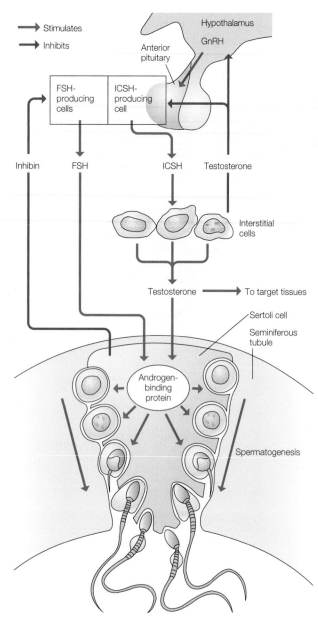

Figure 21–3 Hormonal control of testicular function. Testosterone, FSH, and ICSH participate in a negative feedback loop. The testes also produce a substance called inhibin, which controls GnRH secretion.

Sperm mature because of the effects of testosterone. The continuous control of gonadotropin secretions is regulated by a negative feedback system provided by serum levels of testosterone. Testosterone has other functions, including the development and maintenance of secondary sex characteristics such as deepening of the voice, male hair distribution, and maturing of the external genitalia. Testosterone is an anabolic steroid hormone that influences physical changes during puberty and promotes protein metabolism and skeletal muscle development. Anabolic steroids are now commonly abused by athletes who want to improve and strengthen their bodies, although these substances can cause serious complications to the reproductive structures, liver, and heart.

Infertility

Infertility or sterility may be caused by only male factors, only female factors, or combined factors. These conditions generally occur in the same proportions between males and females. In males, common infertility issues are

- Hormonal abnormalities, due to testicular or pituitary disorders
- Changes in sperm or semen
- Physical obstruction of the sperm, due to congenital problems, scar tissue, or previous infections
- Inability of the sperm to penetrate cervical mucus

The semen is often analyzed to determine specific conditions. Antibodies to the presence of sperm may also influence infertility. Many drugs are now available for erectile dysfunction.

Congenital Abnormalities

Congenital abnormalities of the penis include epispadias and hypospadias. These conditions generally affect the urethral opening (**meatus**). Congenital abnormalities affecting the testes include cryptorchidism, hydrocele, varicocele, and torsion.

Epispadias and Hypospadias

Epispadias refers to a urethral opening on the dorsal (upper) surface of the penis, proximal to the glans (**Figure 21–4**). If the urinary sphincter is affected, the patient may experience *incontinence* (lack of urine control), and infections may occur at the opening. Sometimes this condition is related to *exstrophy of the bladder*, in which the abdominal wall has failed to form across the midline area.

Hypospadias refers to a urethral opening on the ventral (under) surface of the penis (**Figure 21–5**). It is generally more severe if it occurs in the proximal section of the penis, and there may be *chordee* (ventral curvature of the penis). Cryptorchidism may be related to hypospadias. For both epispadias and hypospadias surgical reconstruction may be recommended, in several small stages, to ensure normal sexual function and urinary flow.

Cryptorchidism

Cryptorchidism occurs when a testis fails to descend into the scrotum during the third trimester of pregnancy. Instead, it may remain in the abdominal cavity or descend only to the inguinal canal or above the scrotum (**Figure 21–6**). If the testis is in an abnormal position outside the scrotum, it is called an *ectopic testis*. Often, the testis descends in the first year after birth.

This condition may occur because of hormonal abnormalities, a small inguinal ring, or a shorter spermatic cord. Spermatogenesis is impaired in the undescended testis because of degeneration of the seminiferous tubules. Surgical positioning of the testes in the scrotum before age 2 is advised because this condition may raise the risk of testicular cancer.

Hydrocele

When excessive fluid collects in the potential space between the tunica vaginalis layers, **hydrocele** occurs. This may involve one or both testes and is distinguished by a process known as transillumination (**Figure 21–7**).

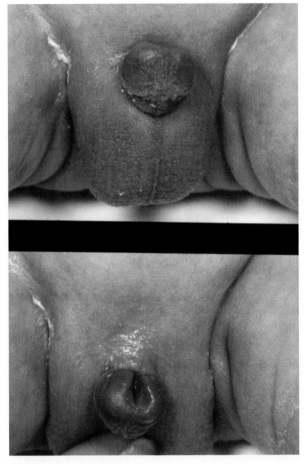

Figure 21–4 Epispadias.

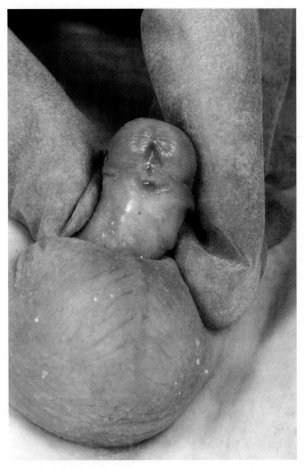

Figure 21–5 Hypospadias.

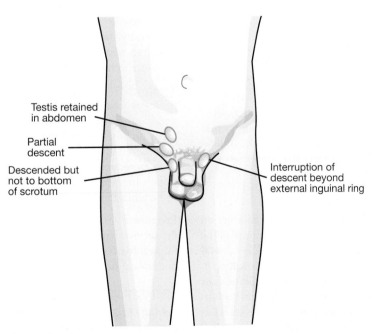

Figure 21–6 Potential sites for cryptorchidism.

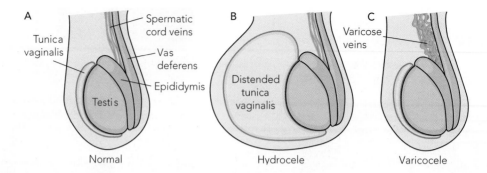

Figure 21–7 (A) Normal tunica vaginalis containing a small amount of fluid. (B) Hydrocele. (C) Varicocele.

Hydrocele may occur in infants congenitally when peritoneal fluid accumulates in the scrotum. This fluid may be reabsorbed over time or may continue to escape from the peritoneal cavity if the proximal processus vaginalis does not close off normally after the testis descends.

Inguinal hernia also may result from an open processus vaginalis. This condition describes a loop of the intestine passing through the abnormal opening, leading to an intestinal obstruction. Surgical repair is usually indicated to avoid the herniation becoming strangulated (constricted, which can cut off blood supply). Causes of hydrocele include infections, scrotal injury, and tumors, although causes may also be unknown. Acquired hydroceles usually occur after middle age, and aspiration may be required because large amounts of fluids may compromise testicular blood supply.

> **RED FLAG**
>
> In hydrocele, fluid usually accumulates more during the day and subsides during the night. More pain and discomfort is caused by increased accumulation of fluid.

Varicocele

A **varicocele** is a mass of dilated veins in the spermatic cord. It usually occurs on the left side, developing often after puberty (also shown in Figure 21–7). A varicocele may result from a lack of valves in the veins, which allows blood to backflow, with increased venal pressure. Usually, a varicocele causes no symptoms. Occasionally, symptoms may include a feeling of heaviness on the affected side because of blood pooling. If extensive, a varicocele is painful, tender, and may lead to infertility because blood flow and spermatogenesis are impaired. When the patient is upright and the affected area is palpated, it may feel like a "bag of worms." This cannot be palpated when the patient is in a recumbent position. Surgical treatment to correct the abnormal veins may be indicated.

Torsion of the Testis

Torsion of the testis describes one of the testes rotating on the spermatic cord. This interrupts the blood supply to the testis, causing swelling of the scrotum (**Figure 21–8A and B**). The veins in the cord are compressed initially, resulting in stoppage of venous blood return from the testis. Blood flow through the arteries may continue, but the condition leads to marked engorgement of the testis with blood. This is soon followed by complete hemorrhagic necrosis of the testis, called a hemorrhagic infarction. Blood flow to the testis must be restored immediately via surgery. This condition may occur spontaneously during puberty or after trauma.

Infections and Inflammation

Infections and inflammation that affect the male reproductive system may be varied, with prostatitis being most significant.

Orchitis

Orchitis is an infection of the testis. It usually requires prompt treatment to alleviate pain and to begin antibiotic therapy.

Signs and Symptoms
One or both testes may be affected by orchitis, which causes swelling, tenderness, and acute pain. Additional symptoms may include chills, fever, general malaise, and nausea or vomiting.

Etiology
Orchitis may be of bacterial or viral origin (such as from the mumps virus). It also may follow epididymitis. Acute orchitis is often related to a sexually transmitted infection. Nearly one-half of all cases will cause atrophy of the affected testicle. If both testicles are affected, sterility results.

Diagnosis
To identify the cause, throat cultures, serologic studies, or urinalysis may be conducted. Clinical history to determine exposure to mumps may be helpful.

Treatment
Bacterial orchitis should be treated immediately with appropriate antibiotics. Unfortunately, there is no specific treatment for mumps orchitis. The patient is usually advised to undertake bed rest and, if severe, to take adrenal steroids to reduce fever and swelling. The scrotum may need to be supported to reduce discomfort. Ice packs may also be beneficial.

Prognosis
Prognosis is based on getting the right diagnosis and treatment for orchitis. Testicular cancer should be ruled out. Mumps orchitis cannot be treated and may result in sterility.

Epididymitis

Epididymitis is inflammation of the epididymis (the excretory duct of the testicles). This condition may cause extreme discomfort during its acute phase.

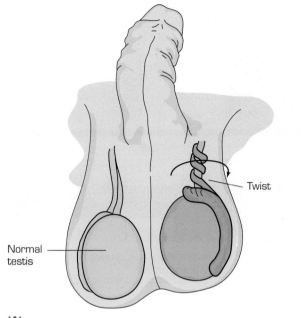

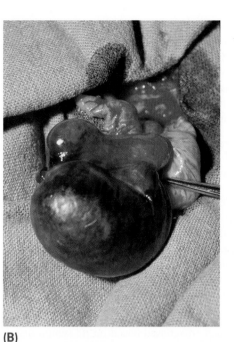

Figure 21–8 Cause and effect of testicular torsion. (A) Rotary twist of testis also twists spermatic cord, interrupting blood supply to the testis. Normally, the epididymis is located along the posterior surface of the testis, but the torsion has rotated the testis and also rotated the epididymis anteriorly. (B) Hemorrhagic infarction of testis caused by torsion.

Signs and Symptoms

Epididymitis may cause fever, pain, and malaise. The epididymis may enlarge, harden, and become tender. The groin may become tender, and pain in the testes can become severe. Walking may be affected due to the scrotum being painful.

Etiology

The most common causes of epididymitis are *Neisseria gonorrheae* and *Chlamydia trachomatis*. Other bacterial causes include *Escherichia coli*, *Staphylococcus*, and *Streptococcus* (see Chapter 22). This condition may also be caused by prostatitis, a urinary tract infection (UTI), and syphilis. A male may be predisposed to the condition because of mumps, tuberculosis, *prostatectomy* (removal of the prostate gland), prolonged use of an in-dwelling catheter, and trauma.

Diagnosis

Epididymitis may be diagnosed by physical examination, urinalysis, urine cultures, and an elevated white blood cell count.

Treatment

Treatment of epididymitis may combine analgesics, antibiotics, rest, and avoidance of spicy foods and alcohol. A scrotal support may be beneficial. Although the condition usually responds well to treatment, scarring may occur, which can lead to sterility. This occurs in more cases of bilateral epididymitis (which means that both epididymides are affected).

Prognosis

Epididymitis usually improves with antibiotics. However, the condition can recur and has the potential to become chronic, causing pain without swelling.

Prostatitis

Prostatitis may be an acute or chronic, bacterial or nonbacterial infection or inflammation. This *ascending infection* (progressing up the urethra) may have multiple causes. The prostate may be protected to some degree from prostatitis because urination and ejaculation "flush" out the tissues. Also, an intact mucous membrane and prostatic secretions help in preventing microbial infection. Because the male reproductive and urinary tracts are closely related, the spread of infection may be promoted. Therefore, prostatitis is related to UTIs. *Prostatodynia* (painful prostate) and prostatitis may be of unknown origin when they are nonbacterial.

When acute bacterial prostatitis occurs, the gland becomes tender and swollen, feeling "soft" upon palpation. Testing of the urine indicates higher quantities of microorganisms, leukocytes, and pus. Expressed prostatic secretions also show microorganisms, but this process may be quite painful and potentially spread infection. When non-

> **RED FLAG**
> The most common complication of prostatitis is a UTI. If untreated, a UTI can progress to prostatic edema, pyelonephritis, urinary retention, epididymitis, and prostatic abscess.

bacterial, prostatitis is indicated by large amounts of leukocytes in the urine and prostatic secretions, without marked enlargement of the prostate. Chronic prostatitis only causes slight enlargement that may be irregular or firm because fibrosis is more extensive. Usually, prostatitis occurs along with a UTI or infections of parts of the reproductive tract.

Signs and Symptoms

Prostatitis, whether acute or chronic, is signified by dysuria, urinary frequency, and urinary urgency. Other symptoms may include low back or abdominal pain. If inflammation of the prostate is severe, urine flow through the urethra may be obstructed, resulting in a decreased urinary stream. Other symptoms may be hesitancy in beginning urination, incomplete bladder emptying, urinary frequency, and nocturia. Systemic symptoms include fever, anorexia, malaise, and muscle aches. If prostatitis is nonbacterial, urinary symptoms may be intermittent, with less marked systemic symptoms.

Etiology
Acute bacterial prostatitis is usually caused by *E. coli*, followed by *Pseudomonas, Proteus,* or *Streptococcus faecalis*. It primarily occurs in young men who have UTIs from intestinal bacterial invasions. It also affects older men who have benign prostatic hypertrophy (BPH). It may be associated with sexually transmitted diseases such as gonorrhea, instrumentation (such as use of catheters), or by spreading through the blood. If chronic, prostatitis is usually related to recurring *E. coli* infections. Sexually transmitted diseases are discussed in detail in Chapter 22.

Diagnosis
Prostatitis is usually diagnosed based on its symptoms. A urine culture confirms the diagnosis and identifies the causative organism. Other tests include complete blood count and transrectal ultrasound.

Treatment
For bacterial prostatitis, antibacterials such as ciprofloxacin are recommended. Follow-up examinations should be conducted to ensure the infection has been completely eradicated. Nonbacterial prostatitis may be treated with anti-inflammatory drugs and prophylactic antibacterials.

Prognosis
Acute prostatitis usually responds well to antibiotics. The chronic form of the disease often recurs, with or without symptoms (usually pelvic pain).

Neoplasms
Common cancerous conditions of the male reproductive system include benign prostatic hypertrophy, prostate cancer, and testicular cancer.

Benign Prostatic Hypertrophy
BPH usually affects older men and is actually hyperplasia of the prostatic tissue. Nodules form to surround the urethra, leading to urethral compression and varying degrees of urinary obstruction (**Figure 21–9**).

This condition is revealed by an enlarged prostate gland, found during a rectal examination. Because the bladder cannot empty completely, there may be frequent infections. Continued obstruction causes dilated ureters, distended bladder, hydronephrosis, and potential renal damage. Surgical intervention is required if significant obstruction and urinary retention develop.

Signs and Symptoms
BPH is initially indicated by obstructed urinary flow, followed by dribbling, hesitancy, and decreased force. Incomplete bladder emptying leads to frequency, nocturia, and recurring UTIs.

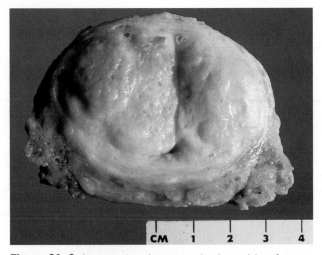

Figure 21–9 Cross-section of prostate, showing nodules of hyperplastic tissue compressing urethra.

Etiology
The cause of BPH is not completely understood. However, the condition seems to be related to a hormonal imbalance associated with aging. When the prostate gland enlarges, it compresses the neck of the bladder or the urethra. This causes obstruction of urinary flow.

Diagnosis
Diagnosis of BPH is based on patient history, symptoms, digital rectal examination, blood tests, prostate-specific antigen (PSA) tests, and urodynamic tests.

Treatment
Usually, only a small amount of cases need intervention, although severe cases may indicate surgery. When surgery cannot be used, drugs that reduce the androgenic effect or alpha-adrenergic blockers such as tamsulosin may be indicated.

Prognosis
Prognosis for BPH is usually good. Medications or surgery are usually successful in treating this condition.

Prostate Cancer
Prostate cancer is the second most commonly diagnosed cancer in men. It usually affects men over age 50, with more than 85 percent of all prostate cancers diagnosed in men older than 65 years of age. African American men have the highest reported incidence rate for prostate cancer at all ages. Asian and Native American men have the lowest rate. Unfortunately, this type of cancer also tends to be diagnosed at a late stage of development. In the United States, prostate cancer is the third leading cause of cancer death. Most prostate cancers are adenocarcinomas that arise from the surface tissue of the prostate gland. Unfortunately, these tumors often metastasize to bones of the pelvis, spine, femur, or ribs relatively early (**Figure 21–10**). In most patients, the cancer has already spread before diagnosis. Other areas of metastasis include the liver, pelvic lymph nodes, adrenal glands, and lungs. **Table 21–2** lists the four stages used to describe prostate cancer.

TABLE 21–2	Stages of Prostate Cancer
Stage	**Description**
A	Small, nonpalpable, encapsulated tumors
B	Palpable tumors confined to the prostate
C	Tumors that extend beyond the prostate
D	Distant metastases are present

Signs and Symptoms

Prostate cancer often causes a hard nodule in the gland's periphery, usually the posterior lobe, that is detectable via rectal examination. Usually, urethral obstruction does not occur initially. As it grows, however, obstruction occurs, with increased urinary problems and infections such as cystitis.

Etiology

The precise cause of prostate cancer is unclear. It may be linked to genetic factors, environmental factors, and hormonal imbalances. **Exogenous** factors are those that originate from outside the body. It has been suggested that dietary patterns, including increased dietary fats, may alter the production of sex hormones and growth factors and increase the risk of prostate cancer.

Diagnosis

Before treatment the disease is usually confirmed via the presence of PSA and elevated prostatic acid phosphatase. Tests must be handled correctly because raised PSA may occur due to infections or BPH. All men over age 45 should be tested annually to check for serum markers, which determine the future treatment and greatly affect outcome. Digital rectal examination is also required for diagnosis. Additional confirmation is via ultrasound and biopsy, with bone scans being useful to detect early metastases.

Treatment

Treatment involves surgery and radiation, and risks as well as benefits must be considered. Such risks are incontinence or impotence as a result of treatment. If the tumor is sensitive

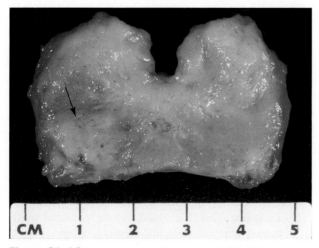

Figure 21–10 A cross-section of resected prostate illustrating a small carcinoma arising from outer prostate glands (arrow).

to androgens, removal of the testes (orchiectomy) or antitestosterone drug therapy may be indicated to reduce hormonal imbalances. The 5-year survival rate of this treatment is 85 to 90 percent.

The role of the physical therapist assistant (PTA) in prostate cancer includes teaching pelvic floor exercises, which can help to decrease incontinence after prostatectomy.

Prognosis

The prognosis for prostate cancer is based on the stage of the disease at diagnosis, the age of the patient, a healthy diet, response to treatment, and various other factors. Approximately one of six American men with prostate cancer dies from the disease. The most important clinical prognostic indicators are the stage of disease, pretherapy PSA level, and Gleason score, which is a scale that indicates the cellular and glandular involvement of prostate cancer.

Testicular Cancer

Testicular tumors are classified as seminomas or nonseminomas. Seminomas are composed of uniform, undifferentiated cells that resemble primitive gonadal cells. The term **differentiation** means increased specialization of cells for certain functions. Most testicular tumors are malignant and arise from germ cells. Testicular cancer is not common in the United States, but its incidence is increasing. It is more common in men between the ages of 20 and 35, and it is the most common solid tumor in young men. Regular monthly testicular self-examination, especially after taking a shower, is recommended to check for unusual hard masses. Instructions on how to perform these self-exams may be found online via the Testicular Cancer Resource Center (http://tcrc.acor.org/tcexam.html). Additional information is available from medical clinics and the American Cancer Society.

Testicular cancer may occur from one or various types of cells. A *teratoma* is made up of various different germ cells. It is derived from one or more germ cell layers combined with an embryonal carcinoma.

Certain malignancies secrete alpha-fetoprotein or human chorionic gonadotropin, which are used as serum markers for diagnosis and follow-up. Testicular neoplasms may spread very early (such as choriocarcinomas) or remain localized for longer periods (such as seminomas). They usually appear first in the common iliac and para-aortic lymph nodes, spreading to the mediastinal and supraclavicular lymph nodes. Later, they may also spread to the liver, lungs, bones, and brain. Staging is based on extent of the primary tumor, amount of lymph nodes involved, and distant metastases.

> **RED FLAG**
>
> Most testicular cancers arise from the germinal epithelium of the testicular tubules and are malignant.

Signs and Symptoms

Testicular tumors are usually hard, painless, and unilateral masses. The testis may feel enlarged or "heavy." A dull ache may then persist in the lower abdomen. Because of inflammation, hydrocele or epididymitis may occur. Also, the breasts of the male may enlarge (**gynecomastia**) because of hormonal secretions from the tumor.

Etiology

Although specific causative factors for testicular cancer are unknown, it is usually familial or may be related to trauma or infection. The main predisposing factor is cryptorchidism (failure of the testicles to descend). If an undescended testis is noted in a child, **orchiopexy** is recommended as soon as possible after birth. There is an increased incidence of testicular cancer in men infected with HIV as well as those with testicular disorders such as Klinefelter's syndrome.

Diagnosis

Most testicular tumors are found in routine checkups or by self-examination. Scrotal ultrasound, computer tomography or chest x-ray (for lung metastasis), abdominal and pelvic computer tomography or magnetic resonance imaging (to check for retroperitoneal lymph node metastasis), and intravenous pyelography (to check for urinary tract involvement) must be done. Serum laboratory analysis of human chorionic gonadotropin and alpha-fetoprotein is also required.

Treatment

Treatment usually involves a combination of surgery, radiation, and sometimes anticancer chemotherapy. If a bilateral orchiectomy is performed, the patient may need hormonal replacement.

> **RED FLAG**
> Extensive surgical resection of the testicle, the spermatic cord, and (sometimes) the regional lymph nodes are required for the treatment of testicular cancer.

> **RED FLAG**
> Nonseminomatous tumors are not radiosensitive, and chemotherapy is the preferred treatment.

The role of the PTA in testicular cancer is to be aware of potential signs and symptoms, which may cause secondary thoracic or lumbar pain radiating around the iliac crest to the groin. The PTA should be aware of the location of superficial lymph nodes. If a mass is observed or there is a "filling in" of a normal concavity, the PT should be consulted regarding palpation of the area to determine if there is a detectable nodule or other indicators.

Prognosis

Prognosis is improved when medical and physical therapies are combined. If orchiectomy is performed, sexual function is usually not affected. Radiation may reduce fertility temporarily, for a few months.

SUMMARY

Male reproductive disorders include a variety of conditions that may result from UTIs, sexually transmitted infections, aging, hormones, and other causes. It is recommended, especially for young men, that regular monthly testicular self-examinations are conducted for early detection of testicular cancer. Cancer of the prostate may be related to androgens in the body and commonly metastasizes to the bones or lungs. Older men often develop BPH, which causes urinary obstruction but is not associated with malignancy. Other conditions, such as torsion of the testis, orchitis, and epididymitis, have the potential to cause sterility of the male.

REVIEW QUESTIONS

Select the best response to each question.

1. Which of the following complications can occur with undescended testes?
   a. infection
   b. gangrene
   c. polyposis
   d. cancer

2. A urethral opening on the dorsal surface of the penis is called which of the following?
   a. hypospadias
   b. epispadias
   c. hydrocele
   d. varicocele

3. The term "prostatodynia" means
   a. enlargement of the prostate
   b. infection of the prostate
   c. inflammation of the prostate
   d. painful prostate

4. The most common cause of acute bacterial prostatitis is which bacteria?
   a. *Escherichia coli*
   b. *Mycobacterium tuberculosis*
   c. *Staphylococcus aureus*
   d. *Streptococcus pneumoniae*

5. The cause of BPH is related to which of the following?
   a. specific diet
   b. hormonal imbalance
   c. having too much sexual intercourse
   d. chronic urinary tract infections

6. Prostate cancer commonly metastasizes to which of the following?
   a. pancreas and thyroid gland
   b. heart and brain
   c. bones and lungs
   d. all of the above

7. The most common malignant tumor of the male reproductive system between ages 25 and 30 years involves
   a. the prostate
   b. the testicles
   c. the penis
   d. none of the above

8. Gynecomastia may be seen in
   a. prostate cancer
   b. hydrocele
   c. benign prostatic hypertrophy
   d. testicular cancer

9. The interstitial "Leydig" cells secrete
   a. estrogen
   b. testosterone
   c. growth hormone
   d. gonadotropic hormone

10. Excessive fluid that collects in the potential space between the tunica vaginalis layers is called
    a. varicocele

b. spermatocele

c. hydrocele

d. cryptorchidism

CASE STUDIES

Karen Coupe, PT, DPT, MSEd

Case 1

An 18-month-old male qualified for early intervention secondary to a diagnosis of Klinefelter's syndrome. The PT evaluation reveals general hypotonia and developmental delays. The primary mode of locomotion is creeping, and the parents report the patient is pulling up to stand but not consistently.

1. Research Klinefelter's syndrome and explain the etiology.
2. The degree of symptoms, in this pathology, depends on the amount of testosterone. Explain the role of testosterone in males.
3. The above patient has low testosterone. Physically, how would this affect the patient? Would this patient require muscle facilitation or inhibition techniques? Is the patient using the appropriate mode of locomotion for his age?
4. What additional pathologies are common with this syndrome?
5. What is the fertility rate for patients with Klinefelter's syndrome?

Case 2

A 65-year-old man was referred to physical therapy 1 day status post right total hip replacement. The patient fell 2 days ago and suffered a femoral neck fracture. Patient medical history: Prostate cancer currently being monitored, osteoporosis secondary to hyperthyroidism, which is currently medication controlled. Prior level of function: Independent in all activities. Current level of function: Bed mobility w/min x1 and v/c's for total hip replacement precautions, transfers with min x1 and v/c's for total hip replacement precautions, ambulates with a front-wheeled rolling walker 20ft x1 with multiple v/c's for gait pattern progression and walker placement distance. Plan of care includes bed mobility, transfer training, gait, and patient education of total hip replacement precautions.

1. Explain the etiology and clinical manifestations of prostate cancer.
2. The patient's prostate cancer is being monitored. Explain what testing is done to monitor this pathology.
3. What are the treatment options for prostate cancer?
4. Based on the signs and symptoms of prostate cancer, will there be any impact on physical therapy treatment?
5. Research the surgical methods for THR. Explain why the THR precautions are based on the surgical approach.

WEBSITES

http://hubpages.com/hub/Epididymitis-A-Common-Infection-Of-The-Male-Reproductive-Tract

http://www.cancer.gov/cancertopics/types/testicular

http://www.medicinenet.com/penis_disorders/article.htm

http://www.ncbi.nlm.nih.gov/pmc/articles/PMC1950215/

http://www.nlm.nih.gov/medlineplus/ency/imagepages/1113.htm

http://www.nlm.nih.gov/medlineplus/malereproductivesystem.html

http://www.pcf.org/site/c.leJRIROrEpH/b.5699537/k.BEF4/Home.htm

http://www.uhmc.sunysb.edu/urology/male_infertility/history_and_physical_exam.html

Female Reproductive System Disorders

LEARNING OBJECTIVES

After completion of the chapter the reader should be able
to

1. Describe the anatomic relation of the structures of
   the external genitalia.
2. List the three layers of the uterus and describe the
   function of the inner layer.
3. Characterize the development of cervical cancer.
4. Define the terms amenorrhea, dysmenorrhea,
   metrorrhagia, and menorrhagia.
5. Differentiate between benign ovarian cysts and
   ovarian cancer.
6. Describe pelvic inflammatory disease.
7. Explain the risk factors for breast cancer and
   the importance of breast self-examinations and
   mammography.
8. Name the organisms responsible for genital
   herpes, gonorrhea, syphilis, and condylomata
   acuminata.

KEY TERMS

Alopecia: Hair loss.
Amenorrhea: Absence of menstrual period in women of
normal reproductive age.
Bacteroides: A type of gram-negative bacteria that are
anaerobic; make up the largest amount of normal
gastrointestinal flora.
Bicornuate: A formation of the uterus wherein the upper
parts remain separate whereas the lower parts are
fused together.
Broad ligament: The wide fold of peritoneum connecting
the sides of the uterus to the walls and floor of the
pelvis.
Budding yeast: A type of fungi that reproduces
asexually, meaning new yeasts grow from others.

KEY TERMS CONTINUED

Chancre: A painless ulcer, usually in the genital area, that is the first sign of a syphilis infection.

Clitoris: A small mass of erectile tissue located at the top anterior part of the vulva; the primary site of female arousal.

Congenital syphilis: A type of syphilis present in utero and at birth, occurring when a child is born to a mother who has secondary syphilis.

Dysmenorrhea: Severe uterine pain during menstruation.

Dyspareunia: Painful sexual intercourse.

Dysuria: Pain or difficulty passing urine.

Endometriosis: A condition wherein uterine tissue forms painful cysts outside of the uterus, such as the pelvic cavity, intestines, and even the lungs.

Follicles: Basic units of female reproduction, composed of primarily round aggregations of cells found in the ovary.

Gardnerella vaginalis: A gram-variable anaerobic bacteria that can cause bacterial vaginosis by disrupting normal vaginal flora.

Human papillomavirus (HPV): A group of over 100 viruses that cause a range of afflictions, including warts and cervical cancer.

Hysterosalpingogram: A radiologic examination of the uterus and fallopian tubes that uses injection of a radiopaque material into the cervix for fluoroscopic viewing.

Hysteroscopy: Inspection of the uterus via endoscopy through the cervix.

Infantile uterus: A uterus that has not attained normal adult characteristics; it may be smaller than normal or not enough sufficient tissue to support a pregnancy.

Labia majora: Major outside pair of lips of the vulva.

Labia minora: Minor inside pair of lips of the vulva.

Lactation: Production and secretion of milk from the mammary glands of the breasts after giving birth.

Leukorrhea: A white or yellowish vaginal discharge normally present in smaller amounts during different points in the menstrual cycle and during pregnancy. A large increase in the discharge may indicate infection.

Mammography: A procedure in which x-rays are passed through the breast and recorded on a photographic film to produce a *mammogram*.

Meatus: A naturally occurring external opening of a canal or duct in the body.

Menarche: First occurrence of a menstrual period, usually between the ages of 9 and 17.

Menopause: Period of natural cessation of menstruation.

Menorrhagia: An increased amount and duration of menstrual flow.

Metrorrhagia: Bleeding between menstrual cycles.

Oligomenorrhea: Abnormally light menstrual periods.

Paget's disease: A rare form of breast cancer that usually affects older women, beginning at the nipple and extending into the areola.

Pap smear: A test commonly used to screen for cancer of the cervix. It is named for George Papanicolaou, the physician who developed the technique.

Pelvic inflammatory disease: Infection of the uterus, fallopian tubes, and other female reproductive structures that is a serious complication of certain sexually transmitted diseases.

Polymenorrhea: Short menstrual cycles of less than 3 weeks.

Prostaglandin: A hormone-like substance that participates in many functions, including muscle contraction and relaxation, blood vessel constriction and dilation, control of blood pressure, and modulation of inflammation.

Rugae: Anatomic folds (wrinkles) of the vagina.

Salpingitis: Inflammation and infection of the fallopian tubes.

Septicemia: An infection of the blood that may be caused by direct injection of bacteria into the blood (as with a contaminated needle) or, more commonly, by an infection anywhere in the body that spreads into the blood.

Stillborn: A fetus that dies within the uterus before birth.

Tubal insufflation: A nonoperative method of evaluating the fallopian tubes by pushing a gas into the cervix and uterus where it is detected by distention and other methods.

Uterine polyps: Growths attached to the inner wall of the uterus.

Vulva: External female reproductive structures that surround the vaginal opening.

Overview

The female reproductive system, which consists of both external and internal genitalia, has both sexual and reproductive functions. The ovaries, fallopian tubes, uterus, and vagina are the main structures of the female reproductive system. In the reproductive life of a female, many diseases and disorders are prone to occur, from sexually transmitted diseases to severe cases of various cancers. Dysfunction of hormone production may lead to various diseases, including infertility.

Menstrual abnormalities and **endometriosis** are common in younger females. Various types of infections may involve one or all organs of the reproductive system, such as **pelvic inflammatory disease** (PID). Females are also susceptible to benign tumors or cysts in the uterus or ovaries, which may lead to malignancies. Cancers of the cervix, uterus, and ovaries are seen in various ages. Breast cancer is the most commonly occurring type of cancer in women, and is the second most common cause of female cancer death.

Anatomy and Physiology of the Female Reproductive System

The external genitalia of females are collectively called the **vulva**. It includes the mons pubis, labia, clitoris, and vaginal orifice. The *mons pubis* is made up of adipose tissue and hair that covers the *symphysis pubis*. The outer fold (**labia majora**) contains the **labia minora**, made up of long folds of thin skin that extend backward and down from the mons pubis, serving to protect the orifices. The **clitoris** consists of erectile tissue, anterior to the urethra, which projects slightly outward. Similarly to the male penis, it is very sensitive to touch.

The *vagina* is the passage through to the reproductive tract. The vaginal orifice (*introitus*) is located between the urethral **meatus** (which lies anteriorly) and the anus (which lies posteriorly) (**Figure 22–1**). The muscular vagina extends up from the vulva to the cervix. The mucosal membrane of the vagina is somewhat folded into **rugae**, which allows it to expand during intercourse (*coitus*) and childbirth. The mucosa is sensitive to hormones and is made up of stratified squamous epithelial cells. The membrane is continuous through the uterus and fallopian tubes. Unfortunately, this allows for infections to spread easily. The mucosa becomes thinner and fragile after menopause with the decline of estrogen secretion.

On either side of the vaginal orifice the greater vestibular (*Bartholin's*) glands secrete mucus as a response to sexual stimulation. This allows the penis to penetrate the vagina during intercourse. The vaginal tissues are kept moist by the

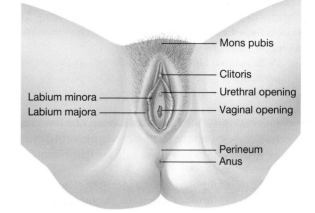

Figure 22–1 The female external genitalia.

Skene's glands near the external urethral meatus. These glands may frequently become infected due to obstruction. They produce the normal vaginal discharge known as **leukorrhea**, which is either clear or whitish and contains mucus and cells that have been sloughed off. Vaginal pH is relatively acidic during reproductive years due to the presence of *Lactobacillus*. This acidity, as well as the epithelial thickness, helps to protect against infections.

The *cervix* is the lower part (neck) of the uterus and is surrounded by the upper part of the vagina. The endocervical canal is the passageway between the *internal os* (which is at the uterine end of the cervix) and the *external os* (at the vaginal end of the cervix). The small external os is an opening containing thick mucus that protects the uterus from ascending bacteria originating in the vagina. The endocervical canal is lined with columnar epithelial cells, whereas the vagina is lined with squamous epithelial cells. The point where these cells change is a common site of cervical dysplasia and cancer. It is called the *squamous-columnar junction* or *transformation zone*.

The muscular, sac-like *uterus* is the structure where the fertilized ovum may be implanted and develop (**Figure 22–2**).

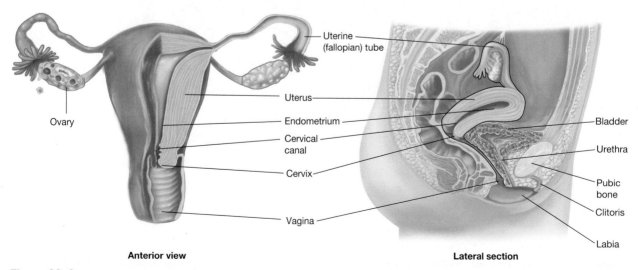

Anterior view   **Lateral section**

Figure 22–2 The female organs of reproduction.

The body of the uterus (*corpus*) is pear-shaped and suspended by ligaments that allow it to expand during pregnancy. The uterus is tipped forward (*anteverted*) to rest on the urinary bladder. Its wall consists of three layers:

- Perimetrium: Outer layer, also known as the *parietal peritoneum*
- Myometrium: Thick middle layer, consisting of smooth muscle
- Endometrium: Inner layer, consisting of a functional layer responsive to hormones during menstrual cycles, as well as an underlying basal layer that regenerates after menses

Near the top of the uterus, just under the *fundus*, is where the fallopian tubes (*oviducts*) originate. The tubes are slender, cylindrical structures attached bilaterally to the uterus. They are supported by the upper folds of the **broad ligament**. The end of the fallopian tube located closest to an ovary forms a funnel-like opening. It has fringed, finger-like projections called *fimbriae* that pick up the ovum after it is released into the peritoneal cavity after ovulation. The ovum continues to move through the fallopian tubes via *cilia* and *peristaltic movements*. Most commonly, an ovum is fertilized by sperm in one of the distal fallopian tubes. After fertilization, it then normally moves to the uterus for implantation into the endometrium.

The *ovaries* are the female gonads, producing one ovum each month during the reproductive years. The structure of an ovary includes several landmarks (**Figure 22–3**), including the female germ cells (immature ova). They are surrounded by differing numbers of cells. Together, the immature ova (oocytes) and cells that surround them are called **follicles**. The onset of this period is called **menarche**, and its ending is called **menopause**. The ovaries, like the uterus, are suspended by ligaments, and lie on either side of the uterus. They also supply female sex hormones (mostly estrogen and progesterone) on a cyclical basis.

In females, the breasts are responsible for **lactation**, which provides milk to the newborn. Increased secretion of estrogen, beginning at puberty, helps to develop the mammary glands (**Figure 22–4**). Each breast is made up of between 15 and 20 lobes that are supported by ligaments. They also contain muscle, fatty tissue, and subunits called *lobules* and *acini*. The basic functional units of breast tissue are the acini, which contain epithelial cells that secrete milk and contracting cells that move the milk through ducts to the nipples. Each breast contains many blood vessels, nerves, lymphatics, and sebaceous glands.

Higher hormone levels cause the breast to increase in vascularity and fullness, also making them more tender during the menstrual cycle. To conduct self-examinations for breast cancer, women should wait until just after menses concludes. This is because hormone levels are lower and the breasts are less nodular and are slightly decreased in size. Regular monthly examinations are vital. They allow for increased accuracy in detecting changes from each previous examination. Postmenopausal women should examine their breasts on the same date every month.

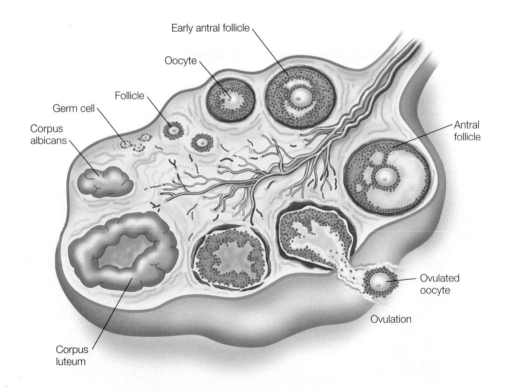

Figure 22–3 Structure of the ovary. This drawing illustrates the phases of follicular development and also shows the formation and destruction of the corpus luteum (CL). Antral follicles give rise to the CL. A fully formed CL and antral follicle would not be found in the ovary at the same time.

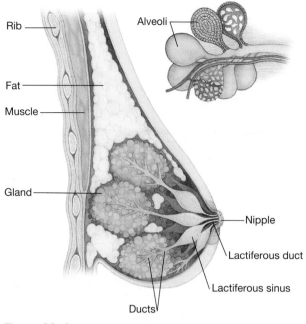

Figure 22–4 The mammary gland.

Female Hormones

During the reproductive years of a woman's life, cyclical patterns govern hormonal secretions, associated endometrial changes, and the release of eggs (ova). The cycle of most normal females is 28 days but may range from 21 to 45 days. **Table 22–1** describes the stages of the menstrual cycle.

When no fertilization occurs, the levels of estrogen and progesterone drop. The endometrium and corpus luteum then degenerate. This causes menstruation and the beginning of another cycle.

During the menstrual cycle, hormonal levels fluctuate greatly. Hormone levels are controlled by interactions of the anterior pituitary, hypothalamus, and ovaries. Estrogen and progesterone give feedback by acting on the anterior pituitary

gland, controlling follicle-stimulating hormone and luteinizing hormone release (**Figure 22–5**).

Infertility

Infertility may relate to one or both partners and to many different causes: hormonal imbalances, structural abnormalities, obstructions, changes in internal environment, and cigarette smoking. Hormonal imbalances may be caused by altered normal body function and also by the use of oral contraceptives before attempting to become pregnant. Structural abnormalities include an abnormally small or divided (**bicornuate**) uterus. Obstructions may be due to infections or *endometriosis*. Vaginal pH may change due to infections or use of *douches*. Sperm may not be able to gain normal access to the fallopian tubes because of abnormally thick cervical mucus or the development of antibodies that actually target the sperm.

Many different tests are available to determine the causes and treatments for infertility. Pelvic examinations, ultrasound, laparoscopy, and computed tomography (CT) scans are all commonly used for this purpose. Uterine and fallopian tube abnormalities may be determined by **hysteroscopy**, **tubal insufflation**, or a **hysterosalpingogram**. Often, a variety of combined factors contributes to infertility.

Menstrual Disorders

Menstrual disorders include menstrual abnormalities, such as **amenorrhea**, **dysmenorrhea**, abnormal menstrual bleeding, and premenstrual syndrome, and endometriosis.

Menstrual Abnormalities

Amenorrhea is the absence of menstruation, which may be a primary or secondary condition. Primary amenorrhea means that menarche has never occurred, usually due to a genetic disorder such as Turner's syndrome. The normal process of menstruation may be influenced by congenital defects affecting the hypothalamus, central nervous system, or pituitary gland. Other factors include congenital uterine hypoplasia (**infantile uterus**) and congenital absence of the uterus.

Secondary amenorrhea is the cessation of menstruation in a previously normal female. It may be caused by a disruption in the hypothalamic-pituitary axis or by the suppression of the hypothalamus by stress, sudden weight loss, eating disorders, strenuous physical exercise, or tumors. Other causative factors include anemia and chemotherapy.

Dysmenorrhea is primary or secondary painful menstruation. Primary dysmenorrhea develops when ovulation begins and has no organic basis. Sometimes the pain can be very severe and may be related to excessive release of **prostaglandin** during endometrial shedding. The prostaglandin can cause ischemia and strong uterine muscle contractions. The pain usually develops 24 to 48 hours before the beginning of menses, lasting for 24 to 48 hours. Other symptoms include headache, dizziness, nausea, and vomiting. The pain may be relieved by exercise, heating pads, and nonsteroidal anti-inflammatory drugs. Dysmenorrhea is often relieved after childbirth.

RED FLAG

In women who are using birth control, oral contraceptives may help to regulate the monthly cycle and reduce dysmenorrhea.

TABLE 22–1 Stages of the Menstrual Cycle	
Stage	**Description**
Menstruation (menses)	Sloughing off of endometrial tissue occurs because an ovum has not been implanted.
Endometrial proliferation	Follicle-stimulating hormone (FSH) is increasingly secreted by the anterior pituitary gland, causing the ovarian follicle to mature.
Secretion of estrogen	This causes proliferation or thickening of the endometrium's functional layer.
Midpoint	As luteinizing hormone (LH) levels rise greatly, ovulation occurs.
Conversion of ovarian follicle into corpus luteum	This increases the production of progesterone.
Preparation for implantation of a fertilized ovum	Progesterone enhances endometrial blood vessel and glycogen-secreting gland development.

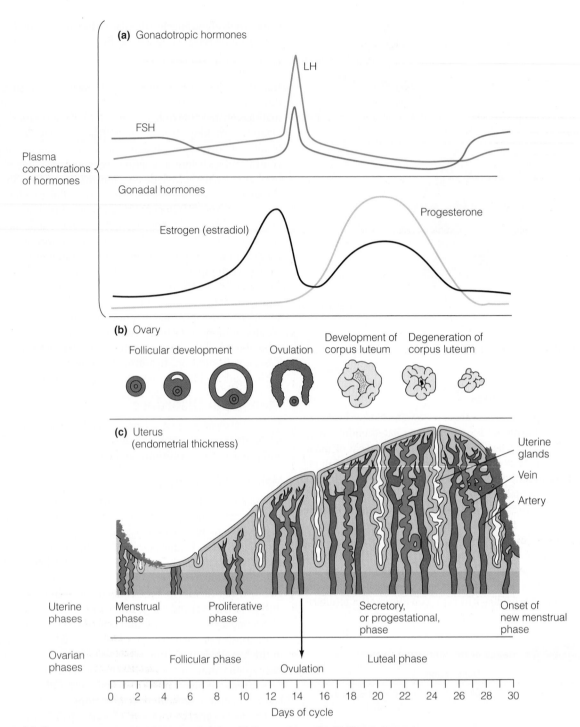

(a) Gonadotropic hormones

LH

FSH

Plasma concentrations of hormones

Gonadal hormones

Estrogen (estradiol)

Progesterone

(b) Ovary

Follicular development — Ovulation — Development of corpus luteum — Degeneration of corpus luteum

(c) Uterus (endometrial thickness)

Uterine glands

Vein

Artery

Uterine phases: Menstrual phase | Proliferative phase | Secretory, or progestational, phase | Onset of new menstrual phase

Ovarian phases: Follicular phase | Ovulation | Luteal phase

Days of cycle: 0 2 4 6 8 10 12 14 16 18 20 22 24 26 28 30

Figure 22–5 The menstrual cycle. (A) Hormonal cycles. (B) The ovarian cycle. (C) The uterine cycle.

Secondary dysmenorrhea is caused by endometriosis, PID, and **uterine polyps** or tumors. *Abnormal menstrual bleeding* is usually caused by lack of ovulation. It may also occur because of hormonal disorders or tumors. The following are examples of abnormal menstrual bleeding:

- **Menorrhagia**: Increased amount and duration of flow
- **Metrorrhagia**: Bleeding between cycles
- **Oligomenorrhea**: Abnormally light menstrual periods
- **Polymenorrhea**: Short cycles of less than 3 weeks

Premenstrual syndrome usually begins about a week before the onset of menses, ending when menses begins. It usually results in breast tenderness, abdominal distention or bloating, irritability, emotional liability, sleep disturbances, depression, headache, fatigue, and weight gain. Mental concentration and activity may improve or

RED FLAG

The climacteric is a normal gradual reduction in ovarian function because of aging. It begins in most women between ages 40 and 50. It results in infrequent ovulation, decreased menstrual function, and, eventually, cessation of menstruation.

diminish. Individual treatment is required, sometimes involving antidepressants or diuretics.

Endometriosis

Endometriosis is a condition in which the functional endometrial tissue is found in ectopic sites (outside the uterus). These sites may include the ovaries, pelvis, posterior broad ligaments, vagina, perineum, intestines, or vulva. It is possible for endometriosis to even affect distant sites (for example, the lungs). The inflammation returns with every cycle, and eventually fibrous tissue forms, which may be palpated. The ectopic endometrium grows during the menstrual cycle's proliferation and secretory stages and then degenerates, sheds, and bleeds. The lack of an exit point for this blood irritates tissues, causing local inflammation and pain. The fibrous tissue may cause adhesions and obstructions of various structures such as the colon or urinary bladder.

Infertility often results whenever the uterus is moved out of its normal position, regardless of the cause. If the fallopian tubes are blocked or the ovaries are covered with tissue, the ovum may not be able to travel to any appropriate areas to be fertilized. Endometrial tissue on an ovary causes the development of a fibrous, sac-like "chocolate cyst" filled with old brown blood (**Figure 22–6**).

Signs and Symptoms

Endometriosis primarily causes dysmenorrhea, with persistent pain lasting through menses and progressing in severity. Other signs and symptoms depend on the location of the ectopic tissue and may include infertility and profuse menses, dysuria, suprapubic pain, and hematuria (bladder). If adhesions develop that affect the vagina and its supporting ligaments, **dyspareunia** may occur.

Etiology

The *ectopic* endometrium occurs because of hormone cycles. Genetic predisposition and depressed immune system function may cause endometriosis, although it is generally of unknown origin.

Diagnosis

Diagnosis of endometriosis requires a laparoscopic examination. Pelvic examination may suggest endometriosis or may be unremarkable. Biopsy at the time of laparoscopy can confirm the diagnosis.

Treatment

Treatments include hormonal suppression of endometrial tissue, pain medications, and surgical removal of ectopic endometrial tissue.

Prognosis

Prognosis depends on the location and severity of endometriotic lesions. Fertility rates range from 30 to 75 percent. Symptoms may be relieved by hormone therapy or pelvic laparascopy.

> **RED FLAG**
> No pharmacologic treatment has been shown to cure endometriosis or to be effective in treating all women who have the condition.

Infections and Inflammation

Infections and inflammation of the female reproductive system are very common, especially in the period of active sexual

MILD

MODERATE

SEVERE

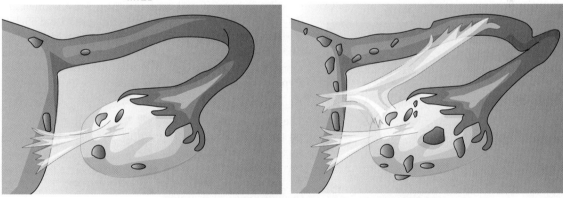

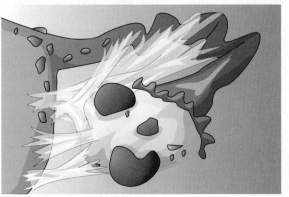

Figure 22–6 Stages of endometriosis.

activity. These disorders and conditions may affect any female reproductive organ. Common infections include vaginitis, cervicitis, endometritis, and **salpingitis**. Most of these may be related to sexually transmitted infections (STIs; diseases), discussed later in this chapter. Infections and inflammation of the female reproductive system may be caused by various microorganisms, including bacteria, viruses, fungi, and protozoa.

Neoplasms

Tumors of the female reproductive tract and organs may be benign or malignant and include myomas, ovarian cysts, fibrocystic breast disease, breast cancer, cancer of the cervix, carcinoma of the uterus, and ovarian cancer.

Cervical Polyps

Polyps are the most common lesions of the cervix. They can be found in women of all ages, although they usually occur during the reproductive years. Polyps are soft, red, velvety lesions. They are usually pedunculated (supported by a stalk) and often found protruding through the cervical opening. They have the potential to become quite large, as shown in **Figure 22–7**. Sometimes, the tip of the polyp erodes and causes bleeding; at this point the only choice for treatment is surgical removal.

Cancer of the Cervix

Cervical cancer is readily detected. If found in the early stages, it is the most easily cured cancer of the female reproductive system. Most cervical cancers are squamous cell carcinomas arising in the transitional zone between different epithelia of

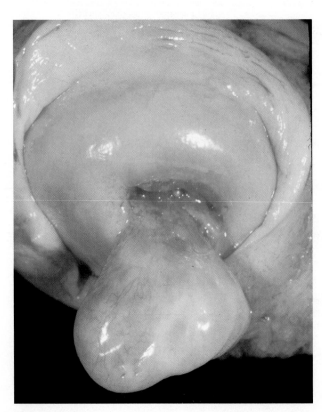

Figure 22–7 Large cervical polyp.

the vagina and uterine corpus. Growth and maturation of cervical squamous epithelium is called *cervical dysplasia* (see Chapter 5). Mild dysplasia may be caused by cervical inflammation. Severe dysplasia usually progresses to in situ carcinoma and, eventually, to invasive carcinoma after a variable period of time. Adenocarcinoma may also occur.

Signs and Symptoms

Cervical cancer usually causes a bloody, watery vaginal discharge that may be heavy and foul smelling.

> **RED FLAG**
> Cervical cancer is of three types: dysplasia, carcinoma in situ, and invasive carcinoma.

Bleeding between menstrual periods, after intercourse, or after menopause may occur. Cervical lesions may be varied in appearance but are usually a mass or ulcer on the surface of the cervix. Other signs and symptoms include pelvic or lower back pain, dysuria, hematuria, or rectal bleeding.

Etiology

Invasive cervical cancer has a long premalignant stage, often lasting for more than 10 years. Risk factors for developing this condition without detection are, first, lack of regular cervical **Pap smear** screening and, second, exposure to oncogenic types of the

> **RED FLAG**
> Preinvasive cancer of the cervix is most commonly seen in women between the ages of 25 and 40.

human papillomavirus (HPV) types 16 or 18. (HPV is discussed later in this chapter.) Females who have had unprotected sex with multiple partners early and frequently in life are at higher risk (**Figure 22–8A and B**). HPV DNA is found in more than 90 percent of invasive cervical cancers. Other risk factors include smoking, early age at first intercourse, multiple sexual partners, low socioeconomic status, history of STIs, and use of oral contraceptives. Most women are diagnosed with cervical cancer between ages 35 and 55, but it is also significant in women who infrequently receive Pap smear tests, such as those over age 65. Cervical intraepithelial neoplasia, the premalignant lesion, involves dysplasia or atypical cervical epithelium changes.

Diagnosis

The most common diagnostic sign is an abnormal Pap smear test result. Biopsy of a cervical lesion confirms diagnosis. Staging is determined through physical examina-

> **RED FLAG**
> African American women and those from lower socioeconomic groups have the highest risk for cervical cancer.

tion, chest x-ray, colposcopy (visual examination of the cervix), intravenous pyelogram, cystoscopy (visual examination of the urethra and bladder), proctoscopy (visual examination of the rectum), and lymph node sampling. Staging of cervical cancer is different from other cancers, relying on clinical evaluation instead of the pathologic features of the tumor.

Treatment

Treatment is based on staging and may include cryoablation (the use of extreme cold to remove tissues), laser therapy, or electrocoagulation. Simple or radical hysterectomy is indicated in extreme cases. For metastasis to the pelvic wall or distant sites, radiation is indicated. Chemotherapy may be used in conjunction with radiation. Patients should receive follow-up physical examinations and Pap smears. The role

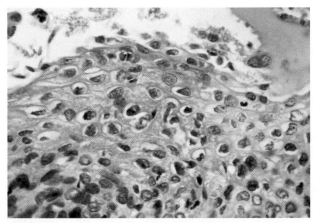

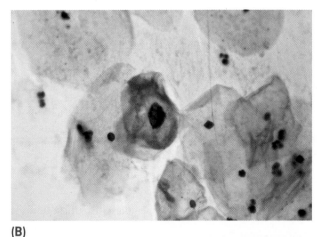

(A)

(B)

Figure 22–8 (A) Cervical epithelial dysplasia caused by papilloma virus. (B) Dyplastic epithelial cell identified in Papanicolaou smear (original magnification X 400).

of the physical therapist assistant (PTA) is to assist patients with activities to promote fitness.

Prognosis

Depending on the stage and spread of cervical cancer, 5-year survival rates are as follows: localized cervical cancer has a 92 percent survival rate, regional cervical cancer has a 58 percent survival rate, and metastasized cervical cancer has a 17 percent survival rate.

Benign Uterine Tumors

A *myoma* is one of the most common types of benign uterine tumors, also called *leiomyomas* or *fibroids*. They are the most common form of pelvic tumor and believed to occur in one of every four to five women over age 35. African American and Asian women are affected more than other groups. Myomas usually develop in the corpus of the uterus. They may be submucosal, subserosal, or intramural (**Figure 22–9**). After menopause many of these tumors tend to shrink. However, surgery may be indicated if signs and symptoms are severe or the tumors do not reduce in size. These benign tumors are not considered precancerous.

Signs and Symptoms

Submucosal or subserosal tumors may develop first as polyps. The submucosal type projects into the uterine cavity, whereas the subserosal type projects outward into the pelvic cavity. They are often asymptomatic until they grow large enough to be palpated and may be indicated by abnormal bleeding. Large tumors put pressure on other structures, leading to changes in urination, constipation, or abdominal fullness. When large, fibroids can interfere with implantation of a fertilized ovum or with pregnancy.

Etiology

These tumors are of unknown origin, occurring during a female's reproductive years, in over 30 percent of patients. They often occur as multiple masses of different sizes that bulge from the uterus (**Figure 22–10**). They depend on hormones and grow more rapidly during pregnancy while decreasing in size after menopause.

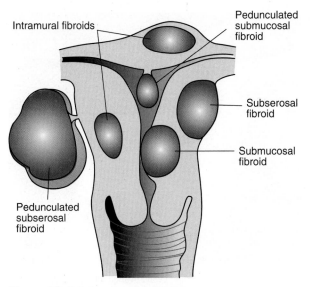

Intramural fibroids

Pedunculated submucosal fibroid

Subserosal fibroid

Submucosal fibroid

Pedunculated subserosal fibroid

Figure 22–9 Leiomyoma classification.

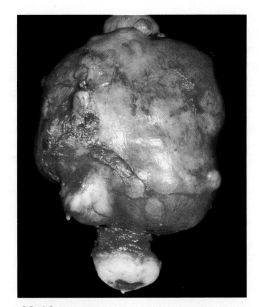

Figure 22–10 Enlarged irregularly shaped uterus containing multiple myomas that bulge from the uterus. The cervix is at bottom of photograph.

Diagnosis

Diagnosis is based on patient history and pelvic examination. Ultrasonography and laparoscopy may also be used. When a nonpregnant woman experiences bleeding, a *dilation and curettage* procedure or endometrial biopsy may be performed to rule out uterine adenocarcinoma.

Treatment

Treatment involves hormonal therapy or surgery. This decision is based on the patient's age and desire to become pregnant. If bleeding continues after tumor removal, hysterectomy (removal of the uterus) is recommended.

Prognosis

Prognosis is excellent due to the benign state of these tumors.

Endometrial Cancer

Endometrial cancer is the most common cancer found in the female pelvis, occurring more than twice as often as cervical cancer. Cancer of the uterus commonly affects women older than 40 years, with most cases occurring between ages 55 and 65. There are no simple screening tests available, but bleeding is an early indicator, especially in postmenopausal women.

Signs and Symptoms

The major symptom of endometrial cancer is abnormal, painless vaginal bleeding or spotting, as this cancer type erodes surface tissues. Later signs of uterine cancer may include cramping, pelvic discomfort, lower abdominal pressure, enlarged lymph nodes, and postcoital bleeding. Pap smear is not an adequate test for this condition; instead, a direct aspiration of uterine cells is used for biopsy.

Etiology

There is a higher risk of uterine cancer in those with a history of increased levels of estrogen. Postmenopausal women should not take high levels of exogenous estrogen. Other possible causes include infertility, previous use of oral contraceptives, obesity, diabetes, and hypertension. Today, the use of estrogen with progestin reduces the risk of hyperplasia.

Diagnosis

Diagnosis is confirmed by endometrial biopsy and hysteroscopy with dilation and curettage. Transvaginal ultrasonography used to measure the endometrial thickness is being evaluated as an initial test for postmenopausal bleeding. It is less invasive than endometrial biopsy and less costly than dilation and curettage.

Treatment

Endometrial cancer is usually treated with surgery and radiation, with a relatively good prognosis. The role of the PTA in endometrial cancer of the uterus involves education about healthy diet, regular exercise, and avoiding carcinogens. Pelvic floor exercises will strengthen muscles and avoid uterine prolapse.

Prognosis

The 5-year survival rate is approximately 90 percent if the cancer is well localized when diagnosed.

Ovarian Cysts and Benign Ovarian Tumors

A wide variety of cysts and tumors may arise from the ovaries. Benign ovarian cysts are common. Ovarian cysts may arise either from ovarian follicles or from the corpora lutea (**Figure 22–11**). Serous cystadenoma and mucinous cystadenoma are the most common benign ovarian tumors. Ovarian fibromas are tumors of the connective tissue composed of collagen and fibrocytes. Cystic teratomas (dermoid cysts) are derived from primordial germ cells. They are made up of various combinations of well-differentiated ectodermal, endodermal, and mesodermal elements. Dermoid cysts may contain hair or teeth (**Figure 22–12A and B**).

Signs and Symptoms

Ovarian cysts may become quite large before becoming symptomatic, usually causing a painless swelling in the lower abdomen or dyspareunia. Menstruation may also be affected, and urinary retention may occur. If a cyst affects hormone production, vaginal bleeding or increased hair growth may occur. If a cyst causes an ovary to twist on its blood supply (a condition known as *torsion*), severe abdominal pain, nausea, and fever can result. Torsion of an ovary may cause a rupture and lead to peritonitis. Solid benign ovarian tumors are asymptomatic unless their size is large enough to cause abdominal enlargement.

Etiology

Physiologic ovarian cysts are caused by normal ovarian function, whereas neoplastic ovarian cysts are not directly related to normal structures of the ovaries. Most are physiologic and related to ovarian follicle growth or a corpus luteum that persists for too long. These cysts are most likely to occur from puberty to menopause. Sexually transmitted diseases or acute infections may also result in inflammatory cysts.

Diagnosis

Ovarian cysts may be discovered during pelvic or rectal examinations. Ultrasonograms allow the indirect viewing of the ovaries. If the cysts are not physiologic, cancer must be ruled out via laparoscopy to directly examine the ovaries. If malignant, surgical removal of the ovaries is indicated.

Treatment

Small ovarian cysts seldom require any treatment and often disappear spontaneously. Large cysts can be drained or

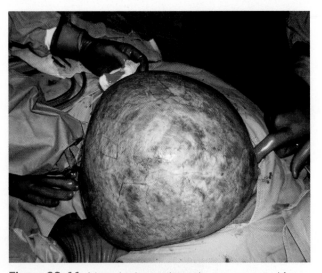

Figure 22–11 A large benign cystic ovarian tumor removed from a pregnant woman. The tumor weighed 35 pounds.

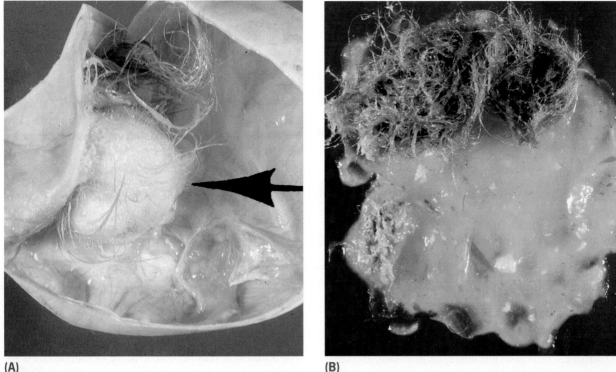

(A)   **(B)**

Figure 22–12 (A) Cystic teratoma (dermoid cyst) of ovary. The cyst is lined by skin containing sweat and sebaceous (oil secreting) glands, and the skin surface is covered by hair. The arrow indicates a nodule in the cyst wall containing fat, muscle, and bone. (B) Contents of cyst, consisting of matted hair and oil derived from skin lining the cyst.

removed. Draining of an ovary or removal of a cyst can usually be performed without affecting the function of the ovary. However, cysts that are drained are more likely to recur than those that are removed. Larger cysts are often resolved by several months of oral contraceptive therapy. Ovarian tumors must be surgically removed. Ovarian tissue that is not affected by a tumor can be left intact if frozen sectional analysis does not reveal malignancy. The role of the PTA is to educate women to avoid heavy physical exercise because this has been linked to rupture of ovarian cysts.

Prognosis
Prognosis is better for ovarian cysts when the patient is still menstruating. There is a higher risk of cancer in postmenopausal women with ovarian cysts.

Ovarian Cancer

Ovarian cancer is the second most common female genitourinary cancer and the most deadly. It is the primary cause of death from reproductive system malignancies in women. The incidence of ovarian cancer is much lower in countries where women bear numerous children, unlike in the United States. The disease is often asymptomatic until it is greatly advanced. Primary ovarian tumors usually develop from epithelial cells.

Signs and Symptoms
Symptoms of ovarian cancer include lower abdominal discomfort, bloating, constipation, irregular menstruation, lower back pain, dyspareunia, or urinary frequency. The most common sign is abdominal enlargement due to fluid accumulation (ascites), which often indicates advanced disease. If digestive disturbances that otherwise cannot be explained are persistent, the patient should be tested for ovarian cancer.

Etiology
The most significant risk factor for ovarian cancer appears to be ovulatory age. Ovarian cancer primarily affects women between the ages of 40 and 65, with etiology mostly unknown. The risk of ovarian cancer may be reduced by pregnancy, prolonged use of oral contraceptives, and tubal ligation. Family history of breast or ovarian cancer increases the risk, as does hereditary nonpolyposis colon cancer.

Diagnosis
There are no reliable screening tests or other early methods of detection for ovarian cancer. It is often diagnosed during palpation, which is part of a routine pelvic examination. If a mass is found, ovarian cancer is usually confirmed by laparoscopic surgery, transvaginal ultrasound, and serum tumor markers such as CA-125 (a cell surface antigen). Staging is based on surgical evaluation, with therapeutic cytoreduction (surgical reduction of tumor volume) performed at this time. Distant metastases may be identified via abdominal or pelvic CT scan.

Treatment
Early-stage ovarian cancer is treated by surgical removal of the ovaries, fallopian tubes, and uterus. If the cancer is diagnosed very early and the patient still wants to have children, only one ovary is removed. Chemotherapy reduces the risk of recurrence. If the disease is advanced, aggressive surgical cytoreduction is performed, in conjunction with chemotherapy. Radiographic tests and serum tests determine the effectiveness of the treatments. Aggressive rechecking

of the patient after treatment is required to determine that there is no recurrence. The role of the PTA is to assist the patient with exercises to improve overall strength, flexibility, and fitness.

Prognosis
Prognosis of ovarian cancer is usually poor due to the lack of any clear early screening test. Average 5-year survival rate is approximately 45 percent.

Fibroadenoma and Fibrocystic Breast Disease
Fibroadenoma is seen in premenopausal women, usually in the third or fourth decade of life. The term *fibrocystic breast disease* describes the most frequent lesion of the breast. It is most common in women 30 to 50 years of age and is rare in postmenopausal women not receiving hormone replacement. It is a very common condition that is characterized by local areas of proliferation of glandular and fibrous tissue in the breast.

Signs and Symptoms
Fibrocystic breast disease causes an uncomfortable feeling in the breasts, and various amounts of lumps or cysts may be palpated. The breasts feel tender on palpation, and some patients experience shooting pains in the breast tissue. Tenderness is usually more intense before menstruation.

Etiology
The causes of fibroadenoma and fibrocystic breast disease are unknown. They develop because of an increase in the formation of fibrous tissue and hyperplasia of epithelial cells in the breast ducts and glands.

Diagnosis
Diagnosis is made by physical examination, biopsy, and ultrasound examination (**Figure 22–13A and B**). A mammogram is used, along with palpation, to give a prompt diagnosis and differentiate this disease from one or more malignant neoplasms.

Treatment
The treatment methods for fibroadenoma are controversial and similar to those used for confirmed breast cancer. They include surgery, radiation therapy, chemotherapy, and hormonal manipulation.

Prognosis
Prognosis for fibroadenoma is excellent, although the condition raises the chance for breast cancer later in life. Continual monitoring of this condition increases the chance for a better prognosis.

Breast Cancer
Cancer of the breast is the most common female cancer. One in eight women in the United States will develop breast cancer in her lifetime. Breast cancer usually arises from the functional unit of breast tissue, known as the terminal ductal lobular unit. Breast carcinoma occurs in both sexes but is a rare tumor in men because their breast tissue is not subject to stimulation by ovarian hormones. However, carcinoma of the breast is very common in women.

Signs and Symptoms
Breast cancer causes a lump, swelling, or breast tenderness. The breast skin may become irritated or dimpled, and the nipple may be painful, ulcerated, or retracted (**Figure 22–14A and B**). The breasts may appear asymmetric. Usually, this condition is revealed by an abnormality on a mammogram, which appears before a lump can be felt.

In advanced stages, the nodule is fixed to the chest wall, with axillary masses and ulcerations developing. In early breast cancer, breast pain is not common.

Etiology
Breast cancer is the most common cancer in American women. It is the second leading cause of cancer death among women 40 to 44 years of age. It is also the second most common fatal cancer in women of all ages, after lung cancer. Breast cancer is 100 times more common in women than men. Risk factors of breast cancer can be classified as

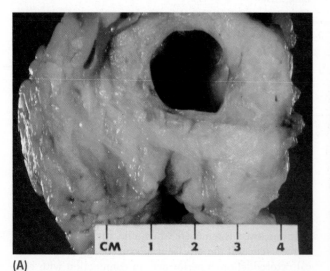

(A)

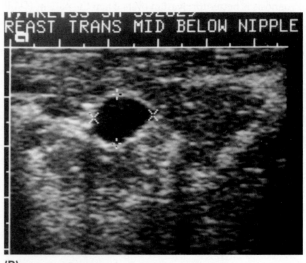

(B)

Figure 22–13 A benign cyst of the breast. (A) A cyst viewed in cross-section. Cyst is filled with fluid that escapes when the cyst is incised. (B) An ultrasound examination of breast, revealing a breast cyst (a dark area near the center of the photograph).

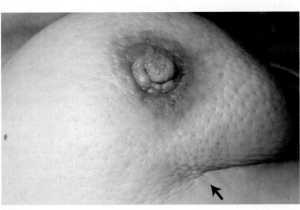

(A)

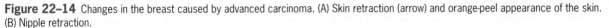

(B)

Figure 22–14 Changes in the breast caused by advanced carcinoma. (A) Skin retraction (arrow) and orange-peel appearance of the skin. (B) Nipple retraction.

hormonal, familial, environmental, and reproductive. However, most breast cancers occur in women whose only risk factors are age and gender.

Prolonged exposure to high concentrations of estrogen increase breast cancer risk. Younger age at menarche, older age at first full-term pregnancy, and older age at menopause are also risk factors. Long-term use of estrogen/progesterone hormone replacement therapy increases risks. Benign breast diseases increase risk, as does prior history of breast cancer. Alcohol use is also related. Although family history is important, only 10 percent of patients have family history of breast cancer. The environmental causes of breast cancer must also be considered. An increased risk of breast cancer is associated with high doses of ionizing radiation. This is especially true if exposure occurs during pregnancy. Breast cancer is rare in Japan, but not in people from Japan who immigrate to the United States and adopt Western eating habits. Ductal carcinoma in situ is a precursor lesion for breast cancer and can potentially lead to **Paget's disease** of the breast.

Diagnosis

More than 90 percent of breast cancers are diagnosed via abnormal mammograms, with the remainder found during physical examination. Diagnostic **mammography** and ultrasound are used to determine needs for biopsy (**Figure 22–15A and B**). A contrast-enhanced magnetic resonance imaging procedure may be required if the breast tissue is dense. Any suspicious lump should be biopsied for definitive diagnosis. After diagnosis, follow-up tests should include physical examination and blood tests. Staging mammography is important for breast-conserving treatment. Advanced cases require CT scans of the abdomen and pelvis, chest x-rays, and bone scans. Prediction of further outcomes can be ascertained via tumor estrogen receptor and progesterone receptor status tests.

Treatment

Treatments include localized excision, radiation, and chemotherapy to prevent progression of the carcinoma. Staging and patient preferences should be considered before treatment.

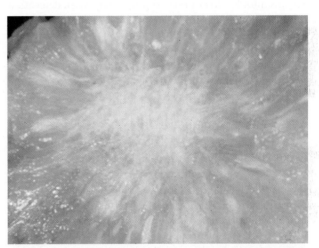

(A)

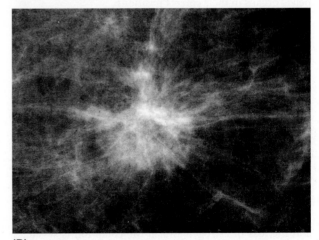

(B)

Figure 22–15 Breast carcinoma. (A) Cross-section of a breast biopsy. The tumor appears as a firm, poorly circumscribed mass that infiltrates the surrounding fatty breast tissue. (B) The appearance of breast carcinoma in a mammogram. The tumor appears as a white area with infiltrating margins. Note that the same criteria used to identify breast carcinoma on gross examination are used to recognize malignancy in the mammogram.

Procedures may include lumpectomy or mastectomy with removal of axillary lymph nodes. Others include radiation therapy, hormone therapy, and chemotherapy. Monoclonal antibodies may be effective against certain tumors, and multiple treatment methods are often used.

The role of the PTA in working with breast cancer patients includes general exercise, especially after surgery, shoulder therapy, walking, and general mobility skills. Instruction as to deep breathing exercises is also helpful.

Prognosis

Prognosis is better than ever in history for breast cancer due to the development of better screening methods and treatments. Prognosis is based on patient and family history, staging and location of tumors, positive or negative tumor receptors, tumor markers, and rates of tumor growth.

Pelvic Floor Dysfunction

Pelvic floor dysfunction is also known as *obstructed defecation*. It results when the external anal sphincter and/or puborectalis muscles do not relax appropriately when defecation is initiated, leading to excessive straining. Pelvic floor muscle exercises are used to teach patients how to coordinate pelvic and abdominal muscles. A high-fiber diet and stool softeners are also indicated. When pelvic floor muscle exercises are not effective, surgery may be used to create a stoma in the abdomen for removal of wastes.

Cystocele and Rectocele

Cystocele is also known as *fallen (prolapsed) bladder*. It occurs in women when the supportive tissue between the bladder and vaginal wall weakens and stretches. This allows the bladder to bulge into the vagina. Cystocele may result from muscle straining during childbirth, from constipation, or from violent coughing or heavy lifting. The condition may lead to other problems after menopause. When extremely severe, surgery may be needed to keep the vagina and other pelvic organs in their correct positions.

A rectocele occurs when the fascia separating the rectum from the vagina weakens. This allows the front wall of the rectum to bulge into the vagina. It is caused by childbirth and other events that put pressure on the fascia. If large, a rectocele may cause a noticeable bulge of tissue into the vagina. Often there are no signs or symptoms, although extreme cases may require surgery.

Uterine Prolapse

Uterine prolapse occurs when pelvic floor muscles stretch and weaken. The uterus loses its normal support and descends into the vaginal canal. The condition often affects postmenopausal women who have delivered multiple children. It is influenced by the effects of childbirth, gravity, straining, and the loss of estrogen. When the condition is severe, a supportive device (*pessary*) may be inserted into the vagina to provide support, or surgical repair of the prolapse may be indicated.

Menopause

Menopause is the permanent cessation of ovarian function. At this point in life a woman's ability to reproduce ends. Most women experience menopause in their early 50s, although onset may vary greatly. Estrogen levels decrease as menopause develops. Nearly all of the 300,000 eggs contained by the ovaries at puberty have been resorbed or shed by the onset of menopause.

Signs and Symptoms

While signs and symptoms vary, menopause commonly causes hot flashes, fatigue, vaginal dryness, anxiety, sleep disturbances, memory loss, mood swings, reduced libido, irritability, and depression. Changes in vaginal pH may lead to increased bladder and vaginal infections. When hot flashes cause perspiration at night, they are called *night sweats*. Some women experience lasting symptoms for years after menopause. Urinary incontinence and various pelvic floor conditions may also develop.

Etiology

Menopause occurs naturally with the aging process as estrogen and other hormones are produced in declining amounts. Hormonal decrease affects many body systems as well as the reproductive system. Menopause can also be brought on by hysterectomy, chemotherapy, radiation, and primary ovarian insufficiency.

Diagnosis

Diagnosis of menopause is based on the obvious signs and symptoms, which are related to patient age. Blood tests that check follicle-stimulating hormone and estrogen levels confirm diagnosis. Further confirmation is made by verifying levels of thyroid-stimulating hormone to rule out hypothyroidism, which can mimic the symptoms of menopause.

Treatment

Treatments for the symptoms of menopause are designed to reduce their severity. Estrogen therapy relieves hot flashes. Medications include antidepressants (in low doses), gabapentin, clonidine, and bisphosphonates. The role of the PTA is to implement exercises designed to improve overall fitness and to promote weight-bearing exercises to offset the effects of osteoporosis related to menopause.

Prognosis

Prognosis for symptom relief in menopause is good because the condition normally resolves itself. However, in some patients severe complications may occur, including osteoporosis, stroke, heart disease, and incontinence.

Sexually Transmitted Infections

STIs (*sexually transmitted diseases*) were formerly called *venereal diseases*. They are among the most common contagious conditions in the United States. STIs are often asymptomatic and therefore easily spread by unknowing participants. Nearly one in four teenagers will get an STI. Some STIs primarily affect the mucocutaneous tissues of the external genitalia. These include chlamydial infection, gonorrhea, syphilis, genital herpes, HPV infection, PID, and trichomoniasis.

Chlamydial Infection

Chlamydial infection (chlamydia) is the most prevalent STI in the United States, with an incidence estimated to be more than twice that of gonorrhea. Approximately 5 million cases are reported annually.

Signs and Symptoms

The signs and symptoms of chlamydial infection resemble those produced by gonorrhea. The most significant difference between chlamydial and gonococcal salpingitis is that chlamydial infections may be asymptomatic. In women, chlamydial infections may cause dysuria, urinary frequency, and vaginal discharge. Seventy-five percent of women and 50 percent of men who have chlamydia have no symptoms. Therefore, most cases are undiagnosed and untreated. For this reason chlamydia is often called "the silent STI." It is the leading cause of PID and a major cause of female sterility.

In both sexes the inguinal lymph nodes are often enlarged, and small transient lesions or skin irritation may be noticed. In newborns the disease may be acquired from the mother, leading to blindness, conjunctivitis, arthritis, or serious infections.

Etiology

Chlamydial infection is caused by the intracellular bacterium known as *Chlamydia trachomatis*, which is usually transmitted by sexual contact. It resembles a virus in that it requires a tissue culture for isolation, but like bacteria it has both RNA and DNA and is susceptible to antibiotics. With the primary infection site being around the genitals, it may also be transmitted via oral or anal contact. Many people carry the disease and transmit it without knowing they are carriers.

Diagnosis

Swab cultures reveal the causative bacterium in the patient's body fluids. Cell scrapings undergo a *Giemsa stain* to test for antibodies, and antigen-specific serologic studies are performed. Nucleic acid probes are now available.

Treatment

Antibiotics are injected into both partners, followed by oral antibiotic therapy. With prompt treatment the infection can be cured and other complications avoided. Follow-up testing is required to ensure the bacterium has been eradicated.

> **RED FLAG**
> Untreated chlamydial infections in women can result in cervicitis, acute salpingitis, endometritis, ectopic pregnancy, irregular menses, infertility, and PID.

Prognosis

If treated early with antibiotics, prognosis of chlamydia is excellent, with no long-term complications. However, delayed treatment or inadequate treatment may lead to cervicitis, urethritis, salpingitis, PID, infertility, ectopic pregnancy, and late postpartum endometritis. Children born to women with chlamydia may develop related conjunctivitis and pneumonia.

Gonorrhea

Gonorrhea is one of the most common STIs in the United States. It may be either local or systemic (disseminated). Local infection involves the mucosal surface of the genitourinary tract, rectum, pharynx, or eyes. Systemic infection occurs due to bacteremia and can lead to multisystem involvement with connective tissue, the heart, and the brain.

Signs and Symptoms

Patients with gonorrhea may be asymptomatic and can therefore unwittingly spread the disease to their sexual partners. Men are more likely to be symptomatic than women. Men may experience a purulent discharge with **dysuria** that can range in severity. The disorder may become chronic, affecting the epididymis and prostate. Rectal infections are common in homosexual men. In women, common symptoms include dysuria, unusual genital or urinary discharge, dyspareunia, pelvic pain, and unusual vaginal bleeding.

Etiology

Sexual transmission often spreads the causative bacterium, *Neisseria gonorrheae*. When a pregnant woman is infected, the newborn can contract the disease when passing through the birth canal. If the hands are contaminated with the bacterium, touching the eyes can lead to the development of conjunctivitis. Risk factors include multiple sex partners and unprotected sexual contact. Gonorrhea is prevalent in younger populations (between the ages of 15 and 29). The highest incidence of infection is in the 20- to 24-year-old age group.

Diagnosis

To diagnose gonorrhea, laboratory cultures of body secretions and microscopic examination of exudate, using a *Gram stain*, are performed.

Treatment

All sexual partners of a patient with gonorrhea must be treated with antibiotics as soon as diagnosis is made. Because many strains of the causative bacterium have become resistant to treatment, follow-up culture studies should be ordered to ensure complete cure. If untreated, gonorrhea can lead to PID, septic arthritis, and **septicemia**.

Prognosis

Prognosis for gonorrhea is good with prompt treatment, which will prevent scarring and infertility. Complications are very similar to those for chlamydia, which may be a concurrent infection.

Syphilis

Syphilis is a chronic STI and has systemic effects over a period of years. Any organ system may become involved. Syphilis is characterized in five stages: incubation, primary, secondary, latency, and late.

Signs and Symptoms

The incubation stage of syphilis begins with the penetration of the infective organism into the skin or mucosa of the body. Within 10 to 90 days the primary stage begins with the appearance of a small, painless red pustule on the skin or mucous membranes. The lesion may appear anywhere on the body where contact with a lesion on an infected person has occurred. However, it is seen most often in the anogenital region. It quickly erodes to form a painless, bloodless ulcer called a **chancre (Figure 22–16A)**. If not treated in its primary stage, syphilis becomes chronic and can involve any organ or tissue.

The second stage occurs about 2 months later, after the spirochetes have increased in number and spread throughout the body. This stage is characterized by anorexia, general malaise, nausea, skin rashes **(Figure 22–16B)**, **alopecia**, bone or joint pain, fever, headaches, mouth sores, and rashes on the palms or soles. The disease remains highly contagious at this stage and can be spread by kissing. Symptoms usually continue from 3 weeks to 3 months and can recur over a period of 2 years.

The third stage may not develop for 3 to 15 (or more) years. It is characterized by soft rubbery tumors called *gummas*. These tumors ulcerate and heal by scarring (**Figure 22–16C**). Gummas may develop anywhere on the body's surface as well as in the eyes, liver, lungs, stomach, or reproductive organs.

The fourth stage may be painless and unnoticed except for gummas, or it may be accompanied by deep pain. Ulceration of the gummas may result in punched-out areas of the nasal septum, larynx, or palate. Late-stage syphilis affects various tissues and body structures, including the central nervous system, myocardium, or heart valves, which may be damaged or destroyed. This may lead to mental or physical disability and premature death. **Congenital syphilis** resulting from prenatal infection may result in the birth of a deformed or blind infant or a **stillborn** child.

Etiology

Syphilis is caused by infection with the *Treponema pallidum* spirochete via sexual or other direct contact with infected lesions or body fluids. It can also be transmitted congenitally during pregnancy.

Diagnosis

A smear must be taken from the primary lesion and examined microscopically to verify the causative bacterium. Antibodies can be detected in the blood serum as well. *T. pallidum* cannot be cultured. Diagnostic tests are based on the detection of specific and nonspecific antibodies that are produced.

Treatment

Syphilis is curable with antibiotic therapy. The treatment of choice for syphilis is penicillin. Long-acting injectable forms of penicillin are used. In patients sensitive to penicillin, tetracycline or doxycycline is used for treatment. Pregnant patients should be desensitized and treated with penicillin. Treatment is most effective early in the course of the disease.

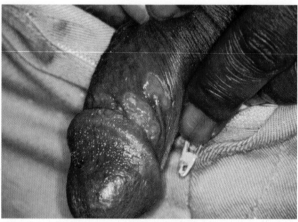

(A)

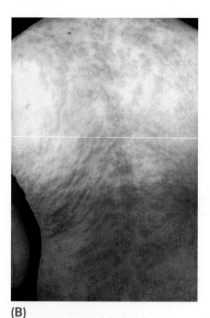

(B)

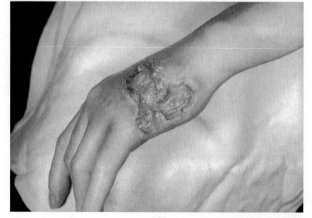

(C)

Figure 22–16 The stages of syphilis. (A) The chancre of primary syphilis as it occurs on the penis. The chancre has raised margins and is usually painless. (B) A skin rash is characteristic of secondary syphilis. (C) The gumma that forms in tertiary syphilis is a granular, diffuse lesion compared with the primary chancre.

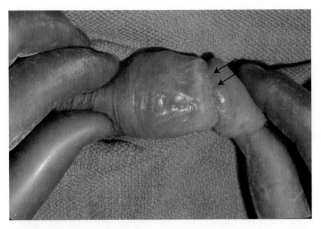

Figure 22–17 Several small superficial herpetic ulcers on shaft of penis behind glans (arrow).

Patients are then monitored with follow-up blood tests for up to a year after treatment.

Prognosis

Syphilis is curable if treated early in its development. Late-stage syphilis can lead to long-term complications, including damage to the skin, bones, heart, blood vessels, and nervous system.

Genital Herpes

Genital herpes is an infection of the skin and mucous membranes at the site of infection (oropharynx or genitalia) where they cause vesicular lesions of the epidermis. They then infect the neurons that innervate the area. Herpes viruses include herpes simplex virus type 1 (HSV-1, usually associated with cold sores) and HSV-2 (usually associated with genital herpes). HSV-1 and HSV-2 are generally similar. They both cause a similar set of primary and recurrent infections. Both may cause genital lesions. Ulcerations are spread by skin-to-skin contact or oral–genital contact, leading to painful genital sores that are similar to cold sores. In men the vesicles usually appear on the glands or shaft of the penis (**Figure 22–17**).

Signs and Symptoms

Genital herpes is a recurrent and incurable disease. Usually, several blister-like lesions are noted on the genitals or around the anus. The painful lesions (ulcers or blisters) usually occur between 2 and 30 days after sexual contact with an infected person. Genital herpes may lead to systemic symptoms that are similar to influenza as well as fever, swollen glands, headache, and painful urination. When sores are present, the condition is infectious. However, certain individuals (referred to as "shedders") can still transmit the virus without having any symptoms themselves. Recurrences can happen for months or years. The virus is hidden in the immune system and remains dormant between outbreaks.

Etiology

Genital herpes is caused by HSV-2. One in six adults carries HSV-2. Open lesions may also aid in transmission of AIDS between carriers of HSV-2 who are positive for HIV.

Diagnosis

Genital herpes is diagnosed via characteristic lesions on the genitalia that are discovered upon physical examination. The HSV-2 virus can be identified and the diagnosis confirmed by an antigen test or tissue culture laboratory techniques.

Treatment

Although not curable, prescription drugs are available that reduce the duration and frequency of outbreaks of genital herpes. The body's own immunity may also lessen the severity of the disease. In females the condition must be monitored because it can lead to cervical cancer. A Pap smear should be given every 6 months. In pregnant women a cesarean section delivery may be indicated to protect the newborn from contracting the virus.

Prognosis

Prognosis is entirely based on the condition of the patient's immune system. Weakened immunity may occur because of fatigue, general illness, immunosuppression, menstruation, stress, and trauma.

Human Papillomavirus (Condylomata Acuminata)

Condylomata acuminata (genital warts) is an infection of the genitals that causes the development of "cauliflower-like" growths in or near the rectum, vagina, or along the penis (**Figure 22–18A and B**).

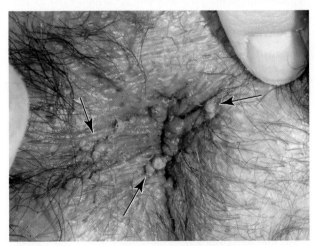

(A)

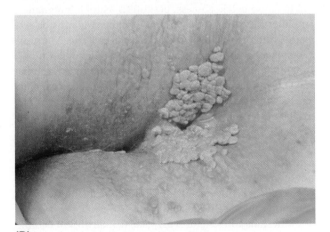

(B)

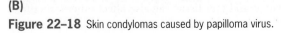

Figure 22–18 Skin condylomas caused by papilloma virus.

Signs and Symptoms

Although usually painless, genital warts may itch or burn. These contagious warts appear between several weeks or months after direct skin-to-skin contact during sexual intercourse. Discomfort varies based on the number, location, and size of the warts.

Etiology

Genital warts are caused by HPV. The virus has an incubation period of 1 to 6 months. One hundred types of HPV have been identified. More than 30 of these affect the anogenital area. Of the high-risk types, type 16 and type 18 appear to be the most virulent. They are associated with most invasive squamous cell cancers. Types 6 and 11 are found in most external genital warts but are usually benign.

Diagnosis

Genital warts are easily identified by their appearance. To rule out carcinoma, a biopsy may be indicated. Also, the warts must be differentiated from the lesions caused by syphilis.

Treatment

Genital warts are treated by chemical agents or surgical removal and commonly recur. Keratolytic agents and antiviral creams are commonly used. Surgical procedures include cryosurgery and electodesiccation (which uses lasers to remove larger warts). Genital warts sometimes resolve on their own. Women with genital HPV infection are at higher risk for cervical cancer. A cesarean section may be required if genital warts occlude the birth canal of a pregnant woman.

Prognosis

The prognosis for genital warts is generally good, although the condition may be passed on to other sexual partners throughout life. Even after treatment the condition may still be transferred. Certain types of genital warts increase a female's chances for cancer of the cervix or vulva.

Pelvic Inflammatory Disease

Pelvic inflammatory disease (PID) is an infection of the reproductive tract, especially of the ovaries (*oophoritis*) and fallopian tubes (*salpingitis*). It includes infections of the cervix (*cervicitis*) and uterus (*endometritis*).

Signs and Symptoms

Whether acute or chronic, PID is common and has the potential to cause pelvic abscess, peritonitis, ectopic pregnancy, and infertility. PID usually begins as either vaginitis or cervicitis, often involving several different bacteria. Microorganisms ascend through the uterus to the fallopian tubes. Inflammation allows more bacteria into the mucosa, tubal walls show edema, and the lumen fills with purulent exudate. This obstructs the tube and restricts uterine drainage. The exudate then drips onto the ovary and surrounding tissue. Peritonitis can develop if the peritoneal membranes cannot localize the infection. If the immune function is not sufficient, abscesses may form, which can be life threatening if not drained via surgery in a short amount of time. Infection can result in septicemia, with septic shock being the most common cause of PID-related death.

Adhesions and strictures may lead to infertility or ectopic pregnancy, and scar tissue can also affect other structures, including the colon. The first symptom of PID is usually lower abdominal pain that gradually increases in intensity. It is usually steady, increasing with walking. The pelvis may feel tender, there may be purulent discharge, and dysuria may occur. Leukocytosis and fever occur with certain causative microorganisms. Increased abdominal distention and rigidity indicate peritonitis.

Etiology

Most PID infections occur because of STIs (such as chlamydiosis or gonorrhea). Causative microorganisms may be varied, including **Bacteroides**, **Gardnerella vaginalis**, *E. coli*, *Pseudomonas*, *Haemophilus influenzae*, and streptococci.

Prior vaginitis or cervicitis often precedes development of a PID, with infection often becoming acute during or just after menses. Intrauterine devices used for contraception may also cause a PID due to contamination by organisms from the lower reproductive tract and other sources. If tissue is traumatized or perforated, inflammation and infection may develop.

Other potential causes of infection include childbirth or abortion. Sometimes, reproductive tract infections can result from bloodborne microorganisms or from peritoneal cavity infections such as appendicitis.

Diagnosis

Diagnosis is via vaginal examination, which may be painful due to swelling and inflammation. A specimen is taken, and Gram staining and sensitivity studies performed. A laparoscopy may be performed to look for an abscess or for hepatic involvement and to confirm diagnosis if the cultures that were taken are negative. Ultrasonography may show possible abscesses or fluid in the *cul-de-sac* (the space above the vaginal apex).

Treatment

Treatment must be aggressive, using various antimicrobials. Because recurrence is common, sexual partners should be treated with antibiotics and have follow-up examinations to ensure the infection has been completely eradicated.

Prognosis

The prognosis for PID is based on how early the condition is diagnosed and treated. PID may cause lifelong reproductive effects if not treated early.

Trichomoniasis

Trichomoniasis is among the most common pathogenic protozoal infections of the lower genitourinary tract in the United States. It affects both females and males and is transmitted primarily by sexual contact. It is considered to be an STI.

Signs and Symptoms

Trichomoniasis is easily spread because most infected patients are asymptomatic. Nearly 15 percent of sexually active people have this disease. Initial symptoms include urethritis, dysuria, and itching. Females may develop a greenish-yellow discharge from the vagina. The discharge may subside on its own, but the infection still remains. Trichomoniasis may become a chronic condition without warning.

Etiology

Trichomoniasis is caused by *Trichomonas vaginalis*, a pear-shaped flagellated protozoan (**Figure 22–19**). It is usually

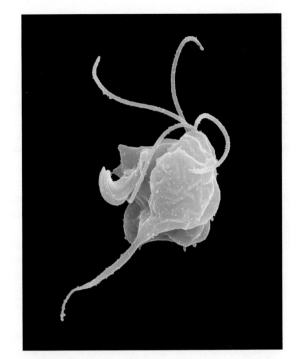

Figure 22–19 *Trichomonas vaginalis*. False-color scanning electron micrograph of a *T. vaginalis* trophozoite. (Bar = 5 μm.)

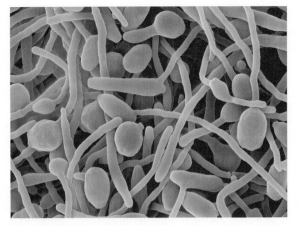

Figure 22–20 False-color scanning electron microscope image of *Candida albicans*. This image shows *C. albicans*, which is the agent responsible for vaginal candidiasis.

transmitted through sexual contact and is often unknowingly spread due to the lack of symptoms.

Diagnosis
Diagnosis is made microscopically by identification of the protozoan on a wet-mount slide preparation.

Treatment
The treatment of choice is oral metronidazole (Flagyl), a medication that is effective against *T. vaginalis*. Sexual partners should be treated to avoid reinfection.

Prognosis
Prognosis is excellent with adequate antibiotic treatment.

Candidiasis
Candidiasis is a non-STI of the reproductive system. *Candida albicans* is also called moniliasis, thrush, or yeast infection. Candidiasis is the second leading cause of vulvovaginitis in the United States. About 75 percent of reproductive-age women in the United States experience one episode in their lifetimes.

Signs and Symptoms
Candida albicans is present in 20 to 55 percent of healthy women without causing symptoms. Alteration of the host vaginal environment is usually necessary before the organism can cause pathologic effects. Although vulvovaginal candidiasis is not usually transmitted sexually, it is still included in the STIs. Candidiasis causes a thick, white, cheesy discharge as well as red, swollen, pruritic mucous membranes. There may be white patches on the vaginal walls, dysuria, or dyspareunia.

Etiology
Candidiasis usually occurs as an opportunistic superficial infection of the skin or mucous membranes. It may also

follow treatment with antibiotics for other bacterial infections. Other causes include decreased immunity, increased glycogen or glucose levels in reproductive system secretions, pregnancy, use of oral contraceptives, or diabetes.

Diagnosis
Candidiasis is diagnosed via a complete gynecologic examination. Accurate diagnosis is made by identification of **budding yeast** filaments, for example, hyphae or spores on a wet-mount slide using 20 percent potassium hydroxide (**Figure 22–20**).

Treatment
Antifungal agents are usually effective in treating candidiasis, but predisposing factors must be addressed to prevent recurrence.

Prognosis
Prognosis for candidiasis is good because the condition is rarely serious. Long-term effects are based on the patient's immune system function.

SUMMARY
The female reproductive system consists of internal paired ovaries, uterine tubes, uterus, and vagina. The genitourinary system as a whole serves sexual and reproductive functions throughout the life cycle. The breast consists of fat, fibrous connective tissue, and glandular tissue that produces milk. Endometriosis is a common cause of dysmenorrhea and infertility.

Cervical cancer is on the increase because of viral sexually transmitted diseases, although early detection via Pap smear improves its prognosis. A frequent opportunistic vaginal infection is known as candidiasis. A complication of a serious bacterial and STI may cause PID. Certain benign and malignant tumors such as cervical polyps, cervical cancer, myomas, endometrial cancer, various ovarian cysts, and ovarian cancer are commonly seen. Certain forms of fibrocystic breast disease require monitoring for malignancies, and routine screening to ensure early detection of breast cancer is recommended. Breast tumors usually occur as single, hard, painless nodules.

REVIEW QUESTIONS

Select the best response to each question.

1. The "silent STI" is known as which of the following?
   a. syphilis
   b. genital warts
   c. gonorrhea
   d. chlamydial infection

2. The absence of the onset of menstruation at puberty is known as which of the following conditions?
   a. metrorrhagia
   b. amenorrhea
   c. dysmenorrhea
   d. menorrhagia

3. Which of the following is the most common route of transmission of trichomoniasis?
   a. urine
   b. sputum
   c. genital secretion
   d. blood

4. Which of the following female reproductive system cancers has the highest 5-year survival rate?
   a. cervical
   b. vaginal
   c. ovarian
   d. uterine

5. The second most common female genitourinary cancer, and the most lethal, is which of the following?
   a. vaginal
   b. cervical
   c. ovarian
   d. uterine

6. Short menstrual cycles of less than 3 weeks are called
   a. menorrhagia
   b. polymenorrhea
   c. oligomenorrhea
   d. menarche

7. The cause of endometriosis is
   a. hormonal dysfunction
   b. cancer of the uterus
   c. virginity
   d. unknown

8. Treatment of cervical cancer is based on staging and may include which of the following?
   a. laser therapy
   b. hysterectomy
   c. cryoablation
   d. all of the above

9. Primary syphilis is marked by a
   a. specific lesion called a gumma
   b. specific lesion called a chancre
   c. rash on the palms
   d. punch-out of the nasal septum

10. Development of "cauliflower-like" growths near the rectum or vagina is characteristic of
    a. syphilis
    b. gonorrhea
    c. genital herpes
    d. condylomata acuminata

CASE STUDIES

Karen Coupe, PT, DPT, MSEd

Case 1

A 45-year-old woman is referred to physical therapy for right shoulder pain and dysfunction. Patient medical history: 6 months status post right modified radical mastectomy followed by chemotherapy and radiation treatment. PT evaluation reveals significant scapular substitution with overhead shoulder motions as well as significant decreases in capsular mobility and shoulder range of motion. Plan of care includes joint mobilization, therapeutic exercise, and instruction in prevention of lymphedema.

1. Explain the etiology, pathogenesis, and clinical manifestations of breast cancer.
2. What is removed with a modified radical mastectomy?
3. Could this patient's shoulder dysfunction be a result of her cancer and subsequent treatments? Explain your answer.
4. Why would this patient require instruction in prevention of lymphedema? What would be some of the instructions for this patient?
5. The plan of care doesn't include any modalities. Explain why the PT may not want any modalities for this patient.

Case 2

A PTA is employed in an outpatient physical therapy clinic that specializes in women's health. As part of community service the clinic conducts free monthly seminars on women's health issues. The director of the facility put the PTA in charge of determining and researching the topics for the next 2 months. The PTA sent topic surveys to community members and found the two most requested topics were sexually transmitted diseases and endometrial cancer.

1. List the types of sexually transmitted diseases. Which is the most common?
2. Explain in layman's terms the clinical manifestations and treatment of each disease.
3. Explain prevention methods for sexually transmitted diseases.
4. Discuss, in layman's terms, the etiology, pathogenesis, and clinical manifestations of endometrial cancer.
5. Explain the treatment options for endometrial cancer.

WEBSITES

http://trichomoniasis.org/

http://www.breastcancer.org/

http://www.cancer.gov/cancertopics/types/ovarian

http://www.cdc.gov/std/pid/stdfact-pid.htm

http://www.emedicinehealth.com/ovarian_cysts/article_em.htm

http://www.merckmanuals.com/home/sec22/ch244/ch244a
.html

http://www.ovariancancer.org

http://www.std-gov.org/stds/std.htm

http://www.suite101.com/content/female-hormones-a41775

http://www.webmd.com/infertility-and-reproduction/guide/
female-infertility

http://www.wrongdiagnosis.com/medical/female_reproductive
_system_disorder.htm

Integumentary System Disorders

LEARNING OBJECTIVES

After completion of this chapter the reader should be able to

1. Describe the major functions of the skin.
2. Identify the components of the dermis.
3. Describe keratinocytes and melanocytes.
4. Compare sweat glands and sebaceous glands.
5. Compare contact dermatitis with eczema and psoriasis.
6. Describe common bacterial and fungal infections.
7. Compare squamous cell carcinoma with malignant melanoma.
8. Describe keratoses and Kaposi's sarcoma.

KEY TERMS

Abscesses: Localized infections that cause pockets of pus.

Apocrine glands: A type of sweat gland whose secretions contain parts of secretory cells.

Athlete's foot: A fungal infection of the foot that usually starts between two toes and spreads to other toes; also known as *tinea pedis*.

Atopic: Pertaining to allergic reactions.

Autoinoculation: Inoculation of a microorganism obtained by contact with a lesion on one's own body, producing a secondary infection.

Basal lamina: Layer of extracellular matrix on which epithelium sits; it is secreted by epithelial cells.

Basement membrane: Layer of extracellular matrix that anchors epithelial tissue to underlying connective tissue.

Blisters: Vesicles or bullae; localized skin swellings containing watery fluid and caused by burns, infection, or irritation.

Boil: Skin abscess; a collection of pus localized deep in the skin.

Bullae: More than one bulla, which is a blister more than 5 mm in diameter with thin walls that is full of fluid.

Callus: A common, usually painless thickening of the stratum corneum at locations of external pressure or friction.

Carbuncles: Deep-seated abscesses that form in hair follicles.

Coalesce: To grow together.

KEY TERMS CONTINUED

Collagen: Primary protein found in bone, cartilage, and connective tissue; it provides strength and support for these structures.

Corns: Horny masses of condensed epithelial cells overlying bony prominences; they result from chronic friction and pressure.

Dermatophytes: Types of fungi that cause parasitic skin diseases.

Dermis: Lowest layer of skin, it is positioned above the subcutaneous fat layer.

Epidermis: Outermost layer of skin.

Erythema: A nonspecific term indicating inflammation and reddening of the skin.

Furuncle: A localized suppurative staphylococcal skin infection that originates in a gland or hair follicle; it is characterized by pain, redness, and swelling.

Hair follicles: Sac-like indentations from which hair grows; they are found in all areas of external skin, even when they no longer produce hair (as in baldness).

Herpetic whitlow: A painful viral (herpes) infection of the hands or fingers.

Impetigo: A bacterial skin infection most commonly seen in children; it is highly contagious.

Kaposi's sarcoma: A skin cancer that most commonly appears in people with damaged immune systems, particularly in those with AIDS.

Keratinocytes: Epidermal cells that synthesize keratin and other white, firmly attached patches that are slightly raised and sharply circumscribed.

Leukoplakia: A precancerous, slowly developing change in a mucous membrane characterized by thickened proteins.

Lichenification: Appearance of flat, scaly lesions on the skin; most commonly due to long-term irritation or inflammation of the skin.

Melanocytes: Melanin-producing cells.

Melanosomes: Cells capable of forming the pigment melanin, from which skin cancer may be derived; this cancer is sometimes referred to as malignant melanoma (an extremely dangerous form of cancer).

Merocrine gland: A gland whose cells secrete a fluid without losing cytoplasm.

Mycoses: Fungal infections.

Onychomycosis: A fungal infection of the nails; also known as tinea unguium.

Paresthesia: An abnormal, usually unpleasant sensation such as numbness, tingling, or prickling.

Pus: An exudate, ranging from white to brown in color, produced during inflammatory pyogenic bacterial infections.

Sebaceous glands: Holocrine glands in the dermis that secrete sebum.

Seborrheic keratoses: Benign, "horny" skin growths related to excessive secretion of sebum.

Sebum: An oily substance secreted by sebaceous glands that helps to keep skin and hair from drying out.

Tinea: A general term used to describe fungal infections of the skin.

Trichophyton: A genus of fungi that infects skin, hair, and nails.

Xerosis: Excessive dryness of the skin, mucous membranes, or eyes.

Overview

The skin, also known as the *integumentum*, is the largest organ of the body. It makes up about 16 percent of body weight and weighs about 9 pounds in an average adult. Its surface area covers between 1.5 and 2 square meters. The skin is the body's first line of defense, protecting the body from environmental agents such as solid matter, gases, liquids, microorganisms, and sunlight. It continually sheds, heals, and regenerates its cells. The skin may also reflect what is occurring inside the body, and a number of systemic diseases cause various skin disorders. Examples include the rash caused by systemic lupus erythematosus and jaundice caused by liver disease. It is therefore important to remember that skin eruptions might not only involve the skin.

Anatomy and Physiology of the Integumentary System

Over most of the body the skin does retain certain similarities. It is composed of three layers: the outer **epidermis**, the inner **dermis**, and the *subcutaneous layer* (**Figure 23–1**). The epidermis and dermis are divided by the **basement membrane**. The subcutaneous tissue is a layer of loose connective and fatty tissues. It binds the dermis to the underlying body tissues.

The epidermis is made up of stratified squamous keratinized epithelium, consisting of five distinct *strata* layers (**Figure 23–2**):

- *Stratum germinativum* (basal layer): The deepest layer, consisting of a single layer of basal cells attached to the **basal lamina**. The columnar basal cells produce new **keratinocytes** that move outward toward the skin surface to replace cells lost during the normal process of shedding.
- *Stratum spinosum*: This layer is formed as keratinocytes move outward. It is two to four layers in thickness. Its cells differentiate as they move outward.
- *Stratum granulosum*: This thin layer (only a few cells in thickness) is made up of granular cells that are the most differentiated type in living skin.

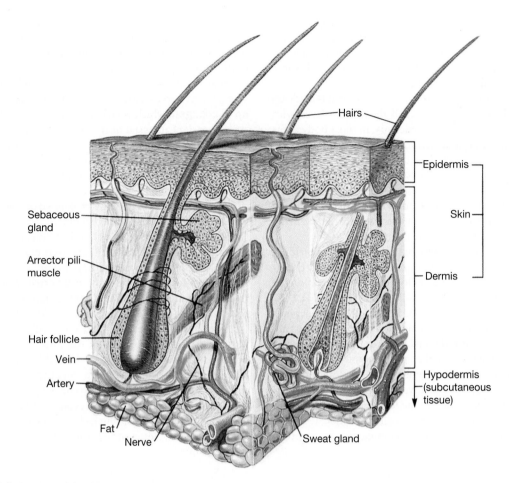

Figure 23–1 Anatomy of the skin.

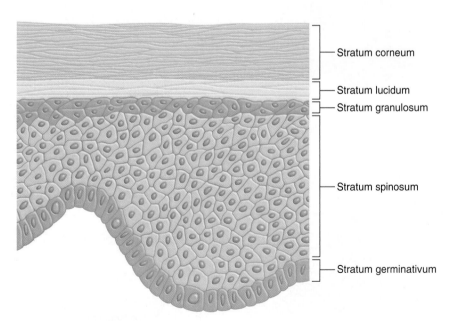

Figure 23–2 The epidermal layers of the skin.

- *Stratum lucidum*: This layer lies slightly superficially to the stratum granulosum. It is thin and transparent, located mostly on the palms of the hands and soles of the feet. It is made up of transitional cells with some functions of lower living cells.
- *Stratum corneum*: The top (surface) layer, it is made up of dead, keratinized cells. It is the thickest layer, with the largest cells of the epidermis. In most body areas the stratum corneum may range from 15 to 25 layers in thickness. However, the palms and soles may be more than 100 layers in thickness.

Keratinocytes take between 20 and 30 days to move from the basal layer to the stratum corneum. The rate of shedding old keratinocytes must be consistent with the rate of producing new keratinocytes to avoid skin anomalies.

Melanocytes are located at or in the basal layer, producing pigment granules called *melanin* (**Figure 23–3**). Freckles and moles are formed from localized concentrations of eumelanin.

The amount of melanin in the keratinocytes determines skin color. In dark-skinned people, larger **melanosomes** are produced and transferred individually to the keratinocytes. In light-skinned people, smaller melanosomes are produced and packaged together in a membrane before transfer to the keratinocytes. There are relatively no melanocytes in the palms of the hands or soles of the feet, regardless of overall skin color. Light-skinned people have less melanocyte as they age, and the skin lightens while becoming more susceptible to skin cancer from ultraviolet light.

The *dermis* is a connective tissue layer separating the epidermis from the subcutaneous fat layer. It serves as the primary source of nutrition for the epidermis. It is made up of the *papillary dermis* and the *reticular dermis*. Both sublayers are made up of cells, fibers, blood vessels, ground substances, and nerves. However, the dermis is primarily made up of **collagen**, which is rich in amino acids and the major stress-resistant material of the skin. Collagenous fibers are tightly bundled in the reticular dermis but loose in the papillary dermis. Hair and glandular structures are embedded in the dermis, continuing into the epidermis. Usually, a dark dermis is more compact and shows less wrinkling over time than a white dermis; hence, lighter skinned people show more wrinkling than darker skinned people.

The *papillary dermis* is thin and consists of collagen fibers and ground substance. It is densely covered with conical projections known as *dermal papillae*. The skin is richly supplied with blood vessels that influence its color and control body heat. The innervation of the skin is complex, with receptors for touch, pressure, heat, cold, and pain widely distributed in the dermis. Flat, encapsulated nerve endings on the palmar surfaces of the fingers and hands and plantar surfaces of the feet are called *Meissner corpuscles*. The deep dermis has small, oval mechanoreceptors called *Ruffini corpuscles* that respond to heavy pressure and joint movement. The sympathetic nervous system also controls the arrector pili muscles, which elevate the hairs on the skin. When these muscles contract, the skin dimples, producing "goose bumps."

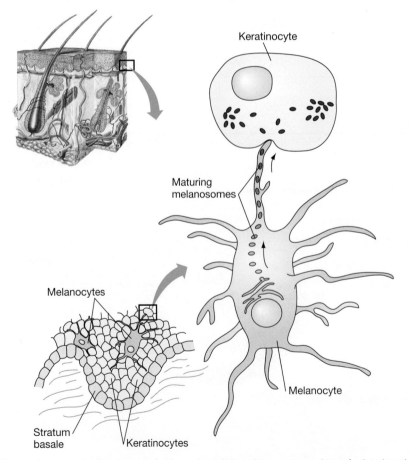

Figure 23–3 Melanocytes produce melanin, the pigment of skin, package it in melanosomes, and transfer it to keratinocytes.

Subcutaneous tissue consists mostly of fat and connective tissues. It supports the vascular and neural structures that supply the outer skin layers. *Skin appendages* include sweat glands, **sebaceous glands**, hair, and nails. *Sweat glands* are either *merocrine* (eccrine) *glands* or *apocrine glands*. Of the sweat glands, each **merocrine gland** is a tubular structure originating in the dermis and opening directly to the skin surface. They are found over the entire body and transport sweat to the outer skin to regulate body temperature. *Apocrine sweat glands* are less numerous, located in the deep dermis, and open through **hair follicles**. They are primarily found in the axillae and groin and secrete an oily substance (**Figure 23–4**). "Body odor" is produced when this substance mixes with skin bacteria.

Sebaceous glands are located everywhere on the body except the palms, soles, and sides of the feet. They secrete **sebum**, a mixture of lipids that includes cholesterol, triglycerides, and wax. Sebum lubricates the hair and skin, preventing evaporation of too much moisture from the stratum corneum to conserve body heat.

The skin is made up of many different types of cells. Its surface is covered with a lipid film layer that contains bactericidal fatty acids. This protects against the entry of harmful microorganisms. The skin also plays a part in *somatosensory* function, regulation of temperature, and the synthesis of vitamin D. It relays impulses via touch, temperature, and pain receptors. Touch receptors detect pressure, dullness, pleasure, and sharpness. Most body heat is generated by deep organs and transferred to the skin. Heat dissipation into the external environment is determined by constriction or dilation of skin arterioles and by evaporation of moisture from the skin surface. The skin has an endocrine function as well, wherein it converts a type of cholesterol into *cholecalciferol*, the inactive form of vitamin D, via ultraviolet light. Vitamin D is essential for normal bone and tooth development.

Skin structures vary greatly in different areas of the body. The skin may be of different thicknesses, have more or fewer sweat glands, and have different amounts and sizes of hair follicles. The skin is thicker on the palms of the hands and the soles of the feet than anywhere else on the body. The dermis is thickest on the back, whereas subcutaneous fat is thickest on the buttocks and abdomen. Hair follicles are more numerous on the scalp, armpits (axillae), and genitalia but very sparse on the abdomen and inner arms. **Apocrine glands** (a type of sweat gland) exist in the axillae and anogenital area but nowhere else.

Skin functions are based on the properties of the epidermis, which covers the body. The epidermis is specialized to form the structures of the glands, hair, and nails. *Keratinocytes* produce *keratin*, a fibrous protein, which is essential for skin protection. *Melanocytes* produce *melanin*, the pigment responsible for skin color, protection against ultraviolet radiation, and tanning. Openings in the epidermis allow the sweat glands to produce water secretions, whereas sebaceous glands produce the oily secretion known as *sebum*.

Hair originates from *hair follicles* in the dermis and is associated with sebaceous glands. The hair structure is made up of the hair follicle, sebaceous gland, hair muscle, and, sometimes, an apocrine gland. Hair is a keratinized structure that pushes up from a hair follicle (**Figure 23–5**). Melanocytes are

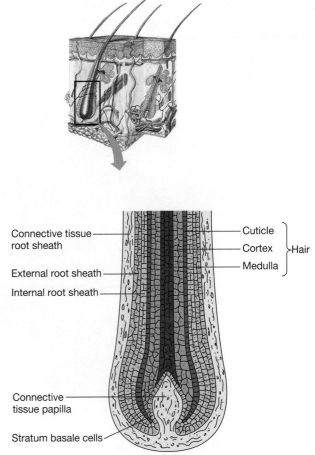

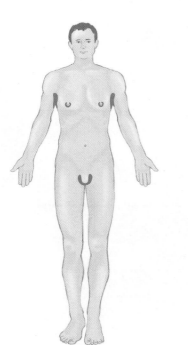

Figure 23–4 The locations of the apocrine sweat glands are shown in red. They include the axilla, areola, pubis, and circumanal region (not shown).

Figure 23–5 A hair follicle.

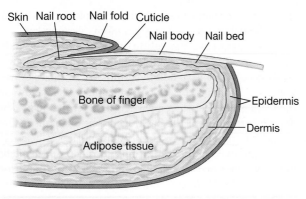

Figure 23–6 Fingernail anatomy.

transferred to the bulb matrix from the bulb, determining hair color. Similar to the skin, darker haired people have larger melanosomes in their hair than lighter haired people.

Nails are plates of hardened keratinocytes that grow outward from a curved *nail groove*. The floor of the groove (*nail matrix*) is the terminal region of the nail plate (**Figure 23–6**). The underlying epidermis is called the *nail bed*. Nails are pushed outward from the nail matrix and are the end product of dead matrix cells. Nails, unlike hair, normally grow continuously and not cyclically. The *nail cuticle* is formed by the stratum corneum. Each nail plate indicates the amount of oxygen in the blood, and nail abnormalities help to diagnose both skin and systemic diseases.

Common Signs and Symptoms

Clinical manifestations of skin dysfunction include the inflammatory reaction of the skin and the formation of lesions. They may also be accompanied by rashes, pruritus, and dryness.

Other common symptoms include pain, edema (swelling), and **erythema**.

Lesions and Rashes

Lesions are any visible, local abnormalities of the tissues of the skin, such as a wound, sore, rash, or **boil**. A lesion may be described as benign, cancerous, gross, occult, or primary. Rashes are defined as cutaneous eruptions and may be associated with childhood disease, diaper irritation, and adverse drug reactions. Lesions and rashes range in size from a few millimeters to many centimeters. They may be white, red, pigmented, or hemorrhagic (purpuric). If repeated scratching or rubbing occurs, the affected area may thicken and become rough and leathery. Skin lesions may be primary or secondary to other disease conditions (**Figure 23–7**).

Blisters are fluid-filled papules or vesicles. They may be caused by friction, skin disorders, or burns. Fluid accumulates, and a noticeable raised area appears on the skin. Blisters usually should not be broken to remove the fluid because this may cause a secondary infection.

A **callus** is a hyperkeratotic skin plaque caused by chronic friction or pressure. Hyperplasia of dead, keratinized cells results in hyperkeratosis and decreased skin shedding (**Figure 23–8**).

Corns (also called *helomas*) are small keratinous thickenings of the skin, usually round in appearance. They often appear on the toes from rubbing or shoes that do not fit properly and are usually painful (**Figure 23–9**).

Pruritus

Pruritus is defined as an "itching sensation" and is a common component of many skin disorders. Pruritus may range from mild to severe and has the potential to disrupt sleep and

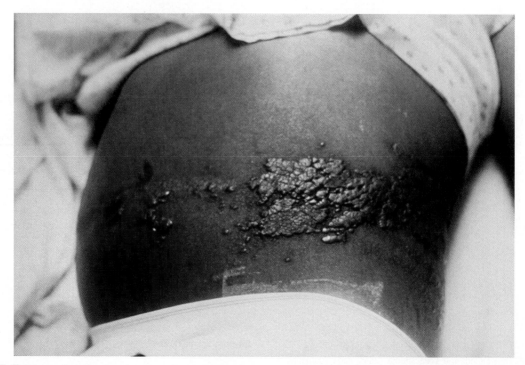

Figure 23–7 Primary skin lesions.

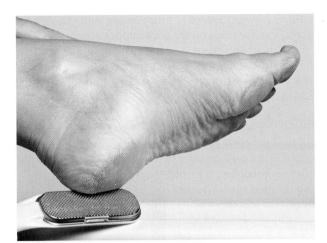

Figure 23–8 Calluses.

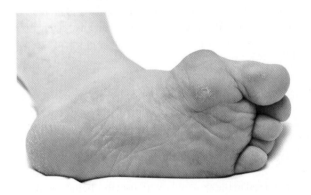

Figure 23–9 Corns.

quality of life. Itching may also be related to internal disorders such as renal or biliary disease or diabetes. Itching basically originates in free nerve endings in the skin.

Dry Skin

Dry skin (**xerosis**) may be associated with aging, skin disorders, or underlying diseases. Usually, dry skin is caused by dehydration of the stratum corneum. The skin may appear rough, scaly, lined, or wrinkled.

Variations in Dark-Skinned People

Although skin cancers may affect light-skinned people more frequently, other conditions are seen in darker skinned people, including those of African, East Indian, or Hispanic descents. Normal variations in darker skin may be mistaken for anomalies. Because of increased melanin, darker skinned people are better protected against skin cancer, premature wrinkling, and skin aging from sun exposure.

Diagnostic Tests

There are a variety of diagnostic tests used for skin conditions. Diagnosis is based on the appearance of the lesions, identification of the specific irritant or allergen with an allergy test, and a medical history. Bacterial infections often require culture and staining of specimens. Biopsies are used to detect malignant tissue changes and provide for surgical removal of skin lesions. Blood tests aid in the diagnosis of allergic or abnormal immune reactions, such as atopic eczema.

Inflammatory Disorders

Inflammatory disorders include burns, contact dermatitis, urticaria, **atopic** dermatitis, psoriasis, and pemphigus.

Contact Dermatitis

Contact dermatitis is a common inflammation of the skin. There are two types: irritant contact dermatitis (**Figure 23–10**) and atopic dermatitis. Irritant contact dermatitis results from a cell-mediated type IV hypersensitivity response, brought about by sensitization to an allergen.

Signs and Symptoms

The skin becomes sensitized upon first exposure to an irritant. When reexposed, symptoms such as pruritic rash occur a few hours later. Location of lesions helps to identify the allergen. Typical allergic dermatitis causes an erythematosus, edematous, pruritic area, often covered with small vesicles. Direct *chemical* irritation causes an inflammatory response from direct exposure to cleaning materials, acids, or insecticides. The skin may be reddened, pruritic, and/or painful.

Etiology

Contact dermatitis occurs via exposure to allergens or direct mechanical or chemical skin irritation. *Allergic dermatitis* may occur from exposure to cosmetics, metals, chemicals, plants, soaps, or other agents.

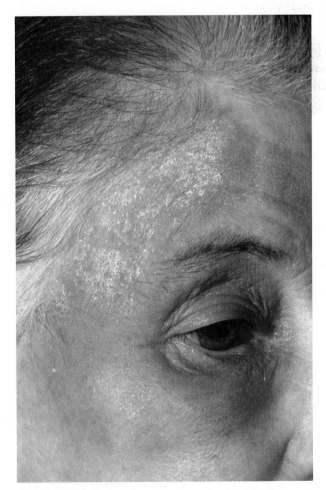

Figure 23–10 Contact dermatitis.

Diagnosis

Diagnosis is based on the appearance of the lesions, identification of the specific irritant or allergen with an allergy test, and a medical history. Patch testing is used to identify allergens. This involves applying a small amount of a suspected antigen to the skin.

Treatment

The irritant must be removed as soon as possible, and the inflamed area may be treated with topical glucocorticoids. Treatment must be focused on alleviating the itching and rash. Cool, wet cloths are effective for treating acute blisters. Oral antihistamines and colloidal oatmeal baths are used to control itching. The role of the physical therapist assistant (PTA) is to assist the patient with physical therapies such as hydrotherapy, as directed by the PT.

Prognosis

Prognosis for dermatitis is generally good, because symptoms can usually be controlled.

Urticaria (Hives)

Urticaria is commonly known as *hives* and results from a type I hypersensitivity reaction. Urticaria manifests as raised erythematous skin lesions (**Figure 23–11**). Common causes include ingestion of substances such as shellfish, certain fruits such as strawberries or tomatoes, and certain drugs such as penicillin or aspirin. Histamine is released, causing hard,

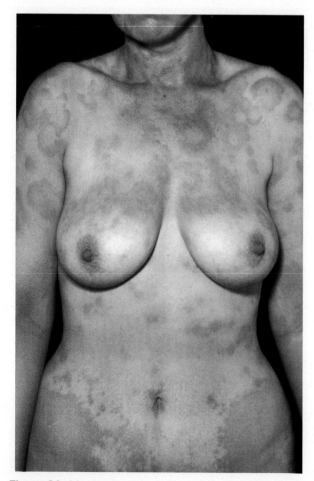

Figure 23–11 Urticaria.

raised, reddened lesions to erupt on the skin. The lesions may occur anywhere on the body and are usually very pruritic. When hives develop in the pharyngeal mucosa, they may obstruct the airway. This is a potentially life-threatening condition because it can cause the laryngopharynx to swell and cause suffocation.

Atopic Dermatitis (Eczema)

Atopic dermatitis often occurs in infancy, although it may continue through adulthood. The term *atopic* means the allergic condition may be inherited. Often, *eczema* occurs in members of the same family, along with allergic rhinitis (hay fever) and asthma. The response to allergens results in chronic inflammation. The allergenic basis for this condition is indicated by eosinophilia and increased serum IgE levels. Atopic dermatitis is a type I hypersensitivity. Approximately 70 percent of cases of atopic allergy start in children younger than 5 years of age.

> **RED FLAG**
> Atopic dermatitis presents differently in various age groups and races.

Signs and Symptoms

When occurring in infants, eczema appears as moist, red, vesicular lesions that are pruritic and covered with a crust. They usually appear symmetrically on the face, neck, extensor surfaces of the arms and legs, and buttocks. In adults the skin appears dry, with thick, leathery, scaly patches, a process known as **lichenification** (**Figure 23–12**). It may be moist and red in the skin folds, with pruritus being common, appearing on the flexor surfaces of the arms and legs as well as the hands and feet. Secondary infections from scratching and viral infections (such as herpes) may occur. Soaps and certain fabrics may irritate areas with lesions. Dermatitis tends to be aggravated by marked changes in humidity and temperature, causing additional outbreaks.

Etiology

Eczema is of idiopathic (unknown) origin but may be related to allergies or family history. In susceptible infants it has been traced to milk, orange juice, or other food sensitivities. Eczema flare-ups are often triggered by anxiety, conflict, or stress. The condition has been proven to be worsened by stress. Extreme climate changes involving temperature or humidity often trigger the condition. In infants, eczema usually subsides by age 2. Eczema gradually improves over time, and the rash may resolve during adolescence. However, it has also been shown to progress into adulthood.

Diagnosis

Eczema is diagnosed through family medical history, skin examination, and testing for specific allergies to determine the underlying cause.

Treatment

Treatment goals for eczema are designed to reduce frequency and severity of eruptions and to relieve itching. Although topical ointments and creams containing cortisone may be helpful, no medications can cure eczema. Medications used for the condition include pimecrolimus, tacrolimus, antihistamines, and certain tranquilizers and other sedatives. The scratching of lesions can trigger secondary bacterial or viral

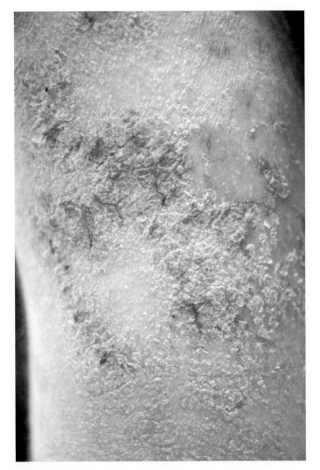

Figure 23–12 Atopic dermatitis.

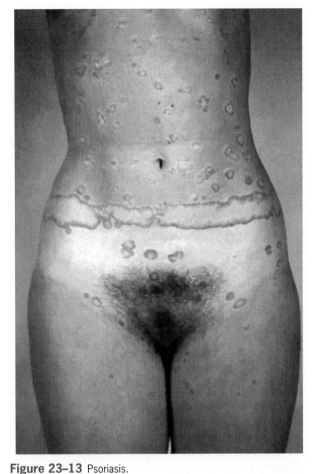

Figure 23–13 Psoriasis.

infections. More serious complications include viral infections, such as that caused by herpes simplex. The role of the PTA is to assist patients with regular physical exercise related to other conditions, bearing in mind that they need to follow infection control principles, depending on the severity of this disease.

Prognosis

Prognosis is good with adequate treatment. Proper management reduces flare-ups and complications such as other infections or scarring.

Psoriasis

Psoriasis is a common, chronic inflammatory skin disorder marked by thick, flaky, red patches of various sizes. It occurs often in the teenage years for the first time and recurs and improves continually. The average age at onset is in the third decade of life, and its prevalence increases with age.

Signs and Symptoms

Psoriasis causes cellular proliferation to increase, leading to dermal and epidermal thickening and increased epidermal shedding. Lesions appear as small red papules that enlarge and form silvery plaques (**Figure 23–13**). The base of each lesion remains red because of vasodilation and inflammation. Psoriasis lesions usually occur on the face, elbows, knees, and scalp and may be associated with psoriatic arthritis.

Etiology

Psoriasis is believed to be genetically determined, although its cause is idiopathic. It is more common in Whites and is suspected to be related to an autoimmune disorder. Hormonal changes, climate changes, emotional stress, and general poor health are believed to contribute to the development of psoriasis.

Diagnosis

Psoriasis is easy to diagnose because of its white, silvery scales. Careful patient history, skin examination, or biopsy may help to determine the condition when the scales are not apparent. Scratching of psoriasis legions reveals the scales.

Treatment

There is no cure for psoriasis. The goal of treatment is to suppress the signs and symptoms of the disease. Treatment depends on its severity and the patient's age, sex, treatment history, and level of treatment compliance. Treatments for psoriasis include glucocorticoids, tar preparations, and, if severe, the antimetabolite *methotrexate*. Exposure to ultraviolet light may also be helpful. The skin should be kept moist and lubricated. Antibiotics may also be

> **RED FLAG**
> Systemic corticosteroids have been effective in treating severe or pustular psoriasis. However, they cause severe side effects such as Cushing's syndrome.

prescribed. The role of the PTA is to follow infection-control principles if required to work with a patient who has psoriasis.

Prognosis

Prognosis is good based on adequate treatment. Management of the condition can reduce the likelihood of becoming a risk factor for nonmelanoma skin cancer.

Pemphigus

Pemphigus is a severe disease of the skin and mucous membranes characterized by thin-walled **bullae** arising from apparently normal skin or mucous membranes. The bullae rupture readily, leaving raw patches. Pemphigus is an autoimmune disorder and has several forms. Autoantibodies disrupt epidermal cell cohesion, causing the formation of blisters. The most common form, *pemphigus vulgaris*, causes the epidermis to separate from the basal layer. Blisters begin to form in the oral mucosa or scalp, spreading over the face and trunk. Vesicles become large and then rupture, leaving *denuded* areas of crusty skin. Treatment includes systemic glucocorticoids and other immunosuppressants.

Acne Vulgaris

Acne vulgaris is an inflammatory disease of the sebaceous glands and hair follicles. It is a disorder of teenagers and young adults that affects more than 80 percent of persons between 11 and 30 years of age. Acne vulgaris is common in adolescents of both sexes. In women, acne may begin earlier and persist longer. However, overall incidence and severity is greater in men.

Signs and Symptoms

Acne vulgaris causes papules (round, elevated elevations of the skin), pustules, and comedones (blackheads and whiteheads). Sometimes boil-like lesions that are deeper in the skin, called *nodules*, can occur. Chronic irritation and inflammation may lead to scarring. Acne vulgaris usually occurs on the face, neck, chest, back, and shoulders (**Figure 23–14**).

Etiology

The cause of acne vulgaris remains unknown, but it has been linked to the hormonal changes that occur in adolescent and affect the sebaceous glands. It may be related to heredity, food

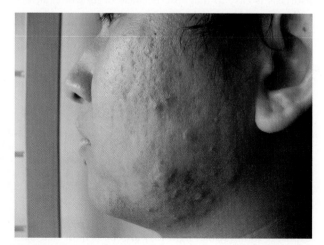

Figure 23–14 Acne vulgaris.

allergies, endocrine disorders, fatigue, psychological factors, and the long-term use of steroid drugs.

Diagnosis

Examination of characteristic lesions and patient history confirm the diagnosis.

Treatment

Treatment for acne vulgaris may require use of topical or systemic antibiotics, or both. Keratolytic agents, used topically, may be adequate for treatment. Medications related to vitamin A help the skin to be drier and to peel more regularly. Although antibiotics are usually helpful, their long-term use may cause side effects. Isotretinoin (Accutane) has shown great success in treatment of acne but is dangerous to use in females during their reproductive years due to high potential of fetal toxicity. Other treatments include low doses of estrogen and combination drug therapies.

Prognosis

Prognosis for acne vulgaris is based entirely on early treatment and ongoing management of the disease. Severe acne can lead to extreme scarring. Complications include skin color changes, depression, and cysts.

Decubitus Ulcers

Decubitus ulcers, also known as *pressure ulcers* or, less commonly, bed sores, are ischemic lesions of the skin and underlying structures caused by unrelieved pressure impairing the flow of blood and lymph. They are localized areas of dead skin affecting the epidermis, dermis, and subcutaneous layers (see Chapter 28).

Signs and Symptoms

Decubitus ulcers cause shiny, reddened skin because of long-term pressure to the affected area. Other signs and symptoms include blisters, erosions, necrosis, and ulceration. When infected, the ulcer becomes foul-smelling, with purulent discharge. Pain may or may not be present.

Ulcers are staged as follows:

- Stage I: Surface reddening; unbroken skin; the ulcer fades when pressure is removed.
- Stage II: Broken or unbroken blisters; lotions to hydrate tissues may prevent further development. Pressure must be removed from the area.
- Stage III: Wound extends through all skin layers; pressure must be relieved and the wound protected from further damage as the skin is already open. It is highly likely to become infected without medical care.
- Stage IV: Involves underlying muscles, tendons, and bones and can produce a life-threatening infection without aggressive medical treatment. Nutrition and hydration are now critical. If the wound is of large diameter, surgical removal of necrotic tissue may be indicated; amputation may become necessary in certain situations.
- Stage V: The wound now involves underlying muscles and bones; surgery or amputation is now indicated.

Etiology

Decubitus ulcers are due to impairment or lack of blood supply to the affected area. They are common in patients who are debilitated, paralyzed, or unconscious. More than 95 percent of pressure ulcers are located on the lower parts of the body, most often over the sacrum and coccygeal areas.

Diagnosis

Visual inspection of the ulcer is sufficient for diagnosis. Culture and sensitivity testing may be required to isolate the causative microorganism.

Treatment

Without treatment, the ulcer progresses from surface skin erosion to complete erosion of all skin layers. It may also involve underlying muscle and bone, with osteomyelitis or gangrene likely to develop. Treatments include absorbable gelatin sponges, antiseptic irrigations, debriding agents, antibiotics, and karaya gum patches. Treatment depends on the severity of the ulcer.

> **RED FLAG**
> Decubitus ulcers can be prevented by frequent position changes, adequate skin care, and frequent skin inspection to detect early signs of skin breakdown.

Prognosis

Prognosis of decubitus ulcer is based on the stage of ulcer development and adequate treatment.

Skin Infections

Skin infections may be of bacterial, viral, fungal, or other sources. The skin may be penetrated through minor cuts, abrasions, or inflamed areas. Serious infections require the culturing of the exudate to identify causative organisms and to determine appropriate treatment.

Bacterial Infections

Bacterial skin infections are common and may be primary or secondary. Primary infections are often caused by resident flora. Secondary infections often develop in pruritic lesions or in wounds. Some are superficial, whereas others are deeper, forming **abscesses**.

Cellulitis (*erysipelas*) is an infection of the dermis and subcutaneous tissue. It is usually secondary to an injury, **furuncle**, or ulcer. Causative organisms are usually *Staphylococcus aureus* or *Streptococcus*. Cellulitis often occurs in the lower trunk and legs, becoming red, swollen, and painful (**Figure 23–15**). Red streaks may appear along lymph vessels proximal to the infected area. Compresses and analgesics are used for treatment, and systemic antibiotics are usually necessary.

Furuncles, also called boils, are infections usually caused by *S. aureus* that begin in hair follicles and spread into the dermis. They often appear on the face, neck, or back and appear initially as firm, red, painful nodules. They eventually develop into large, painful masses with large amounts of purulent exudate (**pus**) draining from them. Boils should not be squeezed because the infection can spread by **autoinoculation**

> **RED FLAG**
> Antibiotic-resistant strains of impetigo are increasing, which is of concern because certain strains can lead to the development of *glomerulonephritis*.

to other areas. If located in the nasal area, squeezing or compressing boils may lead to thrombi or infection spreading to the brain. Collections of boils that **coalesce** to form large, infected masses are called **carbuncles**. They may drain through several sinuses or develop into abscesses.

Impetigo is common in infants and children and is highly contagious. It is primarily caused by *S. aureus* but may also be caused by group A beta-hemolytic streptococci. Lesions begin as small vesicles, usually on the face, and then enlarge and rupture, forming yellow-brown crusty masses (**Figure 23–16**). The lesion below the crusty masses is red and moist, exuding a honey-colored liquid. More vesicles develop around the primary site, and pruritus leads to further spread of the infection. Impetigo is treated with topical or systemic antibiotics, based on the extent of the infection.

Viral Infections

Viral infections of the skin include herpes simplex (cold sores), herpes zoster (shingles), and verrucae (warts). *Herpes simplex* virus type 1 is the most common cause of fever blisters (cold sores), occurring on or near the lips (**Figure 23–17A and B**). Herpes simplex type 2 is related to genital herpes. Primary type 1 infection may be asymptomatic, with the virus remaining latent. When it reactivates, a skin lesion erupts. Lesions may occur when triggered by infections (such as the common cold, hence the name "cold sores"), stress, or exposure to the sun.

Before recurrence there may be a burning or tingling sensation along the trigeminal nerve and on the lips. The lesions are painful and rupture to form a crust, eventually healing

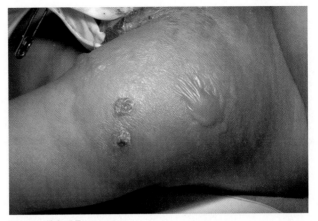
Figure 23–15 Cellulitis.

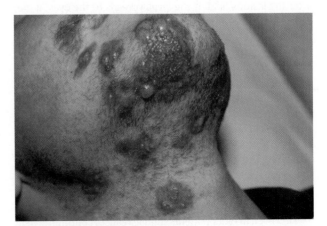
Figure 23–16 Impetigo.

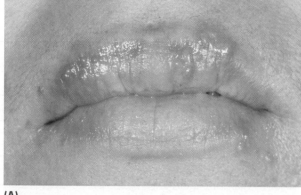

(A)

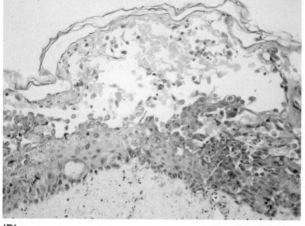

(B)

Figure 23–17 Herpes virus infection. (A) Recurrent oral herpes caused by herpes virus type 1. (B) Section of small herpes blister (vesicle). The superficial skin layer is almost completely destroyed, and a superficial ulcer will form when the surface epithelium sloughs (original magnification X 100).

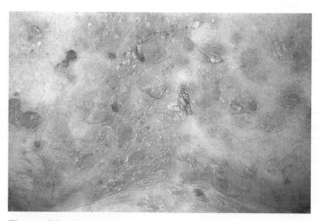

Figure 23–18 Herpes zoster.

in patients who are immune deficient. When the ophthalmic division of the trigeminal nerve is involved, visual impairment can be caused. Shingles is treated with antiviral medications. The shingles vaccine (Zostavax) is recommended for patients over the age of 60.

Verrucae (*warts*) are caused by various human papillomaviruses and include plantar and genital warts. Plantar warts are caused by human papillomavirus types 1 through 4, usually developing in children and young adults. Warts are predominantly harmless but can cause embarrassment due to their unsightly appearance. Plantar warts commonly occur on the soles of the feet, with a similar type occurring on the fingers, hands, or face. They first appear as firm, raised papules, developing rough surfaces (**Figure 23–19**). They may be

on their own within 2 to 3 weeks. Topical antivirals may be used to reduce viral shedding and spreading of cold sores. The virus is spread by direct contact with the fluid from the lesions, which may be present in the saliva for several weeks after the lesions heal. If the virus spreads to the eyes, it can cause *keratitis*. On the fingers it may cause a painful infection called **herpetic whitlow**.

Herpes zoster (*shingles*) may occur in adults years after a primary infection of varicella (chickenpox). It is caused by the varicella-zoster virus. Shingles mostly affects one cranial nerve or one *dermatome*, which is a cutaneous area innervated by a spinal nerve, on one side of the body. It causes pain, **paresthesia**, and a vesicular rash that develops in a unilateral line (**Figure 23–18**). The symptoms may occur on the face along the path of the trigeminal nerve or on the side of the lower trunk, in the hip area, along the path of a lumbar nerve. In most patients the lesions appear for several weeks and then disappear on their own.

However, in older patients shingles causes continuing pain after the lesions disappear. The lesions often spread locally

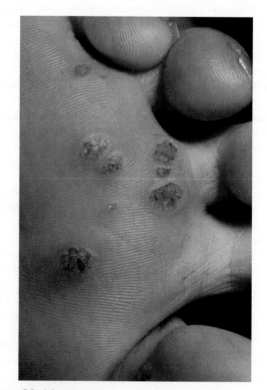

Figure 23–19 Verrucae.

white or tan in color, often occurring in multiples, and spread by viral shedding of surface skin. Plantar warts can be painful when pressure is applied. Although they may resolve on their own after several years, warts usually persist regardless of treatment. Local treatments include laser, liquid nitrogen (which freezes them), and topical medications.

Fungal Infections

Fungal infections are termed **mycoses** and are diagnosed by processing scrapings of the affected skin with potassium hydroxide. Because fungi live off of dead, keratinized epidermal cells (**dermatophytes**), the infections are usually superficial.

Tinea causes several different superficial skin infections and is sometimes called *dermatophytoses* or *ringworm*. Common types include tinea capitis, tinea corporis, tinea pedis, and tinea unguium. *Tinea capitis* commonly infects the scalp, seen mostly in school-aged children (**Figure 23–20**). It can be transmitted by cats, dogs, or humans, appearing as a bald patch due to hair breaking off above the scalp. There also may be erythema or scaling. This condition is treated with oral antifungal agents.

Tinea corporis usually affects nonhairy parts of the body, with rounded red vesicles or papules that have clear centers. This form of tinea is known as "ringworm," even though no "worm" is involved in the condition. The patient may feel a burning or itching sensation. Tinea corporis is treated with topical antifungal medications.

Tinea pedis (**athlete's foot**) is commonly spread from contact with athletic areas and surfaces such as pools or gymnasiums. Caused by various types of **Trichophyton** organisms that may be opportunistic normal flora, it produces a variety of symptoms. It can be spread easily from lesions when there are conditions of excessive warmth and moisture. The skin of the feet and toes becomes inflamed and softened, with painful, pruritic fissures. There may also be a foul odor caused by the infection, and secondary bacterial infections can occur. Topical medications are used to treat tinea pedis.

Tinea unguium (**onychomycosis**) primarily affects the toenails, beginning at the tips. It usually turns each affected nail white and then brown, leading to thickening and cracking of the nails. The infection usually spreads to other nails if untreated. Treatments include topical and systemic antifungal medications.

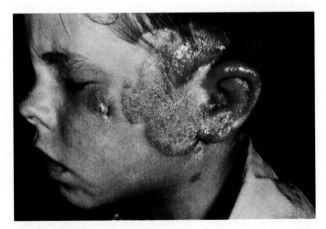

Figure 23–20 Tinea.

Burns

Burns are skin injuries caused by either heat (thermal) or nonthermal sources. A burn triggers an inflammatory reaction and causes tissue destruction. Severity depends on the location on the body and exactly what type of source is involved. The *rule of nines* is used to calculate burn damage in adults and infants, whereas the Lund and Browder chart is used for children (because their body proportions differ from those of adults). **Table 23–1** explains these burn calculations.

Signs and Symptoms

The signs and symptoms of burns are categorized into three levels:

- First-degree burns: Affect the epidermis only, causing pain, erythema, and edema. Examples include mild sunburn and a steam burn without formation of vesicles.
- Second-degree burns (partial-thickness burns): Affect the epidermis and dermis, causing pain, erythema, edema, and blistering. Infections commonly result, and hair follicles or sebaceous glands may be destroyed.
- Third-degree burns (full-thickness burns): Affect all tissue layers, causing white or blackened, charred skin that may be numb. Infections are a major concern, and nerve endings are usually destroyed; hospitalization is required in intensive care or a specialty burn unit (**Figure 23–21**).

> **RED FLAG**
>
> Burns may result in many complications, including local infection, hypovolemia, sepsis, hypothermia, shock, respiratory problems, contractures, and scarring.

Etiology

Burns are caused by thermal or nonthermal sources. Thermal sources include fire, steam, and hot liquids. Nonthermal

TABLE 23-1	Calculations of Burn Damage at Different Ages	
Age Group	**Method Used**	**Calculations**
Adults	Rule of Nines for Adults	9% - head 9% - each upper limb 36% - trunk 1% - genitals 18% - each lower limb
Children	Lund and Browder Chart	13% - head 2% - neck 4% - each upper arm 3% - each lower arm 2.5% - each hand 26% - trunk 1% - genitals 2.5% - each buttock 8% - each upper leg 5.5% - each lower leg 3.5% - each foot
Infants	Rule of Nines for Infants	18% - head 9% - each upper limb 18% - trunk 1% - genitals 13.5% - each lower limb

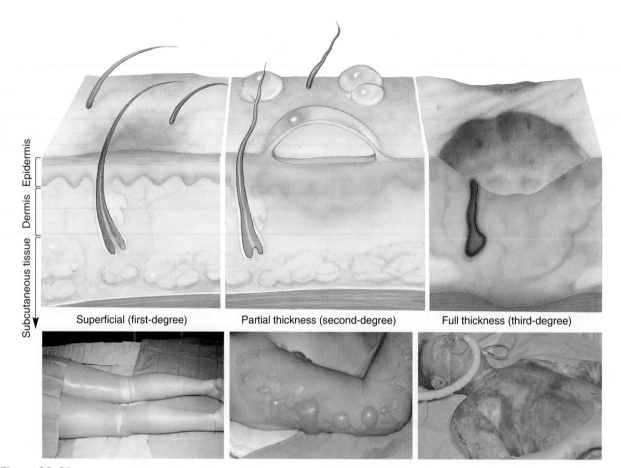

Figure 23–21 Burn classification.

sources include radiation, friction, ultraviolet light, electricity, and chemicals.

Diagnosis

Diagnosis is based on the appearance of the signs and symptoms.

Treatment

Treatment of burns is focused on prevention of infection. First-degree burns usually heal without intervention within 1 week, if kept clean and free of infection. Second-degree burns require bactericidal solutions and debridement of broken blisters or dead skin. Intact blisters should be left alone. Silver sulfadiazine cream and nonadherent, multilayered dressings should be used for up to 1 week. If not immunized as per requirements, a tetanus injection should be given. Analgesics may be used to help relieve pain. If blisters exist, a physician should assess the burn.

For third-degree burns, treatment includes maintaining the patient's airway, fluid replacement, prevention of infection, and the administration of oxygen. For wound healing, debridement of affected tissue and skin grafts are required. Hospitalization is usually indicated.

Prognosis

Prognosis for first-degree burns is usually excellent. For second-degree burns, prognosis is usually good based on the location of the burns and adequate treatment. For third-degree burns, prognosis is varied based on location of the burn and the patient's overall health. Often, third-degree burns may result in scarring, contractures, excision, and amputation. Significant functional impairment may also result.

Skin Tumors

Nearly one of every seven people will develop some form of skin cancer. Overexposure to the sun or to other forms of ultraviolet light is dangerous. Severe sunburns have been proven to increase the risk for skin tumors, with people who have light-colored skin or blond hair showing higher incidence. The following are guidelines for reducing skin cancer:

- Applying "broad-spectrum" sunscreen or sun block with a minimum sun protection factor, or SPF, of 15.
- Covering up exposed skin with clothing.
- Protecting infants and children from exposure and sun damage.
- Reducing sun exposure at midday and early afternoon.
- Remaining in the shade as much as possible.
- Wearing broad-brimmed hats to protect the face and neck.

Keratoses

Keratoses are benign skin lesions usually related to skin damage or aging. *Actinic keratoses* are caused by ultraviolet radiation, usually occurring in fair-skinned people. Lesions appear as pigmented, scaly patches and may develop into squamous cell carcinoma. **Seborrheic keratoses** are caused by proliferation of basal cells, appearing as oval elevations that may be dark in color and either smooth or rough in texture. They often occur on the face or upper trunk.

You should regularly check your skin for keratoses, moles, dark spots, and lesions. Keratoses and certain skin cancers may be treated with creams containing light-sensitive (photodynamic) medications. Tumor cells absorb the medications and can then be destroyed by laser.

Basal Cell Carcinoma

The most common yet least dangerous type of skin cancer is basal cell carcinoma. It begins in the stratum basale, invading the dermis. It causes a small, shiny lesion to appear as a "bump" on the skin. This enlarges to form a central depression with a beaded, pearl-like edge (**Figure 23–22**).

This type of cancer is usually confined to the skin but may do significant localized damage. It is the most common malignant tumor affecting Whites, causing 100,000 new cases per year. It rarely affects African Americans or Asians.

> **RED FLAG**
> The most common cause of basal cell carcinoma is sun exposure, although immunosuppression, genetic predisposition, and certain vaccinations are other possible causes.

Basal cell carcinoma lesions are most often seen in sunny climates in people who are outdoors much of the time. It has a stable growth, with small and large tumors having the same type of structures. It does not metastasize and causes only a small amount of chromosomal damage. This type of cancer is unique in that it usually affects humans and only rarely affects other types of animals. Nodules are usually painless and slowly increase in size, with central ulcerations.

Basal cell carcinoma is diagnosed by clinical examination, histologic studies, and biopsies. Usually, a specimen is removed, frozen, sectioned, and examined for positive margins. If surgical removal cannot be undertaken, radiation therapy is used (but this usually occurs only in people over age 50). Early treatment is usually completely effective.

Squamous Cell Carcinoma

Squamous cell carcinoma is similar to common basal cell carcinoma and has an excellent prognosis when lesions are removed within a reasonable time. This type of skin cancer is painless, malignant, and usually caused by sun exposure. It primarily occurs on the face and neck or other commonly exposed areas of the body (**Figure 23–23**). When occurring in the lower lip or mucous membranes of the mouth, it is usually related to smoking. Squamous cell carcinoma may also be caused by scar tissue, with higher incidence seen in African Americans. Actinic keratoses are also predisposing factors.

When invasive, squamous cell carcinoma arises from premalignant conditions such as **leukoplakia**. It appears as scaly, slightly elevated, semi-red lesions with irregular borders and central ulcerations. The tumors grow slowly in numerous directions, invading surrounding tissues and, eventually, regional lymph nodes. It does not usually metastasize to distant sites.

Signs and Symptoms

Both basal cell and squamous cell carcinoma can appear anywhere on the body, with the face, ears, back, chest, arms, scalp, and backs of the hands being most common. Squamous cell carcinoma lesions are usually crusted or scaly with red, inflamed bases. They also may appear as growing tumors, nonhealing ulcers, or raised, firm papules. Ulcerated lesions may cause pain.

Etiology

Basal cell and squamous cell carcinoma can develop in anyone, but those with a history of chronic sun exposure and fair skin are usually most susceptible. Ultraviolet light can cause mutations in the DNA and suppress the skin's immune system. Other factors include immunosuppression, chronic exposure to arsenic, and therapeutic radiation treatments. Squamous cell carcinoma often results from actinic keratosis and, sometimes, from scar tissue.

Diagnosis

Unusual skin lesions are easy to diagnose by simple visual examination. To confirm diagnosis, a biopsy called a "punch biopsy" is used.

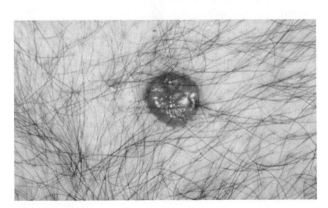

Figure 23–22 Basal cell carcinoma.

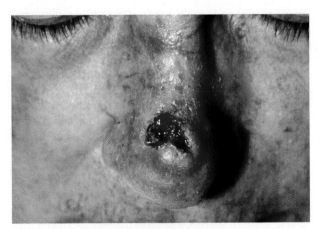

Figure 23–23 Squamous cell carcinoma.

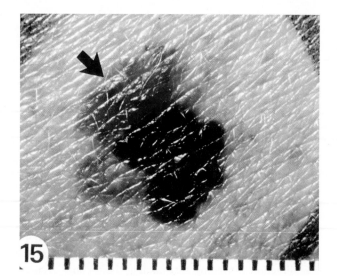

Figure 23–24 Malignant melanoma.

Treatment

In most cases, surgical excision is used for these types of carcinoma. Other treatments include cryosurgery, electrodessication (which uses heat), or radiotherapy. These cancers often trigger recurrences or may lead to malignant melanoma, and these patients should be rechecked every 5 years after treatment.

Prognosis

Prognosis for squamous cell carcinoma depends on how early the cancer was diagnosed. Ninety-five percent of these cancers go into remission if removed quickly.

Malignant Melanoma

Malignant melanoma is a very serious form of skin cancer, developing from melanocytes because of exposure to ultraviolet radiation, genetic factors, and hormonal influence. Melanomas arise in the basal layer of the epidermis or from a mole (nevus). Most nevi do not become malignant. They are actually collections of melanocytes. However, a mole that changes in shape, color, size, or texture or bleeds should be brought to the attention of a physician. Malignant melanoma often appears as multicolored lesions with irregular borders that grow quickly down into tissues (**Figure 23–24**). They metastasize quickly to regional lymph nodes and other organs, and prognosis is often poor. When surgically removed, large amounts of tissue below and surrounding the lesion are also excised to ensure all malignant cells are gone. The additional use of radiation and chemotherapy now provides a 90-percent survival rate over 5 years.

> **RED FLAG**
> A patient with many moles or unusual moles is predisposed to a higher chance of developing melanoma.

Signs and Symptoms

Malignant melanoma can occur anywhere on the skin and are usually indicated by changes in size, color, shape, elevation, surface texture, surrounding skin, sensation, and hardness.

Etiology

Most malignant melanomas result from chronic overexposure to sunlight (ultraviolet light). Risk factors include fair skin, hair, and eyes; living close to the equator or at higher elevations; history of severe sunburn; and use of tanning beds. Family history may also play a part. *Dysplastic nevi* are moles that are greater than one-fifth of an inch in size and have irregular borders or a mixture of colors. Another factor is a weakened immune system.

Diagnosis

An excisional or punch biopsy is typically used to confirm diagnosis after a patient suspects a lesion may be malignant melanoma. Diagnosis is based on tumor thickness and the use of serologic tests. Staging of the melanoma is determined by a full physical exam, chest x-ray, and liver function tests.

Treatment

Usually, complete surgical excision of the lesion, with wide margins, is indicated. Lymph nodes are dissected if they are involved. Chemotherapy or radiation therapy may improve survival rates if the cancer has metastasized. Surgery usually results in skin scarring. If tumors are large, reconstructive skin grafts or flap rotations may be indicated to minimize scarring.

Prognosis

Prognosis for malignant melanoma is based on the stage of the cancer. This can range widely. For example, stage 0 melanoma has a 90-percent survival rate, whereas stage IV melanoma has a survival rate of less than 10 percent.

Four Skin Cancer Warning Signs

- Sores that do not heal
- Lesions that change shape, size, color, or texture, especially with an expanding, irregular surface or circumference
- Newly developing moles or odd-shaped lesions
- Skin lesions that bleed repeatedly, itch, or ooze fluid

Kaposi's Sarcoma

Once a rare type of skin cancer, **Kaposi's sarcoma** has become more common with its association with HIV and AIDS. Previously, it was seen primarily in older men from Mediterranean countries and Eastern Europe. When the immune system is compromised, as in HIV/AIDS, the cancer affects the skin and viscera. Many lesions have shown the presence of *herpesvirus* as well. Malignant cells arise from the endothelium in small blood vessels. Multiple skin lesions appear as purple-colored macules on the face, oral mucosa, scalp, or lower extremities. The lesions begin without pain or itching but progress to large, irregular nodules or plaques that are darker in color. When the immune system is compromised, the lesions spread rapidly over the upper body and may become painful. Kaposi's sarcoma is usually treated with radiation and chemotherapy.

> **RED FLAG**
> The PTA should be aware of the signs and symptoms of skin cancer and Kaposi's sarcoma as he or she works with areas of the patient's body out of sight of the patient, such as the back.

SUMMARY

The integumentary system has many important functions, including protection from the environment and heat regulation. Many skin lesions may result in infection or scar tissue. Lesions are distinguished by their appearance, location, exudates, and the presence of pain or itching. Causes of inflammatory skin disorders include irritants, allergens, hypersensitivities, and heredity. *Staphylococcus aureus* is a bacterium that commonly causes skin infections. Common skin infections include cellulitis, impetigo, cold sores, and shingles. Ultraviolet light may cause a variety of skin tumors, including basal cell carcinoma, squamous cell carcinoma, and malignant melanoma.

REVIEW QUESTIONS

Select the best response to each question.

1. The deepest layer of the epidermis is which of the following?
   a. stratum germinativum
   b. stratum spinosum
   c. stratum granulosum
   d. stratum lucidum
2. Herpes zoster is also called which of the following?
   a. warts
   b. gangrene
   c. impetigo
   d. shingles
3. When exposed to sunlight, the skin is able to convert a type of cholesterol into which of the following?
   a. cholecystokine
   b. cholecalciferol
   c. vitamin A
   d. vitamin K
4. The following are functions of skin *except*
   a. sensory reception
   b. protection
   c. synthesis of vitamin A
   d. regulation of body temperature
5. Athlete's foot is also known as which of the following?
   a. tinea cruris
   b. tinea capitis
   c. tinea pedis
   d. tinea epidermis
6. Atopic dermatitis is also called which of the following?
   a. hives
   b. eczema
   c. pemphigus
   d. shingles
7. Which of the following causes warts?
   a. herpes zoster
   b. herpes simplex
   c. megaloviruses
   d. human papilloma
8. Keratoses may be treated by which of the following?
   a. creams containing light-sensitive medications
   b. cryotherapy
   c. radiation therapy
   d. heat therapy
9. Which of the following causes multicolored lesions with irregular borders?
   a. basal cell carcinoma
   b. squamous cell carcinoma
   c. malignant melanoma
   d. Kaposi's sarcoma
10. Kaposi's sarcoma is usually treated with which of the following?
    a. surgery
    b. laser
    c. blood transfusion
    d. radiation and chemotherapy

CASE STUDIES

Karen Coupe, PT, DPT, MSEd

Case 1

A 17-year-old boy is currently in rehab secondary to an American Spinal Injury Association Classification A (ASIA A) C-7 spinal cord injury suffered in a motor vehicle accident 4 weeks ago. The PTA is working with the patient on bed mobility, transfers, wheelchair mobility, and therapeutic exercise activities. While working on self–range-of-motion instruction the PTA notes nonblanchable erythema on the patient's right calcaneus that does not resolve by the end of the 1-hour treatment session.

1. This patient's right calcaneus presents with what stage of pressure ulcer?
2. Explain how the right calcaneus would present if the patient had the other three stages of pressure ulcers.
3. Based on this patient's diagnoses of ASIA A C-7 spinal cord injury, explain why this patient is susceptible to pressure ulcers.
4. What should be done by medical personnel to prevent pressure ulcers?
5. What type of patient education should be provided for patients who are at risk for pressure ulcers?

Case 2

A PTA is working with a 61-year-old man who suffered a right cerebrovascular accident 2 months ago. Patient medical history: lower extremity cellulitis during his hospital stay is now resolved. The patient is currently being seen in outpatient physical therapy for gait training, balance activities, and strengthening. The patient reports that he has to miss his next therapy appointment because he is having some skin cancer removed from his back. The PTA inquires as to the type of cancer, but the patient doesn't remember.

1. What are the three types of skin cancer?
2. Explain the similarities and differences in the presentation of the three types of skin cancer.
3. What are methods that could be used to help prevent and/or minimize the incidence of skin cancer?
4. Explain the etiology and clinical manifestations of cellulitis.

5. If the patient's cellulitis was active, are there any precautions that should be taken by the PTA?

WEBSITES

http://www.aad.org/public/publications/pamphlets/sun_malignant.html

http://www.buzzle.com/articles/integumentary-system-disorders.html

http://www.dermnet.com/Kaposi-Sarcoma/

http://www.internationaleczema-psoriasisfoundation.org/

http://www.medicinenet.com/skin_cancer_pictures_slideshow/article.htm

http://www.medicinenet.com/skin/focus.htm

http://www.merck.com/mmhe/sec18/ch201/ch201b.html

http://www.nlm.nih.gov/medlineplus/ency/article/003220.htm

http://www.skincancer.org/actinic-keratosis-and-other-precancers.html

http://www.skininfection.com/AboutSkinInfection.html

http://www.wrongdiagnosis.com/sym/skin_tumors.htm

Environmental Hazards

Occupational Disorders and Injuries

LEARNING OBJECTIVES

After completion of the chapter the reader should be able to

1. Identify the risk factors for occupational injuries.
2. Define ergonomics.
3. Explain the two principles of basic ergonomics.
4. Identify the risk factors for occupational asthma.
5. Describe the most prevalent types of musculoskeletal injuries.
6. Define pneumoconiosis, mesothelioma, and hypersensitivity pneumonitis.
7. Describe rubber latex allergy.
8. List four specific substances or conditions that may be related to various cancers.

KEY TERMS

Arsenic: An element that occurs throughout the earth's crust in metal arsenious oxide. Excessive arsenic is stored mainly in the liver, kidneys, gastrointestinal tract, and lungs. Most arsenics are slowly excreted in the urine and feces, which accounts for the toxicity of the element.

Asbestos: A fibrous mineral that can be harmful when inhaled.

Carpal tunnel syndrome: Entrapment and compression of the median nerve in the carpal tunnel causes pain and numbness in the wrist, hands, and fingers.

Human leukocyte antigens: Unique histocompatibility antigens (self-antigens) on the surface of cells, also called major histocompatibility complex antigens.

Mesothelioma: A rare tumor arising from the tissues of the mesothelium that forms a sheet-like cover on the internal organs; it is linked to asbestos exposure.

Pleurisy: Inflammation of the pleura, the double layer of membrane on the outside of the lung and lining the chest wall.

Scleroderma: Pathologic thickening and hardening of the skin.

Silica: A fine, rock dust known to cause lung damage with long-term exposure.

Vitiligo: A benign, generally progressive skin disorder in which irregular, unpigmented white patches form on the exposed skin areas.

Overview

Various types of injury are the leading causes of death for persons aged between 1 and 44 years. Overall, injury is the fourth leading cause of death. Regardless of whether they are intentional or unintentional, injuries are both predictable and preventable. Injury may occur anytime and anywhere, and in the workplace all types of injury must be anticipated. Millions of Americans are injured on the job or because of hazards at work, resulting in approximately $170 billion in costs each year. Males under the age of 25 experience the highest rate of workplace injuries. Nearly half of all these injuries are sprains, lacerations, strains, amputations, avulsions, and soft tissue punctures. The prevalence of technology and computers in the workplace has affected the increase in workplace injuries. Outside the workplace, injuries such as deep vein thrombosis may occur because of regular travel, often for business purposes. Occupational injuries happen in many types of industries, with pulmonary and skin disorders commonly occurring. Exposure to various substances may cause a variety of cancers. Ongoing studies are helping to prevent injuries and illnesses by identifying potential risk factors.

Risk Factors for Occupational Injuries

The Occupational Safety and Health Administration (OSHA) identified risk factors for musculoskeletal occupational injuries. Adults over age 55 who are still in the workplace account for increased amounts of workplace-related injuries. Because aging affects physical work capacity, the potential for workplace injury is heightened when this age group participates in activities that require muscular strength, endurance, and flexibility.

Other risk factors for occupational injuries include psychosocial stress, gender, personality, and preexisting musculoskeletal disorders. Obesity is also a serious concern. Further study is taking place concerning the relationships between work requirements, obesity, and occupational safety and health.

> **RED FLAG**
> Obese workers may be more likely to develop occupational asthma and cardiovascular disease.

Ergonomics

Ergonomics is the study of regular movements required in the workplace and the relationship between people and their physical environment. It has become a branch of industrial engineering, seeking to maximize productivity and minimize worker fatigue and discomfort. It strives to match job requirements with specific workers. Ergonomics integrates engineering, medicine, physical science, and behavior management. Important aspects of ergonomics include posture, body mechanics, biomechanics, and measurements of body size, weight, and proportions in relation to the requirements of the work.

Workers must be able to absorb and dissipate the forces placed on their bodies by their work environment. This enhances productivity while reducing strain and fatigue. Differences in gender, body size, weight, and proportions all play a part in determining the correct ergonomic design of furniture and other equipment used in the workplace. When the design of the workplace is inadequate, workers are more likely to experience injury, pain, stress, impairments, disabilities, and other conditions that relate to lost work productivity. Health and safety hazards can also occur if products are designed without considering the *human factor*.

The basics of ergonomics focus on two principles:
- There is a consistent relationship between certain workplace factors, especially at higher exposure levels, and musculoskeletal disorders
- Specific ergonomic interventions can reduce these injuries and illnesses; interventions include postural education, proper equipment, and use of correct body mechanics

Health care professionals who specialize in ergonomics are called *rehabilitation ergonomists*. They work with those who need changes to their workplaces to safely and productively perform. Improved safety allows workers to be efficient in their movements and activities in the workplace, resulting in increased productivity.

Ergonomist practitioners are certified through the Board of Certified Professional Ergonomists and the Oxford Research Institute. Both organizations are internationally recognized. They offer certifying examinations, and people who are now pursuing ergonomics as a career include not only engineers but psychologists, rehabilitation therapists, and other professionals. The Occupational Injury Prevention and Rehabilitation Society supports accreditation of therapists through the Board of Certified Professional Ergonomists and Oxford Research Institute while recognizing other programs that meet minimum criteria for ergonomic certification.

Occupational Injuries

The most common occupational injuries are musculoskeletal disorders. They involve cumulative trauma disorders because of remaining in static or long-term repetitive positions for prolonged periods of time while using force and forceful repetition and poor posture or incorrect muscle groups. The term *strain* refers to responses to static muscle overload or maintaining constrained postures.

Most occupational injuries occur to the back or upper extremities. Repetitive strain injuries are usually related to manufacturing industries but can occur in any industry or setting. Because much of the U.S. economy now revolves around service industries, the job requirements of employees are resulting in more musculoskeletal injuries.

Musculoskeletal Disorders

Musculoskeletal disorders include both cumulative trauma disorders and repetitive strain injuries. Work-related musculoskeletal disorders are injuries or disorders of muscles, tendons, cartilage, ligaments, or spinal disks that require medical intervention or lost workdays. These disorders do not include traumatic injuries such as slipping, falling, tripping, or other accidents. The disorder must be directly related to the core activities of the worker's job.

Work-related musculoskeletal disorders make up more than one-third of all occupational injuries that result in lost workdays. Risk factors for musculoskeletal disorders are of four types: genetic, morphologic, biomechanical, and psychosocial. The most prevalent types of these injuries are low back injuries and **carpal tunnel syndrome**. This syndrome occurs when the tendon within the wrist tunnel becomes inflamed from repetitive overuse of the hand, wrist, or fingers. This overactivity causes entrapment of the median nerve, which passes through the wrist. The nerve becomes compressed, resulting in pain. Carpal tunnel syndrome accounts for more lost workdays than any other workplace injury (see Chapter 16).

Current studies on carpal tunnel syndrome are ongoing about the relationship between repetition rates, forcefulness of work-related tasks, cellular responses to these tasks, number of strains, and the inflammatory response that results. When continued performance of tasks occurs upon inflamed, injured tissues, a continuing cycle of injury, inflammation, and motor dysfunction occurs.

> **RED FLAG**
> Carpal tunnel syndrome occurs most commonly in women between the ages of 30 and 50 years.

Athletic Injuries

Athletic injuries may have an acute onset or develop from overuse. Acute injuries are due to sudden trauma. Examples include soft tissue injuries (contusions, sprains, and strains) and bone injuries (fractures). Overuse injuries are called chronic injuries. Examples include stress fractures, which are caused by long-term high levels of physiologic stress. Common areas of overuse injuries include the elbow, heel, knee, and shoulder.

In children and adolescents, contact sports pose an increased threat for injury to the growth plates, neck, and spine. Proper coaching and training help to prevent injuries, as do the use of safety equipment and competitions that are based on skill and body size instead of chronologic age. Other factors in preventing injuries include hydration, proper nutrition, and providing enough time to warm up before athletic events.

Joint Injuries

Joint injuries are also called *musculotendinous injuries.* Joints are sites where two or more bones meet. Joints (articulations) are supported by bundles of tough, collagenous fibers (*ligaments*) that attach to joint capsules. Ligaments bind the articular ends of bones together. *Tendons* join muscles to the periosteum of articulating bones. Joint injuries involve mechanical overloading or forcible stretching or twisting.

Strains and Sprains

Strains and sprains are differentiated by the tissues they affect. Strains are complete or partial ligamentous injuries either within the body of a ligament or at the site of attachment to a bone. It is caused by mechanical overloading. Strains are partial or complete disruptions of a muscle, muscle–tendon junction, or tendon. They can be associated with overuse injuries. Pain, stiffness, and swelling usually result. Strains usually occur in the lower back, cervical area of the spine, elbow, shoulder, and feet.

Adolescent athletes are experiencing more mechanical low back strains than ever before. Overuse strains are commonly seen in sports such as track and field, gymnastics, diving, and wrestling. These injuries must be carefully diagnosed because chronic low back pain can indicate a stress fracture. Fractures near the top or bottom vertebrae can cause spinal disks to push into spinal nerve roots. Early detection and treatment protects against future complications. Treatments vary, including stopping activities, application of heat, and massage. During the first 24 hours after injury, cold should be applied to reduce pain and swelling. Once pain and swelling have subsided, posture reduction, use of proper body mechanics, and exercises should be instituted to reduce the risk for reinjury.

A *sprain* involves ligamentous structures surrounding joints, with pain and swelling subsiding more slowly than in strains. Sprains are usually caused by abnormal or excessive joint movements. The ligaments may be partially or completely torn or ruptured (see Chapter 16).

> **RED FLAG**
> Sprains and strains are more likely to see associated bony injuries due to decreased joint flexibility and the prevalence of osteoporosis and osteopenia.

Bone Fractures

A fracture is a break or crack in bone and is the most common types of bone injury. Bones may remain aligned or may be displaced out of position. A fracture occurs when more stress is placed on the bone than it can absorb. Bone fractures are divided into three major categories: those caused by sudden injury, those caused by fatigue or stress, and those that are pathologic in nature. Sudden fractures are most common and may be direct (due to blows or falls) or indirect (due to massive muscle contraction or trauma that is transmitted along the length of the bone). Fatigue fractures are caused by overuse or repetitive stress on the bone. Pathologic fractures occur in bones that have an underlying disease process such as tumors. They may occur spontaneously, with little to no stress or warning (see Chapter 16).

> **RED FLAG**
> Almost 80 percent of all athletes in the United States, at some time in their careers, will experience sprains or strains involving the upper or lower extremities or the spine.

Pulmonary Disorders

Inhaled workplace materials can lead to major chronic pulmonary disorders. Disorders caused by various chemical agents are classified into six groups:

- *Pneumoconioses*: Caused by **asbestos**, **silica**, coal dust (see Chapter 17)
- *Hypersensitivity pneumonitis*: Commonly caused by inhalation of crystalline silica, a component of rock and sand
- *Obstructive airway disorders*: Occupational asthma, often due to inhalation of gases, dusts, fumes, or vapors; work-related asthma has become the most prevalent occupational lung disease in developed countries
- *Toxic lung injury*: Due to toxic chemicals
- *Lung cancer*: Such as **mesothelioma**
- *Pleural diseases*: Such as **pleurisy**, which affects the linings of the lungs

OSHA requires employers to provide safe, healthy work environments free from recognized hazards. Also, the Americans with Disabilities Act of 1990 requires employers to accommodate all workers who have asthma. Episodes of asthma should be documented fully. OSHA and the Americans with Disabilities Act have guidelines addressing many effective, appropriate controls and substitutions that can be incorporated to prevent or eliminate topical and airborne exposures. Pneumoconiosis and hypersensitivity pneumonitis are discussed in detail below.

Pneumoconiosis

Pneumoconiosis is a generic term that means "dusty lungs." It describes a group of lung diseases caused by inhalation of particles of industrial substances over many years. Most commonly, these particles come from coal, iron ore, talc, aluminum, and silica. Asbestosis is a type of pneumoconiosis caused by exposure to asbestos. Each type of pneumoconiosis is described based on its causative agent, for example, silicosis or berylliosis. Most types of pneumoconiosis affect workers in the mining, stone cutting, insulation, metalworking, and farming industries. Related conditions include chronic bronchitis, hypersensitivity pneumonitis, and pulmonary fibrosis.

> **RED FLAG**
> Although widely being phased out, certain brake linings for various types of vehicles still contain asbestos. Workers involved in repair of these vehicles may still be exposed to asbestos.

Risk factors for pneumoconiosis are as follows:

- Type of exposure
- Intensity and duration of the exposure
- Presence of any underlying pulmonary disease
- History of smoking tobacco products
- Size of the particles, and the water solubility of the inhalant

Smokers have a significantly higher risk of contracting lung cancer because of a pneumoconiosis condition. Recently, the cancerous condition known as *mesothelioma* has been more prevalent in the news. It occurs as a result of exposure to asbestos.

> **RED FLAG**
> The oldest known occupational lung disease is silicosis. It usually develops from long-term inhalation of small particles of crystalline free silica (commonly known as *quartz.*)

Dust particles that are not trapped in the nasal passages may be deposited anywhere in the lungs and respiratory tract. Usually, pneumoconiosis develops more than 10 years after initial exposure to a causative agent. Symptoms of pneumoconiosis include chest pain, progressive dyspnea, chronic coughing, and expectoration of mucus. Work-related asthma may occur as an exacerbation of a previously subclinical asthmatic condition. Silicosis may cause loss of appetite, blood to appear in the mucus, general weakness, dyspnea, and obstructive or restrictive lung dysfunction. Asbestosis causes dyspnea, inspiration crackles (on auscultation), and occasionally cyanosis and clubbing of the fingers or toes.

Prevention is critical in the workplace concerning pneumoconiosis. The employer must provide as many safety measures as possible to protect workers, as well as ongoing education. Workers should undergo regular examinations and chest x-rays to determine the extent of their exposure. Asbestos is now ranked as a group A human carcinogen that leads to both mesothelioma and lung cancer.

Diagnosis of pneumoconiosis is made by history of exposure, cytology studies of sputum samples (**Figure 24–1**), lung biopsy, pulmonary function studies, and chest x-rays. Computed tomography and magnetic resonance imaging may also be used. There is no standardized treatment for pneumoconiosis of any type. Symptoms are treated in an attempt to minimize them. For silicosis, corticosteroids may give some relief. When lung neoplasms develop, surgical removal is indicated and may be followed up by radiotherapy or chemotherapy.

Usually, pneumoconiosis is asymptomatic until the disease has become advanced. By that time, prognosis is usually poor. Research studies have shown that neoplasms most often result from exposure to asbestos, radon, chromium, silica, cadmium, nickel, arsenic, and beryllium. Mesothelioma commonly causes neoplasms to develop 30 to 40 years after initial exposure, is highest in people over age 60, and only 9 percent of patients survive for 5 years after diagnosis. The role of the physical therapist assistant (PTA) is to implement a program that may involve respiratory therapy, controlled coughing, postural drainage, breathing exercises, and general segmental bronchial drainage.

Hypersensitivity Pneumonitis

Hypersensitivity pneumonitis, also called *extrinsic allergic alveolitis*, can be caused by exposure to organic dusts or active chemicals and usually affects the alveoli and distal airways. Causative organic compounds include molds, fungal spores, plant fibers, wood dust, cork dust, coffee beans, bird feathers, hydroxyurea (a drug used to treat certain cancers), gram-bacterial endotoxins, and mycobacteria.

Hypersensitivity pneumonitis, regardless of the cause, alters the lungs in specific ways. A combination of T-cell–mediated and immune complex–mediated hypersensitivity reactions occurs. Cigarette smoking aggravates the disease, and **human leukocyte antigens** play an important role in its development. Poorly formed granulomas containing foreign body "giant" cells are seen scattered throughout the

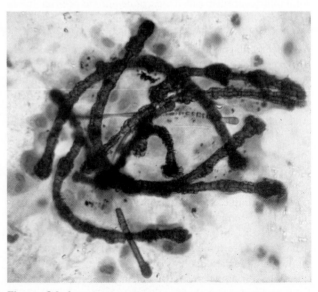

Figure 24–1 Cluster of asbestos bodies in sputum (original magnification X 1,000).

respiratory pathways, with mild fibrosis occurring mostly in the alveolar walls.

Diagnosis is made by history of exposure, pulmonary function studies, clinical manifestations (dyspnea, chills, fever, nonproductive cough), and inflammatory mediators in the sputum. Usually, if a patient is removed from exposure to the causative agent, the condition initially improves. Symptoms return on reexposure and, over time, become chronic. Hypersensitivity pneumonitis may be acute, subacute, or chronic based on exposure. Prognosis is poor with repeat exposure. Other adverse respiratory effects are caused, as is nonreversible interstitial fibrosis.

> **RED FLAG**
> Patients with asthma generally complain of shortness of breath, chest tightness, wheezing, and cough.

Skin Disorders

Approximately 61,000 new cases of occupational skin disorders are reported each year. It is likely that many go unreported. The highest rates of skin disorders are in agriculture and manufacturing. In agricultural workers, contact dermatitis from plants, sunlight, pesticides, and fertilizers is common. Manufacturing workers may also come into contact with substances and chemicals that can cause skin disorders.

Skin disorders may be acute, allergic, or chronic and include contact urticaria, psoriasis, **scleroderma**, **vitiligo** (areas of lack of skin pigment), chlor-acne, actinic skin damage, cutaneous malignancy, and cutaneous infections (see Chapter 23). Agents in the workplace that may damage the skin include irritating chemicals such as solvents, cutting oils, alkalis, detergents, and acids. Arsenic and tar products, in combination with sunlight, may be highly dangerous. Skin cancer in the workplace often results from excessive ultraviolet exposure, usually in people who spend much work time outdoors.

Rubber Latex Allergy

In the health care industry, rubber latex allergy cases have increased because of repeated contact with rubber gloves and other equipment containing latex. The following three types of reactions to latex may occur:

- Immediate (type I) hypersensitivity: Causing urticaria, rhinitis, watery eyes, respiratory distress, and asthma or skin rash
- Irritation or irritant contact dermatitis: Causing dry, crusty, hard bumps; sores; and horizontal cracks on the skin
- Mild-to-severe allergic contact dermatitis: A delayed type IV hypersensitivity that is cell mediated

These responses may occur when items containing latex touch the skin, eyes, mouth, nose, genitals, rectum, or open body areas.

Latex exposure is one of the leading causes of occupational asthma. Once they become sensitized, some health care workers are at risk for severe systemic allergic reactions, which can potentially be fatal. Therefore, anyone with a latex allergy should be treated immediately to avoid inhalation of latex in the air and to avoid the introduction of any latex from clothes or materials.

> **RED FLAG**
> Latex may also be a component of catheters and cause a latex reaction inside the body, in areas such as the bladder.

Occupational Infections

Occupational infections may be caused by exposure to bacteria, fungi, viruses, and protozoa in the workplace. Work activities may involve handling of biologically active organisms, heightening the potential for exposure. Exposure can also occur when coming into contact with infected people, tissue, secretions, or excretions. The most likely occupational infections encountered in therapy practices are herpes simplex, herpes zoster (shingles), viral hepatitis, AIDS, and tuberculosis.

Occupational Burns

Occupational burns may occur in many different industries, but perhaps the predominant type of work is firefighting. With new advances in protective clothing and equipment, the occurrence of burns to firefighters is decreasing. However, tissue injuries may be caused by application of heat, chemicals, electricity, or irradiation. The depth of a burn and extent of tissue injury result from the intensity and duration of exposure to heat or other causative agents. Working as a firefighter may lead to a variety of other chronic conditions over time, including cardiovascular disease, respiratory disease, noise-induced hearing loss, posttraumatic stress disorder, and physical disability. Another concern is carbon monoxide, which is always present at fires.

Occupational burns are also common in the food, metalworking, refining, chemical, and automotive industries. Common burn-causing agents include roofing tar, arc flash explosions (such as during welding), electrical equipment, hot water, cooking oil, molten metal, and flames. Risk factors for burns include lack of smoke detectors, faulty electrical wiring, carelessness when smoking cigarettes or other tobacco products, chemical exposure, radiation exposure, and water heaters (especially when the temperature is set too high).

Occupational Cancer

The causes of various cancers related to occupations are basically divided into two categories: endogenous (genetic) and exogenous (environmental or external). Most cancers likely develop because of multiple environmental, genetic, and viral factors. Chemical agents (including dyes, tar, asphalt, hydrocarbons, oils, arsenic, or nickel) can cause cancer after close, prolonged contact. Physical agents (such as radiation or asbestos) are additional risk factors. Industrial workers are most often affected by chemical agents. Radiation exposure is commonly from natural sources, such as ultraviolet radiation from the sun.

Occupational cancers may affect all tissues and organs of the body. For example, a substantial percentage of cancers of the upper respiratory passages, lungs, bladder, and peritoneum are attributed to occupational factors. Fluids used in metalworking are common in a number of industrial machining and grinding operations. It has recently been discovered that employees working in these operations have an increased risk of cancer of the skin, larynx, pancreas, rectum, scrotum, and urinary bladder. Exposure to various environmental substances has been linked to the development of cancer.

Many different risks for cancer may occur in the workplace. Exposure to the following substances in the workplace may be related to certain types of cancers:

- **Arsenic**: Skin, urinary bladder, and respiratory tract cancers
- *Ultraviolet light*: Skin cancer
- *Vinyl chloride*: Liver cancer
- *Dry cleaning solvents*: Kidney and liver cancer, non-Hodgkin's lymphoma

One notable occupational factor is *asbestos*, which increases the risk of mesothelioma and lung cancer. Before the 1970s, asbestos was used in homes and buildings to insulate ceiling tiles, flooring, and pipe coverings. In Western Europe, the epidemic of mesothelioma in building workers and others born after 1940 did not become apparent until the 1990s. Bladder cancer has been linked to the manufacture of dyes, paint, aromatic amines (such as benzidine), and rubber.

> **RED FLAG**
> Benzol (benzene) inhalation is linked to leukemia in shoemakers and in workers in the explosives, dye, and rubber cement industries.

Exposure to carcinogenic chemicals or radiation may cause alterations or mutations in genetic material (DNA). There is a proven, significant interval between first exposure to a cancer-causing agent and the first manifestation of a tumor. This is referred to as the *induction period, induction-latency period*, or *latency period*.

The length of the induction-latency period may be from 4 to 6 years for radiation-induced leukemias and up to 40 or more years for asbestos-induced mesotheliomas. For most tumors, from 12 to 25 years is common, which may obscure the relationship between remote exposures and newly discovered tumors.

SUMMARY

Many disorders and injuries are related to jobs and occupations. Each type of industry uses its own equipment, substances, and procedures. Any individual occupation therefore may cause specific risks of occupational disorders and injuries. Various risk factors may cause musculoskeletal, pulmonary, or skin disorders. These factors include psychosocial stress, age, gender, personality, preexisting musculoskeletal disorders, and obesity. Commonly, these disorders are job related. There have been many attempts to develop ergonomic furniture and other equipment in the workplace to better support the musculoskeletal needs of employees as they work.

Exposure to different chemicals or even the physical environment results in various pathologic conditions and even cancer. Pulmonary conditions often result from inhaled workplace materials such as asbestos, silica, or coal dust. These conditions include pneumoconiosis (of which there are many types), hypersensitivity pneumonitis, toxic lung injury, and obstructive airway disorders. Skin disorders commonly occur in the agriculture and manufacturing industries, with about 61,000 new cases of occupational skin disorders reported each year. Rubber latex allergy cases are increasing due to repeated contact with rubber gloves and other equipment containing latex.

Many accidents occur during daily life, in any type of activity. Athletic injuries are due to sudden trauma, such as that which may occur during rigorous sporting activities. Joint injuries may be highly debilitating, potentially involving not only the joints (articulations) but also the tendons and ligaments of the body. Strains are stretching injuries that often result from unusual muscle contraction or excessive forcible stretching. Sprains involve ligamentous structures surrounding the joints. Fractures are breaks or cracks in bones. Occupational infections may be caused by exposure to bacteria, fungi, viruses, and protozoa. Occupational burns and cancer may result from exposure to fire, electricity, radiation, dyes, tar, asphalt, hydrocarbons, oils, arsenic, nickel, or asbestos.

REVIEW QUESTIONS

Select the best response to each question.

1. The most common occupational injuries are
   a. respiratory disorders
   b. skin disorders
   c. mental disorders
   d. musculoskeletal disorders

2. Partially or completely ruptured ligaments are called
   a. strains
   b. sprains
   c. tendonitis
   d. bursitis

3. Mesothelioma is linked to exposure of which of the following substances?
   a. nickel
   b. arsenic
   c. asbestos
   d. tar

4. The most prevalent occupational lung disease in developed countries is
   a. occupational asthma
   b. mesothelioma
   c. pleurisy
   d. hypersensitivity pneumonitis

5. Signs and symptoms of pneumoconiosis do *not* include
   a. chest pain
   b. chronic coughing
   c. progressive dyspnea
   d. high fever

6. Arsenic may increase the risk of cancer of the
   a. liver or colon
   b. skin or urinary bladder
   c. spleen or bone marrow
   d. brain or testes

7. The most prevalent types of work-related musculoskeletal disorders are
   a. fracture of the knees
   b. skull fractures
   c. back injuries
   d. rupture of the spleen and ribs

8. Soft tissue injuries in athletic persons include
   a. contusions
   b. sprains
   c. strains
   d. all of the above

9. Each type of pneumoconiosis is described based on its
   a. length of exposure
   b. causative agent
   c. prognosis
   d. treatment

10. Which occupational disorder or injury shows no definitive symptoms?
    a. pneumoconiosis
    b. rubber latex allergy
    c. pleurisy
    d. liver cancer

CASE STUDIES

Karen Coupe, PT, DPT, MSEd

Case 1

A PTA recently accepted a position in a facility where 95 percent of the patients have suffered an on-the-job injury. The PTA was previously employed in an acute care hospital. Although the facility provides a mentoring system, the PTA researches the following questions.

1. What is the age range, variety of injury types, and cost associated with occupational injuries?
2. The facility brochure describes job ergonomics as a benefit of treatment at this facility. Define and give examples of ergonomics.
3. Compare and contrast the difference in the ergonomics of a roofer with those of an administrative assistant in a busy accounting office.
4. The PTA is reviewing various research to ensure her knowledge is up to date. To do so, the PTA needs to know the most common type of occupational injury. What is the most common type?
5. Based on the answer to number 4, what areas of physical therapy practice should be reviewed by the PTA?

Case 2

A PTA is seeing two patients who suffered on-the-job injuries at a privately owned home cabinet and windows company.

The first patient is a 24-year-old male laborer who suffered a lumbar sprain/strain while lifting a large kitchen cabinet into a client's truck. The second patient is a 36-year-old female office manager who suffers from carpal tunnel syndrome. Both patients are having difficulty with their workers' compensation carrier.

1. Research the incidence of occupational spine injuries. How prevalent are these injures? Why do you believe this is true?
2. What could be some typical clinical manifestations of a lumbar sprain/strain? How would this differ from a patient who suffered an L4–5 disk herniation with radiculopathy?
3. The office manager suffers from carpal tunnel syndrome. What is the etiology and clinical manifestations of carpal tunnel syndrome? What are some activities that could predispose this patient to carpal tunnel syndrome?
4. Compare and contrast the ergonomics of both jobs. Based on your answer, consider other possible injury scenarios if the job is performed incorrectly.
5. What is a workers' compensation carrier?

WEBSITES

http://ergonomics.org/articles/overuse/

http://www.aafp.org/afp/2002/0915/p1025.html

http://www.ada.gov/stdspdf.htm

http://www.cdc.gov/ncidod/eid/vol11no07/04-1038.htm

http://www.cdc.gov/niosh/docs/97-141/

http://www.cdc.gov/niosh/topics/cancer/

http://www.nlm.nih.gov/medlineplus/handinjuriesand disorders.html

http://www.osha.gov/SLTC/ergonomics/

http://www.webmd.com/allergies/tc/allergy-to-natural-rubber-latex-topic-overview

http://www.who.int/occupational_health/publications/quantification/en/index.html

http://www.wrongdiagnosis.com/o/occupational_injuries/intro.htm

Psychological Disorders and the Influence of Stress

OUTLINE

LEARNING OBJECTIVES

After completion of the chapter the reader should be able to

1. Describe the limbic system of the brain and its function.
2. Define perceptions, hallucinations, and delusions.
3. Discuss the functions of neuromediators.
4. Compare schizophrenia with bipolar depression.
5. List classifications of anxiety disorders.
6. Explain major depression and dysthymia.
7. Define neuroimaging.
8. Differentiate panic disorder with obsessive-compulsive disorder.

KEY TERMS

Bipolar depression: A disorder in which a person alternates between periods of euphoric feelings and mania and periods of depression.

Cerebral cortex: Layer of the brain known as the "gray matter," it covers the outer portion of the cerebrum and cerebellum.

Delusions: False beliefs or opinions that become "fixed" and unshakable.

Dementia: Loss of brain function because of certain diseases, displaying serious losses in cognitive activity.

Hallucinations: Perceptions of (usually) auditory or visual stimuli that do not exist in reality.

Limbic system: Set of brain structures that support emotion, behavior, memory, and the sense of smell; these structures include the hippocampus, amygdala, thalamus, septum, and limbic cortex.

Neuroimaging: Use of various techniques to image the structures, functions, and pharmacology of the brain; it includes computed tomography scan, magnetic resonance imaging, and many other procedures.

Neuromediators: Neurotransmitters; chemical substances released from synaptic knobs into synaptic clefts; they include acetylcholine, dopamine, epinephrine, norepinephrine, and others.

Schizophrenia: A psychological disorder involving delusions and hallucinations, disorganization, and reduced enjoyment and interests.

KEY TERMS CONTINUED

Sleep Apnea: A sleep disorder characterized by abnormal pauses in breathing or abnormally low breathing; each pause can last for seconds or minutes.

Stress: Inappropriate physiologic response to any demand on the mind or body.

Overview

Psychological disorders are characterized by changes in thoughts, moods, or behaviors that affect normal functioning. Causes of mental disorders may be due to interpersonal relationships, brain structure, **stress**, heredity, substance abuse, and many other factors. The study of mental illness is ongoing, and although significant advancements have been made over time, the human mind is still not completely understood. Widely diverging methods of treatment exist throughout the world, and the results of these methods vary in effectiveness.

Effects of Heredity and Environment

Many studies have shown that both heredity and environment play significant roles in the development of mental illness. It is common for an individual with a condition such as **bipolar depression** to have blood relatives with the same condition. However, some other illnesses develop from a variety of factors and are not simply inherited. Psychological disorders appear in different cultures and across the socioeconomic spectrum. In some cases, development of mental disorders requires certain environmental stressors such as viral illnesses, physical or emotional abuse, and substance abuse.

Brain Structures

Anatomic and biochemical changes in the brain affect behavior and the development of mental illness. The brain is divided into distinct groups of functional neurons. These neurons influence the activity of each other. When certain brain structures are injured or degenerate, the ability to process information and normal cognitive function may be impaired.

Cerebral Cortex

The outermost part of the brain is covered by the **cerebral cortex**. It controls thoughts, motor function, sensory function, speech, and memory. The thalamus is necessary for practically all cortical activity. Damage to the cortex affects brain activity, but even more so if damage also includes the thalamus. **Table 25–1** summarizes the functions of various lobes of the cerebral cortex.

The frontal lobe is the largest lobe and is called the "chief administrator" of the brain (**Figure 25–1**). It is responsible for planning, intellectual insight, judgment, expression of emotion, and problem solving.

The temporal lobe organizes and interprets somatic, auditory, and visual information that is critical to recognize familiar objects, people, locations, and so on. It is also important for appropriate interpretation of social contexts and how to respond to them. The parietal lobe processes and integrates visual, auditory, and tactile input. It also filters out extraneous information. The occipital lobe receives visual information from the eyes and is important for depth perception. Also, association areas in the cerebral cortex help to add meaning and perception to incoming information.

Limbic System

The **limbic system** regulates emotional behavior. It is made up of structures deep inside the brain (**Figure 25–2**). The limbic system links thoughts and autonomic nervous system responses to emotions. One section, the *hippocampus*, encodes, consolidates, and retrieves memories. When the hippocampus atrophies, memory problems result, such as in Alzheimer's disease. Another section, the *amygdala*, is important in emotional function, aggression, fear, and sexual arousal. The hypothalamus plays a critical role in the limbic system by regulating functions related to basic survival needs of the body.

TABLE 25–1 Cerebral Cortex Functions

Lobe	Functions
Frontal	Abstract versus concrete reasoning Aspects of emotional response: blunting Concentration Decision making Making meaning of language Memory and historical sense of self Motivation: volition Purposeful behavior Sequencing Speech organization Speech production
Temporal	Aspects of sexual action and meaning Attention Emotional modulation and interpretation Impulse and aggression control Interpretation and meaning of social context Motivation Visual-spatial recognition
Parietal	Bodily awareness Concept formation Filtration of background stimuli Memory and nonverbal memory Personality factors and symptom denial Sensory integration and spatial relations
Occipital	Possible information-holding area Vision

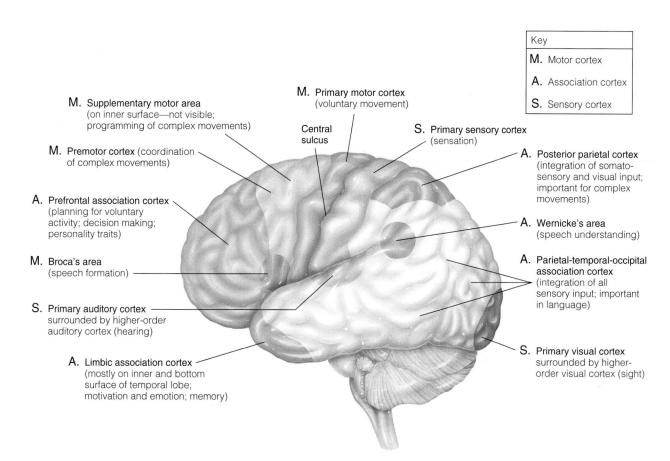

Figure 25–1 Functional regions of the cortex. The cerebral cortex has three principal functions: receiving sensory input, integrating sensory information, and generating motor responses. Special sensory areas handle vision, smell, taste, and hearing.

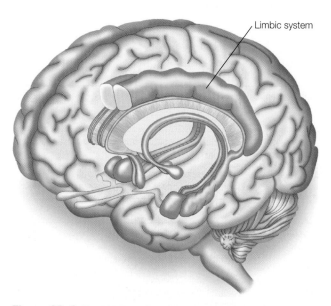

Figure 25–2 The limbic system. The odd assortment of structures shown in green is the limbic system. The limbic system is the seat of emotions such as joy and instincts and is home to other functions as well.

Perceptions

Perception is the conscious awareness of sensory stimuli. It is the final stage of information processing and results in behavior responses to sensations. Information from the body's senses is received by the thalamus. The prefrontal association area tracks where information has been put in long-term memory and integrates memories with sensory input to make decisions. Implicit memory is involved in learning reflexive motor and perceptual skills. Explicit memory is involved with processing facts learned about persons, places, and things. Perception consists of sensory information that is brought in from the outside world and then processed into meaning. The thalamus relays perceptions to the other parts of the brain.

Perception Disorders

Perception disorders are actually disorders of information processing. They include **hallucinations** and **delusions**. Both are common symptoms of many psychiatric disorders but may sometimes occur in healthy persons. Hallucinations and delusions may also accompany other health problems or be side effects of certain drugs.

Hallucinations

Hallucinations are sensory perceptions that do not result from an external stimulus and occur in the waking state. They may seem very real and are different from illusions. They can develop at any time during sensory transmission and can be based on abnormal cortical reception, perception, or interpretation. Hallucinations are classified by the involved structure or function, or etiology. *Release hallucinations* occur when a normal sensory input is blocked. *Ictal hallucinations* are produced by abnormal neuronal discharges. A visual ictal hallucination occurs during the *aura* in people who have epilepsy. Etiologic classifications of hallucinations may be according to disorders of brain structure or function, drug reactions, sensory or sleep deprivation, or psychotic disorders. However, the most common classification method for hallucinations is based on the type of sensation involved. Visual hallucinations are subjective visual experiences in the absence of objective evidence of a corresponding stimulus. Such hallucinations are most likely to be associated with acute organic disorders, such as toxic confusional psychoses, delirium, and focal brain diseases. It may occur with any stage of schizophrenia.

Auditory hallucinations are subjective experiences of hearing voices or other sounds despite the absence of an actual reality-based external stimulus to account for the phenomenon. Auditory hallucinations may involve ringing, buzzing, voices, and music. Auditory hallucinations may also be caused by alcohol withdrawal. When voices are heard, they are hard to localize, as the voices seem to originate inside the head.

Hallucinations of smell and taste are often caused by damage to the olfactory bulb or by tumors at the base of the brain. Also, migraine headaches may cause an aura that consists of smell and taste hallucinations. These hallucinations can also be warning signs of an impending migraine. *Somatosensory* hallucinations occur in phantom limb pain often seen in patients after limb amputations. It is important to understand the phantom pain is "real" pain, not just the perception of pain.

Delusions

Delusions are described as false beliefs that persist regardless of the true facts. Delusions are abnormalities of thought instead of merely perception. They are formed and influenced by an individual's background and may be based on personal, family, and social experiences. Examples of delusions include beliefs of persecution, influence or control of certain events, sickness, grandeur (greatness), poverty, and demonic possession. The causes of delusions are not clearly identified but may result from repeated stress rather than a single situational problem. They have also been associated with sensory deprivation such as hearing loss.

Neuromediators

Today's understanding of mental illness is derived from the understanding of how nerve cells in the brain communicate. Normal nerve cell communication is very rapid. Synapses, the area where two neurons meet, allow synaptic transmission (neurotransmission) to occur. This is accomplished by the release of neurotransmitters (also called **neuromediators**) from the axonal terminal of a neuron (a presynaptic cell).

The following steps are involved in neurotransmission:

- Synthesis of a transmitter substance
- Storage and release of the transmitter
- Binding of the transmitter to receptors on the postsynaptic membrane
- Removal of the transmitter from the synaptic cleft

Classic neurotransmitters include small-molecule transmitters and neuroactive peptides. The neuromediators most often involved in conditions of mental illness are acetylcholine, dopamine, epinephrine, norepinephrine, serotonin, gamma-aminobutyric acid, glutamate, glycine, and aspartate. **Table 25–2** summarizes the effects of neuromediators in the brain.

> **RED FLAG**
> Neuromediators cross synapses and bind to receptors on postsynaptic cells, causing excitatory or inhibitory actions.

TABLE 25–2   **Brain Neuromediators**

Neuromediator	Major Source	Effects
Acetylcholine	Formed in brain synapses; in high concentration in motor cortex and basal ganglia	Excitatory or inhibitory, depending on area of the brain; underactivity is implicated in Alzheimer's disease
Amino acids: gamma-aminobutyric acid, glutamate, glycine, and aspartate	No one major source	Excitatory or inhibitory; implicated in anxiety disorders
Dopamine	Midbrain (substantia nigra and ventral segmental area)	Usually excitatory; involved in motivations, thoughts, emotional regulation; overactivity may be involved in schizophrenia and other psychotic disorders
Epinephrine and norepinephrine	Brainstem (locus ceruleus); derived from dopamine	Excitatory or inhibitory, depending on area of the brain; noradrenergic pathways to cerebral cortex, brainstem, and limbic system; underactivity may be involved in certain types of depression
Serotonin	Brainstem (raphe nucleus); derived from tryptophan	Involved in regulation of attention and complex cognitive functions; pathways to cerebral cortex, brainstem, and limbic system; underactivity may be involved in certain types of depression and obsessive-compulsive disorder

Psychotropic Medications

The first psychotropic medication was chlorpromazine. In high doses this drug was found to calm agitation in patients with schizophrenia and bipolar disorders. It has both tranquilizing and antipsychotic effects. Related drugs in the class of phenothiazines help to reduce or stop delusions, hallucinations, and disordered thoughts.

Typical and atypical antipsychotics are used to treat schizophrenia. Examples of typical antipsychotics are chlorpromazine, haloperidol, and thiothixene. Examples of atypical antipsychotics are clozapine, risperidone, and olanzapine. Atypical antipsychotics work better in treating negative symptoms of schizophrenia.

Antidepressants

Antidepressants alleviate depression by increasing norepinephrine and serotonin activity at postsynaptic membrane receptors. The four common types of antidepressants are monoamine oxidase (MAO) inhibitors, tricyclic compounds, serotonin reuptake inhibitors (SRIs), and the novel (atypical) antidepressants. MAO inhibitors increase concentrations of norepinephrine and serotonin. The tricyclic antidepressants (TCAs) block reuptake of serotonin and norepinephrine. The SRIs inhibit reuptake of serotonin. A subtype, the selective serotonin reuptake inhibitors (SSRIs), selectively targets different neurotransmitters. The atypical antidepressants affect the neurotransmission of serotonin and norepinephrine. All these antidepressant agents are believed to relieve depression by interfering with the reuptake of the neurotransmitter serotonin by the presynaptic nerve cell, thus increasing their free concentration at postsynaptic adrenergic receptors in the central nervous system.

> **RED FLAG**
> Antidepressant effects may not be observed for up to 4 weeks after initiation of treatment.

Neuroimaging

Brain structure and abnormalities can also contribute to mental illnesses. **Neuroimaging** allows the mapping of brain anatomy in great detail. It also helps to estimate brain activity by measuring metabolic rate and brain blood flow. Brain lesions are believed to be correlated with the onset and development of psychiatric manifestations. However, because neuroimaging techniques are not yet applied clinically, they are not used to diagnose mental illnesses. Neuroimaging includes computed tomography (CT) scans, magnetic resonance imaging, magnetoencephalography, positron emission tomography (PET), and single-photon emission CT. PET scans use the infusion of a radioactive substance. Single-photon emission CT is similar to PET but not as expensive. It uses more stable substances and different types of detectors to visualize patterns of blood flow and is useful for diagnosing cerebrovascular accidents and brain tumors.

> **RED FLAG**
> Research has shown that children treated for depression with SSRIs may be at increased risk for suicidal thoughts or actions, according to the U.S. Food and Drug Administration advisory committee.

CT scans allow for three-dimensional views of structures, with extreme detail. Although not diagnosing the type of mental illness, they can suggest a brain-based problem. Magnetic resonance imaging can also distinguish between the gray and white matter of the brain to visualize structural brain abnormalities, which have been studied in patients with dementias, mood disorders, and schizophrenia.

Schizophrenia

Schizophrenia involves a disconnection between thoughts and language and is defined as "splitting of the mind," but it is not the same as a "split personality." It is a chronic and extremely debilitating psychotic disorder. The condition interferes with the ways a person filters environmental stimuli. It affects feelings, perceptions, overall behavior, and thoughts. Schizophrenia usually manifests between ages 17 and 25 but peaks at different ages based on patient gender. It affects men just slightly more than women (1.4 times more prevalent in men).

Schizophrenia peaks between ages 10 and 25 for males and between ages 25 and 35 for females. It seldom occurs before age 10 or after age 60. Risk factors include family history of the disease or of similar schizotypal diseases. Other factors include a birth date in the winter or spring, early history of attention deficit disorder, and influenza infections that occurred in the mother while the patient was a second-trimester fetus.

> **RED FLAG**
> Stressful events appear to initiate the onset of schizophrenia.

Schizophrenia also alters the brain's anatomic structures and biochemistry as well as brain functions. *Positive* or *psychotic* symptoms reflect abnormal behaviors, incomprehensible speech, delusions, hallucinations, and behaviors that are grossly disorganized or even catatonic. Schizophrenics often invent words, make loose associations, cannot stick to their original point of discussion, are incoherent, or use groups of disconnected words, either when speaking or writing.

Schizophrenics usually cannot respond in appropriate ways to their environment. In the early stages of the disorder, the senses may be either enhanced or "blunted." Sounds and colors may seem extremely changed. There may be a "sensory overload" because the patient can no longer screen out external sensory stimuli. Delusions may range from the belief that he or she is being watched or being controlled and manipulated. They may believe they are a historical figure or that they can control the thoughts and actions of others.

Auditory hallucinations, the most common type of hallucination to occur, may seem completely real to the patient. Often, when voices are heard they are perceived as accusatory or vulgar. If visual hallucinations occur, they are usually related to the auditory hallucinations that are perceived.

The *negative symptoms* of the disease include lack of speech (alogia), avolition (lack of motivation to achieve goals), apathy, lack of emotional expression, inappropriate actions, and anhedonia (inability to enjoy things that are normally pleasurable). Patients may also show a blunted response to painful stimuli. Negative symptoms are very difficult to treat. Thought disorders with overlapping positive and negative symptoms may be called *cognitive symptoms*, *disorganized dimension*, or *disorganization symptom cluster* in schizophrenia patients. The patient's mood may be incongruent to his or her environment.

Schizophrenia is subdivided into three types: paranoid, disorganized, and catatonic forms. *Paranoid schizophrenia* involves persecutory or grandiose delusions, auditory hallucinations, intense interactions with others, and lesser amounts of anatomic brain damage. It often begins suddenly, with less obvious negative symptoms. *Disorganized schizophrenia* has many negative symptoms and causes a gradual deterioration of one's personality. For example, the person has withdrawn, inept social skills, with disorganized and incoherent speech. He or she often neglects personal grooming and eventually becomes unable to live alone. Prognosis is worse for this type than for paranoid schizophrenia because the disorganization of the personality progressively worsens. *Catatonic schizophrenia* is very rare and is characterized by decline or increase of psychomotor function, extreme negativism, and peculiar grimacing, posturing, repeating of other people's speech, or imitations of others' movements.

The exact pathogenesis of schizophrenia is unknown and is not associated with any specific brain lesion. Imaging studies often show enlargement of the lateral and third ventricles and a reduction in frontal lobe volume, temporal lobe volume, and whole-brain volume. PET scans reveal reduced metabolic activity in the frontal lobe. Adolescents or young adults often show enlarged ventricles and smaller medial temporal lobes. There may be an increased density of dopamine receptor sites, mostly in the basal ganglia.

A diagnosis of schizophrenia requires that the patient have two or more of the following symptoms consistently for at least 1 month:

- Delusions
- Hallucinations
- Disorganized speech
- Grossly disorganized or catatonic behavior
- Negative symptoms

Also, one or more functions must be greatly impaired compared with the patient's previous life, and signs and symptoms must persist for at least 6 months.

The goals of treatment are to induce remission, prevent recurrence, and improve normal functions. Hospitalization may be needed if the patient is dangerous to others or may self-inflict wounds. It is also indicated if the patient cannot properly care for him- or herself or refuses to eat or drink. Pharmacotherapy and psychosocial interventions can greatly help schizophrenics to live as normally as possible. Psychosocial interventions help the patient to learn about the condition and live independently. Often, family members may also need therapy to help cope with schizophrenia.

The role of the physical therapist assistant (PTA) is to assist the schizophrenic with regular exercise, based on the physical therapy plan of care. Indicated exercises include walking and strength training. Because many medications taken by schizophrenics cause weight gain, it is important for the patient to remain active. If there are no skilled physical therapy needs, these patients often need occupational or recreational therapy services.

Depressive Disorders

Depressive disorders are types of mood disorders. Depression affects about 20 percent of women and 12 percent of men in the United States. Major depression affects twice the amount of women as men. If bipolar disorder exists, men usually begin with the manic phase of the disorder, whereas women usually begin with the depressive phase. About 20 to 40 percent of adolescents who have major depression will develop bipolar disorder within 5 years of incidence. Mood disorders occur in every race with similar percentages, and depression rates are higher among individuals who live at or near the federal poverty level or who are of low socioeconomic status. Genetic factors also play a role, as does environmental, developmental, and biologic factors.

Major Depression and Dysthymia

When depression occurs early in life and its symptoms are frequent, it is more likely that the affected patient will require medications for treatment. After 65 years of age, depression is often a precursor to **dementia**. Patients in this age group should be evaluated for dementia and treated accordingly. *Major depression* is also called *major depressive disorder*. It is characterized by depressed mood, anhedonia (inability to experience pleasure), lack of concentration, feelings of guilt or worthlessness, psychomotor retardation or agitation, hypersonia or insomnia, reduced libido, change in appetite or weight, suicidal ideation, and thoughts of death.

Subclassifications of depression include *melancholic features*, *psychotic features*, and *catatonic features*. Melancholic features include insomnia with early awakening in the morning, worsened depression in the morning, psychomotor agitation or retardation, anorexia (with significant weight loss), increased guilt, anhedonia, loss of interest in activities, and a complete loss of capacity for joy. *Atypical depression* is opposite of melancholic depression. With atypical depression, depression worsens as the day progresses and the patient sleeps excessively and often overeats.

Psychotic features include delusions or hallucinations that may correspond (or not correspond) to mood changes. Catatonic features include excessive mobility or immobility, repetitive speech, extreme negative attitudes, and voluntary movements that seem peculiar. However, these features are only termed chronic if the condition lasts for 2 or more years.

Most women experience some depression after childbirth, and a *postpartum* specifier is included if depression occurs within 6 weeks of childbirth. The mother may be unable to properly care for the infant, may have thoughts about harming the infant, and may experience sleep deprivation, behavior volatility, and manic symptoms.

Dysthymia is a disorder of mood in which the essential feature is a chronic disturbance of mood of at least 2 years' duration. It is basically a milder form of major depression and includes low self-esteem, appetite changes, and sleep and energy problems. Dysthymia may begin insidiously and is chronic. The patient may be unable to separate the condition from normal functioning and may not recognize that he or she has an illness. Dysthymic patients are at risk for developing major depression, substance abuse disorders, and other psychiatric disorders. The role of the PTA is to give the depressed patient as much regular exercise as he or she can tolerate. Overall, regular exercise may help to improve the patient's outlook and increase body fitness.

Bipolar Depression

Bipolar depression is also called *manic-depressive disorder* and includes many different subclassifications. Bipolar depression and its subclassifications are characterized by periods of elation and irritability (referred to as the *manic phase*) that are followed by periods of depression. Unipolar mania, in which no depressive period follows the manic period, is extremely rare. In bipolar depression, the condition can be precipitated by antidepressant medications and therapies such as electroconvulsive treatments.

The manic phase of bipolar depression is signified by extreme changes in mood, decreased need for sleep or food, erratic thoughts, rapid speech, irritability, high distractibility, excessive pleasurable and high-risk activities, and inflated self-esteem. This phase may vary widely in intensity and length. In *cyclothymia*, mild mania and depression may become severely delusional, lasting from hours to weeks. Untreated bipolar episodes may increase in severity with the aging process.

Women are most likely to experience *rapid cycling*, in which four or more extreme mood shifts occur within a 1-year period. The more frequently a patient has extreme mood shifts, the easier it becomes to have recurrences. Many other psychiatric disorders also are subject to this phenomenon. Controlling the occurrences and frequency of mood shifts is critical in helping the patient to maintain quality of life.

Physiologically, there is evidence that these conditions cause a decline in the frontal and temporal lobes of the brain. The amygdala has increased blood flow and oxygen consumption during depressive episodes. This condition may persist for 1 to 2 years after the depression has been managed with medications. Depression involves complex chemical changes within the brain, involving neurotransmitters that include serotonin, norepinephrine, and dopamine.

A critical role in the onset of depression may involve disturbances in the function of the hypothalamic-pituitary-adrenal axis, which is related to the sleep–wake cycle. Many forms of mental illness involve alteration in the sleep–wake cycle, with the normal sleep cycle often being reversed in depression. Circadian rhythms (24-hour cycles of biochemical, physiologic, and behavioral processes) also play a part. *Seasonal affective disorder* is triggered in the winter as the amount of daylight hours shortens. It usually resolves itself as the summer returns and daylight hours are extended.

Treatment for bipolar depression includes antidepressant drugs (usually SRIs, MAO inhibitors, and TCAs), electroconvulsive therapy for extreme cases, lithium, anticonvulsants, phototherapy, and psychotherapy. Phototherapy (light therapy) uses artificial light to produce melatonin and to help balance the catecholamine ("fight-or-flight") systems. Additional therapies include vagal nerve stimulation and transcranial magnetic stimulation. Psychotherapy helps patients and their families deal with the condition and its related stress and to heal disrupted relationships. However, many bipolar patients deny they have the condition and often use other means, such as alcohol or recreational drugs, to mediate their mood changes.

The role of the PTA in working with patients who have bipolar conditions is to include activities that may improve overall wellness and fitness. Physical therapy for the bipolar patient is designed to improve overall mood (indirectly) and also body health. Exercise has been shown to help these patients manage mood swings, and many bipolar patients exercise four to five times per week, with walking, jogging, and cycling indicated regularly. The PTA needs to be aware of medical side effects and educate the patient to stop exercising if they experience these effects.

Anxiety Disorders

Anxiety disorders feature intense fearfulness without a precipitating event, with various manifestations. Anxiety is a normal response to threatening situations, and these disorders are the most prevalent of all psychiatric disorders. They affect nearly 29 percent of all individuals, and affect women more than men. Although there is a familial tendency, a genetic link has not been proven.

Subjective manifestations of anxiety disorders range from heightened awareness to deep fear of impending death or disaster. Objective manifestations include restlessness, palpitations, increased heart rate and blood pressure, dry mouth, sweating, and a desire to escape the impending situation. The five subtypes of anxiety disorders are panic disorder, posttraumatic stress disorder, generalized anxiety disorder, social phobia, and obsessive-compulsive disorder (OCD). All except posttraumatic stress disorder are discussed below.

Panic Disorder

Panic disorder is an acute, psychological reaction manifested by intense anxiety and panic. It affects women more than men and usually causes a variety of symptoms, such as dizziness, fainting, tachycardia, chest pain, palpitations, shortness of breath, feelings of smothering or choking, sweating, nausea, abdominal distress, and psychological symptoms of fear. Panic attacks last from a few seconds to an hour or longer and vary in frequency from several times a day to once a month. Panic disorders are unexpected and not related to external events.

Biologic and environmental factors appear to be related to panic disorder. However, panic disorder occurs without identification of a known underlying organic cause. Most people diagnosed with panic disorder report major life stressors during a 1-year period before a panic attack. Patients who have been physically or sexually abused also experience a higher occurrence of such attacks. Multiple mechanisms and neurotransmitters are involved in initiating panic attacks, primarily gamma-aminobutyric acid, norepinephrine, and serotonin.

RED FLAG
A helpful mode of treatment for those with bipolar depression is to maintain a regular schedule for sleeping and awakening, combined with adequate exercise before mid-afternoon.

Treatment includes behavioral, psychological, and drug therapies. Antidepressants (except bupropion) are effective, and SSRIs are becoming more commonly used even though they have a slower onset of action. Often, multiple medications are required. When treatment is inadequate, the patient often develops phobias (commonly *agoraphobia*, the fear of open spaces), meaning that he or she is unable to leave the security of the home.

The PTA should be aware that individuals with panic disorder can, in some circumstances, experience feelings of panic due to increased heart rate and breathlessness that may occur from exercise. However, in general, moderate exercise is indicated for most patients with this disorder. The PTA must communicate with the PT to assist with physical therapy.

Generalized Anxiety Disorder

Generalized anxiety disorder is characterized by less than 6 months of excessive worrying that is difficult to control. Symptoms include autonomic hyperactivity, muscle tension, becoming easily startled, and an inability to concentrate. Benzodiazepines are very effective in treating this condition. Buspirone may also be used but has a slower onset of action. SSRIs are also used for treatment, along with TCAs and atypical antidepressants. Beta-adrenergic blockers block symptoms of anxiety rather than treating the anxiety disorder itself. The PTA should assist the patient with moderate exercise to help alleviate symptoms of generalized anxiety disorder. The PTA should be aware of any anxiety disorders that may be present in a patient, and how they can affect physical therapy.

Obsessive-Compulsive Disorder

OCD is characterized by repeated thoughts (recurrent obsessions) and repeated acts (recurrent compulsions). To be classified as OCD, behaviors must be repeated excessively and not be related to any environmental condition. The patient usually recognizes that his or her actions are unreasonable but cannot stop doing them. OCD is the 10th most disabling disease worldwide and affects between 2 and 3 percent of the world population. It affects males and females evenly, with higher incidence among family members.

OCD commonly manifests when a patient is in his or her twenties, although it can occur earlier in life. It may result from dysfunction of the prefrontal cortex and basal ganglia. Disorders to rule out before OCD is diagnosed include postencephalitic Parkinson's disease, Huntington's disease, tic disorders, and Syndenham chorea. Diagnosis is based on history and clinical observation. Treatment includes behavioral therapy, cognitive therapy, and medications such as SSRIs or the TCA known as clomipramine. SSRIs are effective in about 50 to 60 percent of OCD patients and given in upper limit dosages that are often very high. The best results often occur with combination therapy of medications and cognitive-behavioral therapy.

The PTA may assist the OCD patient with moderate aerobic exercise, which is usually well tolerated. Strength training, running, and walking are all common modes of exercise for this condition. Again, the PTA must be aware of this condition even though physical therapy will not be initiated for it specifically.

Social Phobia

Social phobia, also called *social anxiety disorder*, is an intense, irrational, persistent fear of being negatively evaluated or scrutinized by other people. Social phobia is diagnosed when symptoms develop during exposure to the feared social situation, when the patient recognizes that his or her fear is irrational, when potentially fearful situations are avoided, and when the symptoms interfere with normal activities. The fear must be present for at least 6 months and not be related to any substance usage.

Social phobia occurs slightly more commonly in females than males, usually beginning between 11 and 19 years of age. It often affects schooling and employment and therefore may result in drug or alcohol problems as coping mechanisms. Treatment of social phobia includes SSRIs, benzodiazepines, and MAO inhibitors. Beta-adrenergic blockers may be useful in certain cases. Behavioral and cognitive therapies are also greatly effective. The PTA may assist the social phobia patient with moderate exercise focused on releasing tension, stress, and anxiety. Again, the PTA needs to be aware of this condition if physical therapy is required for another condition.

Sleep Disorders

Sleep disorders include insomnia and **sleep apnea** as well as other less common disorders. There are several stages of sleep:

- Stage 1—transitional sleep: Occupies 5 percent of sleep time
- Stage 2—deeper sleep: Occupies 50 percent of sleep time
- Stage 3—slow-wave sleep (partial delta brain waves): Occupies 10 percent of sleep time
- Stage 4—slow-wave sleep (mostly delta brain waves): Occupies 20 percent of sleep time

Stages 3 and 4 become shorter with aging. Most adults need between 6 and 8 hours of continuous sleep per night, although younger people need more and elderly people need less. Disorders of sleep can be caused by a number of problems, including functional or organic disorders.

Insomnia

Insomnia is a condition wherein the patient has trouble falling asleep or staying asleep. It causes the patient to feel physically and mentally tired as well as groggy, irritable, anxious, or tense, even after sleep. If chronic, insomnia may require medical intervention. Insomnia may be caused by travel through different time zones, cardiovascular problems, pain, fever, and thyroid conditions.

For diagnosis, sleeplessness must have a duration of more than 1 month and must interfere with occupational, social, or other areas of life. Sleep studies are used, involving the use of polysomnography, which measures rapid eye movement during sleep.

Hypnotics may be prescribed to help the patient achieve adequate sleep.

Regular exercise has been shown to reduce episodes of insomnia. Therefore, the PTA may assist insomniac patients with moderate exercise as directed by the PT. Although the PTA won't see patients specifically for this condition, fatigue and other issues related to sleep deprivation must be considered.

Sleep Apnea

Sleep apnea is defined as intermittent short periods of breathing cessation while asleep. It is considered a potentially life-threatening condition and affects the amount of rest that the patient actually gets while sleeping. Symptoms include temporary cessation of breathing followed by snorting and gasping. Sleep apnea may be related to obesity, airway obstructions, or hypertension and affects men more than women. It is possible for a patient to experience 20 or more episodes of apnea during a single hour. Other causes of sleep apnea may be smoking-related bronchitis, alcohol intake, and sleep deprivation. Onset of sleep apnea usually begins in middle age.

Often, patients appear sleepy while awake, indicating they are not receiving adequate sleep—a common complaint related to apnea. Weight loss is encouraged, with new researching showing that lack of sleep can prevent weight loss. In severe cases that have not responded to other treatments, patients may require use of protriptyline or constant positive air pressure equipment. Surgery may be helpful in removing portions of the uvula, soft palate, and pharynx tissues, but this treatment is only used after all other treatments have failed. The PTA should be aware that sleep apnea affects a patient's ability to participate in physical therapy due to fatigue from lack of sleep.

Coping with Stress

Stress is defined as the response to threatening or challenging events. High levels of stress may cause patients to become ill or to be less likely to recover from an illness. It also may cause an inability to cope with future stressors. The ways in which a patient attempts to lessen stress, through different strategies (such as defense mechanisms), are methods of coping with stress. According to the *general adaptation syndrome*, people go through three phases when faced with stress:

- First phase—alarm and mobilization: This energizes the nervous system as the person becomes aware of the stressor.
- Second phase—resistance: The patient prepares to fight the stressors as they continue, which can cause both physiologic and psychological harm.
- Third phase—exhaustion: If unable to fight continuing stressors, the patient will develop negative physical and psychological symptoms; these may include illness, immunodeficiency, irritability, substance abuse, disorientation, and becoming out of touch with reality.

After these three phases, the patient may avoid contact with stressors as much as possible. Attempts made at this time may be successful in helping the patient to adapt to the stressors when future contact happens. If no successful treatment is given, the patient will repeat the cycle when future contact occurs.

The following are examples of different types of stressors:

- Background stressors: Daily annoyances, including work stressors, traffic jams, waiting in lines, etc. These only slightly impact people but may have intensified results when coupled with other (or multiple) stressors.
- Cataclysmic event stressors: Sudden events that affect many people, such as the 9-11 attacks upon New York and Washington, DC, or Hurricane Katrina's effects on Louisiana.
- Personal stressors: Major personal events such as death of a spouse, losing a job, having a baby, getting married, military deployment, various types of abuse, and moving from one home to another. The reexperiencing of a traumatic event is defined as posttraumatic stress disorder.

SUMMARY

Mental disorders are characterized by alterations in thoughts, moods, or behaviors that interfere with normal activities. There may be many different causes of mental illness, with stress playing a major role. Mental illnesses arise from alterations in neural functioning or from destruction of neurons inside the brain. Schizophrenia is a chronic psychotic disorder of thought and language. Its positive symptoms include abnormal behaviors, delusions, and hallucinations. Negative symptoms of schizophrenia include lack of normal social and interpersonal behaviors and an inability to experience pleasure.

Mood disorders are disorders of emotion instead of thought. They include major depressive disorder, dysthymia, and bipolar depression. Mania is characterized by elation, irritability, high distractibility, and engagement in high-risk pleasurable activities. Depression is characterized by lack of pleasure, feelings of worthlessness and excessive guilt, altered sleep patterns, changes in appetite, and thoughts of death or suicidal ideation. Anxiety disorders include generalized anxiety disorder, panic disorder, OCD, and social phobia.

Common sleep disorders include insomnia and sleep apnea, which can be functional or organic. Insomnia describes an inability to fall asleep or stay asleep. It usually is diagnosed via sleep studies and polysomnography, which measures rapid eye movement during sleep. Sleep apnea is intermittent short periods of breathing cessation while asleep. It is considered potentially life threatening and affects how much rest the patient gets during sleep.

Stress is defined as the response to threatening or challenging events. High levels of stress may cause illness or inability to cope with future stress. Examples of stressors include background stressors (daily annoyances), cataclysmic event stressors (terrorist attacks or hurricanes), and personal stressors (death of a spouse, loss of a job). The general adaptation syndrome describes three phases that people use when faced with stress: alarm and mobilization, resistance, and exhaustion.

REVIEW QUESTIONS

Select the best response to each question.

1. The psychosis characterized by distortions of perception, emotions, thought, and, often, bizarre behavior is referred to as which of the following conditions?
   a. schizophrenia
   b. factitious disorder
   c. bipolar disorder
   d. obsessive-compulsive disorder

2. Anxiety disorders include which of the following?
   a. phobic disorder
   b. personality disorders
   c. major depressive disorder
   d. all of the above

3. The limbic system of the brain regulates which of the following functions?
   a. balance of equilibrium of the body
   b. skeletal muscle contractions
   c. emotional behavior stability
   d. kidney function

4. What is the most common type of hallucination in schizophrenia?
   a. visual
   b. smell
   c. somatosensory
   d. auditory

5. Threatening or challenging events are known as
   a. minor events
   b. stress reducers
   c. stressors
   d. major events

6. An intense, irrational, and persistent fear of being negatively evaluated by others is referred to as which disorder?
   a. obsessive-compulsive disorder
   b. social anxiety disorder
   c. generalized anxiety disorder
   d. panic disorder

7. A disorder characterized by less than 6 months of excessive, hard-to-control worrying is called
   a. obsessive-compulsive disorder
   b. social anxiety disorder
   c. generalized anxiety disorder
   d. panic disorder

8. What part of the brain controls sensory function, motor function, and thought?
   a. thalamus
   b. hypothalamus
   c. brainstem
   d. cerebral cortex

9. The terrorist attacks in New York are an example of what type of stressor?
   a. cataclysmic event stressor
   b. personal stressor
   c. background stressor
   d. psychophysiologic condition

10. If the hippocampus portion of the brain atrophies, the patient will experience problems with which of the following?
    a. vision
    b. speech
    c. memory
    d. language

CASE STUDIES

Karen Coupe, PT, DPT, MSEd

Case 1

A 17-year-old boy was referred to outpatient physical therapy 4 days status post right anterior cruciate ligament (ACL) repair. Patient medical history: Recently diagnosed bipolar disorder. Previous level of function: Independent in all activities, active in basketball, track, and football. Current level of function: Independent ambulation with axillary crutches weight bearing as tolerated right lower extremity. Plan of care includes therapeutic exercise and motor electrical stimulation. The patient's mother confides to the PTA that the patient has progressively lost 8 pounds over the past month and doesn't seem interested in sports. The patient acknowledges he has been sleeping a great deal and doesn't seem to have a lot of energy.

1. What is bipolar disorder? What are the risk factors, genetic predispositions, and age ranges?
2. Compare and contrast clinical manifestations of the depressive phase and the manic phase.
3. Based on the comments by the mother and the patient, the patient is in which phase of bipolar disorder?
4. How could each phase affect the patient during physical therapy treatment? How should the PTA react to these possible changes?
5. How will the physician treat this disorder? Could the treatment have any effect on physical therapy treatment? Should the PTA be aware of any potential side effects of medical management?

Case 2

A 64-year-old woman is currently in inpatient rehabilitation secondary to a left middle cerebral artery cerebrovascular accident. Patient medical history: Anxiety disorder, panic disorder, OCD, and diabetes. Previous level of function: Independent in all activities, but over the past year required at least a once a week assist for general household activities from her husband secondary to bouts of anxiety and panic issues. Husband reports his wife suffers from cleanliness OCD. Current level of function: Minimal to moderate assistance in bed mobility, transfers, and gait due to loss hemiparesis and loss of balance. Plan of care includes strengthening, bed mobility, transfers, gait, and balance activities.

1. Compare and contrast anxiety disorder and panic disorder.
2. During the second treatment session, the patient had a panic attack while working on standing balance activities. What would alert the PTA that this attack was occurring? How should the PTA react to this situation?
3. On the third day of rehab, the patient refuses to leave her room. The patient reports a very strong fear of falling and breaking her hip and no longer wants to

participate in treatment. What is happening with the patient? How should the PTA react to this situation?

4. Monitoring vitals is a common component of treatment. If the patient suffers a panic attack or anxiety disorder, how might the vitals appear?

5. The patient has cleanliness OCD. How might this affect a treatment session? Are there things the PTA could do to help?

WEBSITES

http://psyweb.com/Mdisord/jsp/moodd.jsp

http://www.adaa.org/

http://www.brainsource.com/amazing%20brain.htm

http://www.mentalhealthministries.net/links_resources/other_resources/famouspeople.pdf

http://www.mentalwellness.com/mentalwellness/history.html

http://www.merckmanuals.com/home/sec07/ch098/ch098d.html

http://www.nami.org/template.cfm?section=about_medications

http://www.nimh.nih.gov/health/publications/depression/complete-index.shtml

http://www.schizophrenia.com/

http://www.webmd.com/anxiety-panic/mental-health-causes-mental-illness

http://www.wrongdiagnosis.com/medical/perception_disorder.htm

Substance Abuse

OUTLINE

LEARNING OBJECTIVES

After completion of the chapter the reader should be able to

1. Define the terms *habit*, *tolerance*, *addiction*, and *euphoria*.
2. Compare physical and psychological dependence.
3. Explain the underlying causes of addiction.
4. Describe withdrawal syndromes.
5. Discuss the various classes of substance abuse.
6. Compare marijuana with cocaine.
7. Explain hallucinogens and list two examples.
8. Describe the effects of nicotine on the body.

KEY TERMS

Addiction: Physiologic or psychological dependence on a substance.

Anabolic steroids: Commonly abused hormonal substances that stimulate protein formation, resulting in greater strength and endurance.

Cross-tolerance: Tolerance to similar drugs for which the body has developed a tolerance.

Delirium tremens: The "DTs"; a collection of symptoms resulting from severe withdrawal from alcohol.

DOM: An amphetamine popular at "rave parties," where it is referred to as "STP"; its chemical name is 2,5-dimethoxy-4-methylamphetamine.

Flashbacks: Repeat occurrences of the symptoms of hallucinogens after the actual period of usage is past.

Hallucinogens: Psychedelics; psychoactive substances that can cause serious changes in perceptions of all types.

Hepatotoxin: A substance that is toxic to the liver.

MDA: An amphetamine called the "love drug" because it is believed to enhance sexual desire; its chemical name is 3,4-methylendioxyamphetamine.

MDMA: An amphetamine originally synthesized for research purposes that has since become extremely popular among teens and young adults; its chemical name is 3,4-methylenedioxymethamphetamine but it is commonly called "ecstasy" or "XTC."

Opioids: Chemicals that work by binding to opioid receptors; commonly used for analgesia but cause side effects of sedation, constipation, and respiratory depression.

Overdoses: Ingestions of substances in excessive quantities that may cause serious harm or even death.

Paranoia: An irrational feeling of impending harm from someone or something.

PCP: Phenylcyclohexylpiperidine (commonly called "angel dust" or phencyclidine), it produces a trance-like state that may last for days and results in severe brain damage.

Psychedelics: Substances that alter perception and reality.

Substance abuse: Drug abuse or chemical dependency; use of substances for various effects, which may lead to addiction and dependence.

Synergism: Interaction of several drugs or substances that enhance or magnify their normal effects.

Overview

Substance abuse is also referred to as *chemical dependency*. Nearly 20 million people use illicit drugs, with marijuana use the most common. About 20,000 people die every year from the complications of illicit drug use. For example, alcoholism can lead to cirrhosis of the liver and brain damage. Cocaine is linked to brain and heart damage, whereas anabolic steroid abuse causes hypertension, leading to heart disease. Intravenous drug users often contract hepatitis or HIV, which leads to AIDS. Substance abuse affects the user as well as his or her families and friends. Children of substance abusers are often harmed by the behaviors of their parents.

Substance abuse causes health care treatment problems for users. Medical treatment outcomes can be affected due to adverse drug reactions or interactions, inaccurate diagnostic test results, and aggravation of pathology by illicit drugs and other substances. Health care workers who have abuse problems may have direct access because of the availability of drugs in the health care facility. It is important for health care workers to be able to recognize early signs of drug dependence. There are now many counseling and therapy groups for those affected by substance abuse.

An **addiction** drives a person to continually consume his or her substances of choice repeatedly, while being aware of potential serious consequences. The degree of addiction depends on many different factors and is difficult to predict. The addictive properties of a substance affect how easily it may be discontinued by users.

Terminology

It is important to understand the many terms used to describe substance abuse. Many are similar or overlapping and require clear definition. **Table 26–1** lists commonly used terms relating to substance abuse and their definitions.

Tolerance

Tolerance occurs when the body adapts to a substance after it has been used repeatedly, for varying periods of time depending on the substance. As a result, higher doses are required to achieve the same effects. Drug tolerance is common when using substances that affect the nervous system. It does not develop at the same rate for all drug actions. Drugs that cause nausea and vomiting initially begin to be tolerated. As the body no longer experiences these unpleasant effects, the user "enjoys" the desired effects the drug provides.

Cross-tolerance is tolerance that extends to other drugs similar in chemical structure or effects to the one being abused. For example, heroin causes cross-tolerance to occur when morphine or meperidine (other opioids) are used. Alcoholics may develop cross-tolerance to barbiturates, certain general anesthetics, and benzodiazepines. Tolerance is not the same as immunity or resistance, which refer to the immune system and infections.

Classifications of Substance Abuse

There are many ways to classify abused substances, including *source* and *mode of action*. Commonly abused psychoactive substances, classified under their mode of action, are outlined below:

> **RED FLAG**
>
> **Overdoses** from sedatives and tranquilizers are extremely dangerous, potentially causing cessation of respiration, coma, and death. Benzodiazepines are another class that is widely used but not as dangerous for overdose.

- Central nervous system (CNS) depressants or tranquilizers: Cause a feeling of sedation or relaxation; many are legal but are listed as controlled substances due to their abuse potential.
  - Sedatives and sedative-hypnotics (tranquilizers): Prescribed for sleep disorders and certain types of epilepsy. They include barbiturates and nonbarbiturate sedative-hypnotics. Sedatives are often combined with other commonly abused drugs such as CNS stimulants or alcohol. Many have a long duration of action and cause lethargy, an apathetic attitude, slurred speech, and incoordination.
  - **Opioids** (narcotic analgesics): Prescribed for severe pain, diarrhea, and persistent coughing. They include codeine, morphine, and illegal agents such

TABLE 26–1 Common Terms Related to Substance Abuse	
Term	**Definition**
Addiction	The uncontrollable compulsion to use a substance, often with serious consequences to the user and others. Addiction often results in criminal activities to obtain the substance because judgment is impaired.
Dependence	Physiologic and psychological need for a drug or other substance.
Euphoria	A sense of pleasure ("high") or the altering of perception of reality; decreased awareness of people and environment.
Habit	Practice (often involuntary) of using drugs or other substances at regular, frequent intervals. Common habits include drinking coffee, smoking cigarettes, or using illegal drugs.
Physiologic	A type of dependence wherein the body has adapted to a drug or chemical so that discontinuing the drug results in withdrawal signs (such as tremors or abdominal cramps).
Psychological	A type of dependence wherein the user has a continuing desire to take the drug or substance to function.
Substance abuse (chemical dependency)	The inappropriate or unnecessary (nonmedical) use of drugs or chemicals that impairs the ability to function in some way. The substance is desired to cause euphoria. Drug use interferes with the brain's "reward system," increasing craving for the drug and promoting tolerance and dependence. Substance abuse may include illegal (street) drugs, prescribed drugs, or other readily available substances.
Tolerance	When the body adapts to a substance and needs increased amounts of the substance to achieve the same effect.

as opium and heroin. Effects of oral opioids begin within 30 minutes and can last for more than 24 hours. Parenteral forms produce immediate, intense effects. Symptoms of substance abuse include profound sedation, constricted pupils, respiratory depression, and increased pain threshold. Overdose is extremely dangerous and can lead to death. Addiction can occur rapidly and cause intense withdrawal symptoms.

■ Ethyl alcohol: One of the most commonly abused legal drugs, available in beer, wine, and liquor. Although small quantities have been shown to reduce risk of stroke and heart attack, larger quantities and long-term consumption have devastating effects on all body systems. Alcohol is a depressant that slows the CNS, easily crossing the blood–brain barrier, with effects occurring within 5 to 30 minutes after being consumed. Alcohol is metabolized by the liver slowly, at a rate of about 15 mL/hr (equivalent to one alcoholic beverage serving per hour). Chronic abuse of alcohol leads to cirrhosis of the liver, abnormal blood clotting, nutritional deficiencies, **delirium tremens** (hallucinations, confusion, disorientation, and agitation), anxiety, panic, "crawling" sensations of the skin, and **paranoia**. Withdrawal from alcohol may be life threatening and requires the use of antiseizure medications for treatment.

■ CNS stimulants: Often prescribed for narcolepsy, obesity, and attention deficit hyperactivity disorder. The forms of CNS stimulants commonly abused include amphetamines, methylphenidate, cocaine, and caffeine.

■ Amphetamines and methylphenidate: Effects similar to those of the neurotransmitter norepinephrine. Amphetamines, in high doses, improve self-confidence and cause euphoria, alertness, and empowerment. Long-term use causes anxiety, restlessness, and rage. Due to the negative aspects of amphetamines, they have declined in prescribed uses. Today, illegal laboratories easily produce amphetamines. Methamphetamine is becoming more commonly abused. Its street name is *ice*, and it is usually administered in a powder or crystal form, although it may also be smoked. Another form, methcathinone (street name *cat*), is stronger in its abuse potential. Methylphenidate is mostly used for children with attention deficit hyperactivity disorder, calming them while stimulating alertness. However, older individuals often use methylphenidate in a crushed or dissolved form for inhalation or injection.

> **RED FLAG**
> When methylphenidate is mixed with heroin, the combination is called a *speedball*.

■ Cocaine: Obtained from the leaves of the *coca plant*. When extracted and made into a powder form, the drug is stronger, producing amphetamine-like actions with rapid onset. Cocaine is the second most commonly abused illicit drug in the United States. Although it has medical uses, these have declined with the onset of many safer choices. Cocaine is classified as a schedule II drug. It is usually snorted, smoked, or injected. Small doses cause intense euphoria, analgesia, increased perceptions, and decreased hunger. Larger doses cause sweating, rapid heartbeat, raised body temperature, and dilated pupils. Chronic users develop a runny nose, crusting around the nostrils, and deteriorated nasal cartilage. Withdrawal from amphetamines and cocaine is not as intense as withdrawal from alcohol or barbiturates.

> **RED FLAG**
> Cocaine overdose results in convulsions, dysrhythmias, stroke, or death (because of respiratory arrest).

■ Caffeine: Found naturally in many different plants throughout the world, larger amounts of caffeine are found in coffee, tea, chocolate, soft drinks, and ice cream. Caffeine is added to many over-the-counter pain relievers to increase their effectiveness. It has a strong diuretic effect and can only be metabolized over several hours. This CNS stimulant produces increased alertness, nervousness, restlessness, insomnia, and irritability. It causes bronchodilation, increased blood pressure, higher amounts of stomach acid, and changes in blood glucose levels. Caffeine may lead to physical dependence and tolerance. Withdrawal causes fatigue, headaches, depression, and impaired performance of normal activities.

■ Nicotine: Although sometimes considered a CNS stimulant, it has other unique actions. Nicotine is strongly addictive and carcinogenic when smoked. Cigarette, pipe, or cigar smoke contains over 1,000 chemicals, many of which are carcinogens. When inhaled, nicotine may be effective from 30 minutes to several hours. It causes increased alertness, relaxation, and lightheadedness. Nicotine accelerates the heart rate and increases blood pressure. Smokers have a risk of heart attack that is five times higher than that of nonsmokers. Nicotine also reduces appetite and leads to bronchitis, emphysema, and lung cancer. Severe psychological and physical dependence usually results. Even though tobacco replacement products are available, only 25 percent of smokers remain tobacco-free 1 year after beginning treatment.

■ Cannabinoids: Derived from the hemp plant known as *Cannabis sativa* and include marijuana, hashish, and hash oil. Most cannabinoids are smoked and contain the psychoactive agent called *delta-9-tetrahydrocannabinol*.

■ Marijuana: Also called *grass*, *pot*, *reefer*, *weed*, or *dope*. It is the most commonly used illegal drug in the United States. Marijuana decreases motor activity and coordination and causes disconnected thoughts, paranoia, and euphoria. It increases thirst and appetite and causes telltale "bloodshot" eyes because of its ability to dilate blood vessels. When smoked, marijuana is inhaled very deeply and held within the lungs to intensify effects. It brings up to four times the amount of particulates that tobacco smoking does into the lungs, causing increased risk of lung cancer and respiratory disorders. However, marijuana produces little tolerance or physical dependence. Withdrawal symptoms are extremely mild.

- **Hallucinogens**: Produce altered, dream-like states of consciousness. They are sometimes called **psychedelics**. All hallucinogens are schedule I drugs and have no medical use. The prototype substance for hallucinogens is LSD.

  - Lysergic acid diethylamide (LSD): Common symptoms include laughter, religious revelations, deep personal insights, visions, hallucinations, afterimages (which seem to be projected onto other people as they are moving), unusually bright lights, vivid colors, the hearing of voices, and unusual smells. Sometimes LSD and other hallucinogens cause terrifying experiences, including anxiety, confusion, panic attacks, paranoia, and severe depression. It comes from a fungus that grows on grains such as rye. It is usually administered orally, in capsule, tablet, or liquid form. Often, LSD is dripped onto a special paper containing cartoon images and dried. When a piece or pieces of the paper are ingested, the drug takes effect. Effects of LSD begin within an hour and may last for up to 12 hours. It can lead to psychoses and **flashbacks** but causes little or no dependence.

> **RED FLAG**
> LSD is also called *acid, blotter acid, California sunshine,* and *the beast.*

  - Other hallucinogens: Include mescaline (from the peyote cactus), **MDMA** (also called ecstasy [XTC], an amphetamine that has become popular with teenagers and young adults), **DOM** (popular at "rave parties," where it is known as "STP"), **MDA** (which is believed to enhance sexual desire), **PCP** (also known as "angel dust" or phencyclidine), ketamine (also known as the "date rape" drug or *special coke*), and psilocybin ("magic mushrooms").

Causes of Substance Abuse

The causes of substance abuse are believed to include personality deficits, biologic abnormalities, dysfunctional relationships, psychological imbalances, or any combination of these. Gender may play a role as well, and studies are ongoing about whether smoking and alcohol use lead to later addiction to different drugs. Substance abuse has been linked to disease, easy access to drugs, heredity, stress, increased use of antianxiety drugs, and increased acceptance of the use of alcohol and marijuana.

The media glamorizes substance abuse, leading many young people, via peer pressure, to experiment with various drugs. Many people resort to drug use to cope with anxiety and stress. Younger people are becoming addicted to various substances at alarming rates. Patients who take prescription pain-relieving drugs of all types risk becoming dependent because these drugs are addictive. It is important to educate the public about the causes of substance abuse, related factors, and methods of treatment as well as prevention.

In recent years the abuse of **anabolic steroids** has become more common. Many athletes and bodybuilders use these drugs illegally to boost their athletic performance. Anabolic steroids have many adverse effects, including the reduction of sexual function

> **RED FLAG**
> Anabolic steroids have been shown to cause high blood pressure, mood disorders, liver cancer, and serious damage to the heart.

and changes to normal sex characteristics. Another area of concern is the emergence of "date-rape" drugs, wherein substances such as lorazepam or gamma-hydroxybutyrate are mixed with alcohol to induce a quick, deep sleep. The person given this combination usually has no memory of the events that occurred while under the influence of these drugs.

Recognizing Substance Abuse

It is difficult to recognize the level of substance abuse in many individuals due to differences in how each person tolerates various drugs. Some can only take small amounts of substances without appearing to be "drugged," whereas others have a much higher tolerance level. Because most drugs that are abused are taken orally, there may be no easily visible signs of a person using them. Those who inject drugs will have obvious injection marks on their arms, but these users are in the minority.

In general, substance abuse can be recognized by symptoms such as behavior changes, slowed reflexes, reduced coordination, lethargy or hyperactivity, or slurred speech. Many substance abusers react with anger, embarrassment, or defense techniques when questioned about their usage. A person who "needs" a drink or drug when they feel stress is a likely substance abuser. Other signs of abuse include lack of attentiveness to personal hygiene and appearance, increased excuses for absenteeism from work or other activities, malnutrition, and increased health problems such as anemia or infections.

Health care workers must be able to recognize the signs of substance abuse. For example, requests for pain medications from patients not being treated for pain should be of concern. Drug samples and prescription order forms should be kept away from patients and visitors to the medical office.

Withdrawal Syndrome

Discontinuing a drug to which the body has become physically dependent may cause *withdrawal sickness,* also known as *withdrawal syndrome.* This can range from mild to severe and causes irritability, nausea, vomiting, tremors, high blood pressure, stomach cramps, convulsions, and psychotic episodes. Withdrawal from a drug should be undertaken only under medical supervision.

Often, medically supervised withdrawal from a substance may require the use of other approved medications to lessen the severity of symptoms. For example, alcohol withdrawal commonly involves short-acting benzodiazepines, and nicotine withdrawal usually involves nicotine replacement patches, gums, and other products. Many patients undergoing alcohol or narcotic withdrawal benefit to the greatest extent from substance abuse treatment facilities.

Chronic substance abuse is often based on conditions, surroundings, and other people who also abuse the substance. Contact with other substance abusers after trying to quit on the patient's own initiative often causes him or her to revert to old behaviors. Self-help groups such as Alcoholics Anonymous help recovering users to interact with others who can offer support, counseling, and guidance.

Complications of Substance Abuse

Increased doses of certain drugs may cause toxic effects (overdose) or even death. Combinations of legal or illegal drugs or concurrent use of drugs with alcohol may result in **synergism**, wherein a much stronger reaction occurs than anticipated. Alcohol often plays a major role in drug combination overdoses. Barbiturates and narcotics may depress respirations to a very low level, leading to respiratory failure, cardiac arrest, coma, and death. Certain drugs, when combined with alcohol, are very likely to cause brain damage.

> **RED FLAG**
> Drugs such as "ecstasy" raise the blood pressure to such high levels that brain damage can result.

Many drugs, including alcohol, can harm a developing fetus and cause congenital defects. Fetal alcohol syndrome often causes characteristic facial and physical abnormalities as well as mental deficits. In the third trimester, alcohol consumption usually causes cognitive and behavioral abnormalities in the fetus. Physical and neurologic problems may be numerous as a result of fetal alcohol syndrome. Often, functional capabilities are very different from normal children. Movements may also be impaired because of physical deformity. The physical therapist assistant (PTA) should be aware that behavioral and cognitive problems may impair the child's ability to follow physical therapy instructions and perform exercises adequately.

Cigarette smoking may cause infertility in both males and females and can lead to low birth weight, infant irritability, stillbirth, and miscarriage if smoking continues during pregnancy. Other drugs such as cocaine lead to the newborn becoming addicted and requiring withdrawal therapy. It may also result in developmental defects, premature birth, irregular heartbeat, and increased blood pressure. Often, infants born to women who used cocaine during pregnancy experience fatal heart attacks, other heart abnormalities, or strokes early in life.

Hallucinogens and psychedelic drugs such as LSD may lead to euphoria but also cause acute fear, panic, depression, and increased risk of suicide. Many hallucinogens also cause nausea, increased blood pressure, and tremors. Drug abusers who share needles commonly contract diseases such as hepatitis B and HIV.

> **RED FLAG**
> Chronic alcoholism may also damage the brain and nervous system because of neurotoxicity and malnutrition.

Alcohol abuse leads to cirrhosis of the liver and a variety of other conditions. Alcohol is an irritant, a **hepatotoxin** that causes the accumulation of lipids in liver cells, followed by inflammation and necrosis (alcoholic hepatitis). Beyond this development, fibrosis or scar tissue formation occurs, destroying the liver's ability to function. Signs of developing liver disease may be mild until the condition advances and becomes irreversible. Common signs include confusion, disorientation, loss of motor coordination, altered personality, and amnesia.

Getting Help

When a person overdoses or suffers from toxic effects of any substance, he or she should be treated immediately in an emergency room. Drug rehabilitation centers offer reliable experience in dealing with the withdrawal process. Support includes psychiatric intervention as well as medical treatment, with individualized treatment for addiction. Long-term therapy is usually required, with abstinence from all addictive substances as the goal. Patients with addictions to heroin and similar drugs may require methadone therapy to prevent withdrawal symptoms and lessen the craving for narcotics.

For alcoholics, a drug known as disulfiram is often used. It causes unpleasant reactions if alcohol is used concurrently, even in small amounts. Many people requiring treatment for substance abuse need to have protein and vitamin B deficits addressed. Ongoing behavior modification therapy and counseling are often required. Support groups include Alcoholics Anonymous (for recovering alcoholics) and Al-Anon (for their families).

SUMMARY

Substance abuse affects health care because it can cause inaccuracy of testing, masking or aggravation of disease, and drug interactions. Abused substances include prescription medications, illegal street drugs, alcohol, and household substances. Dependency may be physiologic, psychological, or both. Various abused substances may produce depression or stimulation of the CNS. Physical and behavioral changes are often signs of substance abuse. Overdose or toxicity are frequent outcomes of substance abuse and may lead to the death of the user. Withdrawal from substances should be undertaken only under medical supervision. Substance abuse may also affect children, because many drugs affect the developing fetus. Complications of substance abuse include infections, liver disease, malnutrition, cardiovascular disorders, and CNS damage. Because PTAs may work with patients who are also substance abusers, they need to recognize the signs and symptoms of substance abuse and report these to their PT.

REVIEW QUESTIONS

Select the best response to each question.

1. The need to increase the amount and frequency of a drug is described as
   a. resistance
   b. addiction
   c. tolerance
   d. immunity

2. All the following are symptoms of nicotine withdrawal *except*
   a. weight gain
   b. vomiting
   c. headache
   d. anxiety

3. Marijuana produces effects that occur within minutes of ingestion and last up to
   a. 10 hours
   b. 12 hours
   c. 24 hours
   d. 72 hours

4. The most commonly abused legal substance is
   a. marijuana
   b. oral opioids
   c. barbiturates
   d. alcohol

5. The complications of anabolic steroids include all the following *except*
   a. hypertension
   b. hypotension
   c. liver cancer
   d. mood disorders

6. Fetal alcohol syndrome often causes characteristic facial abnormalities as well as which of the following?
   a. mental retardation
   b. liver disease
   c. pancreatitis
   d. cardiac arrest

7. Cocaine is in which of the five drug schedules?
   a. I
   b. II
   c. III
   d. V

8. All the following drugs cause significant withdrawal symptoms *except*
   a. barbiturates
   b. cocaine and amphetamines
   c. aminoglycosides
   d. opioids

9. Chronic alcoholism is hepatotoxic as well as which of the following?
   a. nephrotoxic
   b. neurotoxic
   c. hemotoxic
   d. ototoxic

10. Dextroamphetamine is commonly called
   a. crack
   b. pot
   c. ice
   d. smack

CASE STUDIES

Karen Coupe, PT, DPT, MSEd

Case 1

A 58-year-old man was hospitalized secondary to a motor vehicle accident where he suffered the following: rib fractures, left tibia fracture, left ulna fracture, and multiple abrasions and contusions. At the time of the accident, the patient's blood alcohol level was 0.13 percent. Patient medical history: Cirrhosis of the liver, chronic gastritis, osteoporosis, and diabetes. The patient has a 32-year history of alcohol abuse and has been in and out of treatment 16 times. The plan of care includes bed mobility, transfers, and gait training with a front-wheeled rolling walker with left upper extremity adaptation.

1. Based on the patient's long-term use of alcohol, what signs and symptoms might the PTA see during physical therapy sessions that indicate withdrawal? Could some potentially be life threatening?

2. This patient has a number of health issues. Explain cirrhosis of the liver and the role of alcohol in this pathology.

3. Could alcohol be the cause of the patient's chronic gastritis? Why or why not?

4. Could alcohol cause diabetes and osteoporosis? Why or why not?

5. Research all the body systems alcohol can potentially affect and list the potential pathologies.

Case 2

A PTA is employed in a pain management clinic that works directly in conjunction with a substance abuse rehabilitation center. The pain management facility treats patients who have chronic musculoskeletal or neurologic pain and are currently undergoing treatment for substance abuse. The PTA is involved in the following situations.

1. A 28-year-old man addicted to OxyContin. The patient was a star college football quarterback who tore his rotator cuff. What are the main effects of the drug used by this patient? What class of drugs does OxyContin fall under? Would this patient suffer withdrawal? Why?

2. A 19-year-old man who had a cocaine addiction. The patient left the rehabilitation center against medical advice. The patient was transported to the emergency department after being found unconscious at home by a friend. Final diagnosis was cocaine overdose and secondary stroke. Explain why cocaine could cause a stroke. Are there other major pathologies that could occur with cocaine use?

3. A large population of patients at the rehabilitation center smoke cigarettes. The PTA is a member of the educational wellness committee and is scheduled to provide an educational program on smoking cessation along with the facility physician. The PTA is going to talk about the physical effects of smoking and the physical benefits of not smoking. What would you include in each of these topics?

4. Reviewing scenarios 1 through 3, how would you differentiate an addiction from a habit? Can both create dependence? Why or why not?

5. Could each of the above scenarios have a physical and psychological dependence? Why or why not?

WEBSITES

http://digestive.niddk.nih.gov/ddiseases/pubs/cirrhosis/

http://www.allbusiness.com/human-resources/workforce-management/520699-1.html

http://www.drugfree.org/intervene

http://www.emedicinehealth.com/substance_abuse/article_em.htm

http://www.medicinenet.com/alcohol_abuse_and_alcoholism/article.htm

http://www.medicinenet.com/drug_abuse/article.htm

http://www.medscape.com/viewarticle/452724_7

http://www.niaaa.nih.gov/Pages/default.aspx

http://www.nlm.nih.gov/medlineplus/cocaine.html

http://www.samhsa.gov/

Fluid, Electrolyte, and Acid-Base Imbalances

LEARNING OBJECTIVES

After completion of the chapter the reader should be able to

1. Define the terms *electrolyte*, *osmotic pressure*, and *acid-base balance*.
2. Differentiate intracellular from extracellular fluid compartments in terms of distribution and composition of water and electrolytes.
3. List the causes of hypokalemia and hyperkalemia.
4. Describe water intoxication and the causes of edema.
5. Explain acid-base balance.
6. Describe the factors that cause acidosis.
7. Differentiate between respiratory alkalosis and respiratory acidosis.
8. Explain the difference between metabolic acidosis and metabolic alkalosis.

KEY TERMS

Acid-base buffer systems: Systems by which a nearly constant pH level of body fluids is maintained.

Acidosis: A clinical state wherein the pH of the blood drops significantly below 7.35.

Acids: Substances that ionize in water to release hydrogen ions.

Alkalosis: A state wherein the pH of the blood rises significantly above 7.4; alkalosis may be due to the side effects of drugs or disease states.

Bases: Substances that ionize in water, releasing hydroxyl ions, having a pH greater than 7.0.

Electrolyte balance: A condition consisting of an equal amount of electrolytes entering and leaving the body.

Electrolytes: Compounds that, in solution, dissociate into positive and negative ions.

Hydrostatic pressure: Pressure of fluids or their properties when in equilibrium.

Hyperchloremia: An excessive concentration of chloride in the blood.

Hyperkalemia: An excessive concentration of potassium in the blood.

Hypernatremia: An excessive concentration of sodium in the blood.

Hypochloremia: A lower than normal concentration of chloride in the blood.

Hypokalemia: A lower than normal concentration of potassium in the blood.

Hyponatremia: A lower than normal concentration of sodium in the blood.

Osmotic pressure: Pressure exerted on a differentially permeable membrane separating a solution from a solvent; the membrane is impermeable to the solutes in the solution and permeable only to the solvent.

pH: A chemical expression that indicates the degree of acidity or alkalinity of a solution.

Transcellular fluid: A portion of the extracellular fluid that includes the fluid within special body cavities.

Water balance: Equivalence of the volume of water entering the body with the volume leaving it.

Water of metabolism: Water produced as a byproduct of metabolism.

Overview

The human body is made up mostly of liquid, which contains various electrolytes dissolved in water. The human body maintains homeostasis by balance between fluid, **electrolytes**, and acids and/or bases. The movement of fluids and electrolytes is regulated between various fluid compartments within the body. Both **hydrostatic pressure** and **osmotic pressure** regulate this movement. The most common water balance disorders include dehydration, edema, and water intoxication. Imbalances of electrolytes are critical and may cause serious conditions to develop, such as hypernatremia, hypocalcemia, hyperkalemia, or hypokalemia.

Distribution of Body Fluids

The human body contains the following fluids: the plasma of the circulating blood, the interstitial fluid between the cells, and the cell fluid within the cells. These fluids can move freely between various compartments. This stabilizes the distribution and composition of body fluids.

Body Fluid Compartments

Most adult males have about 63 percent body water, whereas adult females have only about 52 percent. This is because males have more muscle mass and females more adipose tissue, which has low amounts of water. There are about 40 liters of water in the adult human body. Along with dissolved electrolytes, this water is distributed into an *intracellular fluid (ICF) compartment* and an *extracellular fluid (ECF) compartment*. The ICF compartment includes water and electrolytes that are enclosed by cell membranes.

The ECF compartment includes fluid outside the cells. The fluids in this compartment make up about 37 percent of total body water volume (**Figure 27–1**). This fluid lies within the blood vessels as plasma, tissue spaces as interstitial fluid, and lymphatic vessels as lymph. A certain amount of ECF is separated from other ECF by epithelial layers. **Transcellular fluid** includes the following types of fluid:

- Aqueous and vitreous humors: In the eyes
- Cerebrospinal fluid: In the central nervous system
- Exocrine gland secretions
- Serous fluid: In the body cavities
- Synovial fluid: In the joints

Body Fluid Composition

Body fluids consist of certain amounts of proteins, fats, water, and minerals. These vary among individuals as a result of differences in body density and degree of obesity. ICFs have, in general, high concentrations of magnesium, phosphate, and potassium ions. They have more sulfate and less bicarbonate, chloride, and sodium ions than ECFs. ICFs have higher concentrations of protein than plasma. ECFs have high concentrations of bicarbonate, chloride, and sodium ions. They also have more calcium ions and less magnesium, phosphate, potassium, and sulfate ions than ICF. Blood plasma, an ECF, has much more protein than either lymph or interstitial fluid. **Figure 27–2** shows comparisons of concentrations of electrolytes in ICF and ECF.

Movement of Fluid Between Compartments

Hydrostatic pressure and osmotic pressure regulate the movement of water and electrolytes between fluid compartments (**Figure 27–3**). Fluid leaves the plasma from the arteriolar capillary ends to enter the interstitial spaces via a net outward force (hydrostatic pressure, also known as blood pressure). It returns to plasma from the venular ends of capillaries due to a net inward force (colloid osmotic pressure) from plasma proteins. Hydrostatic pressure inside interstitial spaces forces fluid into lymph capillaries, with lymph circulation returning interstitial fluid to the plasma.

Therefore, similar pressures control fluid movement between the ICF and ECF. Hydrostatic pressure is usually equal and stable, so it is an osmotic pressure change that usually causes any net fluid movements. A decrease of the normally high sodium ion concentrations in ECF causes net movement of water from the ECF to the ICF via osmosis. This causes the cells to swell. The opposite situation causes sodium to increase in the ICF, moving water outward toward the ECF, resulting in shrinking of cells.

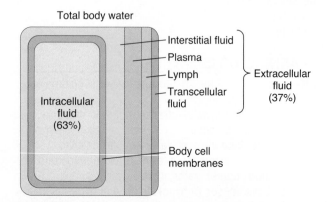

Figure 27–1 Cell membranes separate intracellular and extracellular fluids.

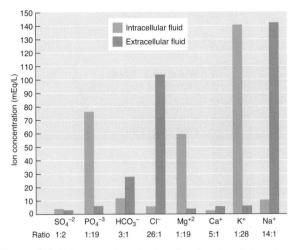

Figure 27–2 Concentration of various ions in extracellular and intracellular fluid.

Source: Adapted from Shier, D. N., Butler, J. L., and Lewis, R. Hole's *Essentials of Human Anatomy & Physiology*, Tenth edition. McGraw-Hill Higher Education, 2009.

Pediatrics and Distribution of Body Fluids

At birth, total body water makes up about 75 to 80 percent of the body weight. By age 1 year, an infant's total body water is approximately 67 percent. Infants have a high metabolic rate and greater body surface area, making them susceptible to significant total body water changes. Dehydration may occur because the kidneys of newborns are not mature until 6 months after birth, and fluids or electrolytes may be lost significantly.

In young children, until the onset of puberty (between 11 and 13 years of age), total body water decreases to between 60 and 65 percent of body weight. By age 13, total body water is close to adult levels, depending on the child's gender. Due to the influence of estrogen, females have greater adipose tissue and less body water than males. Males have increased muscle mass, which requires more body water.

> **RED FLAG**
>
> Infants are at risk for dehydration because their bodies need to have a higher proportion of water to total body weight.

Water Balance Disorders

Common water balance disorders include dehydration, water intoxication, and edema. **Water balance** exists when total water intake equals total water output. Most normal adults take in and lose approximately 2,500 mL of water each day. This breaks down into 60 percent supplied by drinking water or other beverages, 30 percent supplied by moist foods, and 10 percent as a byproduct of oxidative metabolism of nutrients (known as **water of metabolism**). The primary regulator of water input is thirst, which is a homeostatic mechanism usually triggered whenever total body water decreases by as little as 1 percent. Water is normally lost by urine, feces, sweat, evaporation of water from the skin, and breathing. Water balance requires 2,500 mL to be eliminated each day. For example, 60 percent is lost in the urine, 28 percent by evaporation from the skin and lungs, 6 percent in the feces,

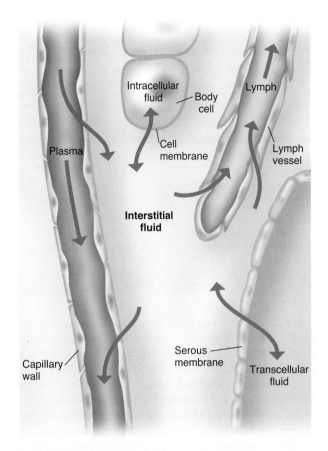

Figure 27–3 Blood plasma has much higher levels of protein than interstitial fluid or lymph.

Source: Adapted from Shier, D. N., Butler, J. L., and Lewis, R. Hole's *Essentials of Human Anatomy & Physiology*, Tenth edition. McGraw-Hill Higher Education, 2009.

and 6 percent in sweat. These percentages may be due to environmental temperature, relative humidity, and physical exercise (**Figure 27–4**).

Dehydration

Dehydration occurs when water output exceeds water intake, which may follow prolonged water deprivation or excess sweating. In dehydration, ECF becomes concentrated, with water leaving the cells via osmosis. Most conditions of dehydration include prolonged diarrhea or vomiting. Fluid intake is usually decreased, resulting in dehydration. Because there is insufficient water for sweat, hyperthermia may develop as the body is unable to regulate its temperature.

In infants, dehydration is a greater risk because their kidneys are less able to conserve water than adults. In the elderly, the sensitivity of the thirst mechanism decreases. Occasionally, debilitated or comatose patients become dehydrated because of inadequate intake of fluid. To treat dehydration, water and electrolytes must sometimes be replaced intravenously. This is essential, because if only water is replaced, the ECF becomes too diluted, causing *water intoxication*.

> **RED FLAG**
>
> In general, any factor that causes intracellular dehydration will cause a sensation of thirst. Examples of metabolic problems that can stimulate thirst include hypernatremia, hyperglycemia, hypercalcemia, and fever.

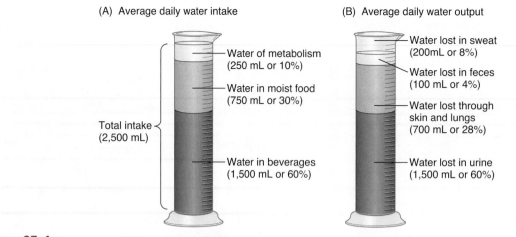

(A) Average daily water intake

Total intake (2,500 mL)
- Water of metabolism (250 mL or 10%)
- Water in moist food (750 mL or 30%)
- Water in beverages (1,500 mL or 60%)

(B) Average daily water output
- Water lost in sweat (200 mL or 8%)
- Water lost in feces (100 mL or 4%)
- Water lost through skin and lungs (700 mL or 28%)
- Water lost in urine (1,500 mL or 60%)

Figure 27–4 Water balance. (A) Major sources of body water, and (B) routes by which the body loses water.

Water Intoxication

Water intoxication may result from administering too much fluid intravenously or when an individual with impaired renal function drinks a large amount of fluid. This condition occurs when the kidneys are unable to excrete efficiently. Overhydration may also alter the concentration of the electrolytes in the ECF, even in a person with normal kidney function.

As water is absorbed from the digestive system, the volume in the ECF increases. Therefore, the sodium ion concentration becomes more diluted. Hyponatremia (lowered sodium ion concentration) may have serious, potentially life-threatening consequences. It may occur in infants who are given water as a supplement to formula or when infant formula is diluted with too much water. Infants under 6 months are at greatest risk for hyponatremia due to immature kidney function.

In infants, water intoxication may cause seizures, although this condition is very rare. As their serum sodium levels drop, the first symptom is a fluttering of the eyes. The ECF becomes hypotonic, and water enters the cells quickly via osmosis, which can lead to coma (due to swelling brain tissues). Water intoxication is treated with restricted water intake and the administration of hypertonic salt solutions.

> **RED FLAG**
> In elderly patients and those with impaired cardiac or renal function, the rate of intravenous fluid administration must be carefully monitored, based on patient response.

Edema

Edema is an abnormal accumulation of ECF inside the interstitial spaces. It may be caused by hypoproteinemia, increased venous pressure, increased capillary permeability, or obstruction of lymphatic vessels. *Hypoproteinemia* may be caused by liver disease, kidney disease, or starvation. This decreases the plasma protein concentration, decreasing plasma colloid osmotic pressure to reduce normal return of tissue fluid to the venular capillary ends. Therefore, tissue fluid accumulates in the interstitial spaces.

Edema may also result from lymphatic obstructions due to cancer, surgery, or parasitic infections, interfering with normal movement of lymph fluid. The osmotic pressure of the interstitial fluid rises, drawing even more fluid into the interstitial spaces. Also, if liver blood flow into the inferior vena cava is blocked, venous pressure increases, and fluid with a high concentration of protein moves from the surfaces of the liver and intestine into the peritoneal cavity. This increases abdominal fluid osmotic pressure, attracting more water by osmosis. This condition is called *ascites*, which is very painful and distends the abdomen greatly.

Because of inflammation, increased capillary permeability may also cause edema. The release of histamine or other chemicals causes vasodilation and increased capillary permeability. Excess fluid is filtered from the capillaries into the interstitial spaces.

Electrolyte Balance

Electrolyte balance occurs when the electrolytes gained by the body equal those lost. Electrolyte balance is regulated by homeostasis. The most important electrolytes for cellular functions are sodium, potassium, calcium, magnesium, chloride, sulfate, phosphate, bicarbonate, and hydrogen ions. Electrolytes are mostly provided by food sources, followed by water and other beverages, and, finally, as byproducts of metabolic reactions.

Usually, response to hunger and thirst provides enough electrolytes for the body, although a severe electrolyte deficiency may produce a craving for salt. Electrolyte output normally occurs by sweating and in the feces, although the majority occurs because of kidney function and the production of urine. Electrolyte balance is maintained in part by the alteration of electrolyte output by the kidneys. For the maintenance of cell membrane potential, muscle fiber contraction, and nerve impulse conduction, positively charged ions such as calcium, potassium, and sodium must be precisely concentrated.

These ions are also regulated by the kidneys and by the hormone *aldosterone*, secreted from the adrenal cortex. Aldosterone increases sodium ion reabsorption in the kidneys' distal convoluted tubules and collecting ducts. It also enhances tubular reabsorption of sodium ions and causes tubular secretion of potassium ions. When calcium ion levels drop below normal, the parathyroid glands secrete parathyroid hormone, which returns calcium concentration in the ECFs to normal. Antidiuretic hormone from the posterior pituitary gland also affects the collecting ducts to reabsorb water from the kidneys to the blood circulation.

Renal tubules passively reabsorb negatively charged ions such as chloride in response to active tubular reabsorption of positively charged sodium ions. Active transport mechanisms that have limited transport capacities regulate, in part, some negatively charged ions (such as phosphate and sulfate). Therefore, if extracellular phosphate ions are low, renal tubules reabsorb phosphate ions. Conversely, if the renal plasma threshold of phosphate is exceeded, excess amounts of phosphate are excreted in the urine.

> **RED FLAG**
> Large amounts of sodium and potassium may also be lost in the urine as a result of prolonged use of diuretics.

Hypernatremia

Hypernatremia exists when serum sodium levels exceed 145 milliequivalents per liter (mEq/L). The normal range of active sodium in the ECF is from 135 to 145 mEq/L. This condition may be caused by a net loss of water or an acute gain in sodium. Hypernatremia causes intracellular dehydration and can lead to hypervolemia and hyperosmolality. This condition is primarily seen in the elderly; however, hospital-acquired hypernatremia occurs in patients of all ages. In adults, a serum sodium concentration greater than 160 mEq/L is associated with a high mortality rate.

High sodium levels are likely to occur with inappropriate administration of hypertonic saline solution or from oversecretion of aldosterone. When sodium levels rise as water levels decrease, fever or respiratory infections often occur. Other causes of water loss in relation to sodium are diabetes insipidus or mellitus, polyuria, diarrhea, and profuse sweating. It also occurs when water intake in insufficient, such as in comatose, confused, or immobilized patients.

In hypernatremia, water is redistributed to the extracellular space, causing intracellular dehydration, thirst, fever, dry mucous membranes, and restlessness. Central nervous system symptoms include hyperactive reflexes (hyperreflexia) and muscle twitching. More serious symptoms include pulmonary edema and convulsions.

Hyponatremia

Hyponatremia occurs when serum sodium concentration falls below 135 mEq/L. This usually causes hypoosmolality, with water movement into cells. Hyponatremia may be caused by sodium loss, dilution of body sodium levels, or inadequate sodium intake. *Pure sodium deficits* are often caused by extrarenal losses caused by diarrhea, vomiting, burns, gastrointestinal suctioning, or use of diuretics. *Inadequate intake* of dietary sodium is possible, although rare, when low-sodium diets are consumed while taking diuretics. *Dilutional hyponatremias* may result when total body water is excessive compared with total body sodium.

When acute renal failure occurs, both total body water and sodium levels are increased, but the total body water levels are higher than the sodium levels. This produces *hypoosmolar hyponatremia*. Conditions such as hyperlipidemia, hyperglycemia, and hyperproteinemia may cause *hypertonic hyponatremia*. Sodium deficits affect the ability of cells to normally depolarize and repolarize. Hyponatremia causes symptoms of confusion, lethargy, apprehension, depressed reflexes, seizures, and coma. *Isotonic hypovolemia* is a related condition, which may cause hypotension, decreased urine output, and tachycardia. Dilutional hyponatremias may cause edema, weight gain, ascites, and distention of the jugular veins.

Hyperchloremia

Hyperchloremia is an abnormally elevated level of chloride ions in the blood. This condition can be related to hypernatremia and metabolic acidosis. Use of an ammonium chloride diuretic can result in hyperchloremia, but this is seen infrequently. There are no specific symptoms associated with hyperchloremia.

Hypochloremia

Hypochloremia is a loss of chloride that usually results from hyponatremia or elevated bicarbonate concentration, such as seen in metabolic alkalosis. It develops with loss of hydrochloric acid and vomiting. When a chloride deficiency exists, it may be accompanied by a sodium deficit that is related to use of diuretics or restricted intake of sodium. Hypochloremia is an important characterization of cystic fibrosis.

Hyperkalemia

Hyperkalemia is an increase in plasma levels of potassium in excess of 5 mEq/L. It usually occurs in unhealthy individuals whose metabolism cannot prevent excess potassium accumulation in the ECF. Hyperkalemia is usually caused by decreased renal elimination, excessively rapid administration, and movement of potassium from the ICF to the ECF. The most common cause is decreased renal function. When chronic, hyperkalemia is usually associated with renal failure. Hyperkalemia can potentially cause heart arrhythmias.

Potassium excretion may be increased by the effects of aldosterone upon the distal tubular sodium-potassium exchange system. Potassium-sparing diuretics can also be causative, as can angiotensin-converting enzyme inhibitors and angiotensin II receptor blockers. Excessive consumption of potassium may also cause hyperkalemia, but this usually cannot affect otherwise healthy individuals. Burns and crushing injuries may also cause potassium to be released into the ECF.

Signs and symptoms of hyperkalemia include nausea, vomiting, intestinal cramps, diarrhea, paresthesias, dizziness, weakness, muscle cramps, electrocardiograph changes, and risk of cardiac arrest. The first symptom associated with this condition is usually paresthesia.

Hyperkalemia is usually treated with calcium gluconate given intravenously, insulin, and glucose. Adequate levels of dietary potassium should be attained. Sodium polystyrene sulfonate may be used to remove potassium ions from the colon.

> **RED FLAG**
> The most serious effects of hyperkalemia affect the heart and include tachycardia, potentially fatal ventricular fibrillation, and cardiac arrest.

Hypokalemia

Hypokalemia (potassium deficiency) occurs when serum potassium concentrations fall below 3.5 mEq/L. Changes in potassium balance may be somewhat gauged by plasma concentration. Usually, lowered serum potassium indicates loss of total body potassium. The causes of potassium deficit are because of inadequate intake, excessive loss (via the gastrointestinal tract, skin, or kidneys), and redistribution between the ICF and ECF compartments.

Inadequate intake of potassium may be prevented by consuming at least 10 to 30 mEq/day. The kidneys are mostly responsible for excessive loss of potassium, allowing 80 to 90 percent of the daily potassium loss via the urine. Renal losses of potassium are heightened by aldosterone and cortisol. Excess secretion of aldosterone by tumor cells causes severe potassium losses. Losses of potassium from the skin and gastrointestinal tract are usually minimal but can become excessive in conditions such as burns and excessive sweating. Redistribution of potassium from the ECF to the ICF compartment can cause a large decrease in potassium plasma concentration. The most common cause of hypokalemia is diuretic therapy (except with the use of potassium-sparing diuretics).

Hypokalemia usually causes muscle weakness, cramps, and irregular heart rhythms. As the kidneys attempt to conserve potassium, their ability to concentrate the urine is impaired. Various gastrointestinal conditions impair potassium intake and exaggerate hypokalemia. When cardiovascular function is affected, postural hypotension is a common result. Other symptoms may be digitalis toxicity during use of this drug and ventricular dysrhythmias. Changes in electrocardiograph readings often occur with this condition, and patients complain of fatigue, muscle cramps during exercise, and weakness.

Hypokalemia is usually treated by increased intake of dietary potassium via dried fruits, meats, fruit juices (especially orange juice), and bananas. Persons receiving diuretic therapy or taking digitalis are usually prescribed oral potassium supplements as a preventative measure. Intravenous potassium may be given when rapid replacement is required or the oral route is not tolerated. This must be handled carefully, as rapid infusion of concentrated potassium can lead to cardiac arrest. Magnesium replacement is related and may also be indicated.

Acid-Base Balance

Electrolytes that dissociate in water and release hydrogen ions are called **acids**. Electrolytes that release ions that combine with hydrogen ions are called **bases**. Homeostasis is maintained when acid and base concentrations in body fluids are controlled. Most hydrogen ions originate as a result of metabolic processes, with small quantities being absorbed directly by the digestive tract. Sources of hydrogen ions are as follows:

- *Aerobic respiration of glucose*, which produces carbon dioxide and water. *Carbonic acid* is formed as carbon dioxide diffuses out of cells and reacts with water in the ECFs. It then ionizes, releasing hydrogen and bicarbonate ions.

- *Anaerobic respiration of glucose*, which produces *lactic acid*, adding hydrogen ions to body fluids.
- *Breakdown (hydrolysis) of phosphoproteins and nucleic acids*, including phosphorus. When oxidized, these substances produce *phosphoric acid*, which releases hydrogen ions when ionized.
- *Incomplete oxidation of fatty acids*, which produces *acidic ketone bodies*, increasing hydrogen ion concentration.
- *Oxidation of sulfur-containing amino acids*, which yields *sulfuric acid*, which releases hydrogen ions when ionized.

Strong acids are defined as those that dissociate to release hydrogen ions more completely. Hydrochloric acid in gastric juice is a strong acid. *Weak acids* are defined as those that dissociate to release hydrogen ions less completely. Carbonic acid, produced when carbon dioxide reacts with water, is a weak acid. Bases release ions, such as hydroxyl ions, that can combine with hydrogen ions. This lowers the hydrogen ion concentration. Therefore, because sodium hydroxide releases hydroxyl ions and sodium bicarbonate releases bicarbonate ions, they are considered to be bases. Strong bases dissociate to release more hydroxyl ions than weak bases.

> **RED FLAG**
> Despite the large amounts of acid produced, the body fluids remain slightly alkaline.

Acid-base buffer systems regulate hydrogen ion concentration in body fluids. They exist in all body fluids, consisting of chemicals that combine with excess acids or bases, helping to minimize pH changes in body fluids. The following are the most important acid-base buffer systems:

- *Bicarbonate buffer system*, which is present in both ICFs and ECFs. It uses bicarbonate ions and carbonic acid to minimize any increase in hydrogen ion concentration of body fluids.
- *Phosphate buffer system*, which is also present in both ICFs and ECFs. When conditions are acidic, monohydrogen phosphate ions react with hydrogen ions to produce dihydrogen phosphate. When conditions are alkaline, dihydrogen phosphate ions release hydrogen ions.
- *Protein buffer system*, which consists of plasma proteins such as albumins and certain cell proteins, including hemoglobin. When pH falls, amino groups accept hydrogen ions. When it rises, carboxyl groups can ionize to release hydrogen ions. Therefore, protein molecules can operate as an acid-base buffer system to minimize pH changes.

In the brainstem, the medullary respiratory center helps regulate hydrogen ion concentration by controlling the rate and depth of breathing. If cells increase carbon dioxide production, carbonic acid production increases. If cells are less active, production of carbon dioxide and hydrogen ions remains lower, and both breathing rate and depth stay close to resting levels (**Figure 27–5**).

Nephrons in the kidneys help to regulate hydrogen ion concentrations by excreting hydrogen ions in the urine. Hydrogen ion concentration regulators each operate at different rates. These chemical buffer systems are sometimes

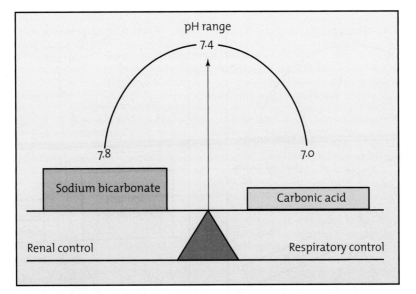

Figure 27–5 "Board-and-fulcrum" concept of normal bicarbonate–carbonic acid relationships.

referred to as the body's first line of defense against changes in pH. The second line of defense consists of physiologic buffer systems and includes respiratory and renal mechanisms.

Acid-Base Imbalance

The pH of arterial blood normally ranges from 7.35 to 7.45, and slight changes to pH levels can result in serious related conditions. A pH level below 7.35 produces *acidosis*, whereas a pH level above 7.45 produces *alkalosis*, both of which can be life threatening. If pH drops below 6.8 or rises above 8.0 for more than a few hours, the patient may not be able to recover. Acidosis is caused by either an accumulation of acids or loss of bases, increasing hydrogen ion concentration. Alkalosis is caused by the reverse situation, decreasing hydrogen ion concentration. **Table 27–1** illustrates the effects of respiratory and metabolic acidosis and alkalosis.

Acidosis

Acidosis is an abnormal increase in hydrogen ion concentration in the body, resulting from an accumulation of an acid or the loss of a base. The two major types are *respiratory acidosis*

and *metabolic acidosis*. Respiratory acidosis is an abnormal condition characterized by a low plasma pH, resulting from reduced alveolar ventilation. Hypoventilation inhibits the excretion of carbon dioxide, which consequently combined with water in the body produces carbonic acid, thus reducing plasma pH. Respiratory acidosis can result from disorders such as airway obstruction, medullary trauma, neuromuscular disease, chest injury, pneumonia, pulmonary edema, and emphysema (**Figure 27–6A**). The body compensates by forming additional bicarbonate from the kidneys and raising the bicarbonate levels in the plasma. This restores the ratios of the two buffer components and shifts pH back toward the physiologic range (**Figure 27–6B**).

Metabolic acidosis is caused by other acids accumulating in body fluids or by a loss of bases (including bicarbonate ions). Renal failure (uremia), ketosis (overproduction of ketone bodies), and lactic acidosis are the three major conditions that cause metabolic acidosis. *Uremia* is the end stage of many kidney diseases. Metabolic acidosis occurs as failing kidneys cannot excrete various acid waste products produced by normal metabolism.

TABLE 27–1 Effects of Respiratory and Metabolic Acidosis and Alkalosis on the Body

Respiratory Acidosis	Respiratory Alkalosis	Metabolic Acidosis	Metabolic Alkalosis
Slow, shallow respirations Respiratory congestion	Hyperventilation	Diarrhea Renal failure Diabetic ketoacidosis	Vomiting Excessive antacid use
Increased partial pressure of carbon dioxide ($PaCO_2$)	Decreased $PaCO_2$	Tissue hypoxia Decreased bicarbonate Rapid, deep respirations	Increased bicarbonate Slow, shallow respirations
Kidneys excrete more hydrogen and reabsorb more bicarbonate	Kidneys excrete less hydrogen and reabsorb less bicarbonate	Kidneys excrete more hydrogen and increase bicarbonate absorption (when not involved)	Kidneys excrete less hydrogen and decrease bicarbonate absorption (when not involved)
High $PaCO_2$ and bicarbonate	Low partial pressure of oxygen (PO_2) and low bicarbonate	Low bicarbonate and $PaCO_2$	High bicarbonate and $PaCO_2$
Compensated pH = 7.35 to 7.4 Decompensated pH < 7.33	Compensated pH = 7.4 to 7.45 Decompensated pH > 7.47	Compensated pH = 7.35 to 7.4 Decompensated pH < 7.33	Compensated pH = 7.4 to 7.45 Decompensated pH > 7.47

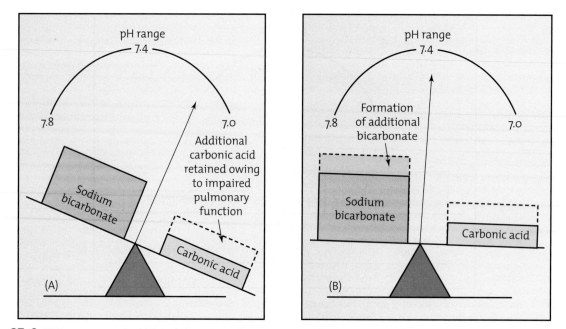

Figure 27–6 (A) Derangement of acid–base balance in respiratory acidosis. (B) Compensation by formation of additional bicarbonate.

Ketosis is caused by overproduction of acid ketone bodies (*acetoacetic acid* and *beta-hydroxybutyric acid*) derived from fat metabolism. Ketosis often occurs in untreated type 1 diabetes because the body cannot use carbohydrates efficiently and must rely on fat as a major energy source. Ketosis also occurs due to starvation and persistent vomiting. *Lactic acidosis* occurs because of shock or severe heart failure. Lactic acid is formed from glucose breakdown in the presence of an insufficient oxygen supply. Reduced pulmonary ventilation may be the result of injury to the respiratory center of the brainstem, obstruction of air passages, or diseases that decrease gas exchange. Metabolic acidosis also may occur in starvation and in uncontrolled diabetes mellitus.

> **RED FLAG**
> Metabolic acidosis is more common in children. Children are vulnerable to acid-base imbalance because their metabolic rates are rapid and ratios of water to total body weight are low.

Symptoms of respiratory acidosis, such as disorientation, drowsiness, labored breathing, cyanosis, and stupor, result from depression of normal central nervous system function. This can lead to coma and death. Metabolic acidosis may be caused by kidney disease, diabetes mellitus, prolonged vomiting, or prolonged diarrhea.

Alkalosis

Alkalosis is an abnormal condition of body fluids characterized by a tendency toward a blood pH level greater than 7.45, as from an excess of alkaline bicarbonate or a deficiency of acid. The two major types are respiratory alkalosis and metabolic alkalosis. Respiratory alkalosis is caused by hyperventilation, resulting from an excessive loss of carbon dioxide and carbonic acid in plasma. This causes an excess of bicarbonate, and blood pH usually increases (**Figure 27–7A**). Compensation occurs because of increased excretion of bicarbonate by the kidneys. This lowers the plasma bicarbonate and restores the ratio of the buffer components toward normal (**Figure 27–7B**).

Metabolic alkalosis is an abnormal condition characterized by the significant loss of acids in the body or by increased levels of alkalinity. Metabolic alkalosis may be caused by excessive loss of hydrogen ions or a gain of bases. Examples of metabolic alkalosis include excessive vomiting and insufficient replacement of electrolytes. Metabolic alkalosis may result from gastric drainage (lavage), prolonged vomiting, and the use of certain diuretics. It can also develop from the ingestion of too many antacids. It causes decreased breathing rate and depth.

Respiratory alkalosis is an abnormal condition characterized by a high plasma pH resulting from increased alveolar ventilation. The consequent acceleration of carbonic acid raises plasma pH. Respiratory alkalosis may occur due to hyperventilation, which can result from anxiety, fever, poisoning, or high altitudes. Symptoms of respiratory alkalosis are agitation, dizziness, lightheadedness, and tingling sensations. When severe, peripheral nerves can trigger impulses, with muscles responding with tetanic contractions. The physical therapist assistant (PTA) should be aware that unexplained confusion, muscle cramps, or other signs and symptoms noted in this chapter can be indicative of serious medical problems and as such should be reported to the PT during or immediately after treatment.

SUMMARY

Water is distributed into an ICF compartment and an ECF compartment. ICF includes water and electrolytes enclosed by cell membranes, whereas ECF includes fluid outside of the cells. Most total body water volume (about 63 percent) is inside the cells. The ECF compartment includes fluid within the blood vessels (plasma), tissue spaces (interstitial fluid), and lymphatic vessels (lymph).

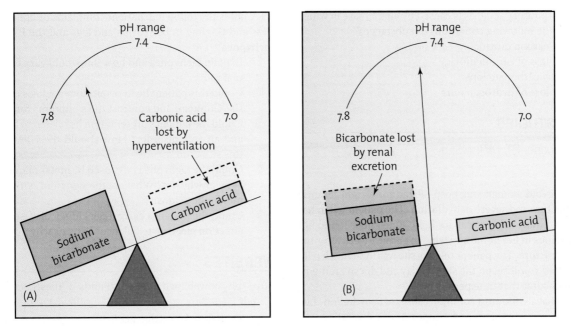

Figure 27–7 (A) Derangement of acid–base balance in respiratory alkalosis. (B) Compensation by excretion of bicarbonate.

Hydrostatic and osmotic pressures regulate water and electrolyte movement between fluid compartments. The most common water balance disorders in humans are dehydration, water intoxication, and edema. Homeostasis regulates electrolyte balance. For cellular functions, the most important electrolytes are sodium, potassium, calcium, magnesium, chloride, sulfate, phosphate, bicarbonate, and hydrogen ions.

Several hormones are involved in the maintenance of water and electrolytes, which include aldosterone, antidiuretic hormone, and parathyroid hormone. Many conditions are related to electrolyte imbalance, including hypernatremia, hyponatremia, hyperkalemia, and hypokalemia. Acid-base imbalance may cause respiratory or metabolic acidosis or alkalosis. These conditions may be regulated by acid-base buffer systems or specific treatments.

REVIEW QUESTIONS

Select the best response to each question.

1. Extracellular fluid consists of which of the following?
   a. interstitial fluid
   b. plasma
   c. lymph
   d. all of the above

2. The electrolytes that dissociate in water and release hydrogen ions are called
   a. bases
   b. acids
   c. neutral
   d. homeostatic

3. The normal pH level of the blood is slightly
   a. neutral
   b. alkaline
   c. acidic
   d. similar to any body fluid

4. Compared with males, females have more adipose tissue and less body water due to the influence of which hormone?
   a. estrogen
   b. aldosterone
   c. parathyroid
   d. antidiuretic

5. Water intoxication in infants is dangerous because of which of the following conditions?
   a. hypotension and collapse
   b. high fever
   c. swelling of brain tissue
   d. urinary retention

6. Hypernatremia may be caused by which of the following mechanisms?
   a. oversecretion of aldosterone
   b. a net loss of water
   c. intracellular dehydration
   d. all of the above

7. Hypochloremia may be seen in which of the following disorders?
   a. pulmonary edema
   b. cystic fibrosis
   c. hypertension
   d. peptic ulcer

8. Hyperkalemia can lead to which of the following complications?
   a. muscle weakness
   b. pulmonary edema
   c. heart arrhythmias
   d. convulsions

9. Which of the following parts of the brain is the center of regulation of hydrogen ion concentration?
   a. hypothalamus
   b. cerebellum
   c. thalamus
   d. brainstem

10. Respiratory acidosis is caused by an increase in which of the following conditions or substances?
    a. carbon dioxide
    b. loss of carbon dioxide
    c. bicarbonate ions
    d. loss of hydrogen ions

CASE STUDIES

Karen Coupe, PT, DPT, MSEd

Case 1

A 92-year-old woman was hospitalized for a right femoral neck fracture and severe dehydration. The patient fell in her home and was unable to call for help. A neighbor found her unconscious in her home and lying in vomit 1 week after the fall and fracture. The patient reports she was in so much pain she started vomiting on the second day and doesn't remember much after that time period.

1. What are the most common causes of dehydration? List the common signs and symptoms of dehydration.
2. After a week on the floor, what would you expect the emergency medical technicians to see when they checked her blood pressure, heart rate and respiration rate? Explain why these changes would occur.
3. Dehydration can cause significant muscle weakness. Explain, physiologically, why this occurs.
4. If a PTA were to check a patient's skin turgor, how would this present in a patient with normal hydration versus a patient with dehydration?
5. What electrolyte imbalances could be present in a patient who is dehydrated?

Case 2

A PTA is working in an outpatient clinic treating a 56-year-old woman for chronic back pain. Patient medical history: Panic and anxiety disorder, early stage chronic kidney disease. While instructing the patient in body mechanics, the PTA notes the following: patient complains of lightheadedness and tingling in both arms and legs and the PTA notes tachypnea.

1. Explain tachypnea and how this would vary from normal rates.
2. Could this patient be in respiratory acidosis or alkalosis? Compare and contrast the symptoms for each.
3. Could the patient's presentation be related to her panic and anxiety disorder? How should the PTA react to this situation?
4. Could the tachypnea be caused by metabolic acidosis? Why or why not? What are the signs and symptoms of metabolic acidosis?
5. Could the patient's early stage kidney disease have an effect on electrolyte balance? Why or why not?

WEBSITES

http://physioweb.med.uvm.edu/Fluids_1_files/Lecture2.pdf

http://www.anaesthesiamcq.com/FluidBook/fl2_1.php

http://www.enotes.com/nursing-encyclopedia/acid-base-balance

http://www.medicinenet.com/dehydration/article.htm

http://www.merck.com/pubs/mmanual_ha/sec3/ch18/ch18d.html

http://www.nlm.nih.gov/medlineplus/edema.html

http://www.nlm.nih.gov/medlineplus/ency/article/001181.htm

http://www.nlm.nih.gov/medlineplus/ency/article/001183.htm

http://www.nlm.nih.gov/medlineplus/ency/article/001187.htm

http://www.wrongdiagnosis.com/medical/chloremia.htm

http://www.wrongdiagnosis.com/medical/kalemia.htm

http://www.wrongdiagnosis.com/medical/natremia.htm

Aging and Disease Processes

LEARNING OBJECTIVES

After completion of the chapter the reader should be able to

1. Define the terms *sedentary*, *apoptosis*, and *sarcopenia*.
2. Compare the changes on the skeleton and integumentary system due to the aging process.
3. Explain the pathophysiology of osteoporosis.
4. Describe the common changes on the brain related to the aging process.
5. Explain the incidence of type 2 diabetes mellitus due to the aging process.
6. List two common disorders of the eyes that may cause blindness.
7. Explain the changes of the digestive system in the elderly.
8. Describe the risk factors of more prevalent cancers related to the aging process.

KEY TERMS

Apoptosis: A type of cell death in which the cell uses specialized cellular processes for self-destruction.
Articular cartilage: Elastic tissue found in the joints.
Ascites: Abnormal accumulation of large amounts of fluid in the abdomen, usually caused by severe liver disease.
Incontinence: Lack of ability to control urination or defecation.
Laminectomy: Surgery to remove the posterior portion (lamina) of the vertebra that covers the spinal canal; also known as decompression surgery.
Meniere's disease: A disorder of the inner ear that causes severe vertigo (dizziness), tinnitus, hearing loss, and a feeling of fullness or congestion.
Neurofibrils: Threads that run through the bodies of neurons and extend into axons and dendrites.
Nocturia: Excessive urination at night.
Osteoblastic: Related to the deposition of calcium into bone via the actions of osteoblast cells.
Osteophytes: Bone spurs, which are bony projections that form along joint margins.
Otosclerosis: Abnormal bone growth in the middle ear that causes hearing loss.
Prostatectomy: Surgical removal of the prostate gland.
Sarcopenia: A loss of skeletal muscle mass that may accompany aging.
Sedentary: Related to a lack of or complete absence of physical activity.
Tinnitus: Perception of sound in the ear when there is no corresponding external sound.
Xerostomia: Dryness of the mouth.

Overview

The aging process refers to the process of growing old. Biological aging partially results from a failure of body cells to function normally or to produce new body cells to replace dead or malfunctioning cells. Normal cell function may be lost through infectious disease, malnutrition, exposure to environmental hazards, or genetic influences. Some body cells normally cease dividing after reaching maturity and exhibit early signs of aging. Sociologic and psychological theories of aging seek to explain other influences caused by the environment, engagement, personality, and non-biologic influences. For example, aging changes affecting cognition and perception include decreased brain weight, diminished enzyme activity in the brain, slowed reflexes, decreased sensory receptors for temperature and pain, weakening of interneuron connections, increased response time, and chronic hypoxia.

Aging

Aging is a continual process that begins at birth. Individuals experience the effects of aging in unique ways. Changes to various organ systems occur in variable order and are based on genetic makeup, health status, and lifestyle. Research into "reversing" the aging process is ongoing, but in actuality this is impossible.

Women tend to live, on average, longer than men. The life span for females averages 80 years in the United States, whereas for men the average is 75 years. Life spans are lengthening with improved nutrition, health care, and quality of living. As we live longer, there is a larger proportion of older adults in the population. As we age, the body generally reduces in function at cellular, tissue, and organ levels. Degenerative age-related changes may predispose people to specific pathologies. These changes are of most concern in the brain and myocardium, which cannot regenerate like other tissues. Aging may be genetically programmed or predetermined (**apoptosis**). Other factors of aging may include the deterioration of body tissues due to life stressors, accumulation of cellular wastes, altered protein or lipid components, and degeneration of collagen and elastin.

Free radicals are reactive chemicals produced during cell metabolism known to damage nucleic acids and cells, potentially leading to cancer and other conditions. Abnormal structures in tissues and organs increase and mitosis (cellular reproduction) slows down. Tissues are not repaired as quickly or as fully as earlier in life. Because neurons and muscle cells cannot replicate, function is reduced. Organs fail as cells become less functional or die.

Effects of Aging

Aging affects every body system, although some systems are affected more than others. The most obvious changes happen to the hair and skin, which tend to lose pigment and become drier and thinner. Changes to the skeleton cause general weakness as bones become more brittle and prone to breakage (osteoporosis). Joint conditions such as arthritis affect movement and flexibility. The major changes of each body system are discussed below.

Integumentary System

Aging causes the skin and mucous membranes to become thin and fragile, with a decreased amount of subcutaneous tissue. As skin cells proliferate more slowly and there are fewer capillaries, wounds take longer to heal and sweat glands begin to atrophy. Sensory receptors are less responsive. As a result of these changes, injuries are more likely. Use of anticoagulants such as heparin causes an increased risk for skin tears and bruising. Wrinkling of the skin is due to reduced amounts of elastic fibers and a toughening of collagen fibers.

Skin *turgor* is the inability of the skin to change shape and return to normal and is determined by hydration and age. Dehydration results in decreased skin turgor, manifested by "lax" skin (lacking in elasticity) that when grasped and raised between two fingers returns to a position level with the adjacent tissue more slowly than normal. For example, elderly people usually lack skin elasticity, and this is an expected part of aging. Marked edema or **ascites** results in increased turgor manifested by smooth, taut, shiny skin that cannot be grasped and raised.

The hands and face may develop dark, flat macules (commonly called "liver spots"), keratoses (rough, raised masses), or skin tags (small projections out from the skin) that may appear on the neck or armpits. These types of skin changes result from thinning of the skin due to aging and excessive exposure to ultraviolet light. The hair turns gray because of reduced amounts of melanocytes and thins because of a decrease in hair follicles.

Musculoskeletal System

Common musculoskeletal changes related to the aging process include *osteoporosis* and osteoarthritis. Reduced muscle strength, reduced flexibility, and slowed or stiffened movements may occur in elderly people. Low-impact regular exercise helps to maintain flexibility and mobility, which slows muscle size decrease and increases muscle strength. Good nutrition is also important to offset changes due to aging. A healthy diet may contain adequate amounts of minerals and vitamins to maintain body structures. **Table 28–1** lists foods with the most benefits for the elderly.

Elderly people may complain of many more musculoskeletal conditions than younger adults. In women the breakdown of the musculoskeletal system accelerates after menopause, resulting in an increased risk of osteoporosis. Calcium is reabsorbed

> **RED FLAG**
> Falling is one of the most common causes of injury in elderly people.

from bones, decreasing bone densities and making bones more brittle. Osteoporosis is seen usually in older women. Muscles decrease in strength and mass due to **sarcopenia** and may even atrophy to a certain degree. Arm and leg muscles appear less toned and appear "flabby." Mild loss of muscle strength places increased stress on joints such as the knees, predisposing a patient to falling or to osteoarthritis. Regular exercise is of vital importance to decrease the effects of aging.

Elderly people may lose height due to spinal curvature and vertebrae compression. Joint flexibility may decrease, although weight training and exercise can maintain flexibility and range of motion. Certain forms of musculoskeletal

TABLE 28–1	Beneficial Foods for the Elderly
Food Group	**Examples**
Fiber	Brown rice Chickpeas (garbanzo beans) Lentils Wheat germ Whole wheat bread Whole wheat cereals Whole wheat crackers
Fruits	Apples Blackberries Black currants Cantaloupes Citrus fruit Kiwifruit Mangos Peaches Raspberries Strawberries
Nuts and seeds (unsalted)	Almonds Brazil nuts Cashews Flax seeds Poppy seeds Pumpkin seeds Sunflower seeds Walnuts
Oily fish	Herring Mackerel Salmon Sardines Trout Tuna
Protein	Beans Cheese Chicken Eggs Lean meat Milk White fish Yogurt
Vegetables	Avocados Broccoli Brussels sprouts Cabbage Carrots Collard greens Kale Leeks Onions Spinach Squash Sweet potatoes Tomatoes

diseases may become partially or totally debilitating, such as osteoarthritis or rheumatoid arthritis. Healing from injuries is slower and pain may be greater. To improve home safety and decrease the risk of falls, elderly people should have their houses "safety checked."

Osteoporosis

Loss of calcium and bone mass, as a result of aging, leads to osteoporosis. It has a higher onset in postmenopausal women and may result in serious consequences, such as fractures of the limbs, pelvis, or spine. Older women should have a routine bone density test to screen for osteoporosis. In elderly men, osteoporosis is also increased by aging. It may be seen more commonly after age 70. The following are risk factors for osteoporosis:

- Decreased estrogen levels due to aging, especially after menopause
- Decreased calcium, vitamin C, and vitamin D intake
- Decreased **osteoblastic** activity, due to use of glucocorticoids
- Decreased weight bearing on the bones due to immobility and **sedentary** or inactive lifestyle
- Hereditary predisposition to osteoporosis

Decreased bone mass and density is caused by reduced new bone deposition. The bones may become porous and brittle, leading to *fractures*. In the spine, spontaneous compression fractures of the vertebrae result in decreased height and *kyphosis*. This leads to a hunchback posture (known as a dowager's hump), shuffling gait, increased fall risk, and breathing difficulties.

To reduce the risk and progression of osteoporosis, recommendations are as follows:

- Administration of bisphosphonates, including the bone resorption inhibitor known as alendronate sodium
- Individualized hormonal therapy, including estrogen/progesterone replacement therapy, selective estrogen receptor modulators such as raloxifene, and synthetic *calcitonin* or parathyroid hormone
- Increased calcium intake with adequate vitamin D
- Weight-bearing exercise, walking, physiotherapy, or rehabilitation programs

Osteoarthritis

Osteoarthritis is defined as degeneration of one or many joints, including subchondral bony sclerosis, loss of articular cartilage, and proliferation of bone spurs (**osteophytes**) and cartilage in the joint (**Figure 28–1**).

Bone spurs or overgrowths often develop at points of stress, causing the **articular cartilage** to become thin and eroded. It is often found in the large, weight-bearing bones (such as the knees, hips, or spine), and results in pain, making

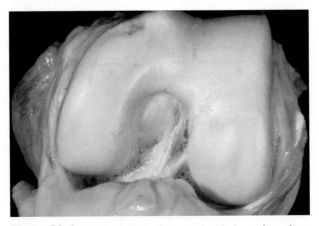

Figure 28–1 Knee joint, illustrating smooth articular surface of femoral condyles.

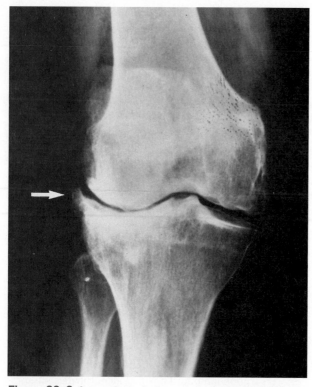

Figure 28–2 Osteoarthritis. Radiograph illustrates increased bone density of femoral condyle (left side of photograph) and adjacent tibia, with overgrowth of bone at margin of tibia (arrow).

mobility and walking difficult. Degeneration of underlying bone or secondary overgrowth of bone frequently occurs in response to the trauma of weight bearing (**Figure 28–2**).

Depending on the severity, surgical treatment is sometimes necessary and may reduce pain and greatly improve the function of a joint. Hip replacement, joint debridement, fusion, and decompression **laminectomy** are some of the surgical procedures used in treating advanced osteoarthritis.

Herniated Intervertebral Disks

With aging, the intervertebral disks undergo a progressive wear-and-tear degeneration of both the nucleus and the annulus. The nucleus of an intervertebral disk becomes denser because its water content is reduced. The annulus of the disk becomes weakened and thinned. When marked compression force is applied to the anterior portion of the disk during flexion of the spine, the nucleus is forced posteriorly against the weakened annulus. Part of the nucleus may be forced into the spinal canal through a weak area or tear in the annulus (**Figure 28–3**). Herniated intervertebral disks cause pressure on spinal nerves and severe back pain. When pressure is not relieved, permanent nerve damage may result.

Neurologic and Sensory Systems

The aging process affects neurologic and sensory systems in many ways. For example, the brain and spinal cord decrease in weight. Nerve cells transmit messages more slowly, and waste products can collect due to the breakdown of these cells. The breakdown of nerves can affect the senses, including

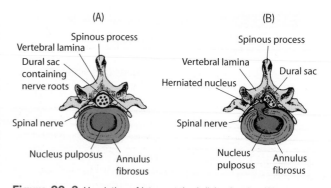

Figure 28–3 Herniation of intervertebral disk, showing (A) a normal disk and (B) a herniated disk.

reduction in reflexes or sensations that leads to problems with movement and safety. All the sensory systems, including hearing, eyesight, taste, and smell, can be affected by aging.

Neurons in the brain are not replaced after birth. Therefore, a natural reduction in brain mass occurs as we age. Although this usually does not affect cognitive function, losses occur in different areas of the brain at different degrees and times, with different outcomes. Maintenance of regular physical exercise and cognitive exercises have been shown to stimulate brain function. Factors such as toxic substances can increase the rate of degeneration.

In the brain, common manifestations due to aging include increased neuronal lipids, myelin sheath loss, and development of abnormal *plaques* and **neurofibrils**. Organic brain syndrome (which includes senile dementia and Alzheimer's disease) is related to increased numbers of abnormal plaques and neurofibrils. Arteriosclerosis and other vascular impairments contribute to neurologic degeneration. Decreased cellular response to *neurotransmitter* chemicals (such as norepinephrine) leads to delays in synaptic transmission in the brain.

Elderly people often have decreased reflexes, short-term memory lapses, and slower response times. However, studies have shown that elderly adults are still able to learn and process new information. Research also supports that adults who remain more mentally active seem to have a less apparent decline of cognitive abilities. This may be slower than earlier in life because in an older individual more information is incorporated and more brain functions are used.

Aging also causes the autonomic nervous system to have slowed adaptation, such as decreased temperature tolerances. Related changes include slower blood circulation, decreased activity levels, and decreased metabolism. The skin may have reduced temperature sensitivity. In the special senses, eye muscles degenerate, which can result in decreased adaptation to light, increased intraocular pressure, and increased likelihood of developing *glaucoma*. As the lens of the eye becomes less transparent, night vision is impaired. *Cataracts* may cause the lens to become opaque and lead to loss of vision (which is able to be restored by removal of cataracts). Other eye changes may include *presbyopia* and vascular changes of the retina. Compensatory measures for vision loss include using enlarged type and pictures to demonstrate techniques for home exercise and other activities.

The physical therapist assistant (PTA) should question the patient about nighttime habits. Night lights in the bathroom can decrease the risk of a fall. Whereas in younger individuals "20/20" vision is most common, by age 65 most people develop reduced vision that is in the area of "20/70." Many elderly people develop arcus senilis (a gray-colored ring at the periphery of the cornea), a visible sign of the affects of aging on the eyes.

Hearing may be diminished because of degenerative inner ear changes, usually beginning with loss of high frequencies followed by loss of lower frequencies. Often, elderly people cannot discriminate between sounds in noisy surroundings. Although many hearing problems can be corrected with hearing aids, their cost (and the stigma attached to using them) influence their use; this situation is declining, however, due to advancements in technology. Men are affected by age-related hearing loss (presbycusis) more than women. Common hearing conditions in older adults include **Meniere's disease**, **otosclerosis**, and **tinnitus**. Compensatory measures for hearing loss include speaking slowly and clearly when addressing elderly patients while facing them so they understand instructions and other information. The use of gestures and written instructions can improve comprehension as well.

The sense of taste can be altered by reduction in salivary secretions or decreased central nervous system perception. The sense of smell may change significantly so that discriminating between different odors becomes more difficult. Changes to both taste and smell may impair both appetite and nutrition.

Endocrine System

Overall, the endocrine system and its hormones change little with aging. Normal amounts of most hormones remain in balance, including pituitary, thyroid, parathyroid, adrenal, and pancreatic hormones. However, as the number of tissue receptors decreases, the body's response to hormonal effects diminishes. This explains the prevalence of type 2 diabetes mellitus in elderly people. In this condition, insulin is produced sufficiently but glucose does not enter the cells because the number or sensitivity of cell receptors is reduced. Type 2 diabetes mellitus must be diagnosed early and managed to prevent serious complications to other body systems. With aging, risks for hypoglycemia and fluid loss also increase. Digestive and metabolic problems become more common because there is less pancreatic and thyroid secretion.

As women enter menopause, the ovaries stop producing estrogen and progesterone. To compensate, the body reacts by increasing the serum levels of follicle-stimulating hormone and luteinizing hormone. As a result, these changes have widespread effects on other body systems. In men, testosterone decreases gradually but the testes do not totally stop functioning. Secondary sex characteristics also change as gonadal secretions are reduced.

Cardiovascular System

Aging causes the myocardium and other tissues to become altered, as collagen fibers and fatty tissue interfere with the heart's ability to contract and conduct normal electrical impulses. Cardiac muscle cells decline in size; therefore, cardiac contractions become weaker. With aging, the left ventricle decreases in size with the decreased demand. It is important to remember that cardiac muscle fibers do not undergo mitosis, meaning they cannot be replaced once lost. Often, heart valves become thicker, less flexible, and less efficient.

Vascular degeneration can cause a decrease in oxygen supply, reducing the ability of the heart to use oxygen. This diminishes cardiac reserve and output, which decreases the heart's maximum output under stress. Because fluid levels decrease in the elderly, it is important for them to consume adequate amounts of fluids to maintain cardiovascular function. Cardiac function can be maintained by regular aerobic exercise.

Because of aging, as the arterial walls lose elasticity and accumulate collagen, they thicken. This limits the amount of expansion of large arteries and obstructs the lumina of smaller arteries. Collectively, this is the beginning of *arteriosclerosis* and elevated blood pressure. Normal blood pressure in a healthy elderly patient is between 90/65 and 130/90 mm Hg. *Cholesterol* and lipids also accumulate in large artery walls (*atherosclerosis*), especially in the presence of elevated blood lipid levels. Blood flow is obstructed by these lipid plaques, leading to the formation of *thrombi*. To lessen the risk of these and other conditions, reduction of cholesterol intake, regular exercise, and dietary changes are recommended.

> **RED FLAG**
> Atherosclerosis commonly leads to angina, heart attacks (myocardial infarctions), peripheral vascular disease (in the legs), and strokes.

Most older adults are at increased risk for hypertension, angina, heart attack, arrhythmias, heart failure, varicose veins, and other cardiovascular problems. Decreased peripheral circulation can result in cool, pale extremities, improper wound healing, and edema in the lower extremities. As circulation changes, the effects of medications also change.

Postural hypotension can cause safety issues. This condition, which can occur at any age, is described as a decrease or drop in blood pressure that occurs when an individual changes from a reclining position to a sitting or standing position. Dizziness may quickly occur, resulting in a fall. Elderly adults should make attempts to "safe check" their homes and implement fall prevention strategies to avoid injuries that may result from postural hypotension. Prevention methods include sitting, lying, or standing slowly. The condition can result from the effects of various drugs, and all medications should be evaluated in relation to postural hypotension. When a patient complains or shows signs of dizziness, the PTA should be ready to assist him or her in lying or sitting safely to avoid falling. All exercise must be stopped immediately. The patient's blood pressure must be taken and recorded.

Total serum iron, total iron-binding capacity, and intestinal iron absorption all decrease with age. Aging causes lymphocytes to decrease in function. The most common blood disorder in the elderly is anemia, usually due to poor nutrition or the inability to absorb nutrients. Anemia often complicates other conditions in older adults. Certain leukemias are more common in elderly people, complicated by decreased gastric motility and impaired circulation, which affects treatment outcomes. Some therapies are therefore less effective as a result.

Immune system function decreases with the aging process. Antibodies are produced in lower quantities, and more infections occur, with longer recovery times. Chronic diseases also cause elderly patients to have higher risks for poor or delayed healing. The incidence of autoimmune disorders is higher. The lymphatic system depends on the vascular system for some of its functions. Therefore, those with impaired circulation or other vascular system diseases experience reduced lymphatic system function as well.

Respiratory System

Respiration becomes reduced in elderly individuals for several reasons. Skeletal changes (such as spinal curves) reduce thoracic movement. The costal cartilage between the ribs and the sternum calcifies to reduce rib movement for lung expansion. Deep breathing and coughing becomes more difficult because of restricted lung movements and expansion. The intercostal muscles can also atrophy and weaken, making breathing difficult.

Residual volume increases, and expiration is reduced. Coughing is not as effective due to weakened trunk and skeletal muscles. As the ability to cough normally is impaired, secretions accumulate, increasing the risk of pneumonia. Pneumonia is the leading cause of death by infection in older adults. Influenza, respiratory infections, and tuberculosis are also of more danger to the elderly than younger patients.

Decreased perfusion and reduced gas exchange in the alveoli is caused by vascular degeneration in the lungs. Usually, oxygen levels are reduced, but carbon dioxide levels remain the same. Regular physical exercise maximizes circulation and ventilation. Breathing exercises and oxygen therapy may also be indicated. However, the inability of the body to meet oxygen demand decreases the length of and tolerance for exercise. Elderly people who are long-term smokers may already have severe respiratory damage, with lung cancer risk heightened.

> **RED FLAG**
> Lung cancer is the second leading cause of death in older adults.

Digestive System

Good nutrition in elderly adults is vital to support general health. Frequently, nutrition is affected when teeth are lost because of *periodontal disease*, reducing the patient's ability to chew and eat normally. As the mucosa in the mouth thins and blood flow is reduced, chewing may become painful. The oral tissues may become irritated by food particles or dentures. Reduced saliva often causes dry mouth (**xerostomia**). Dry mouth may result from certain drugs or because of mouth breathing, which is caused by many respiratory problems. Neurologic conditions or mechanical obstructions such as esophageal cancer may cause dysphagia (swallowing difficulties). In these situations, a liquid diet (liquid or parenteral) may be needed to maintain proper nutrition. Nutritional status may be influenced by the inability to easily leave the house to purchase food, inability to drive a vehicle, or because of lower socioeconomic status.

Lack of physical activity versus excessive intake of carbohydrates and fats can lead to obesity. Obesity can lead to a higher cardiac workload and increases the risk of atherosclerosis and gallstones. Digestive secretions may be reduced and essential nutrient absorption impaired because of atrophy of digestive mucosa and glands. When absorption is impaired, vitamin B_{12} injections and calcium and iron supplements may be indicated.

Peptic ulcers are more likely to develop in elderly people because of thinning of digestive mucosa and decreased mucous secretion. Malignancies in the stomach and colon may also be related to both dietary intake and heredity. Carcinogenic substances in the diet may become more hazardous if constipation exists. Hemorrhoids are a common side effect, which are caused by chronic constipation.

Elderly people more commonly suffer from the complications of chronic hepatitis B or C than younger patients. Cirrhosis in these patients is usually progressive and severe, with a poor prognosis. Cirrhosis is usually related to alcoholism or hepatitis. Elderly adults are more likely to develop bile-related stones. Pancreatic disease may require pancreatic enzyme replacement.

> **RED FLAG**
> Factors that contribute to constipation include excessive use of laxatives, low fiber intake, low fluid intake, and decreased physical activity.

Urinary System

Aging causes reduced kidney function because of degeneration of tubules and blood vessels as well as loss of glomeruli. Due to the aging process, various kidney disorders, or exposure to chemical substances such as medications, the number of glomeruli normally decline by 30 percent (at age 70). As a result, the kidneys may not be able to compensate for rapid acid and electrolyte level changes. Higher than normal levels of certain drugs may also accumulate in the blood because of a reduced capacity to secrete drugs into the urine.

Loss of bladder function, incomplete bladder emptying, and reduced bladder capacity are common problems in older adults. These conditions may lead to **nocturia**, urinary *frequency*, and urinary tract infections. Older women may experience urinary **incontinence** or leaking due to childbirth. Smooth muscle tone of the urinary bladder in women may be decreased by lower levels of estrogen. Incontinence may be caused by a weakened urethral sphincter in combination with a decline in the perception of a full bladder. When incontinence causes incomplete bladder emptying, it can lead to residual urine and frequent infections of the urinary tract and bladder. In elderly men, incontinence can also occur due to spinal cord injury or a benign or malignant prostate gland condition.

Reproductive System

In women menopause usually begins at around age 50, and the ovaries stop responding to follicle-stimulating hormone and luteinizing hormone. Ovulation ceases with menopause, as estrogen and progesterone levels decline. Therefore, the woman can no longer become pregnant. These changes cause a thinning of the mucosa in the vagina and cervix, which become less elastic. As secretions reduce, dryness of the vagina is common in elderly women. All these changes may cause *dyspareunia* and inflammation, which can be treated by estrogen creams.

Hormonal changes also cause women's breast tissue to decrease in volume and "hot flashes" (periodic sweating or vascular disturbances) to occur, as well as headaches, insomnia, and irritability. Menopause may last for several months to several years. About 25 percent of women may experience highly significant symptoms. The symptoms of menopause can occur earlier than normal, as when a younger woman undergoes an oophorectomy (surgical removal of the ovaries).

Men experience far less reproductive changes due to aging. Sperm production reduces, the testes shrink, and prostate secretions decrease. However, older men are usually still able to father children. The most significant problem in elderly men is *benign prostatic hypertrophy*. This condition causes the central part of the prostate gland to enlarge, partially obstructing the urethra and impeding urinary flow. If surgery is required, it may involve **prostatectomy**.

Cancer of both male and female reproductive organs is more prevalent in elderly people. Prostatic, uterine, and breast cancer may be related to changes in hormonal levels. Routine self-examinations, as well as regular medical examination by health care professionals, are indicated to detect cancer in its earlier stages.

Disease Processes Associated with Aging

In the elderly, infections are more common because normal defense mechanisms and tissue healing are impaired. The immune response to fight new microbes is less effective because lymphocytes respond more slowly to antigens and are less active. Also, skin lesions and breakdown of tissues may predispose the elderly to infections. Urinary tract infections increase due to prostatic obstruction in men and a variety of problems (including incontinence, thinner bladder mucosa, and bladder prolapse) in women. More frequent catheterizations or instrumentation also cause more infections.

In elderly people, cancer is more prevalent because the immune system is weaker; also, the elderly have been exposed to more carcinogens over time. Incidence of breast cancer in women and prostate cancer in men increases greatly because of the aging process. In elderly people, autoimmune disorders, degenerative conditions, and slower adaptation to stressors are more common.

The use of several medications by elderly people increases their chance of experiencing adverse drug reactions. Changes in the absorption, distribution, and elimination of drugs also result in negative outcomes. Elderly patients may be confused about dosing instructions, which often results in toxicities and overdoses. Dosages must often be adjusted and combinations of medications carefully evaluated for use in elderly patients.

SUMMARY

The effects of aging are different with every individual. As part of the normal aging process, cell and organ function gradually declines. Hormones (except for the sex hormones) continue to be secreted at normal levels during the aging process. Skin and mucosal membranes thin and have less blood flow. Cancer of reproductive organs is common in both men and women. Arterial degeneration often affects the cardiovascular system. Osteoporosis and other bone disorders are major factors in the elderly. Breathing is reduced, leading to many other conditions. Body movements are usually slower and less controlled. Impairments to the special senses are common. The kidneys do not function as well, and bladder control is often reduced.

REVIEW QUESTIONS

Select the best response to each question.

1. The period of life from old age until death is called which of the following?
   a. kyphosis
   b. apoptosis
   c. senescence
   d. synechia

2. Wrinkling of the skin is due to which of the following?
   a. toughening of elastic fibers
   b. reduced amounts of collagen fibers
   c. increased amounts of elastic fibers
   d. reduced amounts of elastic fibers

3. The following are true to reduce the risk and progression of osteoporosis *except*
   a. increased calcium intake with adequate vitamin D
   b. administration of potassium and sodium chloride
   c. routine physical exercise
   d. individualized hormonal therapy

4. Decreased temperature tolerances in the elderly are caused by which of the following?
   a. inadequate adaptation
   b. decreasing the numbers of cells in the cerebral cortex
   c. inadequate secretion of growth hormone
   d. increasing blood circulation in the skin

5. The following are reasons for decreased respiration in the elderly *except*
   a. costal cartilage between the ribs and the sternum calcifies
   b. deep breathing and coughing becomes more difficult
   c. residual volume decreases
   d. oxygen levels are reduced but carbon dioxide levels are not increased

6. Chronic constipation in the elderly may result in which of the following conditions?
   a. hemorrhoids
   b. ulcerative colitis
   c. volvulus
   d. stomach cancer

7. Women may experience urine incontinence due to which of the following?
   a. using birth control in earlier years
   b. childbirth in earlier years
   c. benign tumor of the uterus
   d. pelvic inflammatory disease

8. Which of the following is the most common cause of impeded urinary flow in elderly men?
   a. impotence
   b. testicular cancer
   c. dyspareunia
   d. benign prostatic hypertrophy

9. Why is it important that elderly people consume adequate amounts of fluids in relation to cardiovascular function?
   a. vascular degeneration can cause a decrease in oxygen supply
   b. diminished cardiac output
   c. usually decreased blood pressure and pulse
   d. fluid levels decrease

10. Organic brain syndrome includes which of the following conditions?
    a. senile dementia
    b. meningitis
    c. Alzheimer's disease
    d. both A and C

CASE STUDIES

Karen Coupe, PT, DPT, MSEd

Case 1

A PTA is working in a pediatric outpatient setting. The PT just evaluated a 10-year-old boy who was born with progeria. The patient complains of general weakness, stiffness, and difficulty walking without losing his balance. The patient presents with alopecia, and bone marrow density tests reveal osteoporosis. The plan of care is for therapeutic exercise, gait training with a front-wheeled rolling walker, and balance activities.

1. What is progeria? Is this a common congenital disorder? Research the types of progeria.
2. Why would a patient at age 10 present with alopecia? Is this a normal age-related change or a complication of his diagnosis?
3. Based on the pathology involved in this diagnosis, what age-related changes will occur in this patient's musculoskeletal system?
4. Why would a 10-year-old patient present with osteoporosis? What risks are associated with this patient having a balance problem?
5. How would the integumentary system of this patient present? Could this presentation make the patient more susceptible to skin tears? Why or why not?

Case 2

A PTA is treating an 85-year-old woman for general strengthening, endurance, gait, and balance activities. The patient has a long history of osteoarthritis in both hips and the right knee and degenerative joint disease in the lumbar spine. The patient currently requires minimal to moderate assistance of her family for all her daily activities due to pain and immobility. The patient is very motivated because she does not want to move from her house into an assisted living facility.

1. How does the patient's osteoarthritis contribute to her lack of independent function? Is this common for her age?
2. During treatment, the patient tells the PTA she used to be 5'2" but now she is 4'11". Explain the reasoning behind her loss in height. Is this a common aging process?
3. Although this patient does not have apparent cardiovascular pathologies, before working on endurance and strengthening exercises, what are important concepts to understand about the cardiovascular system in a geriatric patient? How could this affect the blood pressure and heart rate during exercise? What precautions should the PTA take?
4. After the first bout of exercise, the PTA notes the patient has mild dyspnea. Is this normal based on the patient's level of function? Why or why not? How does the aging process affect the respiratory system? What precautions would the PTA take in this matter?
5. Although this patient does not have any form of dementia, she does occasionally forget what the PTA just instructed her to do. Why would this occur? Is this a normal or abnormal aspect of aging?

WEBSITES

http://merckmanuals.com/home/sec05/ch058/ch058g.html

http://www.aahf.info/sec_exercise/section/respiratory.htm

http://www.ageworks.com/course_demo/513/module3/module3.htm

http://www.associatedcontent.com/article/2998634/obvious_skin_changes_due_to_aging.html

http://www.cumc.columbia.edu/dept/neurology/research/memory.html

http://www.healthinaging.org/agingintheknow/chapters_ch_trial.asp?ch=1

http://www.merckmanuals.com/home/sec26.html

http://www.nlm.nih.gov/medlineplus/ency/article/004000.htm

http://www.psychologytoday.com/blog/sex-sociability/201009/sex-after-60

http://www.rand.org/labor/aging/rsi/rsi_papers/2004_rich.pdf

Effects of Immobility

LEARNING OBJECTIVES

After completion of the chapter the reader should be able to

1. Describe decubitus ulcers (pressure ulcers).
2. Define the terms *atrophy*, *hemiplegia*, *quadriplegia* (*tetraplegia*), and *paraplegia*.
3. Explain how immobility may lead to the development of thrombi in the veins.
4. Describe the effects of immobility on the urinary system.
5. Identify methods that can prevent skin breakdown in patients who are immobilized.
6. Explain the effects of immobility on the tendons and ligaments.
7. Describe the effects of immobility on the cardiovascular system.
8. Define a negative balance of nitrogen (protein deficit) that is caused by inactivity.

KEY TERMS

Contracture: A permanent shortening of a muscle, causing distortion or deformity.
Decubitus ulcers: Skin lesions that result from the pressure of lying in the same position for a long time, especially on a bony prominence.
Extensor: A muscle that extends or straightens a limb or body part.
Flaccidity: Weakness and softness, as of a muscle, with decreased resistance to movement, increased mobility, and greater than normal range of movements.
Flexor: A muscle that, when contracted, acts to bend a limb or joint in the body.
Hemiplegia: Paralysis of one side of the body.
Hypostatic pneumonia: Inflammation of the lungs, with congestion; usually caused by immobility, especially lying on the back.
Immobility: A state of being incapable of movement.
Orthostatic hypotension: A drop in blood pressure after a rapid change of position.
Osteoclastic: Related to the surgical breaking of a bone.
Paraplegia: Paralysis of the legs and lower part of the torso.
Quadriplegia: Complete paralysis of all four limbs; this term is now commonly being replaced with the term *tetraplegia*.
Stasis: Slowing or stopping blood flow or other body fluids.

Overview

Immobility is a lack of movement. It may involve one body part, several parts, or the entire body. There are several different types of paralysis. **Paraplegia** describes paralysis of the lower part of the body (**Figure 29–1**). Paraplegics can maintain use of their arms but not their legs. When one side of the body is paralyzed, the condition is known as **hemiplegia** (**Figure 29–2**). When the trunk and all four limbs are paralyzed, it is termed **quadriplegia** or tetraplegia (**Figure 29–3**). The entire body may be immobile due to an acute illness or coma. The extent and duration of immobilization cause a variety of different effects. When immobilized to any degree, passive exercise or physiotherapy can help to minimize negative effects.

A *supine* posture causes decreased force of gravity on the intestines and urinary tract compared with standing. Lack of bone muscle activity can lead to osteoporosis. Decreased blood circulation can lead to deep vein thrombosis. Other effects of immobilization include changes in metabolism, urinary function, and respiratory function.

Effects on the Skin

When circulation is impaired, cell regeneration is reduced, and the skin breaks down easily. In areas with less muscle or adipose tissue to cushion the body's weight, blood supply is often reduced. However, overweight people have skin breakdown too; any prolonged pressure on the skin can decrease blood supply. The most vulnerable areas of the body to skin breakdown are the sacrum, ischial tuberosities (sitting bones), elbows, and heels. Prolonged pressure (usually 15–20 minutes) in these areas often results in ischemia and tissue necrosis (**Figure 29–4**). This leads to *bedsores* or *pressure sores* (**decubitus ulcers**). The following are additional factors that contribute to skin breakdown and development of decubitus ulcers:

- Anemia
- Edema

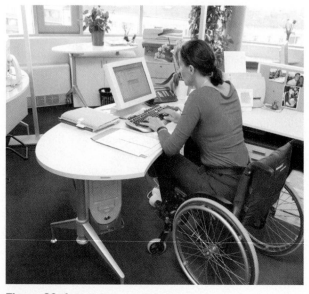

Figure 29–1 Paraplegia.

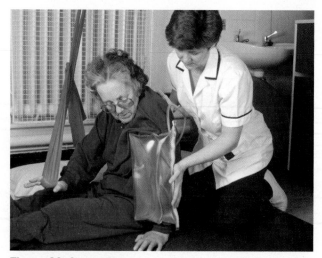

Figure 29–2 Hemiplegia.

- Excessive moisture (from perspiration or urine)
- Inadequate hydration
- Inadequate nutrition
- Inadequate subcutaneous tissue
- Loss of sensation
- Mechanical friction or skin irritation (due to orthotics, braces, adhesive tape, other equipment, or clothing)
- Poor circulation
- Poor personal hygiene

Pressure ulcers may be difficult to heal unless factors such as positioning or nutrition are determined and addressed. Early stage decubitus ulcers first appear reddened but are not open. This is followed by superficial skin breakdown, such as abrasions or blisters. Ulceration then occurs, becoming purple-red in color if skin is deeply damaged.

> **RED FLAG**
> During periods of immobilization, necrosis destroys deeper tissues and results in more serious pressure ulcers and infection.

The patient's position should be frequently changed to avoid prolonged pressure to certain body areas. This helps to maintain adequate blood circulation to the tissues and underlying structures.

The role of the physical therapist assistant (PTA) for the immobilized patient involves implementing a program of gentle range-of-motion exercises, position changes, and patient or

> **RED FLAG**
> Immobilized patients should have their positions changed every 2 hours. Patients in wheelchairs should have their positions changed every 20 minutes.

caregiver education on pressure-relieving methods.

Effects on the Musculoskeletal System

Inactive muscles lose endurance, mass, and strength quickly. Even a short period of time during which a patient has to wear a cast can result in *disuse atrophy*. With atrophy, the muscle fibers shrink and the muscle is smaller. Immobilized joints may shorten and tighten up, increasing the risk of joint contractures. Joints must be correctly positioned when immobilized so abnormal stress can be reduced and abnormal

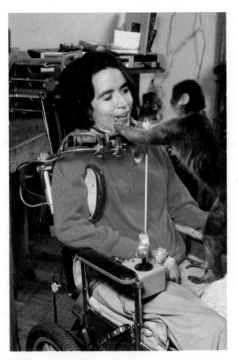

Figure 29–3 Quadriplegia (or tetraplegia).

fixation can be avoided. An example is a "foot drop," caused by improper downward position of the ankles with immobilization, although this can be an issue with wheelchair-bound patients also.

Inactive joints may adopt abnormal positions if flexibility is not maintained via the use of range-of-motion exercises. This is because **flexor** muscles are stronger than their opposing **extensor** muscles. Inactivity causes tendons and ligaments to shorten and lose elasticity, leading to joint contractures. During prolonged immobility, muscle wasting and weakening with decreased flexibility may be seen, as well as other effects, including **contracture** and loss of function.

The effects of immobilization can result in other conditions. Venous return is impaired, causing pooling of blood, edema, and decreased cardiac output. The bones are at risk for osteoporosis, as inactivity causes bones to deteriorate. Bone is living tissue that normally is constantly reformed via osteoblastic activity. Other bone tissue is constantly resorbed via **osteoclastic** activity. When there is a lack of weight bearing on the bones and concurrent lack of muscle activity, bone demineralization occurs. Osteoclastic activities continue even though osteoblastic activities greatly decrease. When this happens, the bone loses mass, leading to *osteoporosis*. Spontaneous bone fractures are then more likely to occur when stress is applied.

As a result of the breakdown of muscles and bones, elevated serum levels of nitrogen wastes such as creatinine occur. Serum calcium is also elevated, and hypercalcemia may result in kidney stones (*renal calculi*) when fluid intake is inadequate, causing overconcentration of urine. High serum calcium levels impede muscle activity, decreasing muscle tone and causing muscle atrophy and weakness. An upper motor neuron lesion may cause **flaccidity**. The role of the PTA includes implementing a program of regular, passive range-of-motion exercises. Passive range of motion prevents or minimizes joint contractures, and active strengthening exercises address atrophy.

Effects on Breathing

With prolonged immobilization, a person requires less oxygen because of decreased metabolism, and the breathing pattern becomes more shallow and slowed. Deep breathing and coughing is more difficult with prolonged immobilization. Chest expansion is restricted by body weight and is also due to weakness of the muscles involved in breathing. Thoracic capacity is reduced and airflow is diminished, thus decreasing gas exchange.

> **RED FLAG**
> Drugs that affect respiration and depress neuromuscular activity include sedatives and opioid analgesics.

Immobilization causes secretions to build up in the airways, thus increasing the risk of pneumonia. These may be difficult to manage due to a diminished coughing mechanism and may require secretion removal techniques. Dehydration and inflammation, due to surgery or testing procedures, may lead to more viscous mucus. Lung expansion is impaired by increased lung fluids, and stasis of secretions encourages serious respiratory complications. Infections such as **hypostatic pneumonia** (which is often related to immobilization) and conditions such as *atelectasis* (lung collapse) may be caused by increased secretions. These conditions can also occur because of aspiration of food or water due to weakness or impairment of swallowing muscles, which occurs more easily in a supine position.

The role of the PTA in immobilized patients with respiratory conditions includes implementing procedures such as positioning (part of postural drainage). Breathing exercises are usually also helpful and are often part of preoperative preparations. Respiration capacity is improved by the use of personal inspirameters.

Effects on the Cardiovascular System

Initial immobilization increases the heart rate and stroke volume. Prolonged immobility reduces cardiac output and venous return. **Orthostatic hypotension** may then occur,

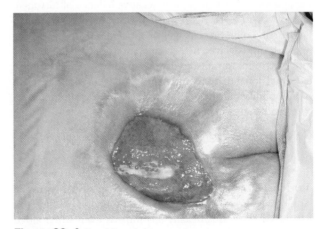

Figure 29–4 Decubitus ulcers.

causing short periods of fainting or dizziness, pallor, sweating, and rapid pulse if body position is changed quickly from a lying position to a sitting position. If a patient who has been immobilized for a long time becomes mobile, there may be a period of several weeks for reflex controls to return to normal.

The pooling of blood in the lower body causes edema and increased capillary pressure. Persistently increasing interstitial fluid, as seen in edema, reduces arterial blood flow and capillary exchange of nutrients to that body region. As a result, the patient has an increased risk of infection, pressure ulcers, and tissue necrosis. The role of the PTA is to implement range-of-motion exercises and low impact exercises such as walking to increase blood flow and improve heart function.

> **RED FLAG**
> To reduce lower extremity edema, an immobilized limb should be elevated. This helps the blood to return to the heart through the inferior vena cava.

Pooling of blood is known as **stasis**, and immobility may cause the formation of thrombi in the veins, typically in the legs. Compression or damage to blood vessels due to pressure may cause blood clots to form. Patients with cancer or dehydration may develop blood clots because of increased blood coagulability. A thrombus that breaks away from the initial site (often because of massage or other movement) may travel to the lungs and result in a *pulmonary embolus*. This is a serious medical condition and requires immediate attention. For periods of immobilization, treatments to avoid emboli conditions include anticoagulant therapy, antiembolic stockings, and gentle range-of-motion or active exercises.

Effects on the Digestive System

Constipation is the major problem associated with immobility. Normal elimination of feces is slowed because of body position and muscle inactivity. Many immobilized patients consume less than adequate amounts of fluid, food, and fiber. Intestinal peristalsis is reduced, and more water is absorbed from the stool. Elderly immobilized patients are most vulnerable to constipation, although all patients are at risk. Laxatives, physical activities, and increased intake of fluids and fiber are very important.

Inactivity also reduces appetite. Decreased food intake usually aggravates depression and fatigue, further decreasing appetite. This can cause a negative balance of nitrogen, known as a *protein deficit*, especially when muscle breakdown is occurring. This protein deficit contributes to low hemoglobin levels and delayed healing of open wounds. Total parenteral nutrition, administered intravenously, may be indicated if normal oral nutrition cannot be maintained. Another result of immobility may be obesity, as it is easy for caloric intake to exceed energy expenditures.

Effects on the Urinary System

In immobilized patients, urinary tract infections may develop due to stasis of urine. Kidney stones (renal calculi) may also develop. Normal drainage of urine into the ureter from the kidneys requires gravity. Horizontal emptying of the bladder into a bedpan is usually incomplete, even when aided by catheterization. Weakness of pelvic floor muscles may affect the normal voiding of urine. If renal calculi form or if catheters are used to drain urine, a bladder infection (cystitis) may develop.

Effects on Children

For children, the effects of immobilization are more serious. Because weight bearing is needed for bone and muscle development, normal growth and development can be delayed or diminished. When the stimulus for bone and muscle development is lost, normal growth is often delayed. However, when the child becomes mobile again, a period of "catch-up growth" may occur. Various immobilizing conditions may cause deformities to develop that involve the hands, feet, hips, or spine.

The role of the PTA with immobilized children includes implementing passive and active range-of-motion exercises, age-appropriate play activities, walking, and other activities to promote normal development. Toys, games, and activities in a playroom setting should be provided if at all possible, with assistance for the child to be able to play with them. Education should be provided to the parents of caregivers of these children as to the activities and movements that are most helpful.

SUMMARY

Immobility can affect one part, several parts, or every part of the body, with temporary or permanent effects. For the integumentary system, skin breakdown and pressure ulcers can result. Because of the lack of gravity and weight bearing, changes can occur to the muscle and bones. The respiratory system shows changes with breathing and coughing mechanisms. Changes to muscle and bone develop quickly, causing many other conditions. Deep breathing and coughing effectiveness may be restricted. In the cardiovascular system, orthostatic hypotension and thromboembolism are serious developments. In the urinary system, reduced peristalsis often leads to constipation and development of infections and renal calculi. For children, immobility can have long-lasting affects on normal growth and development.

REVIEW QUESTIONS

Select the best response to each question.

1. Which cells contribute to the development of osteoporosis?
   a. osteoblasts
   b. osteoclasts
   c. osteocytes
   d. none of the above
2. The following apply to immobility *except*
   a. cardiac output and venous return is increased
   b. cardiac output and venous return is decreased
   c. orthostatic hypotension may occur
   d. the body develops edema and capillary pressure is increased
3. Long-term immobilized patients are highly vulnerable to
   a. diarrhea
   b. nausea and vomiting

c. hemorrhoids

d. constipation

4. Decubitus ulcers are also called

a. gangrene

b. pyemia

c. bed sores

d. pus

5. Paralysis of one side of the body is referred to as what condition?

a. paraplegia

b. hemiplegia

c. quadriplegia (tetraplegia)

d. flaccidity

6. A patient with a cast may experience which of the following conditions?

a. atrophy

b. hypertrophy

c. hyperplasia

d. none of the above

7. A permanent shortening of a muscle that causes deformity is called

a. hypertrophy

b. dystrophy

c. exfoliation

d. contracture

8. The slowing or stopping of the flow of blood is known as

a. hypostatic pneumonia

b. orthostatic hypotension

c. stasis

d. none of the above

9. The effects of immobilization on the urinary system include which of the following?

a. urinary tract infections

b. renal calculi

c. hypertrophy of the prostate

d. both A and B

10. Paralysis of lower limbs is called which of the following?

a. flaccidity

b. paraplegia

c. hemiplegia

d. quadriplegia (tetraplegia)

CASE STUDIES

Karen Coupe, PT, DPT, MSEd

Case 1

An 18-year-old girl suffered an American Spinal Injury Association Classification A (ASIA A) T-12 spinal cord injury and a traumatic brain injury secondary to a motor vehicle accident. The patient was in a coma for 4 days and on a ventilator for 1 week. Patient medical history: Unremarkable. The patient is currently being treated in an inpatient rehabilitation center. She recently developed a pressure ulcer over the sacrum.

1. Based on the level of injury, is this classified as a tetraplegia (quadriplegic) or paraplegia injury? Compare and contrast the difference in the two levels of injury.

2. Explain what is meant by coma. Does the patient have eye opening? Can the patient respond to your verbal instructions?

3. The patient was on a ventilator. As the patient was weaned off the ventilator, what would you expect to observe?

4. This patient is currently working on wheelchair mobility and therefore is no longer ambulatory. What will occur to the skeletal system below the level of injury? Why does this occur?

5. Why would this patient be susceptible to pressure ulcers? Explain methods to prevent pressure ulcers.

Case 2

A 29-year-old man was referred to physical therapy secondary to a right ankle fracture with subsequent open reduction internal fixation. The patient was non–weight bearing (NWB) for 2 weeks followed by 4 weeks of weight bearing as tolerated in a cam walker boot and axillary crutches. Prior level of function: Independent in all activities. PT evaluation reveals poor skin mobility with some surgical scar adherence, decreased ankle range of motion, decreased muscle strength with atrophy present. Plan of care is for therapeutic exercise and gait training activities.

1. Based on the period of immobilization, are the changes in skin mobility expected? What are some methods used in physical therapy to improve skin mobility?

2. The PT evaluation shows a decrease in ankle range of motion. Why would this occur? What structures have lost mobility?

3. Part of the plan of care includes therapeutic exercise. When the PTA begins stretching, what precautions should be taken based on the length of immobilization?

4. Why would this patient present with atrophy and loss of muscle strength? Based on the injury, what muscles would you suspect to be involved? What type of therapeutic exercise would be used to address this problem?

5. The patient was initially NWB and then progressed to WBAT. Using Wolff's law, compare and contrast the difference in NWB for 6 weeks versus NWB for 2 weeks.

WEBSITES

http://emedicine.medscape.com/article/190115-overview

http://findarticles.com/p/articles/mi_m0FSS/is_1_14/ai_n17208303/

http://symptoms.wrongdiagnosis.com/cosymptoms/immobility/skin-problems.htm

http://www.associatedcontent.com/article/6124/caregiving_tips_for_the_bedridden.html?cat=5

http://www.mayoclinic.com/health/bedsores/DS00570

http://www.mayoclinic.com/health/orthostatic-hypotension/DS00997

http://www.niams.nih.gov/Health_Info/Bone/Osteoporosis/Conditions_Behaviors/bed_rest.asp http://www.nlm.nih.gov/medlineplus/ency/article/003188 .htm

http://www.nlm.nih.gov/medlineplus/paralysis.html

http://www.tpub.com/content/armymedical/md0916/ md09160042.htm

http://www.wrongdiagnosis.com/t/thromboembolism/intro .htm

Reference Laboratory Values

Test	Normal Range
Complete blood count	
RBC count	M: 4.5–6.0 million/cc
	F: 4.0–5.5 million/cc
Hematocrit	M: 40–50%
	F: 35–45%
Hemoglobin	M: 14–18 g/dL
	F: 12–16 g/dL
RBC indices	
MCV	80–95 μm^3
MCH	27–31 pg
MCHC	32–36 g/dL
RDW	11–15%
WBC count	5,000–10,000/mm^3
Granulocytes	
Neutrophils	2,500–8,000/mm^3
Eosinophils	50–500/mm^3
Basophils	25–100/mm^3
Agranulocytes	
Lymphocytes	1,000–4,000/mm^3
Monocytes	100–700/mm^3
Platelet count	150,000–400,000/mm^3
Coagulation tests	
Coagulation factors	
I (Fibrinogen)	200–400 mg/dL
II (Prothrombin)	80–120%
D–Dimer	<250 mcg/L
EDPs	<10 mcg/mL
Platelet count	150,000–400,000/mm^3
PT	11–15 sec
PTT	60–80 sec
aPTT	25–40 sec
Thrombin time	10–13 sec

Test	Normal Range
Chem 7, chem 12, chem 20, hepatic function panel, renal function panel, abdominal pain panel	
ALP	30–100 units/L
ALT (SGPT)	5–40 units/L
Amylase	50–190 units/L
AST (SGOT)	5–40 units/L
Bilirubin—total	0.1–1.25 mg/dL
Direct	0.1–0.3 mg/dL
Indirect	0.2–1.0 mg/dL
Blood urea nitrogen	8–20 mg/dL
Ca++—total	9–11 mg/dL
Ionized	4.25–5.25 mg/dL
Lipid profile	
High-density lipoprotein	M: >45 mg/dL
Low-density lipoprotein	F: >55 mg/dL
Very-low-density lipoprotein	60–180 mg/dL
Total cholesterol	25–50%
Triglycerides	<200 mg/dL
	M: 40–60 mg/dL
	F: >35–135 mg/dL
Cardiac profile	
CPK–MB/CPK relative index	<2.5%
CPK—total	WM: 60–320 units/L
Glucose	WF: 50–200 units/L
LDH—total	BM: 130–450 units/L
LDH–1	BF: 60–270 units/L
Troponin 1	70–110 mg/dL
	100–190 units/L
	14–26%
	Negative
Electrolyte panel	
Na+	135–145 mEq/L
K+	3.5–5 mEq/L
Cl	91–110 mEq/L
CO_2	20–30 mEq/L

Test	Normal Range
Toxicology—toxic levels	
Drug serum screen	
Alcohol	
Intoxicated	0.1–0.4%
Stuporous	0.4–0.5%
Comatose	>0.5%
Acetaminophen	>250 mcg/mL
ASA	>300 mcg/mL
Barbitals	
Sedatives	>10 mcg/mL
Anticonvulsant	>40 mcg/mL
Carboxyhemoglobin	>20%
Dilantin	>20 mcg/mL
Lead	> 40 mcg/mL
Lithium	>2.0 mEq/L
Drug urine screen	
Amphetamine	>3 mcg/mL
Diet suppressants	>15 mcg/mL
Dextroamphetamine	>50 mcg/mL
Phenmetrazine	
Methamphetamine	>40 mcg/mL
Mercury	>100 mcg/day
Cerebrospinal fluid	
Pressure	70–200 mm H_2O
Color	Clear
Protein	10–45 mg/dL
Glucose	45–78 mg/dL
WBCs—total	<5 cells/mm^3
Neutrophils	0–4%
Lymphocytes	60–80%
Monocytes	20–50%
Urinalysis	
Volume	750–1,800 cc/day
pH	4.6–8.0
Appearance	Clear
Color	Amber
Specific gravity	1.003–1.030
Osmolality	250–1,000 mOsm/L
Albumin	10–100 mg/day
Amylase	<17 units/h
Calcium	<250 mg/day
Creatinine	0.75–1.5 g/day
Glucose	<500 mg/day
Potassium	25–125 mEq/day
Protein	0–8 mg/dL
Sodium	40–200 mEq/day
Urea nitrogen	10–20 g/day
Uric acid	250–750 mg/day

BF, Black female; BM, Black male; F, female; M, male; RBC, red blood cell; WBC, white blood cell; WF, White female; WM, White male.

Normal Vital Signs

	0–1 Year	1–6 Years	6–11 Years	11–16 Years	Adults
Blood pressure, mm Hg					
Systolic	60–95	80–100	80–120	94–136	90–120
Diastolic	50–65	50–70	50–80	58–88	60–80
Temperature, °F					
Oral	96–99.5	98.5–9.5	97.5–99.6	97.6–99.6	97.6–99.6
Rectal	99–100	99–100	98.5–99.6	98.6–100.6	98.6–100.6
Pulse, beats/min	80–160	75–130	70–115	55–110	60–100
Respirations, breaths/min	26–40	20–30	18–24	16–24	12–20

Temperature Conversion Chart

Fahrenheit Temperatures	Celsius Temperatures
32 degrees	0 degrees
95 degrees	35 degrees
96 degrees	35.5 degrees
96.8 degrees	36 degrees
98.6 degrees	37 degrees
99.6 degrees	37.5 degrees
100.4 degrees	38 degrees
102.2 degrees	39 degrees
104 degrees	40 degrees
212 degrees	100 degrees

Answer Key

Chapter 1

Answers

1. B
2. D
3. C
4. B
5. D
6. B
7. D
8. D
9. A
10. C

Chapter 2

Answers

1. B
2. D
3. C
4. D
5. C
6. B
7. D
8. A
9. D
10. B

Chapter 3

Answers

1. A
2. C
3. B
4. D
5. D
6. C
7. A
8. C
9. D
10. B

Chapter 4

Answers

1. C
2. A
3. B
4. D
5. B
6. C
7. A
8. B
9. D
10. A

Chapter 5

Answers

1. B
2. A
3. C
4. A
5. C
6. D
7. A
8. B
9. D
10. A

Chapter 6

Answers

1. A
2. D
3. B
4. C
5. A
6. B
7. D
8. B
9. A
10. D

Chapter 7

Answers

1. D
2. B
3. C
4. D
5. A
6. C
7. B
8. C
9. D
10. A

Chapter 8

Answers

1. D
2. B
3. A
4. B
5. C
6. D
7. B
8. A
9. C
10. D

Chapter 9

Answers

1. B
2. C
3. A
4. D
5. A
6. C
7. A
8. D
9. B
10. C

Chapter 10

Answers

1. C
2. D
3. B
4. D
5. A
6. C
7. B
8. D
9. A
10. D

Chapter 11

Answers

1. B
2. C
3. A
4. D
5. B
6. B
7. D
8. A
9. C
10. D

Chapter 12

Answers

1. A
2. D
3. A
4. D
5. D
6. D
7. B
8. B
9. A
10. C

Chapter 13

Answers

1. A
2. A
3. D
4. B
5. D
6. B
7. A
8. C
9. D
10. C

Chapter 14

Answers

1. C
2. D
3. A
4. B
5. D
6. C
7. B
8. A
9. D
10. B

Chapter 15

Answers

1. A
2. B
3. D
4. C
5. B
6. D
7. B
8. A
9. C
10. B

Chapter 16

Answers

1. D
2. B
3. A
4. D
5. C
6. A
7. D
8. B
9. C
10. A

Chapter 17

Answers

1. D
2. A
3. B
4. C
5. D
6. B
7. C
8. B
9. A
10. A

Chapter 18

Answers

1. D
2. B
3. D
4. C
5. B
6. A
7. C
8. A
9. B
10. C

Chapter 19

Answers

1. C
2. D
3. B
4. A
5. A
6. B
7. D
8. C
9. A
10. D

Chapter 20

Answers

1. D
2. C
3. B
4. D
5. A
6. C
7. B
8. A
9. C
10. A

Chapter 21

Answers

1. D
2. B
3. D
4. A
5. B
6. C
7. B
8. D
9. B
10. C

Chapter 22

Answers

1. D
2. B
3. C
4. A
5. C
6. B
7. D
8. D
9. B
10. D

Chapter 23

Answers

1. A
2. D
3. B
4. C
5. C
6. B
7. D
8. A
9. C
10. D

Chapter 24

Answers

1. D
2. B
3. C
4. A
5. D
6. B
7. C
8. D
9. B
10. A

Chapter 25

Answers

1. A
2. A
3. C
4. D
5. C
6. B
7. C
8. D
9. A
10. C

Chapter 26

Answers

1. C
2. B
3. C
4. D
5. A
6. A
7. B
8. C
9. B
10. C

Chapter 27

Answers

1. D
2. B
3. B
4. A
5. C
6. D
7. B
8. C
9. D
10. A

Chapter 28

Answers

1. C
2. D
3. B
4. A
5. C
6. A
7. B
8. D
9. D
10. D

Chapter 29

Answers

1. B
2. A
3. D
4. C
5. B
6. A
7. D
8. C
9. D
10. B

Glossary

Chapter	Term	Definition
18	Abdominocentesis	Surgical puncture of the abdomen via a needle to withdraw fluid.
5	Abrasion	Scraping away of the skin.
9	Abscess	A localized pocket of pus in a solid tissue.
23	Abscesses	Localized infections that cause pockets of pus.
18	Achalasia	A disorder of the esophagus that prevents normal swallowing.
12	Achlorhydria	Lack of hydrochloric acid in the stomach.
18	Achlorhydria	Absence of hydrochloric acid in the stomach's gastric secretions.
3	Achondroplasia	A type of dwarfism that is usually a sporadic mutation.
16	Achondroplasia	A genetic condition that results in abnormally short stature.
15	Achromatic vision	Total color blindness, wherein the patient can see only white, gray, and black.
27	Acid-base buffer systems	The systems by which a nearly constant pH level of body fluids is maintained.
4	Acidosis	A condition of excessive acid in the body fluids.
27	Acidosis	A clinical state wherein the pH of the blood drops significantly below 7.35.
27	Acids	Substances that ionize in water to release hydrogen ions.
17	Acini	Clusters of cells with a "berry-like" appearance, such as the alveoli of the lungs.
4	Acne	A skin condition characterized by inflammation of the oil-producing glands and ducts, commonly occurring during adolescence.
20	Acromegaly	Abnormal, continued growth of parts of the body that begins after puberty.
9	Acute	Of rapid onset and relatively short duration.
17	Acute bronchitis	Inflammation of the large bronchi, usually caused by viruses or bacteria, that lasts for several days or weeks.
17	Acute rhinitis	Acute inflammation of the nose and nasal membranes.
26	Addiction	Physiologic or psychological dependence on a substance.
18	Adenocarcinoma	A cancer of the epithelia originating in glandular tissue.
9	Adhesions	Bands of scar tissue that join two surfaces that are normally separated.
16	Adhesions	The union of two opposing tissue surfaces, as in the sides of a wound.
18	Adhesions	Conditions of body tissues that are normally separate growing together.
17	Adult respiratory distress syndrome (ARDS)	A serious reaction to various types of injuries to the lung.
11	Afterload	The force against which cardiac muscle shortens.
14	Akinesia	Impaired body movement.

Chapter	Term	Definition
19	Albuminuria	The presence of albumin in the urine.
20	Aldosterone	A hormone that increases reabsorption of water and sodium and the release of potassium in the kidneys.
27	Alkalosis	A state wherein the pH of the blood rises significantly above 7.4; alkalosis may be due to the side effects of drugs or disease states.
6	Alleles	Alternative forms of a gene that occupy a corresponding position on homologous chromosomes.
22	Alopecia	Hair loss.
15	Amblyopia	"Lazy eye"; characterized by poor or indistinct vision in an eye that is relatively normal; not the same as "strabismus."
22	Amenorrhea	Absence of menstrual period in women of normal reproductive age.
14	Amnesia	Lack of memory about specific events.
6	Amniocentesis	An obstetric procedure in which small amounts of amniotic fluid are removed for laboratory analysis. It is usually performed between the 16th and 20th weeks of gestation to aid in the diagnosis of fetal abnormalities.
3	Amniotic fluid	A liquid produced by and contained within the fetal membranes during pregnancy.
18	Amylase	An enzyme that breaks starch down into sugar.
26	Anabolic steroids	Hormonal substances that are commonly abused; they stimulate protein formation, resulting in greater strength and endurance.
5	Anaerobic	Without air; lacking oxygen.
10	Anaphylaxis	A severe and acute type I hypersensitivity reaction, with potentially life-threatening symptoms.
18	Anastomoses	Surgical or pathologic connections between several vessels or tubular structures.
7	Anemia	A decrease in the normal number of red blood cells or less than the normal quantity of hemoglobin.
1	Angiogram	An x-ray image produced by angiography, which involves injecting a radiopaque substance into the blood vessels.
7	Angiogenesis	The growth of new blood vessels from preexisting vessels.
11	Angioplasty	Repair of a narrowed blood vessel via surgery or other angiographic procedures
16	Annulus	A ring-like structure or part.
6	Anomaly	A congenital malformation, such as the absence of a limb.
9	Anorexia	Lack or loss of appetite for food.
5	Anoxia	A total lack of oxygen.
11	Anoxia	A total lack of oxygen in tissue.
4	Antenatal	Occurring before birth.
17	Anthracosis	Any lung disease related to inhalation of coal or carbon.
13	Antigens	Specific invading substances or structures that the body senses as "foreign."
10	Antimicrobial	Preventing or inhibiting microbial infection.
7	Antineoplastic	Inhibiting or combating the development of cancer.
8	Antiseptics	Agents that can be applied to the skin to destroy pathogens.
19	Anuria	Complete suppression of urine formation and excretion.
12	Aplastic anemia	The type of anemia in which bone marrow does not produce sufficient new cells to replenish blood cells.
4	Apnea	Absence or severe reduction in breathing.
17	Apnea	Suspension of external breathing.
23	Apocrine glands	A type of sweat gland whose secretions contain parts of secretory cells.
5	Apoptosis	The process of programmed cell death.

Chapter	Term	Definition
28	Apoptosis	A type of cell death in which the cell uses specialized cellular processes for self-destruction.
18	Appendicitis	Inflammation of the appendix.
14	Arachnoid	The middle layer of the meninges, covering the brain and spinal cord.
24	Arsenic	An element that occurs throughout the earth's crust in metal arsenious oxide. Excessive arsenic is stored mainly in the liver, kidneys, gastrointestinal tract, and lungs. Most arsenics are slowly excreted in the urine and feces, which accounts for the toxicity of the element.
17	Arterial blood gases	Blood tests performed by using blood from an artery; the tests are used to determine blood pH, partial pressure of carbon dioxide and oxygen, and bicarbonate levels.
1	Arteriogram	X-ray image produced by arteriography, which involves injecting a radiopaque substance into the arteries.
11	Arteriosclerosis	Hardening of the arteries.
16	Arthritis	Inflammation of one or more joints.
16	Articular	Related to joints (articulations).
28	Articular cartilage	The elastic tissue that is found in the joints.
17	Asbestosis	A chronic inflammatory, fibrotic condition that affects the lungs; it is due to inhalation and retention of asbestos fibers.
24	Asbestos	A fibrous mineral that can be harmful when inhaled.
18	Ascites	Accumulation of fluid in the peritoneal cavity.
28	Ascites	Abnormal accumulation of large amounts of fluid in the abdomen, usually caused by severe liver disease.
5	Asphyxial injuries	Harmful events caused by lack of oxygen for breathing.
20	Asphyxiation	Suffocation; the inability to breathe normally.
17	Asthma	A common chronic inflammatory disease of the airways characterized by variable, recurring airflow obstruction and bronchospasm.
15	Astigmatism	A refractive error of the eye in which there is a difference in the degree of refraction in different areas of the eye.
14	Astrocytomas	A type of common primary childhood brain tumor.
11	Asystole	The absence of contractions of the heart, also known as "cardiac standstill."
4	Atelectasis	Lack of gas exchange within the alveoli.
16	Atelectasis	The lack of gas exchange within alveoli, due to alveolar collapse or fluid consolidation.
11	Atheroma	Athermatous plaque; a plaque-like deposit of material in the coronary arteries.
11	Atherosclerosis	A type of arteriosclerosis wherein fatty deposits collect along the walls of arteries that may harden and eventually block them.
23	Athlete's foot	A fungal infection of the foot that usually starts between two toes and spreads to other toes; also known as tinea pedis.
5	Atrophy	Wasting away of tissue due to disease, poor nutrition, or disuse.
7	Atypical	Not common in form, as in the symptoms of a disease.
11	Auscultation	A diagnostic technique of listening for sounds within the body.
10	Autoantibodies	Antibodies that attack the body's own tissue.
18	Autodigestion	The digestion of the body's own tissue by its enzymes.
8	Autoclaving	The process of using an "autoclave," a device that combines intense pressure and high temperatures to sterilize equipment and other items.
23	Autoinoculation	The inoculation of a microorganism obtained by contact with a lesion on one's own body, producing a secondary infection.
1	Autopsy	Medical examination of a dead body to discover the cause and manner of death.

Chapter	Term	Definition
6	Autosomes	Chromosomes that are not sex chromosomes and appear as a homologous pair in a somatic cell.
16	Avulsion fracture	One in which part of the bone is torn away.
8	Bacteria	Single-celled microorganisms that do not need living tissue to survive.
22	Bacteroides	A type of gram-negative bacteria that are anaerobic and make up the largest amount of normal gastrointestinal flora.
2	Bariatrics	The branch of medicine that deals with the treatment of obesity and its complications.
23	Basal lamina	The layer of extracellular matrix on which epithelium sits; it is secreted by epithelial cells.
23	Basement membrane	A layer of extracellular matrix that anchors epithelial tissue to underlying connective tissue.
27	Bases	Substances that ionize in water, releasing hydroxyl ions, having a pH greater than 7.0.
13	Bence-Jones protein	A monoclonal globulin protein found in the blood or urine that is often suggestive of multiple myeloma.
22	Bicornuate	A formation of the uterus wherein the upper parts remain separate, whereas the lower parts are fused together.
4	Bilirubin	A pigment released into the blood after the destruction of old or damaged red blood cells.
7	Biopsies	Medical tests that involve the removal of cells or tissues for examination.
1	Biopsy	A surgical procedure wherein a piece of tissue is removed for further diagnostic study. Some biopsies require general anesthesia, whereas others are minor procedures done with local anesthesia or even no anesthesia at all.
25	Bipolar depression	A disorder in which a person alternates between periods of euphoric feelings and mania and periods of depression.
3	Blastocyst	A thin-walled, hollow structure that contains the inner cell mass (embryoblast) from which the embryo arises.
15	Blepharitis	Chronic inflammation of the eyelid.
9	Blister	A small pocket of fluid within the upper skin layers.
23	Blisters	Vesicles or bullae; localized skin swellings containing watery fluid and caused by burns, infection, or irritation.
19	Blood urea nitrogen (BUN)	The amount of nitrogen in the blood in the form of urea, which is used to test renal function.
13	B lymphocytes	Those lymphocytes that play a central role in the humoral immune response, creating antibodies against specific antigens.
23	Boil	A skin abscess, a collection of pus localized deep in the skin.
11	Bolus	A single, relatively large dose of a drug.
16	Bone mass density	A measure of the amount of bone tissue in a certain volume of bone.
19	Bowman's capsule	The glomerular capsule; a cup-shaped structure around the glomerulus of each nephron in the kidneys that serves as a filter.
4	Bradycardia	A slower than normal heart rate.
14	Brain	The main component of the nervous system along with the spinal cord, it is protected by and contained within the skull.
6	Brainstem	The lower extension of the brain, where it connects with the spinal cord.
14	Brainstem	The portion of the brain divided into the midbrain, pons, and medulla that contains nerves and helps control respiration, swallowing, wakefulness, and other activities.
22	Broad ligament	The wide fold of peritoneum connecting the sides of the uterus to the walls and floor of the pelvis.
17	Bronchiectasis	Localized, irreversible dilation of part of the bronchial tree.

Chapter	Term	Definition
10	Bronchoconstriction	Narrowing of the breathing tubes of the lungs.
4	Bronchopulmonary dysplasia	A condition in premature infants wherein the lung tissue develops abnormally and is characterized by inflammation and scarring.
17	Bronchoscopy	A method of visualizing the inside of the airways by inserting a bronchoscope through the mouth or nose and, sometimes, via a tracheostomy.
11	Bruit	An abnormal sound heard during auscultation; it results from blood flowing through a narrow or partially occluded artery.
22	Budding yeast	A type of fungi that reproduces asexually, meaning that new yeasts grow from others.
21	Bulbourethral glands	Mucous glands at the base of the penis that secrete into the penile urethra.
23	Bullae	More than one bulla, which is a blister more than 5 mm in diameter with thin walls, that is full of fluid.
16	Bunion	A structural anomaly of the bones and joint between the foot and big toe.
16	Bursitis	Inflammation of the bursa, which are small fluid-filled pads that act as cushions among bones, joints, muscles, and tendons.
7	Cachexia	Wasting syndrome, which includes loss of weight, muscle atrophy, fatigue, weakness, and significant loss of appetite.
23	Callus	A common, usually painless thickening of the stratum corneum at locations of external pressure or friction.
18	Caput medusae	Distended, engorged pariumbilical veins, radiating from the umbilicus across the abdomen, to join the systemic veins.
23	Carbuncles	Deep-seated abscesses that form in hair follicles.
11	Cardiomegaly	Enlargement of the heart.
11	Cardiomyopathy	Chronic disease of the heart muscle wherein it is abnormally enlarged, thickened, or stiffened.
15	Carotenoids	Organic pigments with nutritional value that are found in vegetables and fruits such as carrots, sweet potatoes, spinach, kale, collard greens, and tomatoes.
16	Carpal tunnel syndrome	A painful condition in which the medial nerve becomes pressed or squeezed at the wrist.
24	Carpal tunnel syndrome	Entrapment and compression of the median nerve in the carpal tunnel causes pain and numbness in the wrist, hands, and fingers.
16	Cartilage	Stiff, semi-inflexible connective tissue found throughout the body.
15	Cataract	A clouding of the crystalline lens of the eye or its envelope.
19	Catheterization	Inserting a tube into a body cavity, duct, or vessel.
14	Cauterize	To burn with electricity; used to stop bleeding from tissues.
14	Central nervous system	The brain and spinal cord; it communicates with the organs and body systems via the peripheral nervous system.
14	Cephalgia	Headache.
14	Cerebellum	The portion of the brain that helps to control fine motor movements and coordination.
25	Cerebral cortex	The layer of the brain known as the "gray matter," it covers the outer portion of the cerebrum and cerebellum
14	Cerebrum	The primary portion of the brain, divided into two lobes, each of which have specialized lobes.
22	Chancre	A painless ulcer, usually in the genital area, that is the first sign of a syphilis infection.
9	Chemical mediators	Substances released as part of the inflammatory response that bring about vascular and cellular changes; example histamine.
9	Chemotaxis	Movement that is based on specific chemical factors affecting a cell or organism.
18	Cholecystectomy	Surgical removal of the gallbladder.
18	Cholecystitis	Inflammation of the gallbladder.
18	Cholelithiasis	The formation of gallstones due to hardening of bile components.

Chapter	Term	Definition
14	Chorea	Continuing and rapid complex body movements.
15	Choroid	The middle, vascular layer of the eye, containing connective tissue; also known as the "choroid coat" or "choroidea."
7	Chromosomes	Organized structures of DNA and proteins found in cells.
9	Chronic	Of slow onset and relatively long duration.
17	Chronic bronchitis	A chronic inflammation of the bronchi in the lungs; it is defined as a persistent cough that produces sputum and mucus lasting for between 3 months and 2 years.
17	Chronic obstructive pulmonary disease	A condition that refers to both chronic bronchitis and emphysema, in which the airways become narrowed.
18	Cirrhosis	A result of chronic liver disease characterized by replacement of liver tissue by fibrosis, scar tissue, or regenerative nodules.
3	Cleavage	The process of mitotic cell divisions that produces a blastula from a fertilized ovum.
22	Clitoris	A small mass of erectile tissue located at the top anterior part of the vulva; the primary site of female arousal.
16	Closed fracture	A broken bone underneath intact skin.
17	Clubbing	A deformity of (usually) the fingers and fingernails usually related to various conditions of the lungs and heart.
23	Coalesce	To grow together.
4	Colic	Painful spasms in the colon, usually affecting infants.
9	Collagen	The protein portion of the white, shiny, nonelastic fibers of the skin, tendons, bone, cartilage, and all other types of connective tissue.
23	Collagen	The primary protein found in bone, cartilage, and connective tissue; it provides strength and support for these structures.
18	Colorectal	Referring to the colon and rectum.
16	Comminuted fracture	A broken bone that is splintered or crushed into a number of pieces.
10	Complement	A protein that helps antibodies to clear pathogens from the body.
16	Complete fracture	One involving the entire cross-section of a bone.
16	Compound fractures	Those in which the bone or bones stick through the skin; it is also known as an "open fracture."
16	Compression	Pressing together.
16	Compression fracture	A fracture caused by pressing together, often seen in vertebral fractures due to osteoporosis.
16	Computed tomography	An x-ray procedure that combines many images via computer to generate cross-sectional or three-dimensional views.
22	Congenital syphilis	A type of syphilis present in utero and at birth, occurring when a child is born to a mother who has secondary syphilis.
15	Conjunctivitis	"Pink eye"; an acute inflammation of the conjunctiva (the outermost layer of the eye and innermost layer of the eyelids).
18	Constipation	A symptom of infrequent, hard to pass bowel movements.
29	Contracture	A permanent shortening of a muscle, causing distortion or deformity.
9	Contractures	Shortenings of specific structures.
5	Contusion	A bruise; an injury with no break in the skin, characterized by discoloration, pain, and swelling.
14	Convulsions	Abnormal muscle contractions.
12	Cooley's anemia	Beta thalassemia major; it occurs when similar gene defects affect production of the beta globin protein, with both parents having the defective gene.
15	Cornea	The transparent front part of the eye that covers the iris, pupil, and anterior chamber.
23	Corns	Horny masses of condensed epithelial cells overlying bony prominences; they result from chronic friction and pressure.

Chapter	Term	Definition
11	Coronary artery disease	A condition characterized by blockage of the blood vessels (coronary arteries) that supply the heart muscle.
6	Cranium	The part of the skull that encloses the brain.
19	Creatinine clearance test	A test that gauges the volume of blood plasma that is cleared of creatinine over a unit of time; it helps to determine the glomerular filtration rate.
20	Cretinism	Severely stunted physical and mental growth due to untreated congenital hypothyroidism.
26	Cross-tolerance	Tolerance to drugs similar to a drug for which the body has developed a tolerance.
15	Cryotherapy	The local or general use of low temperatures to decrease cellular metabolism and other activities; when done as a surgical treatment, it is known as "cryosurgery."
21	Cryptorchidism	Failure of one or both testicles to descend into the scrotum.
8	Culture	A substance (medium) used to grow microorganisms (usually bacteria or viruses) for the purpose of further examination or study.
17	Cyanosis	A blue coloration of the skin and mucous membranes due to higher than normal levels of deoxygenated hemoglobin in blood vessels near the skin surface.
12	Cyanotic	A bluish discoloration of the skin and mucous membranes resulting from inadequate oxygenation of the blood.
19	Cystitis	Inflammation of the urinary bladder.
19	Cystogram	A visualization of the urinary bladder via use of a catheter, radiocontrast agent, and x-rays.
19	Cystoscopy	Endoscopy of the urinary bladder via the urethra.
10	Cytotoxic	Destructive or toxic to cells.
15	Daltonism	The more common form of color blindness, wherein the patient cannot distinguish between the colors red and green.
29	Decubitus ulcers	Skin lesions that result from the pressure of lying in the same position for a long time, especially on a bony prominence.
16	Debridement	The act of removing dead, contaminated, or adherent tissue or foreign material.
18	Defecate	To eliminate feces from the digestive tract via the anus.
11	Defibrillation	The process of using an electronic device to shock the heart to stop rapid, irregular heartbeat and restore normal rhythm.
1	Degeneration	Deterioration of tissue to a less functionally active form.
18	Delirium tremens	An acute episode of delirium usually caused by withdrawal from alcohol.
26	Delirium tremens	The "DTs"; a collection of symptoms resulting from severe withdrawal from alcohol.
25	Delusions	False beliefs or opinions that become "fixed" and unshakable.
25	Dementia	Loss of brain function because of certain diseases, displaying serious losses in cognitive activity.
18	Dental caries	Tooth decay or "cavities."
18	Dental plaque	A natural biofilm that may develop on teeth, becoming hardened and discolored; it often leads to dental caries.
7	Deoxyribonucleic acid (DNA)	A nucleic acid that contains genetic instructions needed for development and normal functioning of living organisms.
11	Depolarization	The reduction of a membrane potential to a less negative value.
23	Dermatophytes	Types of fungi that cause parasitic skin diseases.
23	Dermis	The lowest layer of skin, it is positioned above the subcutaneous fat layer.
20	Diabetes inspidus	A condition of excessive thirst and secretion of large amounts of severely diluted urine, most commonly caused by a deficiency of antidiuretic hormone.
20	Diabetes mellitus	Commonly known as "diabetes"; a condition of abnormally high blood sugar, either due to inability of the body to produce enough insulin or because body cells do not respond to the insulin that is produced.

Chapter	Term	Definition
20	Diabetic ketosis	A condition wherein, as a result of diabetes, the body has elevated levels of ketone bodies in the blood; these bodies are formed when glycogen stores in the liver are depleted.
19	Dialysis	The provision of an artificial replacement for lost kidney function in people who have renal failure.
9	Diapedesis	The outward passage of red or white blood cells through the intact walls of the capillaries.
12	Diapedesis	The outward passage of blood cells through intact vessel walls.
11	Diaphoresis	Sweating.
14	Diencephalon	The portion of the brain that houses the thalamus and hypothalamus.
7	Differentiation	The process by which a less specialized cell becomes a more specialized cell type.
21	Differentiation	Increased specialization of cells for certain functions
15	Diplopia	Double vision; the simultaneous perception of two images of the same object.
8	Disinfectants	Agents used to destroy microorganisms or their toxins.
16	Diskectomy	Surgery to remove part or all of a spinal disk.
16	Dislocation	A separation of two bones where they meet at a joint.
16	Displaced fracture	A fracture in which the two ends of a broken bone are separated from each other.
18	Diverticulitis	Inflammation of one or more of the pouches (diverticula) that form because of diverticulosis.
18	Diverticulosis	A common digestive disease, usually in the large intestine, wherein pouches form on the outside of the colon.
26	DOM	An amphetamine popular at "rave parties," where it is referred to as "STP"; its chemical name is 2,5-dimethoxy-4-methylamphetamine.
16	Dowager's hump	An abnormal curvature of the spine that appears as a rounded hump in the upper back.
16	Dual-energy x-ray absorptiometry	A means of measuring bone mineral density via two x-ray beams with different energy levels.
3	Ductus arteriosus	The shunt that connects the pulmonary artery to the aortic arch in developing infants.
21	Ductus deferens	The duct that carries sperm from the epididymis to the ejaculatory duct.
14	Dura mater	The outermost layer of the meninges, covering the brain and spinal cord.
20	Dwarfism	Abnormally short stature due to a variety of conditions, most commonly abnormally low amounts of human growth hormone.
18	Dysentery	An inflammatory condition of (usually) the large intestine that consists of severe diarrhea containing mucus and/or blood, fever, and abdominal pain; untreated dysentery may lead to death.
22	Dysmenorrhea	Severe uterine pain during menstruation.
22	Dyspareunia	Painful sexual intercourse.
14	Dysphagia	Difficulty swallowing.
18	Dysphagia	Difficulty swallowing.
14	Dysphasia	Impaired ability to use and understand language.
17	Dysphonia	An impaired ability to produce normal vocal sounds.
5	Dysplasia	The development of abnormal cells.
12	Dyspnea	Increased efforts to breathe.
17	Dyspnea	Shortness of breath.
19	Dysuria	Painful urination.
22	Dysuria	Pain or difficulty passing urine.
18	Edema	Swelling of body tissues because of fluid accumulation.
4	Egocentric	Concerned with the "self" rather than society.

Chapter	Term	Definition
11	Ejection fraction	The fraction of the total ventricular filling volume that is ejected during each ventricular contraction.
1	Electrocardiogram	A printed readout of the electrical activity of the heart.
15	Electrocholeography	Recording of the electrical activity produced when the cochlea is stimulated.
1	Electroencephalogram	A printed readout of the electrical activity of the brain.
27	Electrolytes	Compounds that, in solution, dissociate into positive and negative ions.
27	Electrolyte balance	A condition consisting of an equal amount of electrolytes entering and leaving the body.
1	Electromyogram	A printed readout of the electrical activity of skeletal muscles.
16	Electromyography	A technique for evaluating and recording the physiologic properties of muscles while they alternately contract and rest.
15	Electronystagmography	A test used in evaluating the vestibulo-ocular reflex.
3	Embryo	The developing offspring, from the 2nd through 8th weeks of pregnancy.
3	Embryoblast	The inner cell mass, from which the embryo arises.
17	Emphysema	Long-term, progressive lung disease that primarily causes shortness of breath; it causes the airways to become unable to hold their functional shape when exhaling.
17	Empyema	A collection of pus within an anatomic cavity.
18	Enamel	The hard white substance covering the crown of a tooth.
19	Encephalopathy	Any disorder or disease of the brain.
8	Endemic	Occurring only in a specific area or population of the world.
5	Endogenous	Occurring from within the body.
22	Endometriosis	A condition wherein uterine tissue forms painful cysts outside of the uterus, such as the pelvic cavity, intestines, and even the lungs.
1	Endoscopy	A procedure that allows the viewing of internal body structures, through the use of tubular devices with cameras and other equipment attached.
18	Enteritis	Inflammation of the small intestine.
23	Epidermis	The outermost layer of skin.
21	Epididymis	A coiled structure in the testis for the storage and transport of sperm to the vas deferens.
14	Epidural	Between the skull and dura mater.
14	Epilepsy	A chronic brain disease caused by intermittent electrical activity, involving seizures or convulsions.
21	Epispadias	An abnormal urethral opening on the upper surface of the penis
10	Erythema	Redness of the skin, often caused by inflammation.
23	Erythema	A nonspecific term indicating inflammation and reddening of the skin.
9	Erythrocyte sedimentation rate	The rate at which red blood cells precipitate within 1 hour; an erythrocyte sedimentation rate test provides a nonspecific measurement of inflammation.
12	Erythrocytosis	Secondary polycythemia, which involves increased erythrocytes in response to prolonged hypoxia and increased erythropoietin secretion.
19	Erythropoiesis	The process by which red blood cells (erythrocytes) are produced.
12	Erythropoietin	A hormone secreted by the kidneys that stimulates the production of erythrocytes in the red bone marrow as a response to insufficient oxygen.
18	Esophageal varices	Extremely dilated submucosal veins in the lower esophagus.
20	Euphoria	A profound sense of well-being.
18	Exacerbation	Irritation; generally refers to a worsening of any condition.
5	Exogenous	Occurring from a source outside the body.
21	Exogenous	Originating from outside the body.
20	Exophthalmos	An outward protrusion of the eyeballs.

Chapter	Term	Definition
6	Expression	The indication of a physical or emotional state through facial appearance or vocal intonation.
29	Extensor	A muscle that extends or straightens a limb or body part.
9	Exudate	Fluid, cells, or other substances that slowly escape from blood vessels and are deposited on tissues or tissue surfaces.
3	Fertilization	The union of a male sperm and a female ovum; also called conception.
3	Fetus	The developing offspring, from the 8th week until birth.
9	Fibrinogen	A soluble plasma glycoprotein formed in the liver that is converted (by thrombin) into fibrin during blood coagulation.
9	Fibrinous	Inflammation resulting in a large increase in vascular permeability that allows fibrin to pass through the blood vessels.
9	Fibroblasts	Cells that synthesize the extracellular matrix and collagen and play an important role in wound healing.
13	Filarial parasites	Long, round, threadlike worms that may invade lymphatic structures and vessels, soft tissues, and skin; they are most common in tropic and subtropic regions.
29	Flaccidity	Weakness and softness, as of a muscle, with decreased resistance to movement, increased mobility, and greater than normal range of movements.
26	Flashbacks	Repeat occurrences of the symptoms of hallucinogens after the actual period of usage is past.
29	Flexor	A muscle that, when contracted, acts to bend a limb or joint in the body.
22	Follicles	The basic units of female reproduction, composed of primarily round aggregations of cells found in the ovary.
4	Fontanels	Spaces covered by tough membranes between the bones of an infant's cranium, sometimes referred to as "soft spots."
3	Foramen ovale	The second shunt in a fetal heart; it allows blood to enter the left atrium from the right atrium.
16	Fracture	A separation of a bone into two or more pieces; a fracture may be partial or complete.
9	Fracture callus	A temporary formation of fibroblasts and chondroblasts at the site of a bone fracture as the bone attempts to heal itself.
19	Frequency	The need to urinate more often than usual.
3	Full-term	A fetus that has reached 37 weeks of development and is essentially able to survive outside of the womb.
18	Fulminant	Occurring quickly, with extreme severity.
8	Fungi	Single-celled or multiple-celled microorganisms that can change shape and grow well in warmth or moisture.
23	Furuncle	A localized suppurative staphylococcal skin infection that originates in a gland or hair follicle; it is characterized by pain, redness, and swelling.
5	Gangrene	A condition involving a large amount of necrosis (body tissue death).
22	Gardnerella vaginalis	A gram-variable anaerobic bacteria that can cause bacterial vaginosis by disrupting normal vaginal flora.
18	Gastritis	Inflammation of the lining of the stomach.
18	Gastroenteritis	An inflammation of the gastrointestinal tract, involving the stomach and small intestine, which results in extreme diarrhea.
6	Genotype	The complete genetic constitution of an organism or group, as determined by the specific combination and location of the genes on the chromosomes.
20	Gigantism	Abnormal, continued growth of parts of the body that begins before puberty.
18	GI hemorrhage	Bleeding in the gastrointestinal tract.
18	Gilbert's syndrome	The most common hereditarily linked cause of raised bilirubin levels, resulting in jaundice.

Chapter	Term	Definition
18	Gingivitis	Inflammation of the gum tissue.
15	Glaucoma	A disease of the optic nerve, involving increased intraocular pressure and potentially progressing to blindness.
14	Gliomas	A common type of primary brain tumor.
19	Glomerulonephritis	Inflammation of the glomeruli (small blood vessels) in the kidneys.
12	Glossitis	Inflammation or infection of the tongue.
4	Glucagon	A pancreatic hormone that increases blood sugar; it has the opposite effect of insulin.
4	Glucometer	Also called a "glucose meter"; a medical device that measures the approximate concentration of glucose in the blood.
18	Gluten-induced enteropathy	A pathologic intestinal condition brought about by a reaction to the proteins gliadin and glutenin (which collectively form gluten).
4	Glycogen	A starch-like substance composed of linked glucose molecules that act as an emergency supply of glucose.
10	Glycoproteins	Molecules made up of sugars and amino acids.
20	Glycosuria	Presence of glucose in the urine.
16	Gout	Metabolic arthritis; a disease caused by a buildup of uric acid.
9	Granulation tissue	Perfused, fibrous connective tissue that replaces the fibrin clot in wounds that are healing.
9	Granuloma	A roughly spherical mass of immune cells that forms when the immune system perceives substances that are foreign and not able to be eliminated.
3	Grasp reflex	A pathologic reflex induced by stroking the palm, with the result that the fingers flex in a grasping motion. In newborns and young infants the tonic grasp reflex is normal.
20	Graves' disease	An autoimmune disorder involving overactivity of the thyroid; excessive production of thyroid hormones results in hyperthyroidism and thyrotoxicosis.
16	Greenstick fracture	A broken bone common in children wherein the break is incomplete and usually healed easily; it is especially common in children with rickets.
18	Gynecomastia	The development of abnormally large mammary glands in males, causing breast enlargement.
21	Gynecomastia	Abnormal enlargement of breast tissue in men.
22	Hair follicles	Sac-like indentations from which hair grows; they are found in all areas of external skin, even when they no longer produce hair (as in baldness).
25	Hallucinations	Perceptions of (usually) auditory or visual stimuli that do not exist in reality.
26	Hallucinogens	Psychedelics; psychoactive substances that can cause serious changes in perceptions of all types.
20	Hashimoto's thyroiditis	An autoimmune disease in which the thyroid gland is destroyed by various immune processes; it often results in either hypo- or hyperthryoidism.
12	HbF	Fetal hemoglobin; the main fetal oxygen transport protein.
12	Hemarthrosis	A bleeding into joint spaces.
18	Hematemesis	The vomiting of blood.
18	Hematochezia	The passage of a maroon-colored stool.
12	Hematocrit	The proportion of cells (mostly red blood cells) in blood.
5	Hematoma	Blood loss into a tissue, organ, or other confined space.
12	Hematopoiesis	The development of blood cells.
7	Hematopoietic	Related to hematopoiesis, the formation of blood cellular components.
19	Hematuria	The presence of red blood cells in the urine.
14	Hemiparesis	Weakness on one side of the body.
29	Hemiplegia	Paralysis of one side of the body

Chapter	Term	Definition
18	Hemochromatosis	An iron overload from a hereditary and/or primary cause.
1	Hemophilia	The body's inability to control normal blood clotting or coagulation.
11	Hemoptysis	Spitting up blood.
9	Hemorrhagic	Related to bleeding, or bloody in appearance.
18	Hemorrhoids	Normal structures in the anal canal that may become pathologic when swollen or inflamed.
18	Hepatic encephalopathy	A condition caused by liver failure wherein the patient exhibits confusion, altered levels of consciousness, followed by coma and, potentially, death.
18	Hepatitis	Inflammation of the liver.
12	Hepatomegaly	Enlargement of the liver.
18	Hepatomegaly	An enlarged liver.
26	Hepatotoxin	A substance that is toxic to the liver.
23	Herpetic whitlow	A painful viral (herpes) infection of the hands or fingers.
13	Heterophil	A neutrophil that can recognize an antigen other than the one it is expected to attack.
6	Heterozygous	An organism whose somatic cells have two different allomorphic genes on the same location of each pair of chromosomes.
18	Hiatal hernia	Protrusion of the upper stomach into the thorax through a weakness or tear in the diaphragm.
20	Hirsuitism	Excessive hair growth on parts of the body that usually only experience minimal or complete lack of hair growth.
11	Holter monitor	A portable device used for recording cardiac activity over 24 hours or longer; the patient wears it throughout the day and keeps a journal of stressful events, which is compared with the monitor's record.
1	Homeostasis	The regulation and stabilization of a normal internal body environment.
6	Homozygous	Having two identical alleles at corresponding locations on homologous chromosomes.
24	Human leukocyte antigens	Unique histocompatibility antigens (self-antigens) on the surface of cells, also called major histocompatibility complex (MHC) antigens.
22	Human papillomavirus (HPV)	A group of over 100 viruses that cause a range of afflictions, including warts and cervical cancer.
10	Humoral	Pertaining to, or derived from, a body fluid.
21	Hydrocele	A fluid-filled cavity or duct that may occur in the scrotum.
19	Hydronephrosis	Distention and dilation of the renal pelvis and calyces of the kidney.
2	Hydrostatic weighing	Underwater weighing; a method to determine the mass density of a body.
27	Hydrostatic pressure	The pressure of fluids or their properties when in equilibrium.
4	Hyperbilirubinemia	Higher than normal amounts of bilirubin in the blood.
27	Hyperchloremia	An excessive concentration of chloride in the blood.
20	Hypercortisolism	High levels of cortisol in the blood, leading to Cushing's syndrome.
9	Hyperemia	The increase of blood flow to different body tissues.
4	Hyperinsulinemia	A condition of abnormally high levels of insulin in the blood due to either excessive secretion from the pancreas or by decreased metabolism of insulin.
27	Hyperkalemia	An excessive concentration of potassium in the blood.
4	Hyperlipidemia	A condition of excessive levels of any specific fat or fats in the blood.
27	Hypernatremia	An excessive concentration of sodium in the blood.
15	Hyperopia	Farsightedness (long-sightedness or hypermetropia); it occurs often when the eyeball is too short or the lens cannot become round enough. This causes the individual to be able to see far-off objects more clearly than close-up objects.
20	Hyperparathyroidism	Overactivity of the parathyroid glands, resulting in excess parathyroid hormone.
3	Hyperplasia	An abnormal increase in cells that causes enlargement of a tissue or organ.

Chapter	Term	Definition
5	Hyperplasia	An increase in the amount of normal cells in a tissue or organ.
5	Hypertrophy	Enlargement or overgrowth of an organ or body part due to hyperplasia.
19	Hypervolemia	Fluid overload; a condition of too much fluid in the blood.
27	Hypochloremia	A lower than normal concentration of chloride in the blood.
12	Hypochromic	Paler than normal (cells).
10	Hypogammaglobulinemia	An immune disorder characterized by a reduction of gamma globulins.
4	Hypoglycemia	Abnormally low blood sugar.
20	Hypoglycemia	Lower than normal levels of blood glucose.
3	Hypokalemia	Lower than normal potassium in the blood.
27	Hypokalemia	A lower than normal concentration of potassium in the blood.
27	Hyponatremia	A lower than normal concentration of sodium in the blood.
20	Hypoparathyroidism	Underactivity of the parathyroid glands, resulting in lower than normal levels of parathyroid hormone.
10	Hypoproteinemia	An abnormally low level of protein in the blood.
29	Hypostatic pneumonia	Inflammation of the lungs, with congestion; usually caused by immobility, especially lying on the back.
4	Hypotonia	A state of low muscle tone.
11	Hypovolemia	A decrease in the volume of blood plasma, which decreases overall blood volume.
4	Hypoxemia	Low concentration of oxygen in the blood.
17	Hypoxemia	Decreased partial pressure of oxygen in the blood.
5	Hypoxia	Low concentration of oxygen in a tissue or lack of an adequate supply of oxygen.
17	Hypoxia	A deprivation of adequate oxygen supply.
22	Hysterosalpingogram	A radiologic examination of the uterus and fallopian tubes that uses injection of a radiopaque material into the cervix for fluoroscopic viewing.
22	Hysteroscopy	Inspection of the uterus via endoscopy through the cervix.
1	Iatrogenic	Pertaining to a disease or condition caused by a physician's treatment. For example, side effects of drugs are sometimes referred to as iatrogenic conditions.
1	Idiopathic	Pertaining to a disease or condition of unknown cause.
18	Ileus	A disruption of normal, propulsive gastrointestinal activity due to nonmechanical causes.
29	Immobility	A state of being incapable of movement.
16	Impacted fracture	A broken bone in which one broken end is wedged into the other broken end.
23	Impetigo	A bacterial skin infection most commonly seen in children; it is highly contagious.
3	Implantation	The process by which a fertilized egg implants in the uterine lining.
19	In and out catheterization	A temporary procedure wherein a catheter is removed as soon as urine is drained from the urinary bladder.
16	Incomplete fracture	A fracture that does not extend through the full transverse width of a bone.
28	Incontinence	Lack of ability to control urination or defecation.
17	Induration	An area of soft tissue or organ hardening.
19	Indwelling catheter	A catheter placed into the urinary bladder for longer periods of time.
22	Infantile uterus	A uterus that has not attained normal adult characteristics; it may be smaller than normal or not enough sufficient tissue to support a pregnancy.
9	Infection	The colonization of a host organism by a foreign microorganism.
5	Inflammation	Redness, pain, and swelling due to infection or other causes.
9	Inflammation	A normal body defense mechanism that localizes and removes harmful agents; it is signified by swelling, redness, heat, pain, and occasional loss of function.
17	Influenza	The "flu"; a viral infection that causes chills, fever, muscle pains, sore throat, coughing, severe headache, weakness, fatigue, and general malaise.

Chapter	Term	Definition
18	Inguinal hernia	A protrusion of the abdominal cavity contents through the inguinal canal.
14	Insomnia	A chronic inability to sleep or to remain asleep throughout the night.
9	Interferons	Blood proteins that have antiviral effects.
10	Interleukins	Proteins called lymphokines that help to regulate the immune system.
16	Interphalangeal	Between the phalanges (fingers or toes).
19	Interstitial cystitis	A urinary bladder disease characterized by pain during urination, urinary frequency, urgency, and pressure in the bladder and/or pelvis.
18	Intestinal obstruction	Bowel obstruction that may be mechanical or functional; it can occur in any section and is a medical emergency.
18	Intestinal polyps	Abnormal growths of intestinal tissue.
19	Intravenous pyelogram (IVP)	A radiologic procedure used to visualize abnormalities of the urinary system.
18	Intrinsic factor	A glycoprotein produced in the stomach that is required for the absorption of vitamin B_{12}.
18	Intussusception	A condition wherein part of the intestine has folded into another section of the intestine.
15	Iridotomy	Also known as "laser iridotomy," it is a surgical procedure used to treat angle-closure glaucoma; the procedure involves making a hole in the iris to change its configuration.
15	Iris	The colored portion of the eye; it controls the diameter and size of the pupil.
18	Irritable bowel syndrome	Spastic colon; a functional bowel disorder characterized by abdominal pain, discomfort, bloating, and altered bowel function.
5	Ischemia	A temporary reduction of blood supply to an organ or tissue because of an obstruction of a blood vessel.
11	Ischemia	Insufficient supply of blood to an organ, usually because of a blocked artery.
18	Islets of Langerhans	Regions of the pancreas that contain its endocrine cells.
9	Isoenzymes	Enzymes that differ in amino acid sequence but catalyze the same chemical reaction.
1	Isotopes	Substances that emit characteristic radiation, used to label various substances to determine their uptake and excretion.
18	Jaundice	A yellowish discoloration of the skin, sclera, and mucous membranes due to various liver conditions.
16	Joints	Articulations; connections that allow motion between two bones.
23	Kaposi's sarcoma	A skin cancer that most commonly appears in people with damaged immune systems, particularly in those with AIDS.
5	Karyolysis	Complete dissolution of a cell's chromatin as a result of the actions of deoxyribonuclease (DNase).
6	Karyotype	A diagrammatic representation of the chromosome complement of an individual or species in which the chromosomes are arranged in pairs in descending order of size and according to the position of the centromere.
23	Keratinocytes	Epidermal cells that synthesize keratin and other white, firmly attached patches that are slightly raised and sharply circumscribed.
19	Kidneys-ureter-bladder (KUB)	A diagnostic medical imaging technique of the abdomen.
16	Kyphosis	Hunchback; an abnormal backward curvature of the spine, resulting in a "humped" appearance of the upper back.
22	Labia majora	The major outside pair of lips of the vulva.
22	Labia minora	The minor inside pair of lips of the vulva.
5	Laceration	A torn wound with ragged edges.
22	Lactation	The production and secretion of milk from the mammary glands of the breasts after giving birth.

Chapter	Term	Definition
16	Laminectomy	Surgical removal of the posterior arch of a vertebra.
28	Laminectomy	Surgery to remove the posterior portion (lamina) of the vertebra that covers the spinal canal; also known as decompression surgery.
1	Laparoscope	A device used for minimally invasive procedures that require small incisions; it allows internal body structures to be viewed either by an attached camera or a remote camera that is connected by cabling.
17	Laryngitis	Inflammation of the larynx.
13	Larvae	Juvenile forms of various types of animals, including insects.
15	Lens	The transparent, bioconvex structure that works with the cornea to refract light that is focused on the retina.
4	Lethargy	A state of drowsiness, sluggishness, or indifference.
7	Leukemia	A cancer of the blood or bone marrow characterized by an abnormal increase of white blood cells.
9	Leukocytes	White blood cells; they defend the body against infectious disease and foreign materials and include five types: neutrophils, eosinophils, basophils, lymphocytes, and monocytes.
12	Leukocytes	White blood cells.
8	Leukocytosis	An increase in white blood cells in the blood.
12	Leukocytosis	An increase in circulating white blood cells.
8	Leukopenia	A decrease in white blood cells in the blood.
12	Leukopenia	A decrease in leukocytes, often caused by certain viral infections, radiation, and chemotherapy.
23	Leukoplakia	A precancerous, slowly developing change in a mucous membrane characterized by thickened proteins.
22	Leukorrhea	A white or yellowish vaginal discharge normally present in smaller amounts during different points in the menstrual cycle and during pregnancy. A large increase in the discharge may indicate infection.
23	Lichenification	The appearance of flat, scaly lesions on the skin; most commonly due to long-term irritation or inflammation of the skin.
16	Ligaments	Sheets or bands of tough, fibrous tissue connecting bones or cartilages at a joint, or supporting an organ.
11	Ligate	To tie or bind with a ligature.
25	Limbic system	The set of brain structures that support emotion, behavior, memory, and the sense of smell; these structures include the hippocampus, amygdala, thalamus, septum, and limbic cortex.
19	Lipoid nephrosis	The earliest stage of childhood nephrotic syndrome.
19	Lithotripsy	The use of shock waves to break up stones in the urinary system.
16	Longitudinal fracture	A fracture that follows the long axis of a bone.
16	Lordosis	An abnormal forward curvature of the spine in the lumbar region; also known as "saddle back" or "hollow back."
13	Lymph nodes	Masses of lymphoid tissues that create lymphocytes, remove noxious agents, and are believed to help produce antibodies.
8	Lymphadenopathy	Any disease of the lymph nodes.
12	Lymphadenopathy	Disease of the lymph nodes.
13	Lymphocytopenia	A deficiency of lymphocytes.
13	Lymphocytosis	An unusually large concentration of lymphocytes in the blood; it is often seen during allergic reactions or infections.
13	Lymphomas	Neoplastic growths of lymphoid tissue.
5	Lysis	The breaking down of cells.

Chapter	Term	Definition
9	Macrophages	Large phagocytic cells produced in the bone marrow that are initially released from the marrow as monocytes. Macrophages are widely distributed throughout the body and may lodge in the walls of blood vessels or in connective tissue.
4	Macrosomia	Also known as "big baby syndrome," it is sometimes referred to as "large for gestational age" (LGA). Macrosomia describes a fetus that weighs more than 8.8 pounds.
15	Macula	Also known as the "macula lutea," it is the yellow spot near the center of the retina; it is responsible for central vision.
15	Macular degeneration	A medical condition that usually affects older adults, resulting in a loss of vision because of damage to the retina.
16	Magnetic resonance imaging	A method of viewing the internal body structures by combining magnets with powerful pulses of radio waves; offers fewer health risks than other techniques.
12	Malabsorption	A state caused by abnormal absorption of food nutrients across the gastrointestinal tract.
18	Malabsorption syndrome	A condition that arises from abnormality in absorption of food nutrients across the gastrointestinal tract.
9	Malaise	A feeling of general discomfort or uneasiness.
18	Malaise	A feeling of general discomfort or uneasiness.
22	Mammography	A procedure in which x-rays are passed through the breast and recorded on a photographic film to produce a mammogram.
1	Mammogram	An x-ray of the breast used to detect tumors and other abnormalities.
10	Mast cells	Cells in connective tissue that contain histamine and heparin, which are released during allergic reactions or in response to inflammation or tissue injury.
26	MDA	An amphetamine called the "love drug" because it is believed to enhance sexual desire; its chemical name is 3,4-methylendioxyamphetamine.
26	MDMA	An amphetamine originally synthesized for research purposes that has since become extremely popular among teens and young adults; its chemical name is 3,4-methylenedioxymethamphetamine, but it is commonly called "Ecstasy" or "XTC."
21	Meatus	The external urethral orifice.
22	Meatus	A naturally occurring external opening of a canal or duct in the body.
6	Meiosis	The division of a sex cell as it matures into two and then four haploid cells. The nucleus of each receives one half of the number of chromosomes present in the somatic cells of the species.
6	Melanin	The natural pigment that gives color to the hair, skin, and irises of the eyes.
23	Melanocytes	Melanin-producing cells.
23	Melanosomes	Cells capable of forming the pigment melanin, from which skin cancer may be derived; this cancer is sometimes referred to as malignant melanoma (an extremely dangerous form of cancer).
18	Melena	Black, "tarry" feces associated with gastrointestinal hemorrhage.
10	Memory cells	Those that protect the body if an invading antigen returns by "remembering" the previous occurrence.
22	Menarche	The first occurrence of a menstrual period, usually occurring between the ages of 9 and 17.
28	Meniere's disease	A disorder of the inner ear that causes severe vertigo (dizziness), tinnitus, hearing loss, and a feeling of fullness or congestion.
14	Meninges	Membranes that cover the brain and spinal cord that are divided into three layers: the dura mater, arachnoid, and pia mater.
14	Meningiomas	A common type of primary brain tumor in adults that usually originate in the dura mater of the meninges.
22	Menopause	The period of natural cessation of menstruation.
22	Menorrhagia	An increased amount and duration of menstrual flow.
23	Merocrine gland	A gland whose cells secrete a fluid without losing cytoplasm.

Chapter	Term	Definition
24	Mesothelioma	A rare tumor arising from the tissues of the mesothelium that forms a sheet-like cover on the internal organs; it is linked to asbestos exposure.
2	Metabolic syndrome	A combination of medical disorders that increase the risk of developing cardiovascular disease and diabetes.
16	Metacarpophalangeal	Relating to the bones and joints of the hand.
5	Metaplasia	A reversible replacement of one differentiated cell type with another mature differentiated cell type.
7	Metastasis	The spread of a disease from one organ or body part to another that is not adjacent.
16	Metatarsophalangeal	Relating to the bones and joints of the foot.
22	Metrorrhagia	Bleeding between menstrual cycles.
11	Microcirculation	The flow of blood or lymph through the smallest vessels of the body (usually the venules, capillaries, and arterioles).
12	Microcytic	Unusually small (cells).
7	Micrometastases	Multiple metastases that are too small in size to be detected.
8	Microorganisms	Organisms visible only under a microscope, including bacteria, fungi, protozoa, and viruses.
1	Microscopic	Requiring a microscope to be seen.
6	Mitosis	The separation of chromosomes in a cell nucleus into two identical sets in two cell nuclei.
10	Monocytes	Large leukocytes that have only single nuclei.
8	Monocytosis	An increase in the number of monocytes circulating in the blood; monocytes are important for immunity.
10	Monokines	Cytokines (cell-signaling protein molecules) produced by monocytes and macrophages.
4	Morbidity	A state of illness or disease.
12	Morphology	The size and shape of cells.
4	Mortality	Death, or the state of being subject to dying.
3	Morula	The round mass of blastomeres that results from cleavage of the fertilized ovum; it forms the blastula.
18	Motility	The ability to move spontaneously and actively, which requires energy.
11	Murmurs	Blowing sounds heard when listening to the heart or blood vessels with a stethoscope.
16	Muscular dystrophy	Actually a group of inherited disorders in which strength and muscle bulk gradually decline.
8	Mutate	Change of a microorganism, either spontaneously or because of environmental conditions or medications.
10	Mutate	To produce a change in the base pair sequences of chromosomal molecules.
6	Mutation	An unusual change in a gene or a gene sequence.
7	Mutations	Sudden changes in the nature of genes as opposed to gradual genetic changes that develop over the course of generations.
23	Mycoses	Fungal infections.
4	Myelinated	Covered with myelin, which is a substance composed of various fats, proteins, and cholesterol.
12	Myelotoxins	Toxins that destroy bone marrow cells.
11	Myocardium	The middle, thickest layer of the heart, composed of cardiac muscle.
15	Myopia	"Nearsightedness," a refractive error wherein the eyeball is too long or the cornea is too steep; it causes far-off objects to appear blurred, whereas close-up objects are clear.
20	Myxedema	A specific type of cutaneous and dermal edema secondary to increased deposition of connective tissue components; it is related to hypothyroidism and Graves' disease.

Chapter	Term	Definition
5	Necrosis	The premature death of living cells and tissue.
6	Neonates	Infants between birth and 28 days of age.
5	Neoplasia	The abnormal proliferation of body cells.
19	Nephrectomy	Removal of a kidney.
20	Nephrogenic	Originating in the kidneys.
19	Nephrons	The filtering units of the kidneys.
14	Nervous system	The brain, spinal cord, and nerves; it is subdivided into the central and peripheral nervous systems.
28	Neurofibrils	Threads that run through the bodies of neurons and extend into axons and dendrites.
19	Neurogenic bladder	Dysfunction of the urinary bladder due to a nervous system disease that relates to the control of urination.
25	Neuroimaging	The use of various techniques to image the structures, functions, and pharmacology of the brain; it includes computed tomography, magnetic resonance imaging, and many other procedures.
25	Neuromediators	Neurotransmitters; chemical substances that are released from synaptic knobs into synaptic clefts; they include acetylcholine, dopamine, epinephrine, norepinephrine, and others.
8	Neutropenia	An abnormally low number of neutrophils in the blood; neutrophils are the most important type of white blood cells.
9	Neutrophils	The most abundant type of leukocytes; after trauma, they move quickly to the area as part of the acute inflammatory response.
19	Nocturia	The need to urinate during the night, interrupting sleep.
28	Nocturia	Excessive urination at night.
16	Nondisplaced	Not displaced; this type of fracture means the bone is cracked but its pieces are still in normal alignment.
8	Nosocomial	Occurring as a result of hospital (or other institutionalized) medical treatment; nosocomial infections are often caused by microorganisms becoming resistant to commonly used antimicrobial agents.
16	Oblique fracture	A break that occurs at an angle across the bone, usually the result of a sharp, angled blow.
12	Occult	Hidden, such as when bleeding occurs internally.
18	Occult blood	Blood that is present but not visibly apparent.
22	Oligomenorrhea	Abnormally light menstrual periods.
19	Oliguria	Decreased production of urine.
7	Oncology	The medical specialty that deals with tumors and cancers.
23	Onychomycosis	A fungal infection of the nails; also known as tinea unguium.
16	Open fractures	Those that involve the bone protruding through the skin (see compound fractures).
15	Ophthalmic	Referring to ophthalmology, the branch of medicine that focuses on the eyes; ophthalmologists differ from optometrists in that they are both medically and surgically trained.
26	Opioids	Chemicals that work by binding to opioid receptors; commonly used for analgesia but causing side effects of sedation, constipation, and respiratory depression.
10	Opportunistic	Able to take effect due to a lack of immune function.
21	Orchiopexy	Surgical descent of the testes into its normal position within the scrotum.
6	Organogenesis	The formation and differentiation of organs and organ systems during embryonic development.
17	Orthopnea	Shortness of breath that occurs when the patient is lying flat.
29	Orthostatic hypotension	A drop in blood pressure after a rapid change of position.

Chapter	Term	Definition
27	Osmotic pressure	Pressure exerted on a differentially permeable membrane separating a solution from a solvent; the membrane being impermeable to the solutes in the solution and permeable only to the solvent.
16	Osteoarthritis	Degenerative arthritis; the type caused by the breakdown and eventual loss of the cartilage of one or more joints.
28	Osteoblastic	Related to the deposition of calcium into bone via the actions of osteoblast cells.
29	Osteoclastic	Related to the surgical breaking of a bone.
16	Osteomalacia	Softening of the bones, usually due to demineralization.
16	Osteomyelitis	An infection of the bones caused primarily by bacteria.
28	Osteophytes	Bone spurs, which are bony projections that form along joint margins.
16	Osteoporosis	A decrease in bone density and strength that commonly results in fractures.
15	Otalgia	Ear pain or an "earache."
28	Otosclerosis	Abnormal bone growth in the middle ear that causes hearing loss.
26	Overdoses	Ingestions of substances in excessive quantities that may cause serious harm or even death.
2	Ozone	A compound made up of three oxygen atoms that in the lower atmosphere is an air pollutant harmful to the respiratory system.
22	Paget's disease	A rare form of breast cancer that affects usually older women, beginning at the nipple and extending into the areola.
22	Pap smear	A test commonly used to screen for cancer of the cervix. It is named for George Papanicolaou, the physician who developed the technique.
7	Palliative	Improving patient comfort but not treating the underlying condition.
12	Pallor	Paleness of the face.
18	Palmar erythema	Reddening of the palms.
18	Pancreatitis	Inflammation of the pancreas, which may be acute or chronic.
12	Pancytopenia	A reduction in the number of red blood cells, white blood cells, and platelets.
12	Panhypoplasia	The inability of the bone marrow to produce red blood cells, white blood cells, and platelets.
18	Paralytic obstruction	Paralytic ileus; obstruction of the intestine due to paralysis of the intestinal muscles.
26	Paranoia	An irrational feeling of impending harm from someone or something.
14	Paraplegia	Paralysis of the lower part of the body.
29	Paraplegia	Paralysis of the legs and lower part of the torso.
9	Parenchymal cells	Types of cells that are functional elements of organs, such as the hepatocytes.
23	Paresthesia	An abnormal, usually unpleasant sensation such as numbness, tingling, or prickling.
8	Pathogenicity	The capacity of microorganisms to cause disease.
2	Pathogens	Infectious agents that cause disease in their hosts.
8	Pathogens	Disease-causing microbes, commonly called "germs" and "bugs."
16	Pathologic	Related to or caused by disease.
26	PCP	Phenylcyclohexylpiperidine (commonly called "angel dust" or phencyclidine), it produces a trance-like state that may last for days and results in severe brain damage.
22	Pelvic inflammatory disease	Infection of the uterus, fallopian tubes, and other female reproductive structures that is a serious complication of certain sexually transmitted diseases.
6	Penetration	A stage in which genetic material enters a host cell.
18	Peptic ulcer	An ulcer of the gastrointestinal tract that is usually acidic and extremely painful.
9	Perforation	A complete penetration of the wall of a hollow organ.
18	Perforation	A small hole or tear.
11	Perfusion	Delivery of oxygen and other nutrients to the tissues by the blood.

Chapter	Term	Definition
18	Periodontal disease	Any condition involving bacterial plaque, the gums, teeth, and the immunoinflammatory mechanisms of the patient.
18	Peristalsis	A symmetric contraction of muscles that moves substances through a body structure, such as food through the intestines.
18	Peritonitis	Inflammation of the peritoneum (the mucous membrane that lines the abdominal cavity and viscera).
9	Permeability	The capacity of a blood vessel to allow ions, water, nutrients, or cells to move in and out of the vessel.
12	Petechia	Pinpointed skin hemorrhages.
27	pH	A chemical expression that indicates the degree of acidity or alkalinity of a solution.
15	Phacoemulsification	A procedure used in modern cataract surgery wherein the eye's internal lens is emulsified with an ultrasonic handpiece; the emulsified cataract is then aspirated from the eye.
9	Phagocytosis	Cell-eating; the engulfing of solid particles by a cellular membrane.
17	Pharyngitis	Inflammation of the throat or pharynx.
6	Phenotype	The complete observable characteristics of an organism or group, including anatomic, physiologic, biochemical, and behavior traits.
12	Phlebotomy	The act or practice of opening a vein by incision or puncture to remove blood.
15	Photocoagulation	A type of laser surgery used to treat many eye disorders; a laser is used to cauterize small ocular blood vessels, lowering the risk of severe vision loss.
15	Photophobia	A symptom of excessive sensitivity to light and the aversion to sunlight or areas of bright lighting.
11	Plaque	A deposit of hardened material lining a blood vessel.
12	Plasma	The clear yellowish fluid that remains after the cells are removed.
10	Plasmapheresis	The removal, treatment, and return of components of blood plasma from the blood circulation.
12	Plethoric	Characterized by an overabundance of blood.
17	Pleural effusion	Excess fluid that accumulates in the pleural spaces that surround the lungs.
17	Pleurisy	Inflammation of the pleura; it causes sharp pain when breathing in.
24	Pleurisy	Inflammation of the pleura, the double layer of membrane on the outside of the lung and lining the chest wall.
17	Pneumoconioses	Occupational, restrictive lung diseases that are caused by inhalation of various types of dust.
17	Pneumothorax	A collection of air or gas in the pleural cavity between the lung and chest wall.
19	Polycystic kidney disease	A genetic kidney disorder wherein multiple, fluid-filled cysts form, greatly enlarging kidney size.
3	Polycythemia	Increased numbers of erythrocytes in the blood circulation.
6	Polygenic	Pertaining to or dominated by several different genes.
22	Polymenorrhea	Short menstrual cycles of less than 3 weeks.
18	Polyp	A fleshy growth.
20	Polyuria	Excessive elimination of urine.
18	Portal hypertension	High blood pressure in the portal vein and its tributaries.
4	Precipitous delivery	Birth of an infant after less than 3 hours of labor; it usually involves intense contractions and pain for which there is not adequate time to relieve.
15	Premenstrual edema	Fluid retention and tenderness of the breasts occurring shortly before the onset of menstruation.
15	Presbyopia	"Old eye"; a progressively diminished ability to focus on close-up objects due to aging.
1	Probability	The likelihood that something will occur.
17	Productive cough	A cough that produces phlegm.

Chapter	Term	Definition
7	Prognosis	A prediction of the course and outcome of a disease.
7	Prophylactic	Used to prevent rather than to treat or cure.
10	Prophylactic	Preventing the spread of disease.
22	Prostaglandin	A hormone-like substance that participates in many functions, including muscle contraction and relaxation, blood vessel constriction and dilation, control of blood pressure, and modulation of inflammation.
28	Prostatectomy	Surgical removal of the prostate gland.
19	Proteinuria	The presence of excess serum proteins in the urine.
8	Protozoa	Single-celled microorganisms that may live independently, on dead matter, or inside (or upon) living hosts.
10	Pruritic	Itchy.
26	Psychedelics	Substances that alter perception and reality.
17	Pulmonary abscess	A collection of pus inside lung tissue.
17	Pulmonary edema	Fluid accumulation in the lungs.
17	Pulmonary embolism	A blockage of the main artery of the lung, or one of its branches, by a thrombus (blood clot) from elsewhere in the body.
9	Purulent	Containing pus, which is a white, yellow, green, or brown exudate produced by dead and/or living cells that travel into intercellular spaces around infected cells.
23	Pus	An exudate, ranging from white to brown in color, produced during inflammatory pyogenic bacterial infections.
19	Pyelitis	Inflammation of the renal pelvis of the kidney.
19	Pyelonephritis	An ascending urinary tract infection that has reached the renal pelvis of the kidney.
9	Pyrexia	Fever, which may be mild or severe.
9	Pyrogens	Substances that induce a fever.
19	Pyuria	Pus in the urine.
14	Quadriplegia	Paralysis of the arms and legs. Also called "tetraplegia."
29	Quadriplegia	Complete paralysis of all four limbs; this condition is now commonly referred to as tetraplegia.
19	Radical cystectomy	Surgical removal of all or part of the urinary bladder.
1	Radioactive	Capable of giving off alpha, beta, or gamma rays.
16	Radiologic	Related to radiology, the branch of medicine that uses radiation for the diagnosis and treatment of disease.
1	Radiopaque	Not allowing the passage of x-rays or other types of radiation.
17	Rales	Clicking, crackling, or rattling noises of the lungs when breathing in.
7	Recurrence	Return of a disease state.
18	Reflux esophagitis	Inflammation of the esophagus caused by abnormal "reflux" of stomach acid into the esophagus, causing heartburn.
15	Refraction	The deviation of light waves entering the eye; a "refractive test" may be used to determine the eye's "refractive error" and the best corrective lenses to be prescribed.
9	Regeneration	The regrowth of tissue so that normal function returns.
18	Regional enteritis	Crohn's disease; an inflammatory disease of the intestines that may affect any part of the gastrointestinal tract, causing pain, vomiting, diarrhea, weight loss, and other symptoms.
7	Remission	The state of absence of disease activity in patients with a chronic illness.
18	Remission	The state of absence of disease activity in patients with a known, incurable chronic illness.
13	Remissions	Disappearances of diseases as a result of treatment.
19	Renal calculi	Kidney stones.

Chapter	Term	Definition
19	Renal failure	The failure of the kidneys to adequately filter toxins and waste products from the blood.
11	Repolarization	The restoration of a resting potential across a membrane.
11	Resected	Cut out part or all of an organ or other body structure.
8	Resident flora	Indigenous or "normal" microorganisms that live on the skin and inside most areas of the body; also called "resident microbiota."
12	Reticulocyte	An immature red blood cell.
15	Retina	The light-sensitive tissue lining the inner surface of the eye.
15	Retinal detachment	A disorder in which the retina peels away from the choroid, leading to loss of vision and potential blindness.
4	Retinopathy	Any degeneration of the blood vessels supplying the retina of the eye that is not caused by inflammation.
15	Retinopathy	Noninflammatory damage to the retina.
15	Retrobulbar	Related to the area behind the globe of the eye.
10	Retrovirus	Any virus containing RNA that replicates in targeted host cells.
16	Rheumatism	An older term used to describe a variety of painful conditions affecting the muscles, bones, joints, and tendons. Examples of rheumatic conditions include bursitis and tendinitis.
16	Rheumatoid arthritis	An autoimmune disease that causes chronic inflammation of the joints.
17	Rhinorrhea	"Runny nose"; a discharge or flow of nasal fluids.
17	Rhonchi	Harsh, rattling sounds usually caused by bronchial secretions.
22	Rugae	The anatomic folds (wrinkles) of the vagina.
22	Salpingitis	Inflammation and infection of the fallopian tubes.
28	Sarcopenia	A loss of skeletal muscle mass that may accompany aging.
9	Scar	An area of fibrous tissue that replaces normal skin or other tissue after injury or disease.
25	Schizophrenia	A psychological disorder involving delusions and hallucinations, disorganization, and reduced enjoyment and interests.
15	Sclera	The outer, white portion of the eye.
24	Scleroderma	Pathologic thickening and hardening of the skin.
11	Sclerosing	Hardening, as of a body part.
4	Scoliosis	A lateral or "side-to-side" curvature of the spine, often in the form of an "S" shape.
16	Scoliosis	An abnormal curvature of the spine to the left or right, causing a twisting of the vertebrae.
21	Scrotum	The pouch of skin comprising the part of the male external genitalia that contains the testes.
23	Sebaceous glands	Holocrine glands in the dermis that secrete sebum.
15	Seborrhea	A chronic, inflammatory skin disorder that affects the sebaceous glands of the head and trunk.
23	Seborrheic keratoses	Benign, "horny" skin growths related to excessive secretion of sebum.
23	Sebum	An oily substance secreted by sebaceous glands that helps to keep skin and hair from drying out.
10	Secondary	Not primary; a condition that develops as the result of a primary condition.
28	Sedentary	Related to a lack of or complete absence of physical activity.
7	Seeding	A final cancer process wherein the disease spreads via body fluids or membranes.
14	Seizure	A sudden attack that is commonly indicative of a convulsive seizure.
8	Seizures	Symptoms of brain abnormalities that often cause convulsions; they occur because of sudden, abnormal electrical activity in the brain.

Chapter	Term	Definition
21	Seminal vesicles	A pair of sac-like glandular structures that lie posterolateral to the urinary bladder in the male and function as part of the reproductive system.
21	Seminiferous tubules	Tubules in the testes where the sperm cells form.
3	Sepsis	A potentially serious systemic inflammatory response affecting numerous parts of the body, commonly caused by septicemia (the presence of pathogenic microorganisms in the bloodstream).
8	Sepsis	The presence of various pus-forming (and other) pathogenic organisms, or their toxins, in the blood or tissue.
8	Septicemia	An overwhelming systemic infection that may occur when pathogens circulate and reproduce in the blood; septicemia is a common type of sepsis.
18	Septicemia	Pathogenic microorganisms in the bloodstream, leading to sepsis.
22	Septicemia	An infection of the blood that may be caused by direct injection of bacteria into the blood (as with a contaminated needle), or more commonly by an infection anywhere in the body that spreads into the blood.
9	Serous	Watery in appearance; resembling or producing serum.
12	Serum	The fluid and solutes that remain after the cells and fibrinogen are removed.
2	Shaken baby syndrome	A form of physical child abuse occurring when a person violently shakes an infant or small child; it creates a whiplash-type motion that causes acceleration-deceleration injuries of the brain.
14	Shingles	An acute infection caused by the varicella-zoster virus; causes a painful rash and sharp stabbing pains along the path of sensory nerves.
24	Silica	A fine rock dust known to cause lung damage with long-term exposure.
17	Silicosis	A type of occupational lung disease caused by inhalation of crystalline silica dust; a type of pneumoconiosis.
16	Simple fracture	An uncomplicated closed fracture (the bones do not pierce the skin).
20	Simple goiter	A goiter that has spread through the entire thyroid, with "goiter" defined as a swelling in the thyroid.
17	Sinusitis	An inflammation of the paranasal sinuses.
14	Sleep apnea	A condition that involves more than five periods of interrupted breathing, each lasting for at least 10 seconds, during every hour of sleep; it affects nearly one-third of adults in the United States.
25	Sleep apnea	A sleep disorder characterized by abnormal pauses in breathing or abnormally low breathing; each pause can last for seconds or minutes.
2	Somatoform	A mental disorder characterized by physical symptoms that suggest physical illness or injury.
16	Spasms	Painful, involuntary muscle contractions.
21	Spermatic cord	Collectively, the spermatic vessels, nerves, lymphatic vessels, and ductus deferens extending between the testes and proximal end of the inguinal canal.
21	Spermatogenesis	Formation and development of spermatozoa.
18	Spider angiomas	Central reddish spots with spider-like reddish extensions on the skin; they consist of dilated blood vessels and may indicate liver disease.
6	Spina bifida occulta	The type of spina bifida that does not involve herniation of the meninges or the contents of the spinal cord.
14	Spinal cord	The portion of the nervous system that runs from the brain through the vertebral column, stopping near the tailbone; it transmits motor and sensory impulses.
16	Spinal orthosis	Orthopedic appliances or apparatuses used to support, align, prevent, or correct spinal deformities or to improve functioning.
16	Spiral fracture	A torsion fracture in which the bone has been twisted apart.
10	Splenectomy	Removal of the spleen.
12	Splenomegaly	Enlargement of the spleen.

Chapter	Term	Definition
18	Splenomegaly	Enlargement of the spleen.
16	Spondylolisthesis	The anterior displacement of a vertebra or the vertebral column in relation to the vertebrae below.
16	Sprain	Injury to a ligament or ligaments caused by stretching beyond normal capacity or tearing.
17	Sputum	Secretions expelled from the respiratory tract, such as mucus or phlegm (mixed with saliva).
8	Staining	The process of using a dye (e.g., Gram stain) to color cells and subcellular structures to facilitate microscopic examination.
3	Startle reflex	A reflex response to a sudden unexpected stimulus. The reaction may be accompanied by physiologic effects, including increased heartbeat and respiration, closing of the eyes, and flexion of the trunk muscles.
29	Stasis	Slowing or stopping blood flow or other body fluids.
17	Status asthmaticus	An acute exacerbation of asthma that is resistant to standard bronchodilators and steroid treatments.
16	Stellate fracture	A bone fracture in which the lines of the break radiate from a point into numerous fissures.
10	Stem cells	Undifferentiated cells that can grow into any type of body cells.
9	Stenosis	Narrowing of structures such as tubes or ducts.
8	Sterilization	The process of completely eradicating pathogens from equipment, surfaces, etc.
22	Stillborn	Dying within the uterus before birth.
12	Stomatitis	Oral mucosa ulcers.
15	Strabismus	A condition in which the eyes are not properly aligned with each other.
16	Strain	An injury caused by overuse or overexertion, commonly called a "wrench" of a body structure.
5	Strangulation	Compression of the throat that leads to unconsciousness via lack of oxygen; it may lead to cerebral ischemia, asphyxia, and death.
25	Stress	Inappropriate physiologic response to any demand on the mind or body.
16	Stress fractures	Those caused by prolonged, repeated, or abnormal stress to bones.
16	Striations	Stripes or streaks of differently colored tissue.
11	Stroke	Sudden death of brain cells in a localized area, due to inadequate blood flow.
14	Subdural	Between the dura mater and the arachnoid layer.
16	Subluxation	An incomplete or partial dislocation.
26	Substance abuse	Drug abuse or chemical dependency; use of substances for various effects, which may lead to addiction and dependence.
3	Sucking reflex	Involuntary sucking movements of the circumoral area in newborns in response to stimulation.
5	Suffocation	The process of being asphyxiated.
15	Suppurative	Causing the formation or discharge of pus.
19	Suprapubic catheter	A catheter used to drain urine from the bladder by insertion through the abdominal wall just above the pubic bone.
4	Surfactant	A lipoprotein-based substance secreted in the lungs that reduces the surface tension of fluids that coat the lung.
12	Syncope	Fainting.
26	Synergism	The interaction of several drugs or substances that enhance or magnify their normal effects.
12	Tachycardia	Higher than normal heart rate.
17	Tachypnea	Rapid breathing.

Chapter	Term	Definition
16	Temporomandibular joint syndrome	An incorrect alignment of the lower jaw to the skull that causes pain, nausea, and many other symptoms.
16	Tendinitis	Inflammation of a tendon or tendons.
16	Tendons	Fibrous cords of connective tissue that attach muscles to bones or cartilage.
16	Tennis elbow	Inflammation of the elbow structures caused by repeated, forceful contractions of the wrist muscles of the outer forearm.
6	Teratogenic	Capable of causing the formation of one or more developmental abnormalities in the fetus.
18	Testicular atrophy	Diminished size of the testicles of the male, sometimes accompanied by loss of function.
21	Testosterone	The primary male hormone; it is produced mainly in the testes and is secreted into the blood.
14	Tetanus	An acute, potentially fatal infection of the central nervous system.
16	Tetany	An abnormal condition of painful muscle cramps, spasms, and numbness.
23	Tinea	A general term used to describe fungal infections of the skin.
15	Tinnitus	The perception of sound within the ear when there is no corresponding external sound.
28	Tinnitus	The perception of sound in the ear when there is no corresponding external sound.
12	Thrombocytopenia	The presence of relatively few platelets in the blood.
11	Thromboembolism	Obstruction of a blood vessel with thrombotic material carried by the blood from another site in the body.
11	Thrombosis	Formation or presence of a thrombus.
11	Thrombus	A stationary blood clot along the wall of a blood vessel.
10	Thymus	The lymphoid gland located near the sternum that is essential in the development of immunity before puberty.
13	Thymus	A lymphatic gland that shrinks as the body ages; it serves primarily to begin the body's immunity during childhood.
20	Thyroid cancer	A malignant neoplasm that can be treated with radioactive iodine or by surgical resection; in fewer cases, chemotherapy or radiotherapy are used.
10	Titer	The concentration of a substance in a solution as determined by titration (the process of adding amounts of different solutions to create a specific chemical reaction).
15	Tonometric	Related to the measurement of tension or pressure; in ophthalmology it is used to determine intraocular pressure.
16	Tophi	Deposits of sodium urate that develop in fibrous tissue around joints; commonly seen in gout.
11	Toxic	A state of being poisoned or poisonous.
8	Toxins	Poisonous substances (often proteins) produced by living cells or organisms; toxins are capable of causing diseases and other harm to the body.
27	Transcellular fluid	A portion of the extracellular fluid that includes the fluid within special body cavities.
14	Transient ischemic attack (TIA)	An episode of cerebrovascular insufficiency, usually due to partial occlusion of a cerebral artery.
4	Transient tachypnea	Temporary, abnormally rapid breathing.
19	Transurethral resection	The passage of a cystoscope into the bladder through the urethra, and a resectoscope that removes tissue for biopsy as well as burns away any existing cancer cells.
16	Transverse fracture	A fracture that occurs at right angles to the longitudinal axis of a bone.
23	Trichophyton	A genus of fungi that infects skin, hair, and nails.
6	Trisomy	The presence of a third chromosome of one type in a cell that would normally have two of the same chromosomes.
3	Trophoblast	Also called the "trophoderm"; it is the outermost layer of cells of the blastocyst that attaches the fertilized ovum to the uterine wall, providing nutrition to the embryo.

Chapter	Term	Definition
20	Tropic	Targeting endocrine glands; such as in "tropic hormone" from the anterior pituitary gland.
22	Tubal insufflation	A nonoperative method of evaluating the fallopian tubes by pushing a gas into the cervix and uterus where it is detected by distention and other methods.
21	Tunica vaginalis	The serous membrane surrounding the testis and epididymis.
15	Tympanic membrane	The "eardrum"; it separates the external ear from the middle ear and transmits sounds from the air to the auditory ossicles.
18	Ulcerative colitis	A form of inflammatory bowel disease that includes ulcers in the colon.
9	Ulcers	Sores or lesions that result from erosion to areas of organs or tissues.
11	Ultrasonography	The imaging of deep body structures by recording the echoes of pulses of ultrasonic waves directed into the tissues.
1	Ultrasound	The use of ultrasonic waves to form images of interior body organs.
4	Unconjugated	Not commonly united with a compound or compounds.
8	Unicellular	Having or consisting of one cell.
19	Urgency	A sudden, compelling urge to urinate.
19	Urinalysis	A variety of tests performed upon the urine to test a variety of substance levels.
19	Urinary incontinence	The involuntary excretion of urine.
19	Urine culture and sensitivity (C&S) test	A test used to diagnose urinary tract infections; it usually takes between 24 and 48 hours to culture any bacteria that are present.
22	Uterine polyps	Growths attached to the inner wall of the uterus.
21	Varicocele	Distended or swollen veins in the spermatic cord of males.
18	Varicosities	Enlarged varicose veins.
9	Vasodilation	Widening of blood vessels.
11	Vasospastic	Related to or an agent that produces spasms of the blood vessels.
4	Vertex	Cephalic; a type of presentation during childbirth wherein the infant's head comes through the pelvis of the mother before the rest of his or her body.
15	Vertigo	A type of dizziness wherein there is a feeling of motion when a person is actually stationary.
10	Vesicles	Small, raised skin lesions that usually contain fluid.
8	Virulence	The degree of pathogenicity of a specific microorganism.
8	Viruses	The smallest type of microorganism; viruses must have living hosts to replicate.
24	Vitiligo	A benign, generally progressive skin disorder in which irregular, unpigmented white patches form on the exposed skin areas.
18	Volvulus	A bowel obstruction in which a loop of the bowel has twisted upon itself.
22	Vulva	The external female reproductive structures that surround the vaginal opening.
27	Water balance	Equivalence of the volume of water entering the body with the volume leaving it.
27	Water of metabolism	Water produced as a byproduct of metabolism.
17	Wheezing	Continuous, harsh whistling sound produced during exhalation.
23	Xerosis	Excessive dryness of the skin, mucous membranes, or eyes.
28	Xerostomia	Dryness of the mouth.
2	X-ray absorptiometry	A means of measuring bone mineral density that uses two x-ray beams with different energy levels.
3	Zygote	The cell formed by fertilization, before the occurrence of cleavage.

Index

Figures and tables are indicated by an italic *f* or *t* following the page number.

Credits

Chapter 1
1-2, 1-3, 1-4, 1-5A,B, 1-6, 1-8, 1-9, 1-10, 1-11 Courtesy of Leonard V. Crowley, MD, Century College; 1-12 Courtesy of Belinda Thresher

Chapter 3
3-1A,B Courtesy of Leonard V. Crowley, MD, Century College; 3-5 Courtesy of the Carnegie Institution of Washington; 3-6 Courtesy of Leonard V. Crowley, MD, Century College

Chapter 4
4-1 © NMSB/Custom Medical Stock Photo; 4-2 © Marcin Okupniak/Dreamstime.com; 4-3 Courtesy of Leonard V. Crowley, MD, Century College

Chapter 5
5-2A,B, 5-3A,B, 5-4 Courtesy of Leonard V. Crowley, MD, Century College

Chapter 6
6-1 © SPL/Custom Medical Stock Photo; 6-4 © John Radcliffe Hospital/Photo Researchers, Inc.; 6-5 © Joe McDonald/Visuals Unlimited; 6-7 © REUTERS/Associazione Luca Coscioni/Landov; 6-9A,B, 6-10, 6-12A,B, 6-13, 6-14 Courtesy of Leonard V. Crowley, MD, Century College; 6-15 Courtesy of Dr. Robert Gorlin; 6-16, 6-17, 6-18 Courtesy of Leonard V. Crowley, MD, Century College; 6-19 © Wellcome Trust/Custom Medical Stock Photo; 6-20 © Nucleus Medical Art/Visuals Unlimited; 6-21A,B Courtesy of Leonard V. Crowley, MD, Century College; 6-22 © J. Pat Carter/ AP Photos; 6-23 © Wellcome Images/Custom Medical Stock Photo; 6-25 © Visuals Unlimited

Chapter 7
7-1A,B, 7-2A,B, 7-3A,B Courtesy of Leonard V. Crowley, MD, Century College; 7-4 © BioMedical/ShutterStock, Inc.

Chapter 8
8-1A,B Courtesy of Leonard V. Crowley, MD, Century College; 8-3C Courtesy of CDC; 8-4, 8-5 Courtesy of Leonard V. Crowley, MD, Century College; 8-6A © 1987 American Society of Clinical Pathology and ASCP Press.; 8-6B Courtesy of CDC; 8-8 © Alexander Raths/ShutterStock, Inc.; 8-9 © Comstock/Thinkstock; 8-10A,B Courtesy of Leonard V. Crowley, MD, Century College

Chapter 9
9-1, 9-2, 9-3, 9-4, 9-5, 9-6 Courtesy of Leonard V. Crowley, MD, Century College

Chapter 10
10-5 Courtesy of Leonard V. Crowley, MD, Century College; 10-9 © Dr. Ken Greer/Visuals Unlimited; 10-10 Courtesy of Leonard V. Crowley, MD, Century College; 10-11B Courtesy of Louisa Howard, Dartmouth College, Electron Microscope Facility; 10-14 © Dr. P. Marazzi/Photo Researchers, Inc.

Chapter 11
11-8 © Alexander Raths/ShutterStock, Inc.; 11-9 © Jaimie Duplass/ShutterStock, Inc.; 11-10, 11-11, 11-12, 11-13 Courtesy of Leonard V. Crowley, MD, Century College; 11-15 © James Cavallini/BSIP/age fotostock; 11-17, 11-19 Courtesy of Leonard V. Crowley, MD, Century College; 11-20 © CNRI/Photo Researchers, Inc.; 11-21 © Audie/ShutterStock, Inc.; 11-22 © Medical-on-Line/Alamy Images; 11-23 © Medicimage/Visuals Unlimited

Chapter 12
12-2A © David M. Phillips/Visuals Unlimited; 12-2B © Sashkin/ ShutterStock, Inc.; 12-3 © Donna Beer Stolz, Ph.D., Center for Biologic Imaging, University of Pittsburgh Medical School; 12-4 © John D. Cunningham/Visuals Unlimited; 12-5A,B, 12-6A,B Courtesy of Leonard V. Crowley, MD, Century College; 12-8 (photo) © Phototake, Inc./Alamy Images; 12-10B Courtesy of Janis Carr/CDC

Chapter 13
13-2 © Donna Beer Stolz, Ph.D., Center for Biologic Imaging, University of Pittsburgh Medical School; 13-3A,B Courtesy of Leonard V. Crowley, MD, Century College; 13-4 Courtesy of Robert Krasner; 13-5, 13-6A,B, 13-7, 13-8, 13-9, 13-10 Courtesy of Leonard V. Crowley, MD, Century College

Chapter 14
14-6, 14-7, 14-8A,B, 14-9 Courtesy of Leonard V. Crowley, MD, Century College; 14-10 © Ted S. Warren/AP Photos; 14-11A,B © Scott Camazine/Photo Researchers, Inc.; 14-13, 14-14 Courtesy of Leonard V. Crowley, MD, Century College

Chapter 15

15-4 © Courtesy of John T. Halgren, M.D./University of Nebraska Medical Center; 15-5A © Science Photo Library; 15-5B © Science Photo Library/Custom Medical Stock Photo; 15-6 © Chris Barry/Visuals Unlimited; 15-7 © Medical-on-Line/Alamy Images; 15-8 Courtesy of Christopher J. Rapuano, M.D.; Cornea Service, Wills Eye, Professor, Jefferson Medical College of Thomas Jefferson University, Philadelphia, PA; 15-11 Courtesy of the National Eye Institute/NIH; 15-12 © Medical-on-Line/Alamy Images; 15-13 © Kokel/BSIP/age fotostock; 15-14 © Justin Paget/ShutterStock, Inc.; 15-16 Courtesy of Andrew Heaford and Richard Smith, University of Iowa

Chapter 16

16-5 Courtesy of Leonard V. Crowley, MD, Century College; 16-6 © DR LR/age fotostock; 16-7 Courtesy of Leonard V. Crowley, MD, Century College; 16-8 © Medical-on-Line/Alamy Images; 16-9 © CNRI/Photo Researchers, Inc.; 16-10, 16-12, 16-13A,B, 16-14A,B,C Courtesy of Leonard V. Crowley, MD, Century College; 16-16A © Medical-on-Line/Alamy Images; 16-16B, 16-17, 16-18 Courtesy of Leonard V. Crowley, MD, Century College; 16-19 © Alexander Bark/ShutterStock, Inc.; 16-21A © Carolina K. Smith, M.D./ShutterStock, Inc.; 16-21B © Andres Rodriguez/ShutterStock, Inc.; 16-24 Courtesy of Leonard V. Crowley, MD, Century College; 16-25 (photo) © Robert O. Brown Photography/ShutterStock, Inc.; 16-27A,B Courtesy of Leonard V. Crowley, MD, Century College; 16-28 © Javier Larrea/age fotostock

Chapter 17

17-2B © David M. Phillips/Photo Researchers, Inc.; 17-4A,B Courtesy of Leonard V. Crowley, MD, Century College; 17-7 © Dr. P. Marazzi/Photo Researchers, Inc.; 17-8 Courtesy of Ben J. Marais and Robert P. Gir; 17-9 Courtesy of CDC; 17-13, 17-15A,B Courtesy of Leonard V. Crowley, MD, Century College; 17-17 Courtesy of Michael-Joseph F. Agbayani; 17-18 © Medical-on-Line/Alamy Images; 17-19 Courtesy of Leonard V. Crowley, MD, Century College; 17-20 © PHT/Photo Researchers, Inc.; 17-21A © University of Alabama at Birmingham Department of Pathology PEIR Digital Library (http://peir.net); 17-21B Courtesy of National Cancer Institute

Chapter 18

18-5A (inset) Courtesy of Douglas Burrin/USDA ARS; 18-5B,C © John D. Cunningham/Visuals Unlimited; 18-5D © David M. Phillips/Visuals Unlimited; 18-7, 18-8A,B, 18-9, 18-10, 18-11A,B, 18-12A,B,C, 18-13, 18-14, 18-16, 18-17, 18-18A,B, 18-20, 18-21, 18-22, 18-23B, 18-24 Courtesy of Leonard V. Crowley, MD, Century College

Chapter 19

19-2 © Blamb/ShutterStock, Inc.; 19-3A,B, 19-5A,B, 19-6 Courtesy of Leonard V. Crowley, MD, Century College; 19-9 © Dr. Gladden Willis/Visuals Unlimited; 19-10 © Medical-on-Line/Alamy Images

Chapter 20

20-6 © AP Photos; 20-7 © Ken Greer/Visuals Unlimited; 20-8A © Science Photo Library; 20-8B © Science Photo Library/Custom Medical Stock Photo; 20-9, 20-10, 20-11A,B, 20-12A,B Courtesy of Leonard V. Crowley, MD, Century College

Chapter 21

21-4, 21-5 © Wellcome Images/Custom Medical Stock Photo; 21-8B, 21-9, 21-10 Courtesy of Leonard V. Crowley, MD, Century College

Chapter 22

22-7, 22-8A,B, 22-10, 22-11, 22-12A,B, 22-13A,B, 22-14A,B, 22-15A,B, 22-16A,B,C, 22-17, 22-18A,B, Courtesy of Leonard V. Crowley, MD, Century College; 22-19 © Dr. Dennis Kunkel/Visuals Unlimited; 22-20 © Phototake/Alamy Images

Chapter 23

23-7 Courtesy of CDC; 23-8 © Anneka/ShutterStock, Inc.; 23-9 © Marcel Jancovic/ShutterStock, Inc.; 23-10 © Dr. Zara/age fotostock; 23-11 © Wellcome Images/Custom Medical Stock Photo; 23-12 Courtesy of Paul Matthews; 23-13 © Susan Lindsley/CDC; 23-14 © Arthur Ng Heng Kui/ShutterStock, Inc.; 23-15 © CDC/Allen W. Mathies, MD/California Emergency Preparedness Office (Calif/EPO), Immunization Branch; 23-16 © Cavallini James/age fotostock; 23-17A,B Courtesy of Leonard V. Crowley, MD, Century College; 23-18 © Dr. Dancewiez/CDC; 23-19 © Phototake Inc./Alamy Images; 23-20 Courtesy of CDC; 23-21(photo left) © Amy Walters/ShutterStock, Inc.; (photo middle) Courtesy of Rhonda Beck; (photo right) © John Radcliffe Hospital/Photo Researchers, Inc.; 23-22, 23-23, 23-24 Courtesy of National Cancer Institute

Chapter 24

24-1 Courtesy of Leonard V. Crowley, MD, Century College

Chapter 28

28-1, 28-2 Courtesy of Leonard V. Crowley, MD, Century College

Chapter 29

29-1 © Gina Sanders/ShutterStock, Inc.; 29-2 © Simon Fraser/Hexham General Hospital/Photo Researchers, Inc.; 29-3 © Rita Nannini/Photo Researchers, Inc.; 29-4 © Tierbild Okapia/Photo Researchers, Inc.

Page xxii (photo of author) Courtesy of Garrett Wade

Unless otherwise indicated, all photographs and illustrations are under copyright of Jones & Bartlett Learning or have been provided by the authors.